Contents

To my late father, Gilbert Ivor Jenkins

Foreword

The trend in professions relating to sport and exercise, including physical education, has been to move from general issues towards more specialized concerns with respect to the scientific knowledge available. Scientific technology has advanced to the stage that human movement can be analyzed using three-dimensional high-speed digital video analysis and athletic potential can be determined using biochemical analysis.

Much of what students learn has a strong interrelationship that requires a common base of theoretical knowledge and practical application. Terminology is often a barrier in the study of human movement, especially in the scientific disciplines. Dr. Jenkins' *Sports Science Handbook* brings a clear focus of how Kinesiology, Sport & Exercise Science, Physical Education, and Health interrelate and provides a framework of commonality in which to discuss key concepts. It is an impressive collection of diligently researched and useful references.

I believe that this book will become highly regarded in the USA, as well as many other nations, and it will be heavily used as an authoritative reference book. It is a must for every university library; for departments related to health, physical education and sports science; and especially for professors and students in these fields.

DANNY R. MIELKE, Ed.D.; M.P.H.; C.H.E.S.
Professor, Eastern Oregon University

Preface

As a boy, growing up in the UK, my dreams included playing rugby for Wales and winning the British Open golf championship. I didn't fulfill those dreams, but I did become a good all-round sportsman. I was obsessed with playing sport, but eventually my motivation turned to finding out why I was unable to emulate my heroes. It was the urge to understand the processes involved in skill acquisition, performance enhancement and injury prevention that drove me to study sports science, and to pursue it as my vocation. Having completed my undergraduate degree, I was inspired by my father's book, *Oil Economist's Handbook*, to produce a similar book for sports science.

When the first edition of *Sports Science Handbook* was published, I was in the midst of my doctoral studies at the University of Oxford, with a thesis entitled, "Conscious and Unconscious Control in Highly Learned Motor Actions." My research was carried out on the PGA European Tour, at the same time as I worked as a caddie. My theoretical, empirical and experiential insights made me realize why I was never going to win the British Open.

After completing my doctoral work in 1994, I became a lecturer in sports science at St. Mary's University College, specializing in psychology and also teaching courses in research methods and statistics. At the University of Surrey (Guildford), an opportunity arose to lead the development of a new sports science program designed specifically for part-time adult learners. At Surrey, I learned much from colleagues, such as Dr. Joe Millward in nutritional science, and Nicky Gilbert in dietetics, who contributed to my courses. Subsequently, at the University of Wales (Swansea), I led the development of a new sports science degree for full-time students. My understanding of chemistry was enhanced through developing a course on exercise metabolism with Dr. Tony Wellington. Basic knowledge in chemistry is important for being able to gain a thorough understanding of many questions in exercise science. I also led the development of a state-of-the-art motion analysis laboratory, and gained new perspectives on biomechanics by working with colleagues in physics and engineering. By 2001, I had delivered or developed courses in most of the subdisciplines related to sports science.

Between 1997 and 2001, I was also an Associate Coach for the English Golf Union, working in the Winter Coaching Program for Potential Boy Internationals in the South Region. I worked with the professional golf teachers, Steve Rolley and Gary Smith, providing education and training on fitness, diet and psychology. Most of the boys dreamed of winning the British Open, and my corpus of knowledge from sports science, as well as my research on golf, should increase the probability that at least one of these boys will fulfill that dream.

Having worked in the USA since 2002, I am currently working as a Visiting Lecturer at Pepperdine University. Two of the coaches at Pepperdine are Dr. Marv Dunphy, who was Head Coach of the gold-medal winning USA Volleyball team at the 1988 Olympic Games; and Paul Westphal, who was a successful NBA coach after a stellar career as a player with the

University of Southern California and the Boston Celtics. During one of his coaching classes in 2004, which I sat in on, Dunphy conducted an interview with Westphal, who was asked whether it was more important for one of his players to get a degree or to be drafted for the NBA. Westphal replied, "There's a politically correct answer, but I'm not going to give it. I want to see the young man succeed and fulfill his dreams." For some student-athletes, making a good college team and getting a degree is the fulfillment of a dream; an end in itself. For other student-athletes, college is a stepping-stone for, say, becoming an NBA player or an Olympian.

Consider the case of Matt Leinart, who was quarterback of national football champions University of Southern California in 2005 and also the recipient of the Heisman Trophy. Rather than enter the 2005 NFL Draft, with the prospect of making millions of dollars, Leinart decided to stay at the University of Southern California for his final year of eligibility, which would also allow him to achieve the final 18 credits required for his sociology degree. Leinart said he thought his decision "made a statement to college football – maybe to student-athletes about school being more important" than money (*Los Angeles Times*, 15 January 2005).

My involvement in providing education and training for NCAA Division I athletes has largely been through teaching a health and life skills course, based on the NCAA program, "Challenging Athletes' Minds for Personal Success" (CHAMPS). Objectives of the CHAMPS program include: supporting the efforts of every student-athlete toward intellectual development and graduation; using athletics as a preparation for success in life; respecting diversity; and enabling student-athletes to make meaningful contributions to their communities.

Following my experience in adapted physical education at Eastern Oregon University and also in golf coaching for the Special Olympics, I was inspired to develop an adapted physical activity program at Pepperdine. This program provides opportunity for persons with developmental disabilities, such as Down syndrome, to participate in golf and aquatics. The life skills of many students from my CHAMPS classes at Pepperdine have enabled the Adapted Physical Activity program to be a success.

The major addition of information on disabilities and health for this edition of the *Sports Science Handbook* reflects my work in this area over the last four years. The desire to understand the relevant psychology and physiology was driven by the practical experience. Consider these words from the reflective journal of a student on the Adapted Aquatics Program at Eastern Oregon University:

"I worked with a girl who has autism, cerebral palsy, and a Dandy-Walker cyst. I never knew that an individual could have so many disorders. She walks around school with a walker, and according to the aide, she maneuvers it very well. She also controls her upper body better than most people with cerebral palsy, and she does not drool. As I learned from talking to the aide, my girl feeds herself and she also lets people know what she wants by using cue cards. She is also very capable of maneuvering herself in her wheelchair, as I found out when she raced us, while we were on scooters. Although my girl has all these disorders and handicaps, she is a very unique and wonderful person. All the days she is in a good mood, she is a blast. She smiles and laughs a lot. She even grunts a little. In the pool, she is usually very active and cooperative and seems to be having fun. On the days she is not in a very good mood, you just try to make it fun. Working with my girl was exciting, memorable and fulfilling."

Using the Book

A feature of the *Sports Science Handbook* is that the language used in scientific journals is maintained as much as possible, in order to gain an understanding of terminology and concepts. Development of the book has been driven by a 'top-down' approach in which overviews of important areas are compiled, before detail is added. Many entries provide a concise and comprehensive coverage of a particular subject matter. Within these entries, some scientific terms are highlighted in bold and are defined. Most of the scientific terms that are not highlighted in bold are defined in a separate entry, but the author has avoided use of a signifier (such as an asterisk) for highlighting the terms that are defined in a separate entry. No hard and fast rules were used to determine where scientific terms are defined, but an attempt has been made to make the book user-friendly. The book is largely a 'review of authoritative reviews;' thus to avoid unnecessary cluttering of the text, citations in the text are minimized. Instead, a bibliography is provided at the end of the entry and further bibliographies attached to cross-referenced terms or to entries for relevant subdisciplines. There is also a general bibliography, which includes textbooks that were used extensively by the author when compiling this latest edition of the *Sports Science Handbook*.

The *Sports Science Handbook* provides concise and up-to-date overviews of subject matter and clarifies confusing issues. It can be used, for example, to distinguish: ability vs. skill; cellulite vs. stretch marks; cholesterol vs. lipoprotein; convulsion vs. seizure; creep vs. stress relaxation; force vs. work; hypnosis vs. meditation; learning disability vs. mental retardation; medial tibial stress syndrome vs. shin splints; negative reinforcement vs. punishment; power vs. strength; reflex vs. stereotypy; stretch reflex vs. stretch-shortening cycle; and torque vs. torsion.

The book can be used as a source of reference for introductory or foundation courses that are concerned with: (i) the nature and scope of kinesiology and its various professional applications; (ii) key concepts and terminology within the subdisciplines; (iii) the historical and philosophical foundations of the field; and (iv) the use of historical knowledge to understand current issues, controversies and future directions.

Readership

The book will be useful to students throughout their academic career as a handbook for work on essays, projects, laboratory reports, exam revision, and thesis ideas. Teachers in high

schools, community colleges and universities will find much useful and interesting information in the *Sports Science Handbook* to supplement material from their textbooks. Sports
coaches will find the book useful for clarifying and building upon what they learn from coach
education courses. With respect to the cause and prevention of sports injuries, the book will
be a useful cross-disciplinary source of reference for physicians and allied health professionals. For professionals in the health and fitness industry, the book will be especially useful for
the coverage of diseases and disabilities; and also for the wealth of information that relates
to exercise and nutrition. Librarians should find the *Sports Science Handbook* valuable when
needing to provide their readers with a starting point for answering questions that relate to
physical fitness and health, and hot topics in sport such as doping and dietary supplements.

Acknowledgements

To Dr. Danny Mielke, who provided me with the initial opportunity to work in the USA as a sabbatical replacement, Assistant Professor in the Department of Physical Education and Health at Eastern Oregon University in La Grande for the academic year 2001-2002; and to whom I am indebted for mentoring and inspiration in many aspects of sport, physical education, and health in the USA. It is most appropriate that Dr. Mielke has kindly written the foreword for this edition of the *Sports Science Handbook*.

To Dr. Peggy Anderson, also of the Department of Physical Education and Health at Eastern Oregon University, for facilitating my work in the Adapted Aquatics Program with Mr. Bill Durand of the Union-Baker School District, before she took leave for her sabbatical year. Working in this program has been the most rewarding experience of my career. I am grateful to Mr. Durand for enabling me to learn so much from his expertise in adapted physical education; and to the PE students at Eastern Oregon University, who were so devoted to their work. I am also grateful to Dr. Jim Sheehy and Dr. Gary Lillard of the Grand Ronde Child Center for our many discussions about behavioral conditions, such as attention-deficit hyperactivity disorder; and to Brian Fischer and Lonnie Myers for my work with Special Olympics Golf in La Grande.

To Dr. Caroline Vos Strache, who brought me to Pepperdine University in Malibu for 2002-2003 as her sabbatical replacement to coordinate the major in Physical Education.

To Dr. Doug Swartzendruber, who made me welcome for an extended period of employment as a Visiting Lecturer in the Natural Science Division at Pepperdine and who supported my efforts to develop an adapted physical activity program for persons with developmental disabilities.

To Mike Anderson, my colleague in Physical Education at Pepperdine, for making my life easy when it came to matters of academic administration.

To Kimberlee Rodriguez of the Athletics Department at Pepperdine, for our many discussions about the lives of student-athletes and for encouraging students to take my classes.

To my students at Pepperdine University, who read and provided comments on entries that were being prepared for this edition, especially Morgan Matthies and Joey Parker; and, specifically, to students in my History & Philosophy class, whose feedback convinced me to embed the chronology items in the main part of the book rather than in a separate section: Nelson Caraballo, Jasmine Clarendon, Amber Coffman, Teiosha George, Amber Heydel, Terrance Johnson, Marvin Lea, Glen McGowan, Derek Mills, Leslie Pacheco, Ali Pavoni, Maytal Shvartz, and Ashley Swanson.

To my publisher, Bill Hughes, for his confidence in the vision of this book for the US market.

To my family and friends for continual support and encouragement; and especially to my wife, Chrys, who provided limitless patience, as well as guidance and assistance on editing; and spurred me to write a preface explaining why the book is a vocational project.

Introduction

Kinesiology

The *Sports Science Handbook* has now adopted a subtitle that includes the term 'kinesiology,' which can be defined as the study of movement or, more generally, the study of physical activity (Newell, 1990). In 1993, the American Academy of Physical Education (AAPE) changed its name to the American Academy of Kinesiology and Physical Education (AAKPE).

While the term 'kinesiology' has become accepted in higher education, the term 'physical education' is the correct name for the teaching of exercise and sport activities (and related theoretical knowledge) in elementary and high schools, because it has long been understood by society (Spirduso, 1990).

The American Academy of Kinesiology and Physical Education (AAKPE) provides information about doctoral programs that focus on the study of physical activity. Based on a survey of programs at 61 doctoral institutions (69 departments) by the AAKPE, the most frequently used terms in departmental titles are: kinesiology (22), exercise and/or sport(s) science(s) (21), health (14), physical education (6) and human performance (5). The widespread use of the term 'kinesiology' is shown also by the fact that eight of the eleven "Big Ten" Schools in the USA now have a department (or division) with 'kinesiology' in its name. None of these schools has a department with 'physical education' in its name, but the Department of Kinesiology at the University of Indiana is in the School of Health, Physical Education & Recreation. The term 'sport & exercise science,' or simply 'exercise science,' is now often used by departments that embrace contexts other than sport, especially those concerned with health. Only one of the "Big Ten" schools (University of Iowa) has 'exercise science' in the name of a department, but three other schools have named programs or majors at undergraduate level in 'exercise science.' The University of Michigan defines the scope of its major in 'movement science' as being biomechanics, physiology and motor control, but the University of Wisconsin-Madison uses a broader definition of 'movement science' and also has a major in 'exercise science.' The Exercise Science option at Wisconsin-Madison prepares students for graduate study in exercise physiology, cardiac rehabilitation, sport psychology, or biomechanics; whereas the Movement Science option prepares students for graduate study in motor behavior, motor control/learning, motor development, sport psychology, or biomechanics. What the University of Wisconsin-Madison calls 'movement science' is called 'exercise science' at the University of Indiana (Bloomington) and the University of Iowa. Ohio State University uses 'exercise science' to refer to the field of health-related fitness (fitness evaluation/exercise prescription), but Penn State University calls this 'movement science.'

The chronology of name changes at Michigan State University, one of the "Big Ten" schools, is a good reflection of historical trends and the fact that 'kinesiology' is perhaps the best 'catch-all' term for university departments to use in their name: Department of Physical Culture and Athletics (1899); Department of Physical Training (1916); Department of Physical Education (1921); Department of Physical Education, Health and Recreation (1944); Department of Health, Physical Education and Recreation (1954); Department of Health and Physical Education (1981); School of Health Education, Counseling Psychology and Human Performance (1985); Department of Physical Education and Exercise Science (1990); and Department of Kinesiology (1998).

Physical Education as an Academic Discipline

Central to historical accounts of the development of kinesiology from physical education are the University of California, Berkeley and the University of California, Los Angeles (UCLA). In the early 1940s, the Executive Committee of the College of Letters and Science at the University of California (Berkeley) completed a review of the physical education department and concluded that its curriculum was lacking in academic content. As a result, the physical education department proposed a new major that met the College's criteria for academic standards. Elsewhere, physical education continued to be regarded as an area of teaching rather than an academic discipline. Many physical educators argued that academic theory, empirical research and scholarship are of little use to those engaged in the practice of teaching children and youths in schools.

In the early 1960s, James Conant studied the education of the nation's teachers and recommended that graduate programs in physical education be abolished due to lack of academic credibility. In 1962, the Fisher Bill was passed in the state of California. It created a single-subject teaching credential that limited a teacher to a specific subject field. Physical education was identified as a nonacademic area, but it could be classified as an academic area if certain criteria were met. Following the Fisher Bill and Conant's report, physical education departments in universities and colleges underwent academic reform.

In the 1950s, the Physical Education Department at the University of California, Los Angeles (UCLA) offered one of the finest teacher preparation programs in the USA (Smith, 1999). The first research facility, the Human Performance Laboratory, was dedicated in 1958. With the establishment of California's Master Plan for Higher Education in 1960, most teacher preparation programs for University of California undergraduates were discontinued. Consequently, the School of Applied Arts at UCLA was disestablished. The Physical Education Department was transferred to the Life Science Division in the College of Letters and Science, and the tenured faculty members designed new educational programs in the science of human movement. A revised physical education major, involving primarily one of three allied fields of study – physiology, psychology or sociology – was approved in 1962. This major became a model for adoption by other universities, especially after the State Board of Education approved it in 1965 as being equivalent to that of an academic subject-matter major. Camille Brown, a professor of physical education at UCLA, was described by *Quest* as "an accomplished conceptual synthesizer who works in the areas of human movement theory and physical education curriculum." The Kinesiology Department at UCLA was established in 1972 and was the first of its kind in the USA. In 1990, however, the Kinesiology Department at UCLA became the Physiological Science Department, when it was decided to decrease the scope of the department's research and education programs and focus primarily on physiology.

The American Alliance for Health, Physical Education, and Recreation (AAHPER) formed a panel in 1963 to address the professional preparation of physical education teachers and it publicly refuted the views of James Conant. In 1964, Franklin M. Henry spoke at the annual meeting of the National College Physical Education Association for Men (NCPEAM) on: "Physical Education – An Academic Discipline." Henry proposed that physical education must not only become a credible academic discipline, but also it must preside over the profession (practice) of physical education. Henry defined an academic discipline as an organized body of knowledge that is theoretical and scholarly, without any requirement of practical application, as distinguished from technical and professional knowledge (Henry, 1978).

In the history of physical education, a distinction is made between 'education of the physical' and 'education through the physical.' Charles McCloy was a champion of 'education of the physical,' in which the purpose of physical activity is to develop the physical body. Jesse F. Williams advocated 'education through the physical,' in which the purpose of sport and physical education is to build character. Following Franklin M. Henry's address in 1964, there was a shift away from both 'education of the physical' and 'education through the physical' towards a disciplinary-oriented approach in higher education.

Subdisciplines

For three years in the mid 1960s, the "Big Ten" directors met to discuss "The Body of Knowledge in Physical Education." Five subdisciplines were covered at all three meetings: history/philosophy of sport; exercise physiology, motor learning/sport psychology; biomechanics; and sport sociology. These subdisciplines represented much of what, at the time, was considered to be the body of knowledge for "the study of human movement (Thomas, 1990). By 1980, all the leading graduate programs in kinesiology across the USA were based on a subdisciplinary model (Swanson and Massengale, 1997).

Interdisciplinary and Cross-disciplinary

The subdisciplines have typically maintained their interdisciplinary connections (e.g. exercise physiology to physiology and biochemistry), but they have not sufficiently developed the cross-disciplinary connections (e.g. exercise physiology to biomechanics to psychology) that would broaden the impact of knowledge and research (Newell, 1990; Sharp, 2003). An example of an attempt to promote the cross-disciplinary approach can be found in the Department of Kinesiology at University of Illinois (Urbana-Champaign). The academic programs are organized around five clusters of core concepts related to the study of human movement: (i) Biodynamics of Physical Activity ("the study of work output, energy, and efficiency of movements as it relates to the nature of exercise stress, the mechanics of human movement, and fitness throughout the human lifespan"); (ii) Social Science of Physical Activity ("the study of the antecedents and consequences of involvement in physical activity and sport as well as the impact that physical activity and sport have upon individuals, society and culture"); (iii) Coordination, Control and Skill ("the study of the mechanisms and processes involved in the acquisition and performance of human motor skills"); (iv) Pedagogical Kinesiology ("the study of the organizational and instructional concepts essential for the efficient and effective conduct of physical activity programs, particularly those that relate to physical education and sport contexts"); and (v) Therapeutic Kinesiology ("the study of movement as a therapeutic vehicle for health and wellness, particularly the prevention and rehabilitation of injury, disease or movement dysfunction").

References

American Academy of Kinesiology and Physical Education. AAKPE Doctoral Program Information. 3 June 2004. Http://www.aakpe.org/

Brown, C. (1967). The structure of knowledge of physical education. *Quest* (monograph IX), 53-67.

Conant, J. (1963). *The education of American teachers*. New York: McGraw-Hill.

Department of Kinesiology (2000). College of Applied Life Studies. University of Illinois at Urbana-Champaign. Http://www.kines.uiuc.edu/overview

Dunn, J.M. (2001). Honoring the past – embracing the future. *Quest* 53(4), 495-506.

Estes, S.G. and Mechikoff, R.A. (1999). *Knowing Human Movement*. San Francisco, CA: Benjamin Cummings

Henry, F. (1964). Physical education as an academic discipline. *Journal of Health, Physical Education, and Recreation* 35(7), 32-33, 69.

Henry, F. (1978). *The academic discipline of physical education. Quest* 29, 13-29.

McCloy, C.H. (1940). *Philosophical basis for physical education*. New York: F.S. Crofts & Co.

Newell, K.M. (1990). Physical education in higher education: Chaos out of order. *Quest* 42(3), 227-242.

Newell, K.M. (1990). Physical activity, knowledge types, and degree programs. *Quest* 42(3), 243-268.

Newell, K. (1990). Kinesiology: The label for the study of physical activity in higher education. *Quest* 42(3), 269-278.

Sharp, R.L. (2003). Doctoral education: The mixture perspective. *Quest* 55, 82-85.

Smith, J.L. (1999). University of California: In Memoriam. Donald Thomas Handy, Kinesiology: Los Angeles. Http://dynaweb.oac.cdlib.org:8088/dynaweb/uchist/public/inmemoriam/inmemoriam1999/@Generi c..._

Swanson, R.A. and Massengale, J.D. (1997). Exercise and sport science in 20th century America. In: Massengale, J.D. and Swanson, R.A. (eds). *The history of exercise and sport science*. pp1-14. Champaign, IL: Human Kinetics.

Spirduso, W.W. (1990). Commentary: The Newell epic – A case for academic sanity. *Quest* 42, 297-304.

Thomas, J.R. (1990). The body of knowledge: A common core. In: Corbin, C.B. and Eckert, H.M. (eds). *The evolving undergraduate major*. pp5-12. Champaign, IL: Human Kinetics.

Williams, J.F. (1930). Education through the physical. *Journal of Higher Education* 1, 279-282.

Wrynn, A. (2003). Contesting the canon: Understanding the history of the evolving discipline of kinesiology. *Quest* 55(3), 244-256.

Zeigler, E.F. and McCristal, K.J. (1967). A history of the Big Ten Body-of-Knowledge Project in physical education. *Quest* 9, 79-84.

Survey of the eleven "Big Ten" Schools, December 2004

Department of Exercise Science. University of Iowa. Http://uiowa.edu/~exsci

Department of Health and Kinesiology. Purdue University. Http://www.sla.purdue.edu/academic/hk

Department of Kinesiology. College of Applied Life Studies. University of Illinois at Urbana-Champaign. Http://www.kines.uiuc.edu/

Department of Kinesiology. College of Education. Michigan State University. Http://edweb6.educ.msu.edu/kin.

Department of Kinesiology. College of Health and Human Development. Penn State University. Http://www.hhdev.psu.edu/kines/

Department of Kinesiology. School of Education. University of Wisconsin-Madison. Http://www.education.wisc.edu/kinesiology

Department of Kinesiology. School of Health, Physical Education and Recreation. Indiana University (Bloomington). Http://www.indiana.edu/~kines/

Division of Kinesiology. University of Michigan. Http://www.kines.umich.edu

Division of Kinesiology. College of Education and Human Development. University of Minnesota. Http://education.umn.edu/Kin

School of Physical Activity and Educational Services. College of Education. Ohio State University. Http://www.coe.ohio-state.edu/paes

Department of Physical Therapy & Human Movement Sciences. Feinberg School of Medicine. Northwestern University. Http://www.nupt.northwestern.edu

General Bibliography

American College of Sports Medicine (2001). *ACSM's resource manual for Guidelines for exercise testing & prescription*. 4th ed. Philadelphia, PA: Lippincott Williams & Wilkins.

Anderson, M.K., Hall, S.J. and Martin, M. (2004). *Foundations of athletic training: Prevention, assessment and management*. 3rd ed. Philadelphia, PA: Lippincott, Williams and Wilkins.

Anshel, M.H. (2003). *Sport psychology: From theory to practice*. 4th ed. San Francisco: Benjamin Cummings.

Antonio, J. and Stout, J.R. (2001). *Sports supplements*. Philadelphia, PA: Lippincott Williams & Wilkins.

Brown, S.P. (2000). *Introduction to exercise science*. Philadelphia, PA: Lippincott Williams & Wilkins.

Coakley, J. (2004). *Sports in society. Issues and controversies*. 8th ed. Boston, MA: McGraw-Hill.

Cox, R.H. (2002). *Sport psychology: Concepts and applications*. 5th ed. Boston, MA: McGraw-Hill.

Eitzen, D.S. and Sage, G.H. (2003). *Sociology of North American sport*. 7th ed. Boston, MA: McGraw-Hill.

Enoka, R.M. (2002). *Neuromechanics of human movement*. 3rd ed. Champaign, IL: Human Kinetics.

Gallahue, D.L. and Ozmun, J.C. (2002). *Understanding motor development. Infants, children, adolescents, adults*. 5th ed. New York, NY: McGraw-Hill.

Germann, W.J. and Stanfield, C.L. (2001). *Principles of human physiology*. San Francisco, CA: Benjamin Cummings.

Gill, D.L. (2000). *Psychological dynamics of sport and exercise*. 2nd ed. Champaign, IL: Human Kinetics.

Guyton, A.C. and Hall, J.E. (2000). *Textbook of medical physiology*. 10th ed. Philadelphia, PA: W.B. Saunders Co.

Hall, S.J. (2003). *Basic biomechanics*. 4th ed. Boston, MA: WCB McGraw-Hill.

Hamill, J. and Knutzen, K.M. (2003). *Biomechanical basis of human movement*. 2nd ed. Philadelphia, PA: Lippincott Williams & Wilkins.

Hamilton, N. and Luttgens, K. (2002). *Kinesiology. Scientific basis of human motion*. 10th ed. Madison, WI: Brown & Benchmark.

Harries, M. et al. (1998). *Oxford textbook of sports medicine*. 2nd ed. Oxford: Oxford University Press.

Haywood, K.M. and Getchell, N. (2004). *Life span motor development*. 4th ed. Champaign, IL: Human Kinetics.

Horn, T. (2002, ed). *Advances in sport psychology*. 2nd ed. Champaign, IL: Human Kinetics.

Housh, T.J. and Housh, D.J. (2000, eds). *Introduction to exercise science*. Boston, MA: Allyn and Bacon.

Houston, M.E (2001). *Biochemistry primer for exercise science*. 2nd ed. Champaign, IL: Human Kinetics.

Insel, P., Turner, R.E. and Ross, D. (2004). *Nutrition*. 2nd ed. Sudbury, MA: Jones and Bartlett.

Irvin, R., Iversen, D. and Roy, S. (1998). *Sports medicine. Prevention, assessment, management and rehabilitation of athletic injuries*. 2nd ed. Boston, MA: Allyn & Bacon.

Kamen, G. (2001). *Foundations of Exercise Science*. Philadelphia, PA: Lippincott, Williams and Wilkins.

Kreighbaum, E. and Barthels, K.M. (1996). *Biomechanics: A qualitative approach*. 4th ed. Needham Heights, MA: Allyn and Bacon.

Leonard, W. (1998). *Sociological perspectives of sport*. 5th ed. San Francisco, CA: Benjamin Cummings.

Levangie, P.K. and Norkin, C.C. (2001). *Joint structure and function: A comprehensive analysis*. 3rd ed. Philadelphia, PA: F.A. Davis Company.

Le Veau, B.F. (1992). *Williams and Lissner's biomechanics of human motion*. 3rd ed. Philadelphia, PA: W.B. Saunders.

Marieb, E.N. (2002). *Anatomy and physiology*. San Francisco, CA: Benjamin Cummings.

Mathews, C.K., Van Holde, K.E. and Ahern, K. (2000). *Biochemistry*. 3rd ed. San Francisco, CA: Benjamin/Cummings.

McArdle, W.D, Katch, F.I. and Katch, V.L. (2004). *Exercise physiology. Energy, nutrition, and human performance*. 5th ed. Philadelphia, PA: Lippincott Williams & Wilkins.

Mechikoff, R.A. and Estes, S.G. (2002). *A history and philosophy of sport and physical education. From ancient civilization to the modern world*. 3rd ed Boston, MA: McGraw-Hill.

Nieman, D.C. (2003). *Exercise testing and prescription.* 5th ed. Boston, MA: McGraw-Hill.

Payne, V.G. and Isaacs, L.D. (2005). *Human motor development. A lifespan approach.* 6th ed. Boston, MA: McGraw-Hill.

Plowman, S.A. and Smith, D.L. (2003). *Exercise physiology for health, fitness and performance.* 2nd ed. San Francisco, CA: Benjamin Cummings.

Polidoro, J.R. (2000). *Sport and physical activity in the modern world.* San Francisco, CA: Benjamin Cummings.

Powers, S.K. and Dodd, S.L. (2003). *Total fitness and wellness.* 3rd ed. San Francisco, CA: Benjamin Cummings.

Powers, S.K. and Howley, E.T. (2004). *Exercise physiology. Theory and application to fitness and performance.* 5th ed. Boston, MA: McGraw-Hill.

Rasch, P.J. (1989). *Kinesiology and applied anatomy.* 7th ed. Philadelphia, PA: Lea & Febiger.

Robergs, R.A. and Roberts, S.O. (2000). *Fundamental principles of exercise physiology.* Boston, MA: McGraw-Hill.

Rose, D.J. (1997). *A multilevel approach to the study of motor control and learning.* San Francisco, CA: Benjamin Cummings.

Safran, M.R., McKeag, D.B. and Van Camp, S.P. (1998). *Manual of sports medicine.* Philadelphia, PA: Lippincot-Raven.

Schmidt, R.A. and Wrisberg, C.A. (2004). *Motor learning and performance.* 3rd ed. Champaign, IL: Human Kinetics.

Schmidt, R.A. and Lee, T.D. (1999). *Motor control and learning. A behavioral emphasis.* 3rd ed. Champaign, IL: Human Kinetics.

Sherill, C. (2004). *Adapted physical activity, recreation, and sport: Crossdisciplinary and lifespan.* 6th ed. Boston, MA: McGraw-Hill.

Sherry, E. and Wilson, S. (1998). *Oxford handbook of sports medicine.* 2nd ed. New York: Oxford University Press.

Siedentop, D. (2004). *Introduction to physical education, fitness and sport.* 5th ed. Boston, MA: McGraw-Hill.

Silva, J.M. and Stevens, D.E. (2002, eds). *Psychological foundations of sport.* Boston, MA: Allyn & Bacon.

Stryer, L, Berg, J. and Tymoczko, J. (2002). *Biochemistry.* 5th ed. New York: W.H. Freeman.

Swanson, R.A. and Spears, B. (1995). *History of sport and physical education in the United States.* 4th ed. Boston, MA: WCB/McGraw-Hill.

Tortora, G.J. and Grabowski, S.R. (2003). *Principles of anatomy and physiology.* 10th ed. New York: John Wiley and Sons.

Vander, A., Sherman, J. and Luciano, D. (2001). *Human physiology. The mechanisms of body function.* 8th edition. Boston, MA: McGraw-Hill.

Van Raalte, J.L. and Brewer, B.W. (1996). *Exploring sport and exercise psychology.* Washington, DC: American Psychology Association.

Wann, D.L. (1997). *Sports psychology.* Upper Saddle River, NJ: Prentice Hall.

Williams, J.M. (2001, ed). *Applied sport psychology: Personal growth to peak performance.* 4th ed. Boston, MA: McGraw-Hill.

Wilmore, J.H. and Costill, D.L. (2004). *Physiology of sport and exercise.* 3rd ed. Champaign, IL: Human Kinetics.

Winnick, J.P. (2000, ed). *Adapted physical education and sport.* 3rd ed. Champaign, IL: Human Kinetics.

Wuest, D.A. and Buecher, C.A. (2003). *Foundations of physical education, exercise science, and sport.* 14th ed. Boston, MA: McGraw-Hill.

A

ABDOMINAL CAVITY   The hollow space that contains the abdominal viscera. The **abdominal wall** refers to the layers of muscle between the skin and the abdominal cavity.

ABDOMINAL INJURIES   The abdominal muscles, most commonly the *rectus abdominis*, may incur a strain as a result of direct trauma such as sudden twisting or hyperextension of the spine. Complications arise when the epigastric artery or intramuscular blood vessels are damaged, leading to hematoma formation. If hollow viscera are damaged, their contents can leak into the abdominal cavity and cause severe hemorrhage, peritonitis and shock. Baseball catchers wear torso protection from compressive forces to prevent contusions of the abdominal wall.

See also HERNIA; SOLAR PLEXUS CONTUSION.

ABDOMINAL OBESITY   Upper-body obesity. Android-type obesity. It is associated with visceral fat storage, including an increase in intra-abdominal fat (mesenteric and omentum fat).

Evidence from research on twins has suggested there may be specific genetic determinants of central abdominal fat, independent of overall obesity.

According to the American Heart Association, a person is considered to be upper-body (android) obese when the waist-to-hip ratio is greater than 0.95 (men) and greater than 0.88 (women). The **waist-to-hip ratio** is the ratio of waist girth to hip girth. The waist girth is measured at the narrowest point during relaxed standing (without 'pulling in the stomach'). The hip girth (over the buttocks) is measured at the widest point. In men, waist-to-hip ratio correlates with increasing fatness, because of the tendency to store excess fat in the abdominal region. In women, waist-to-hip ratio correlates poorly with fatness, because of the heterogeneity of fat storage in women. The proportion of intra-abdominal fat progressively increases with age.

Women tend to be lower-body (gynoid-type) obese and men tend to be upper-body (android-type) obese, but there are many men who are lower-body obese and women who are upper-body obese. It is not clearly understood why some people are upper-body obese and some people are lower-body obese. Fat distribution is partly determined by the regional activity of the enzyme lipoprotein lipase. Females possess larger amounts of lipoprotein lipase. The areas of greatest lipoprotein lipase are (female) hip, thigh and breast; and (male) intra-abdominal. There are age-related variations in lipoprotein lipase and this plays a role in the development of upper-body obesity in middle-aged females. In women, compared to men, the enzyme is markedly more active in the femoral fat regions. In pre-menopausal women, this activity is greater in femoral fat than in breast or abdominal fat. Women with upper-body obesity have much higher levels of male hormones, such as testosterone, compared to women with lower-body obesity.

Abdominal obesity is a more serious risk factor than total body obesity for cardiovascular disease, diabetes, hypertension, hypertriglyceridemia (excessive fat in the blood) and low HDL cholesterol.

Obese subjects with visceral fat accumulation more frequently demonstrate impairment of glucose and lipid metabolism than those with subcutaneous fat accumulation. Visceral fat obesity is present in almost 90% of obese patients with ischemic heart disease. Even in nonobese subjects, visceral fat accumulation is correlated with glucose intolerance, hyperlipidemia and hypertension. 40% of nonobese subjects with coronary artery disease have increased visceral fat. Intra-abdominal fat has been shown to have high activities of both lipogenesis and lipolysis. Its accumulation can therefore induce high levels of free fatty acids, a product of lipolysis, in portal circulation. Excess free fatty acids may cause the enhancement of lipid synthesis and gluconeogenesis, as well as insulin resistance, resulting in hyperlipidemia, glucose intolerance and hypertension, and finally atherosclerosis. Matsuzawa et al. (1995) proposed a disease entity, **visceral fat syndrome**, which may increase susceptibility to atherosclerosis due to multiple risk factors induced by visceral fat accumulation.

Limited evidence suggests that exercise-induced weight loss is associated with decreases in abdominal obesity as measured by waist circumference or imaging methods.

Abdominal protrusion ('pot belly;' 'beer belly') arises when the intra-abdominal fat pushes the abdominal muscles into a taut position. Abdominal protrusion is not always associated with abdominal obesity. There are a number of other causes, such as enlargement of the spleen, liver or ovaries. When abdominal protrusion is severe, and the viscera drop into a new position, it is known as **visceroptosis (splanchnoptosis)**. The stomach, liver, spleen, kidneys, and intestines may all be displaced, resulting in adverse effects upon their various functions. Lordosis caused by weakness of the abdominal muscles may also be a cause of potbelly, though it is not thought to be the usual cause. Weak abdominal muscles also allow the hip flexors and lumbar extensors to tilt the pelvis downward, increasing the lumbar curve. Abdominal protrusion is normal in the young child and usually accompanied by lordosis. The protruding abdomen characterizes paralysis or muscle weakness that results from spinal cord injuries.

In general, even a huge potbelly does not show the outlines of bloated fat cells (i.e. cellulite), because abdominal skin is thicker and less taut than the skin covering the pelvis, buttocks and thighs.

See also under DEHYDROEPIANDRO-STERONE; METABOLIC SYNDROME.

Bibliography

Avery, C.S. (1991). Abdominal obesity. *The Physician and Sportsmedicine* 19(10), 137-143.

Buemann, B. and Tremlay, A. (1996). Effects of exercise training on abdominal obesity and related metabolic complications. *Sports Medicine* 21(3), 191-212.

Elia, M. (2001). Obesity in the elderly. *Obesity Research* 9(4S), S244-S248.

Matsuzawa, Y. et al. (1995). Pathophysiology and pathogenesis of visceral fat obesity. *Obesity Research* 3(2S), 187-194.

Matsuzawa, Y. et al. (1995). Pathophysiology and pathogenesis of visceral fat obesity. *Annals of the New York Academy of Sciences* 748(1), 399-406.

Ross, R. and Janssen, I. (1999). Is abdominal fat preferentially reduced in response to exercise-induced weight loss? *Medicine and Science in Sports and Exercise* 31(11), S568-S572.

Ross, R. and Janssen, I. (2001). Physical activity, total and regional obesity: Dose-response considerations. *Medicine and Science in Sports and Exercise* 33(6S), S521-S527.

Stamford, B. (1991). Apples and pears. Where you 'wear' your fat can affect your health. *The Physician and Sportsmedicine* 19(1), 123-124.

Vogel, J.A. and Friedl, K.E. (1992). Body fat assessment in women. Special considerations. *Sports Medicine* 13(4), 245-269.

ABDOMINOPLASTY Tummy tuck. It is a major surgical procedure to remove excessive skin and fat from the middle and lower abdomen to tighten the muscles of the abdominal wall. The procedure can dramatically decrease the appearance of a protruding abdomen, but produces a permanent scar.

Bibliography

American Society of Plastic Surgeons. Http://www.plasticsurgery.org

ABILITY A relatively stable trait or characteristic, which underlies performance and is largely unmodified by practice. Biological forces are primarily responsible for determining a person's basic abilities. Although it used to be commonly believed that some people possess 'general motor ability,' it is now thought that each skill depends on a large number of specific, separate motor abilities. Abilities are the building blocks of skills, as well as limiting factors in, the acquisition of skills.

Fleishman (1972) identified the following categories of perceptual motor ability: multi-limb coordination (ability to coordinate movements of a number of limbs simultaneously); control precision (ability to make rapid and precise movement adjustments of control devices involving single arm-hand or leg movements, and making adjustments in response to visual stimuli); response orientation (ability to make a rapid selection of controls to be moved or the direction to move them in); reaction time (ability to respond rapidly to a signal when it appears); speed of arm movement (ability to rapidly make a gross, discrete arm movement where accuracy is minimized); rate control (ability to time continuous anticipatory movement adjustments in response to speed and/or direction changes of a continuously moving target or object); manual dexterity (ability to make arm-hand movements to manipulate fairly large objects under speeded conditions); finger dexterity (ability to make controlled manipulations of tiny objects involving primarily the fingers); arm-hand steadiness (ability to make precise arm-hand positioning movements where strength and speed are minimized); wrist-finger speed (ability to make rapid and repetitive movements with the hand and fingers, and/or rotary wrist movements when accuracy is not critical); and aiming (ability to rapidly and accurately move the hand to a small target).

It is not known whether timing is a general ability that underlies skilled performance, or whether there are various types of timing abilities that are specific the requirements of particular skills.

See MOTOR SKILL.

Bibliography

Fleishman, E.A. (1972). On the relationship between abilities, learning, and human performance. *American Psychologist* 27, 1017-1032.

Fleishman, E.A. and Quaintance, M.K. (1984). *Taxonomies of human performance*. Orlando, FL: Academic Press.

Magill, R.A. (2004). *Motor learning and control. Concepts and applications*. 7th ed. Boston: MA: McGraw-Hill.

ABRASION Scrape. An acute injury resulting from shearing forces between the epidermis or mucosa and another surface (e.g. athletic track), with the result that the granular and keratinized skin cells are abruptly removed from the underlying dermis.

'**Turf burn**' develops when an athlete, such as a football player, slides an exposed area of skin across artificial turf. Because the artificial turf has a lower coefficient of friction than natural grass, especially when wet, the athlete slides a greater distance, thus generating heat and producing an injury that is part abrasion and part burn.

Bibliography

Basler, R.S., Hunzeker, C.M. and Garcia, M.A. (2004). Athletic skin injuries. Combating pressure and friction. *The Physician and Sportsmedicine* 32(5), 33-40.

ABSORPTION The movement of chemicals produced by the digestion of food from (mainly) the intestine into the blood stream for transportation to body tissues. Unabsorbed food is eliminated as feces.

ACCELERATION The time rate of change of velocity or the time rate of change of speed. The SI unit is meters per second per second (m/s^2). The US Customary units are feet per second per second or inches per second per second. $1 \text{ ft}/s^2 = 0.3048 \text{ m}/s^2$. It is possible to have positive velocity and negative acceleration (**deceleration**), and the reverse.

Simulation models have shown that for a 100 m sprint, the best pacing strategy is an all-out effort, even if this causes a strong decrease in velocity at the end of the race. Two phases can be distinguished in a 100 m race: an acceleration phase and maximum running phase. Sprinting requires a high acceleration during the start and maintenance of a high velocity after the start. The shorter the time that is necessary to cover the sprinting distance, the more important the initial acceleration during the start. This is because of the relative time lost during the first meters covered at submaximal velocities.

See ANGULAR ACCELERATION; CENTRIPETAL ACCELERATION; NEWTON'S LAWS.

Chronology

•1987 • At the World Athletics Championships in Rome, cameras and timing equipment covered every 10 m segment of the 100 m race in order to establish the top speed man can reach in running. Ben Johnson and Carl Lewis were both found to reach 26.3 mph. Johnson peaked at around 60 m and slowed hardly at all. Lewis continued to accelerate until 90 m. Johnson's style was characterized by a high step rate, while Lewis' style was characterized by a large stride length (maximum of 2.74 m). Johnson won the race in a world record time of 9.83 secs (to

Lewis' record-equalling 9.93 secs). Johnson lost the title and the record when he failed a drug test at the 1988 Olympics.

Bibliography

van Ingen Schenau, G.J., de Koning, J.J., and de Groot, G. (1994). Optimization of sprinting performance in running, cycling, and speed skating. *Sports Medicine* 17(4), 259-275.

ACCELEROMETER   A device used to directly measure acceleration. Most accelerometers are simply force transducers designed to measure reaction forces associated with a given acceleration. A mass is accelerated against a force transducer that produces a signal voltage that is proportional to the force. Since the mass is known and constant, the voltage is also proportional to the acceleration.

Bibliography

Winter, D.A. (1990). *Biomechanics and motor control of human movement.* 2nd ed. New York: Wiley.

ACCESSORY BONES   *See under* OSSICLES.

ACCLIMATION   *See under* STRESSORS.

ACCLIMATIZATION   *See under* STRESSORS.

ACCOMMODATION   *See under* COGNITIVE DEVELOPMENT; VISION.

ACCOUSTOMYOGRAPHY   Phonomyography. The technique of recording muscle sounds. Skeletal muscle makes sounds when it contracts at a frequency that is below the normal capacity of the human ear (c. 40 Hz). The mean frequency is about 10 Hz at low forces and increases to about 22 Hz during a maximal voluntary contraction. These sounds are probably due to the lateral movements of muscle fibers as they contract. Like electromyography, accoustomyography is directly related to muscle force under isometric conditions, but in a quadratic, not linear, relation.

Electromyography and accoustomyography vary independently of one another as torque increases and then decreases. Accoustomyography is more variable than electromyography.

Bibliography

Enoka, R.M. (2002). Neuromechanics of human movement. 3rd ed. Champaign, IL: Human Kinetics.

ACE INHIBITORS   *See* ANGIOTENSIN-CONVERTING ENZYMES INHIBITORS.

ACETALDEHYDE   An aldehyde formed from the oxidation of ethanol.

ACETOACETATE   *See under* KETONE BODIES.

ACETONE   *See under* KETONE BODIES.

ACETYLCHOLINE   A substance secreted at many nerve endings when nerve impulses arrive there. For nerve fibers that end at a synapse and at neuromuscular junctions, acetylcholine acts as a transmitter substance, allowing the nerve impulse to be passed on. After being secreted, acetylcholine is rapidly broken down into acetate and choline by the enzyme cholinesterase.

The release of acetylcholine has a direct vasodilatory action (coupled to nitric oxide formation and guanylyl cyclase activation). The release of acetylcholine can stimulate the release of kallikrein from glandular tissue that acts upon kininogen to form kinins (e.g. bradykinin).

Acetylcholine deficiencies are linked with a number of neurological disorders, such as tardive dyskinesia (involuntary facial grimaces and body jerking), Huntington's chorea, Friedrich's ataxia and Alzheimer's disease.

See also NEUROTRANSMITTER; NICOTINE.

ACETYL CO-ENZYME A   Acetyl CoA. The acetylated form of co-enzyme A. A two-carbon (acetyl) molecule made active by the attachment of coenzyme A. It is involved in the Krebs cycle, fatty acid oxidation and in other metabolic reactions.

See AEROBIC ENERGY SYSTEMS.

ACHIEVEMENT MOTIVATION THEORY   A theory of motivation to account for behavior in situations where an individual knows that his/her performance will be evaluated in terms of some criterion or standard of excellence, resulting in either success or failure. The theory proposes that individuals have one of two primary motives, either to approach success or to avoid failure. Individuals who tend to approach success are classed as having a high need for achievement; whereas individuals who tend toward avoiding failure are classed as having a low need for achievement. A person with a high need for achievement has the following characteristics: an attraction to situations in which he or she takes personal responsibility for finding solutions to problems, a tendency to set moderate achievement goals and to take 'calculated risks,' and a desire for concrete feedback as to how well he is doing.

See also COMPETITION; GOALS.

Bibliography

McClelland, D.C., Atkinson, J.W. and Lowelli, E.L. (1953). *The achievement motive*. New York: Appleton-Century-Crofts.

Roberts, G.C. (1992, ed). *Motivation in sport and exercise*. Champaign, IL: Human Kinetics.

ACHILLES TENDON   Calcaneal tendon. Formed by the merging tendons of the *gastrocnemius* and *soleus* muscles, it is the largest and strongest tendon in the human body. It inserts onto the calcaneus (heel bone) and is encased by a paratenon sheath.

Being a long tendon that is in series with muscles containing short fibers, the Achilles tendon is well adapted for energy storage and release. When a person jumps, the fascicle length of these muscles stay relatively constant and the tendon recoils at a high velocity to produce the movement.

Inflammation of the paratenon is usually an overuse injury that may become chronic (especially in older adults). Risk factors for inflammation of the tendon or paratenon include poor flexibility, overpronation, change in shoe (e.g. lower heels), increase in training intensity/duration (especially if it includes hill running), change in playing surface, and running on cambered surfaces. **Achilles tendinosis** is internal degeneration of the tendon itself. The tendon becomes thickened and painful, with scar tissue being formed.

Complete rupture (tear) of the Achilles tendon usually occurs 4 to 5 cm proximal to the calcaneal insertion (where the blood flow is poorest), through regions of pre-existing tendon degeneration. A partial rupture of the Achilles tendon can lead to scar formation that is liable to cause inflammation. Indirect mechanisms of Achilles tendon rupture include sudden dorsal flexion of a plantar-flexed foot (e.g. a cricket fielder leaning back and planting his rear foot as he throws) and pushing off a weight-bearing foot while extending the knee joint of the same leg (e.g. a basketball player making a rapid change of direction); direct mechanisms include a taut tendon being struck by a blunt object (e.g. a hockey stick).

Two bursae surround the Achilles tendon: (superficially) the subcutaneous bursa and (deep) the retrocalcaneal bursa. The **subcutaneous bursa** lies between the skin and the posterior surface of the Achilles tendon. It is vulnerable to pressure from shoes and may thus become inflamed, resulting in **Haglund's disease** ('calcaneal bump;' 'pump bump'). The **retrocalcaneal bursa** lies between the Achilles tendon and the calcaneus. It may become inflamed as a result of either external pressure or a partial tendon rupture. Excessive compensatory pronation is the usual cause of retrocalcaneal bursitis. Risk factors include pes cavus.

See also RUNNING INJURIES; SEVER'S DISEASE.

Chronology

•1575 • Ambroise Paré reported Achilles tendon rupture as a clinical entity. It remained uncommon until the 1950s, from whence its increase has probably been due to the increased popularity of recreational sports among middle-aged people.

ACHILLES TENDON REFLEX   'Ankle-jerk' reflex. Triceps surae reflex. The middle of the Achilles tendon is tapped with a reflex hammer, stretching the *gastrocnemius* and *soleus* muscles, which should respond by reflexively contracting and extending the foot.

ACHONDROPLASIA   *See under* DWARFISM.

ACID   A proton donor. The 'strength' of an acid is its tendency to donate a proton, i.e. the extent to which

it dissociates into ions. Strong acids, such as hydrochloric acid, completely give up their protons. Moderate-to-weak acids do not dissociate completely.
See ACID-BASE BALANCE.

ACID-BASE BALANCE The equilibrium of acids and bases in the body. Acidosis and alkalosis are disruptions of acid-base balance and may be either respiratory or non-respiratory (metabolic) in origin. The ability of muscles to do work is affected by a disruption of the acid-base balance through one or more of the following processes: a slowing of glycolysis, a direct effect on the contractile elements of muscle, and an impairment of nerve impulse propagation. Acid-base balance is maintained by buffering.
See LACTIC ACID; SODIUM BICARBONATE.

Bibliography
Hultman, E and Sahlin, K. (1980). Acid-base balance during exercise. *Exercise and Sport Sciences Reviews* 8, 41-128.

ACIDEMIA A condition in which there is an excess of hydrogen ions in the blood.

ACID MALTASE DEFICIENCY Glycogenosis type 2. Pompe's disease (infantile form). A carbohydrate processing disorder that causes slowly progressive weakness, especially of the respiratory muscles and those of the hips, upper legs, shoulders and upper arms. Cardiac problems may occur in the childhood form, but is less common in adults. It is inherited as an autosomal recessive trait.

ACIDOSIS An excess of hydrogen ions in both blood and other body fluids. **Respiratory acidosis** is caused by failure to eliminate carbon dioxide as quickly as it forms; there is an increase in the partial pressure of carbon dioxide in arterial blood. Causes include conditions that impair gas exchange or lung ventilation such as rapid, shallow breathing, and narcotic or barbiturate overdose. **Metabolic acidosis** is caused by excessive production or ingestion of acid other than carbonic acid, or by loss of base. It can be caused by diets high in protein, because protein catabolism produces phosphoric acid and

sulfuric acid. Other causes include severe diarrhea, renal disease, untreated diabetes mellitus, starvation, excess alcohol ingestion, and a high concentration of potassium ions in the extracellular fluid.
See also ACIDEMIA.

ACL Anterior cruciate ligament.
See under KNEE LIGAMENTS.

ACNE An inflammatory disease of the hair follicles and sebaceous glands. Common acne is also known as **acne vulgaris**, in which lesions occur most frequently on the face, chest and back. The cause is unknown, but it has been suggested that many factors play an etiologic role, including stress, hereditary factors, hormones, drugs and bacteria.
Acne mechanica is a skin condition that results from chronic friction and pressure. It is often seen in athletes, and works with other factors (e.g. occlusion and heat) under athletic apparel such as football helmets. Inflammatory papules (pimples) and pustules (pimples with pus) that sometimes progress to cysts and nodules are seen under protective padding or less bulky equipment. It is particularly prevalent among football players, probably because the maximum bulk of their protective padding comes into contact with dense areas of sebaceous areas of the body, such as the face, shoulders and upper back. A clean T-shirt under shoulder pads helps to prevent football acne.
See also under ORAL CONTRACEPTIVES.

Bibliography
Basler, R.S., Hunzeker, C.M. and Garcia, M.A. (2004). Athletic skin injuries. Combating pressure and friction. *The Physician and Sportsmedicine* 32(5), 33-40.

ACROMIALE An anatomical landmark that is the most superior and lateral point of the acromion process of the scapula when the subject is standing erect with arms relaxed and hanging vertically.

ACROMIOCLAVICULAR JOINT *See under* SHOULDER GIRDLE.

ACROPODION Akropodion. It is an anatomical landmark that is the most anterior point on the toe of the foot when the subject is standing. This may be the first or the second phalanx.

ACTH   Adrenocorticotropic hormone. *See* CORTICOTROPIN.

ACTIN   A protein found in the thin filaments of skeletal muscle fibers and important for muscle contraction.

ACTION POTENTIAL   *See under* NEURONS.

ACTIVE RECOVERY   Low-intensity aerobic exercise that facilitates recovery from anaerobic exercise, partly by increasing the rate of removal of blood lactate. The rate of lactate removal by the liver appears to be the same whether an individual is resting or exercising. Since blood flow is increased during exercise, oxidation of lactate by skeletal and cardiac muscles is also increased. Although active recovery is best for lactate removal, it can delay glycogen resynthesis by further depleting glycogen stores. Active recovery helps to guard against potential deleterious effects of the post-exercise increase in plasma catecholamines. It also helps to prevent blood pooling in the extremities that occurs because of venous return falling too abruptly. This may result in hyperventilation, or even shock. This decreases carbon dioxide levels and can cause muscle cramps. During exercise, venous return occurs mainly through the action of the muscle pump. **Passive recovery** involves procedures such as stretching and massage.

ACTIVE TRANSPORT   The energy dependent transport of molecules or ions across a cell membrane against a concentration gradient (i.e. 'uphill'). The transport is active rather than passive, because energy from metabolism is required. **Vesicular transport** includes exocytosis, endocytosis, pinocytosis and phagocytosis. **Exocytosis** (emiocytosis) is the bulk transport of materials such as undigested food, excretory material or secretory materials out of the cell by encasing them within membranes, and forming a vacuole that is transported to the cell surface.

Endocytosis is cellular uptake of material by the indentation and pinching off of its membrane to form a vesicle that carries material into the cell. In **bulk-phase endocytosis**, the plasma membrane sinks beneath an external fluid droplet containing small solutes. This occurs in most cells and is most important for the intake of solutes by absorptive cells of the kidney and intestines. In **receptor-mediated endocytosis**, an external substance binds to membrane receptors and coated pits are formed. This is the means of intake of some hormones, cholesterol, iron and other molecules. **Pinocytosis** is the process by which cells internalize fluid and macromolecules; the cell membrane invaginates and forms a pocket around the substance. **Phagocytosis** is a form of active transport where particles or fluids are engulfed by the cell.
     See also CALCIUM PUMP; PROTON PUMP; SODIUM-POTASSIUM PUMP.

ACUTE   Of abrupt onset or short duration. The opposite of acute is chronic.

ACUTE PHASE PROTEINS   Proteins produced and secreted from the liver. Acute phase proteins such as C-reactive protein are stimulated by proinflammatory cytokines and are so named because they increase rapidly during an infection.

ADAPTATION   *See under* COGNITIVE DEVELOPMENT; STRESSORS.

ADAPTED PHYSICAL ACTIVITY   *See under* DISABILITY; PHYSICAL EDUCATION.

ADDICTIVE   A term used in reference to a substance (usually a drug) that is habitually taken. Deprivation of this substance leads to withdrawal symptoms and an urge to take the substance again.
     See also EXERCISE DEPENDENCE; SUBSTANCE-RELATED DISORDERS.

ADDISON'S DISEASE Adrenal hypoplasia. A rare disorder characterized by chronic, usually progressive, inadequate production of cortisol and aldosterone by the adrenal cortex.

See also under OVERTRAINING.

Bibliography

National Institute of Neurological Disorders and Stroke. Http://ninds.nih.gov

ADDUCTOR MUSCLE STRAIN An injury that results from strain of the adductor muscles (muscles that draw the leg towards the midline of the body). It is caused by sudden abduction and occurs in sports where cutting, sidestepping or pivoting is required. It is most commonly an overuse injury involving inflammation of the paratenon that is caused by repetitive tensile force. Acute injuries are common in soccer where the adductor muscles lengthen to prevent hyperabduction during a kicking action. The *adductor longus* is the most frequently injured of the adductor muscles. Ruptures of the *adductor longus* may be partial or complete. Partial ruptures usually occur in the muscle itself, or in its attachment at the pubic bone. Complete ruptures are usually located at the muscle's attachment into the femur, but can also occur at its origin.

ADENINE A nitrogenous, purine base found in DNA and RNA.

ADENOCARCINOMA A malignant tumor that develops in epithelial cells in the lining or inner surface of an organ. Breast and prostate cancer are types of adenocarcinoma.

ADENOIDS Lymphatic tissues located high on the posterior wall of the pharynx. The adenoids trap and destroy pathogens in air that enter the nasopharynx.

ADENOSINE A nucleoside composed of adenine and ribose. It can be derived from the breakdown of adenosine triphosphate (ATP). Once formed, adenosine can be used for ATP resynthesis or catabolized via the purine catabolic pathway to ultimately yield uric acid. Exercise produces increased rates of ATP breakdown, enhancing extracellular and blood levels of adenosine. A decrease in ATP breakdown leads to a net reuptake of adenosine by the cell and a decrease in extracellular and blood adenosine levels. Adenosine stimulates ventilation in humans by increasing tidal volume and inspiratory flow rate while decreasing expiratory duration. One of the long-term adaptations to increased adenosine levels may be neovascularization. Research on mice has found that increased adenosine levels enhance erythropoiesis by inducing the kidneys to increase the manufacture of the hormone erythropoietin. Since adenosine levels are dependent on the rate of ATP use, it follows that intense exercise with high levels of ATP use per unit time should not only lead to increases in adenosine levels, but also to enhanced erythropoiesis and neovascularization.

Adenosine provokes bronchoconstriction in asthmatics, but not in nonasthmatics. This process appears to be mediated by activation of mast cells, because it can be blocked by antihistamines and inhibitors of mass cell activation.

Adenosine is an inhibitor neuromodulator affecting norepinephrine, dopamine and serotonin activity. Blockade of adenosine receptors appears to be involved in the action of methylxanthines such as caffeine and theophylline. Theophylline is used in the treatment of chronic asthma, because it is a modest bronchodilator.

See also ISCHEMIA.

Bibliography

Feoktistov, I. and Biaggioni, I. (1996). Role of adenosine in asthma. *Drug Development Research* 39, 333-336.

Simpson, R.E. and Phillis, J.W. (1993). Adenosine and the adaptation to exercise. *Sports Medicine* 15(4), 219-224.

ADENOSINE DIPHOSPHATE ADP. *See under* ADENOSINE TRIPHOSPHATE.

ADENOSINE MONOPHOSPHATE AMP. A purine monophosphate, AMP is an activator of phosphorylase and phosphofructokinase (PFK), which are the important allosteric enzymes that increase the rate of glycogenolysis (and therefore glucose 6-phosphate production) and of the fructose 6-phosphate to fructose 1,6-bisphosphate reactions, respectively. AMP in exercising muscle is related to exercise intensity. AMP also leads to an increase in the concentration of malonyl CoA that depresses the entry of long-chain carboxylic acids into muscle mitochondria.

See under AMMONIA; GLYCOLYSIS.

ADENOSINE MONOPHOSPHATE KINASE
An enzyme that is a member of a metabolite-sensing protein kinase family that functions as a metabolic 'fuel gauge' in skeletal muscle. During exercise, adenosine monophosphate kinase becomes activated in skeletal muscle in response to changes in cellular energy status (e.g. increased ratios of adenosine monophosphate to ATP and creatine to phosphocreatine) in an intensity-dependent manner, and serves to inhibit ATP-consuming pathways, and activate pathways involved in carbohydrate and fatty-acid metabolism to restore ATP levels. Adenosine monophosphate kinase plays this key role during sessions of acute exercise, but it is also an important component of the adaptive response of skeletal muscles to endurance exercise training because of its ability to alter muscle fuel reserves and expression of several exercise-responsive genes.

Bibliography
Aschenbach, W.G., Sakamoto, K. and Goodyear, L.J. (2004). '5 adenosine monophosphate-activated protein kinase, metabolism and exercise. *Sports Medicine* 34(2), 91-103.

ADENOSINE TRIPHOSPHATE   ATP. A
nucleotide composed of a purine (adenine), ribose and three phosphates. It is the main currency of energy exchange in the cells of the human body. ATP is used for motion, active transport, biosynthesis and signal amplification. ATP is broken down to ADP by hydrolysis using ATPase as an enzyme. In the process, energy (7 to 12 kilocalories) is released when each high-energy bond is broken. If a compound's free energy for hydrolysis is equal to or greater than that of ATP, then it is a 'high-energy' compound; if its free energy for hydrolysis is less than that of ATP, then it is not a 'high-energy' compound. **Cytosolic phosphorylation potential** is the ratio of ATP concentration to ADP concentration.

ATP must be recycled continuously by each cell,

because stored ATP will last only for a few seconds during work of maximum intensity. ATP turnover at rest is about 28 g/min, but can be as high as 500 g/min during vigorous exercise. ATP is resynthesized using either aerobic or anaerobic energy systems. In order to be useful as an energy currency, the concentration of ATP in the cell must be kept far from equilibrium so that the ratio of ATP to ADP is normally greater than 50.

During vigorous exercise, the rate of ATP hydrolysis is high. Although muscle efficiently resynthesizes ATP from ADP, there is an increase in ADP concentration when compared to rested muscle. The enzyme adenylate kinase (AMP kinase; myokinase) catalyses the reaction of two ADP molecules to form one AMP and one ATP. This keeps the ADP in check.

AMP is deaminated by the enzyme adenylate deaminase, and is converted to inosine monophosphate (IMP) and ammonia. Working in concert with the adenylate kinase reaction in skeletal muscle during vigorous exercise, the irreversible adenylate deaminase reaction drives the reversible adenylate kinase reaction to the right, to decrease ADP. This reaction also maintains a high cytosolic phosphorylation potential that is important for the hydrolysis of ATP. The ammonia that results from the adenylate deaminase reaction is a base and is ionized to ammonium. This keeps the muscle from becoming too acidic. The ammonium ion stimulates the process of glycolysis by activating one of the rate-controlling enzymes. The adenylate deaminase reaction is only important during vigorous exercise.

Muscles become rigid and stiff soon after death (**rigor mortis**) because ATP resynthesis is ceased. Consequently, myosin cross bridges and actin remain attached and muscle cannot return to a relaxed state.

See also under EFFICIENCY; ELECTRON TRANSPORT CHAIN; MUSCLE CONTRACTION.

Chronology
•1929 • ATP and ADP were discovered independently by Karl Lohmann of Germany and by two American scientists.
•1935 • Vladimir Engelhart of Russia noted that muscle contractions require ATP.

•1941 • Fritz Lipmann of the USA had showed that ATP is the main bearer of chemical energy in the cell. He coined the phrase "energy-rich phosphate bonds."

•1961 • Peter Mitchell of the UK showed that cell respiration leads to differing concentrations of hydrogen ions inside and outside the mitochondrial membrane. This is known as the chemiosmotic hypothesis.

•1964 • Paul D. Boyer of the USA proposed that ATP is synthesized through structural changes in the ATP synthase enzyme.

•1997 • Richard Cross of the USA showed that parts of the ATP synthase rotate during the synthesis and hydrolysis of ATP.

ADENYLATE CYCLASE   It is an enzyme that catalyzes the conversion of ATP to cyclic AMP.

ADENYL CYCLASE   An enzyme that catalyzes the synthesis of cyclic AMP.

ADENYLATE DEAMINASE   *See under* ATP.

ADEQUATE INTAKE   *See under* DIETARY REFERENCE INTAKE.

ADH   Anti-diuretic hormone. *See* VASOPRESSIN.

ADIPOCYTE   Fat cell. *See under* CONNECTIVE TISSUE; FAT.

ADIPOSE TISSUE   *See under* CONNECTIVE TISSUE; FAT.

ADOLESCENT AWKWARDNESS   *See under* GROWTH.

ADP   *See* ADENOSINE DIPHOSPHATE.

ADP-ATP TRANSLOCASE   *See under* MITOCHONDRIAL MEMBRANE SHUTTLES.

ADRENAL GLANDS   Suprarenal glands. Endocrine glands that are located in pairs near each kidney. The inner part of the gland, the **medulla**, secretes epinephrine and norepinephrine. The outer part of the gland, the **cortex**, secretes steroid hormones and is not part of the autonomic nervous system. Activity of the cortex is controlled by corticotropin.

ADRENALINE   *See* EPINEPHRINE.

ADRENERGIC   *See under* EPINEPHRINE.

ADRENOCORTICOTROPIC HORMONE   *See under* CORTICOSTEROIDS.

ADSORPTION   The surface retention of solid, liquid or gas molecules, atoms or ions by a solid or liquid as opposed to absorption (the penetration of substances into the bulk of the solid or liquid).

AEROBIC   Utilizing oxygen.

AEROBIC CAPACITY   The total amount of energy that is available from the aerobic energy systems.
    See under AEROBIC ENERGY SYSTEMS.

AEROBIC DANCE   More commonly known as 'aerobics,' aerobic dance is a form of fitness training, which became popular when Jane Fonda's 'Work-out' tape appeared in 1982. It involves exercise of large muscle groups in continuous rhythmic activity to music. The original 'aerobics' programs consisted of various dance forms in combination with callisthenic-type exercises, such as jumping and ballistic stretching. There have been concerns about joint injury from high-impact aerobics that occur especially to the lower leg as a result of ballistic movements and impact with hard floor surfaces. More recent innovations, therefore, have included water aerobics, low impact aerobics and step aerobics. In low-impact aerobics, at least one foot is in contact with the floor at all times. Step aerobics ('step') involves stepping up and down from a platform, with exercise intensity being varied by changing the platform height and the use of propulsion. There are many combinations of high- and low-impact aerobics. Footwear is important for injury prevention in aerobic dance; the shoe should be able to slide without sticking, but not slip unexpectedly.
    See also PHYSICAL FITNESS.

Bibliography

Garrick, J.G. and Requa, R.K. (1988). Aerobic dance. A review. *Sports Medicine* 6, 169-179.

Stamford, B. (1989). Low impact aerobics. *The Physician and Sportsmedicine* 17(3), 264.

Williford, H.N., Scharff-Olson, M. and Blessing, D.L. (1989). The physiological effects of aerobic dance. A review. *Sports Medicine* 8(6), 335-45.

AEROBIC DRIFT *See* OXYGEN DRIFT.

AEROBIC ENDURANCE The ability to persist in exercise that is predominantly aerobic. It is determined primarily by aerobic capacity. *See under* AEROBIC ENERGY SYSTEMS.

AEROBIC ENERGY SYSTEMS This involves the synthesis of ATP by oxidative phosphorylation, which is the coupling of phosphate with adenosine diphosphate (ADP) to produce adenosine triphosphate (ATP) through the transfer of electrons from NADH and $FADH_2$ to oxygen. $FADH_2$ and NADH are the reduced forms of FAD and NAD^+, which are oxidizing-reducing coenzymes. Carbohydrates and lipids are used as substrates for oxidative phosphorylation.

Hawley and Hopkins (1995) proposed that the oxidation of carbohydrates and lipids should be regarded as the basis of two functionally distinct aerobic systems: the **aerobic glycolytic system** (which oxidizes carbohydrate for high-intensity endurance events) and the **aerobic lipolytic system** (which oxidizes lipids to provide most of the energy for longer, less intense endurance and ultra-endurance events). These systems have substantially different metabolic pathways. In the aerobic lipolytic system, a set of cytoplasmic and membrane-bound enzymes is responsible for the beta-oxidation of lipids to fatty acyl CoA, the transport of fatty acyl CoA into mitochondria, and its conversion to acetyl CoA. In the aerobic glycolytic system, a separate set of enzymes controls the conversion of intramuscular and extramuscular carbohydrates to pyruvate and then to acetyl CoA. Once the acetyl CoA stage has been reached, the pathways for oxidation are the same for both systems. The relative contribution of each system to the energy required for exercise depends on the intensity and duration of the exercise, and these contributions can be modified selectively by training or other interventions.

By asserting that there are two functionally separate aerobic power systems, it is inferred that there are two qualitatively different kinds of prolonged, maximal exercise: '**endurance**' (lasting less than 4 hours, performed at greater than 70% of maximal oxygen uptake and powered by aerobic glycolysis) and '**ultra-endurance**' (longer, lower-intensity exercise powered by aerobic lipolysis). This implies that different training and dietary programs are necessary to optimize performance in 'endurance' and 'ultra-endurance' events.

Bibliography

Hawley, J.A. and Hopkins, W.G. (1995). Aerobic glycolytic and aerobic lipolytic power systems. A new paradigm with implications for endurance and ultra-endurance events. *Sports Medicine* 19(4), 240-250.

AEROBIC POWER The maximum amount of energy that can be produced, per unit of time, from (predominantly) aerobic energy.

AEROBIC TRAINING Utilization of the aerobic energy systems to improve aerobic power, aerobic capacity and aerobic endurance. The threshold for obtaining a training effect from aerobic exercise is usually about 50 to 55% of maximal oxygen uptake. The length of time per session that is necessary to produce an aerobic training effect is not known, but seems to depend on factors such as exercise intensity, total work done, training frequency and initial fitness level. Exercise intensity seems to be the key factor in improving aerobic power, since increasing intensity up to, or near, 100% of maximal oxygen uptake produces the greatest improvements across all frequencies, durations, program lengths and initial fitness levels.

According to the American College of Sports Medicine (1998), sedentary or unfit people should perform aerobic exercise 3 to 5 days a week at 40 or 50% to 85% of maximum oxygen uptake reserve or maximum heart rate reserve. Exercise should be done for 10 to 60 minutes per day; 10-minute bouts can be accumulated throughout the day. An optimal level of strength should be developed when following an endurance-training program. This allows a muscle group to work at lower percentages of its maximum capacity and thus significantly increase absolute endurance.

According to the American Heart Association, for health benefits to the heart, lungs and circulation, a person should perform any vigorous activity for at least 30 minutes most days of the week at 50 to 75% of maximum heart rate. The greatest potential for decreased mortality is in sedentary people who become moderately active (exercising at 40 to 60% of maximal oxygen uptake).

Persons who get 30 minutes of moderate-intensity exercise per day are likely to achieve additional health benefits if they exercise more (Blair et al, 2004).

See DETRAINING; ENDURANCE; OXYGEN UPTAKE; TAPERING; TRAINING FOR DISTANCE RUNNING.

Bibliography

American College of Sports Medicine (2000). *ACSM's guidelines for exercise testing and prescription.* 6th ed. Philadelphia, PA: Lippincott Williams and Wilkins.

American Heart Association. Http://www.americanheart.org

Blair, S.N., LaMonte, M.J. and Nichaman, M.Z. (2004). The evolution of physical activity recommendations: How much is enough. *American Journal of Clinical Nutrition* 79(5), 913S-920S.

Pollock, M.L. et al. (1998). The recommended quantity and quality of exercise for developing and maintaining cardiorespiratory and muscular fitness, and flexibility in healthy adults. *Medicine and Science in Sports and Exercise* 30(6), 975-991.

Shephard, R.J. and Astrand, P.O. (1992, eds). *Endurance in sport. Encyclopaedia of sports medicine. Vol. II. An IOC Medical Commission publication.* Oxford: Blackwell Scientific Publications.

Wenger, H.A. and Bell, J.G. (1986). The interactions of intensity, frequency and duration of exercise training in altering fitness. *Sports Medicine* 3, 346-356.

AEROSOL *See under* AIR POLLUTION.

AFFERENT NEURON Sensory neuron. It is any neuron that transmits impulses toward the central nervous system. *See under* NERVOUS SYSTEM.

AFTERLOAD *See under* CARDIAC CYCLE.

AGE *See under* GROWTH.

AGENESIS Failure of development.

AGGRESSION The intent to injure another person or oneself. Such intent often manifests itself in verbal abuse, even if it does not result in actual physical violence. Examples of aggressive acts in sport are: a '**bean ball**' (a baseball thrown deliberately by the pitcher at the batter's head), a '**clothes line**' tackle (a football tackle in which the ball carrier is hooked from one side, or behind by an arm around the neck) and '**raking**' (deliberately trampling with cleated boots over an opponent who is lying on the ground). Aggressive roles in sport include the '**enforcer**' in ice hockey (a player who is skilled at intimidating and actually fighting with opponents). Aggression in sport has resulted in legal action. **Intimidation** involves the use of verbal and nonverbal behavior that threatens violence or is aggressive.

Hostile aggression is said to occur when the primary reinforcement sought via the act of aggression is inflicting harm on someone. **Instrumental aggression** is defined as the use of aggression as a means to a non-aggressive end, such as winning money in boxing.

There have been three major theories proposed to explain aggression: Instinct theory, Frustration-Aggression Displacement theory and Social Learning theory. **Instinct (Catharsis) theory** proposes that humans have an innate drive to aggress and that 'bottled-up' emotions can be released through aggressive behavior.

Frustration-Aggression Displacement theory proposes that aggression is caused by frustration (the blocking of instrumental goal attainment by someone or something). If a frustrated person cannot act out the aggression on the instigator of the frustration, then the frustrated person will attempt to displace the aggression onto another person. Frustration and aggression may be linked by anger. Frustration may lead to anger, but anger may or may not lead to aggression. In sport, the sources of frustration include: losing by a large margin; losing to an inferior opponent; and playing poorly.

Social Learning theory proposes that aggressive behavior is learned through modeling (observational learning) and reinforcement. If a person is positively reinforced (or not negatively reinforced) for being aggressive, then that person is likely to be aggressive in the future. Males demonstrate more aggressive tendencies than females. Sport socialization may legitimize aggressive behavior that violates rules for males, but not for females.

Based on the premise that black is regarded as the color of evil and death in most cultures, Frank and Gilovich (1988) asked the following question: Are professional football and ice hockey teams who wear black uniforms more aggressive than those who wear non-black uniforms? An analysis of the penalty records of the National Football League and the National Hockey League showed that teams with black uniforms in both sports ranked near the top of their leagues in penalties throughout the period of study. Also, when a team switched from non-black to black uniforms, there was an immediate increase in penalties. These findings may be attributed to the biased judgments of referees and/or to the increased aggressiveness of the players themselves.

Varca (1980) hypothesized that home and away teams differ in the type, rather than the level, of aggressive behavior. It was found that home teams outperformed visiting teams in terms of 'functional aggression' (i.e. rebound, blocked shots and steals), but visiting teams displayed more 'dysfunctional aggression,' committing more fouls.

There is evidence that officials make more subjective decisions against visiting teams or in favor of home teams. Lehman and Reifman (1987) reasoned that officials might feel more pressure from fans to be lenient toward the home teams' star players, because these players are most likely to lead the home team to victory. Using archival data from games involving the Los Angeles Lakers for the 1984-5 season, it was indeed found that significantly fewer fouls were called on star players at home; no such differences were found for non-stars players.

Brust et al. (1992) found that body checking accounted for 86% of all injuries that occurred during games. Consequently, the American Academy of Pediatrics (AAP) recommends limiting body checking in hockey players of 15 years of age and younger as a means to decrease injuries. Good sportsmanship programs have been shown to decrease injury and penalty rates.

For discussion about the International Society of Sport Psychology's stand on aggression and violence in sport, see Tenenbaum et al. (1997, 2000) and Kerr (1999, 2002).

See also under VIOLENCE.

Chronology

•1978 • In the National Basketball Association, a third referee was added in order to curb the escalation of violent play.

•1997 • The National Coalition Against Violent Athletes was formed in response to the growing number of violent crimes committed by athletes in many sports. The organization is based solely on the fact that athletes should be held to the same standards and laws as the rest of society.

•1999 • Tony Limon, a high school basketball player in San Antonio, Texas, intentionally elbowed an opponent in the face, causing facial damage that required plastic surgery. Limon was sentenced to five years in prison for aggravated assault.

•2000 • Michael Costin, a little league hockey coach, died after being savagely beaten by a parent, Thomas Junta. Costin (6 feet, 156 lb) and Junta (6 feet 1 inch, 270 lb) argued over what Junta described as rough play during hockey drills. In a Massachusetts court, Junta received a sentence of 6 to 10 years in a state prison after being convicted of involuntary manslaughter (unintentional killing as a result of a battery in which the defendant knew, or should have known, that a human life was endangered).

Bibliography

American Academy of Pediatrics (2000). Safety in youth ice hockey: The effects of body checking. RE9835. *Pediatrics* 105(3), 657-658.

Bennett, J.C. (1991). The irrationality of the catharsis theory of aggression as justification for educators' support of interscholastic football. *Perceptual and Motor Skills* 72(2), 415-418.

Berkowitz, L. (1989). The frustration-aggression hypothesis:

Examination and reformulation. *Psychological Bulletin* 106, 59-73.

Brust, J.D. et al. (1992). Children's ice hockey injuries. *American Journal of Diseases of Children* 146, 741-747.

Frank, M.G. and Gilovich, T. (1988). The dark side of self and social perception: Black uniforms and aggression in professional sports. *Journal of Personality and Social Psychology* 54(1), 74-85.

Husman, B.F. and Silva, J.M. (1984). Aggression in sport: Definitional and theoretical considerations. In: Silva, J.M. and Weinberg, R.S. (eds). *Psychological foundations of sport*. pp246-260. Champaign, IL: Human Kinetics.

Kerr, J.H. (1999). The role of aggression and violence in sport: A rejoinder to the ISSP Position Stand. *The Sport Psychologist* 13(1), 83-88.

Kerr, J.H. (2002). Issues in aggression and violence in sport: The ISSP Position Stand Revisited. *The Sport Psychologist* 16(1), 68-78.

Lehman, D.R. and Reifman, A. (1987). Spectator influence on basketball officiating. *Journal of Social Psychology* 127, 673-675.

Silva, J.M. (1984). Factors related to the acquisition and exhibition of aggressive sport behavior. In: Silva, J.M. and Weinberg, R.S. (eds). *Psychological foundations of sport*. pp261-273. Champaign, Illinois: Human Kinetics.

Tenenbaum, G. et al. (1997). Aggression and violence in sport: An ISSP position stand. *The Sport Psychologist* 11, 1-7.

Tenenbaum, G. et al. (2000). Aggression and violence in sport: A reply to Kerr's rejoinder. *The Sport Psychologist* 14, 325-326.

Varca, P. (1980). An analysis of home and away game performances of male college basketball teams. *Journal of Sport Psychology* 2, 245-257.

Widmeyer, W.N. (1984). Aggression-performance relationship in sport. In: Silva, J.M. and Weinberg, R.S. (eds). *Psychological foundations of sport*. pp174-286. Champaign, IL: Human Kinetics.

Widmeyer, W.N. et al. (2002). Explanation for the occurrence of aggression in sport: Theories and research. In Silva, J.M. and Stevens, D.E. (eds). *Psychological foundations of sport*. 2nd ed. pp352-379. Boston, MA: Allyn & Bacon.

AGILITY   The capacity to change direction of movement rapidly without loss of balance. It is a combination of speed, strength, reaction time, balance and neuromuscular coordination. It is demonstrated in movements such as stopping, shuttle sprints and sidestepping.

AGING   This is the continuous process of development in an adult. It leads to a progressive loss of adaptive capabilities and capacity to function as in the past.

There are two major theories of aging: Error theories and Program theories. **Error theories** are based on the premise that with aging it becomes more difficult to repair damage caused by internal malfunctions or external assault to the body, and that the immune system loses effectiveness in combating infection and destroying abnormal body cells. **Program theories** suggest that there is an internal clock that starts ticking at conception and is programmed to run only for so long.

The effects of aging are similar to those that accompany physical inactivity. Connective tissues lose elasticity, causing a loss of flexibility. The loss of minerals in bones can lead to osteoporosis. Part of the decrease in bone density observed in older adults is due to disuse rather than the aging process itself. In the elderly, the femoral neck is the most common fracture site.

The typical weight gain with aging is due to increasing levels of body fat. There may be little benefit in encouraging weight loss in extreme old age (short life expectancy), especially when there are no obesity-related complications or biochemical risk factors, and when strong resistance and distress arise from changes in lifelong habits of eating and exercise. In contrast, weight loss in the elderly can decrease morbidity from arthritis, diabetes and other conditions, decrease cardiovascular risk factors, and improve wellness. Sarcopenia appears to be the major factor in the age-related loss of muscle strength.

Sarcopenia is age-related decrease in muscle mass. With increasing age, human skeletal muscles gradually decrease in volume, mainly due to a decreased number of motor units and muscle fibers, in addition to a decreased size of fast twitch muscle fibers. By the seventh or eighth decade of life, maximal voluntary contractile strength is decreased on average by 20 to 40% for both men and women. The loss of function is generally less in the arms than in the legs. It is not known whether this is due to an inherent biological difference or a reflection of differential changes in activity patterns between the arms and legs. Resistance training programs can substantially slow down or reverse the aging process, if the training stimulus is of sufficient intensity and duration. Impairment in strength development may result when aerobic training is added to resistance training, but can be avoided with training limited to 3 days per week. Resistance training in older adults increases power, decreases difficulty of performing daily tasks, enhances energy expenditure, and promotes participation in spontaneous physical activity. It is a myth that older adults should prefer machines to free weights. Brill et al. (1998) found that free weights in an elderly population (73 to 91 years) promoted beneficial adaptations in several functional performance measures (e.g. balance, stair climbing). Strength and muscle mass are increased following resistance training in older adults through a poorly understood series of events that appears to involve the recruitment of satellite cells to support hypertrophy of mature muscle fibers. Other factors include the increased ability to neurally activate motor units and increased high-energy phosphate availability.

Reaction and movement times decrease with age, probably due to aging-related changes in the central nervous system.

Muscle blood flow during exercise is lower due to a decrease in the ratio of capillaries to muscle fibers. Maximal stroke volume is lower due to a decrease in both heart volume and quantity of cardiac muscle. Aerobic training lowers resting heart rate, and decreases levels of heart rate and plasma catecholamines at the same absolute submaximal workload. Maximal heart rate is lowered due to decreased stimulation of the sympathetic nervous system. Peripheral resistance and blood pressure are increased due to loss of elasticity in the blood vessels. Baroreceptor control of peripheral vascular resistance is preserved better than arterial baroreceptor control of the heart.

The loss of elasticity in the lungs causes decreased elastic recoil of the lungs and an increased energy cost of breathing. The increase in the size of the alveoli causes a decrease in pulmonary diffusion capacity and an increase in dead space. The decrease in the number of lung capillaries causes a decrease in the ventilation-perfusion ratio. In most cases, however, the demand put on the pulmonary system does not exceed its capacity to meet that demand.

Maximal oxygen uptake usually declines 8 to 10% per decade after 25 years of age for both males and females. This may be due to decreases in the size and number of mitochondria, muscle oxidative enzyme activity and muscle capillarization.

Vigorous endurance training elicits a proliferation of muscle capillaries, an increase in oxidative enzyme activity and a significant improvement in maximal oxygen uptake. It also has a beneficial effect on age-related diseases such as Type II diabetes, coronary artery disease, hypertension, osteoporosis and obesity. Anaerobic glycolysis is slower due to decreased lactate dehydrogenase, but glycolytic capacity does not seem to be decreased. Aging does not appear to decrease capacity to perform normal activity at high altitude. Aging is associated with a decreased capacity to adapt to exercise in the heat, mainly because sweating capacity decreases with aging. There is a decrease in the antioxidant capacity of tissues, reflected in a decreased level of plasma GSH. In the fifth decade of life, the body's defence mechanisms begin to weaken. Changes are most notable in T-cell function.

Older adults are more prone than other adults to both acute and overuse injuries related to sport and exercise. Most of the sports injuries sustained by older adults are associated with aging processes. The lower extremities are more susceptible to injury than the upper extremities. Based on epidemiological data, former athletes have more degenerative changes in their joints and spine compared with control populations. At old age, however, their good muscle function related to high physical activity level seems to compensate for the effects of degenerative changes on function.

Studies of former athletes have shown that the functional profiles of former athletes and their age-matched counterparts are not significantly different once the athletes have ceased training and their physical activity has fallen to a level comparable to that of their age-matched counterparts. After lifelong athletic training, many veteran athletes have a functional capacity that is comparable to that of younger, sedentary individuals. Maximal oxygen uptake declines at a rate of 10% per decade in men and women regardless of activity level. High-intensity exercise may decrease this loss by up to 50% in young and middle-aged men, but not in older men, if maintained long term. Middle-aged and older women do not seem to be able to decrease loss rates in maximal oxygen uptake to less than 10% per decade. This may be related to estrogen status. The age-related decline in maximal oxygen uptake seems to be due to both central and peripheral adaptations, primarily decreases in maximal heart rate and lean body mass. Exercise training does not influence declines in maximal heart rate.

Older adults recover balance with less speed, because of less accurate feedback regarding the position of body parts. Falls account for more accidental deaths in the elderly than do any other factor. Half of the elderly who fall never regain functional walking. Half of the elderly hospitalized from hip fracture die within a year. Maintenance of a physically active lifestyle helps to prevent falling.

Around 40 years of age, less light reaches the retina of the eye and persons lose the ability to accommodate near objects (**presbyopia**). With age, there is also increased risk of eye diseases, such as cataracts (loss of transparency of the lens of the eye or of its capsule).

Increased amount and thickening of cerumen can block the external auditory canal affecting the transmission of sound waves to the middle and inner ears. **Presbycusis** is hearing loss with age. It can result from membrane changes and loss of cells in the auditory nerve or other organs that are instrumental in transmitting or interpreting sound waves. In addition, decreased blood flow to various parts of the ear may contribute to presbycusis. Older adults may also experience tinnitus.

Effects of aging on the genitourinary system include decreased bladder capacity, increase in quantity of residual urine, uninhibited bladder contractions (detrusor hyperreflexia), delay in desire to urinate and urine production occurring mainly at rest. Instead of sensing bladder filling at about half

capacity, as younger people do, many older adults first feel the need to void at or near bladder capacity. In men up to the age of 40 years, the prostate grows slowly and few voiding problems occur. After the age of 40 years, growth of the prostate gland accelerates due to a change in the balance of hormones in aging men. As the prostate enlarges, the base of the bladder can become distorted and obstructing tissue can cause increasing urethral resistance. **Prostatism** is a condition marked by symptoms of frequency and urgency of voiding, and also nocturia (excessive urination at night).

The '**Last-In-First-Out**' **theory** has been used to explain the phenomenon of slowing with age for relatively simple versus complex movements. The neuromuscular capability to perform simple movement acts, such as reflexive movement or other integrated movements that fall into the category of spatial transposition, is developed early in life and appears to somewhat resist decline with aging. The more complex, goal-directed movements are not developed until later in life and start to decline in people as young as 30 years.

See also DEMENTIA.

Bibliography

Aoyagi, Y. and Shephard, R.J. (1992). Aging and muscle function. *Sports Medicine* 14(6), 376-396.

Brill, P.A. et al. (1998). Clinical feasibility of a free-weight strengthening program for older adults. *Journal of the American Board of Family Practitioners* 11(6), 445-451.

Dempsey, J.A. and Manohar, M. (1992). The pulmonary system and endurance. In: Shephard, R.J. and Astrand, P.O. (eds). *Endurance in sport.* pp61-71. Oxford: Blackwell Scientific Publications.

Deschenes, M.R. (2004). Effects of aging on muscle fiber type and size. *Sports Medicine* 34(12), 809-824.

Doherty, T.J. (2003). Invited review: Aging and sarcopenia. *Journal of Applied Physiology* 95(4), 1717-1727.

Elia, M. (2001). Obesity in the elderly. *Obesity Research* 9(4S), S244-S248.

Ferrari, A.U., Radaelli, A. and Centola, M. (2003). Invited review: Aging and the cardiovascular system. *Journal of Applied Physiology* 95(6), 2591-2597.

Hawkins, S.A. and Wiswell, R.A. (2003). Rate and mechanism of maximal oxygen consumption decline with aging: Implications for exercise training. *Sports Medicine* 33(12), 877-888.

Hunter, G.R., McCarthy, J.P. and Bamman, M.M. (2004). Effects of resistance training on older adults. *Sports Medicine* 34(5),

329-348.

Johnson, B.D. and Dempsey, J.A. (1991). Demand versus capacity in the aging pulmonary system. *Exercise and Sport Sciences Reviews* 19, 171-210.

Joyner, M.J. (1993). Physiological limiting factors and distance running: Influence of gender and age on record performances. *Exercise and Sport Sciences Reviews* 21, 103-133.

Kallinen, M. and Marku, A. (1995). Aging, physical activity and sports injuries. An overview of common sports injuries in the elderly. *Sports Medicine* 20(1), 41-52.

Kenney, W.L. and Hodgson, J.L. (1987). Heat tolerance, thermoregulation and aging. *Sports Medicine* 4, 446-456.

Kretzschmar, M. and Muller, D. (1993). Aging, training and exercise. *Sports Medicine* 15(3), 196-209.

Kujala, U.M. et al. (2003). Sports career-related musculoskeletal injuries: Long-term health effects on former athletes. *Sports Medicine* 33(12), 869-875.

Mazzeo, R.S. et al. (1998). American College of Sports Medicine position stand: Exercise and physical activity for older adults. *Medicine and Science in Sports and Exercise* 30(6), 992-1008.

Mazzeo, R.S. and Tanaka, H. (2001). Exercise prescription for the elderly: Current recommendations. *Sports Medicine* 31(11), 809-818.

Payne, V.G. and Isaacs, L.D. (2005). *Human motor development. A lifespan approach*. 6th ed. Boston, MA: McGraw-Hill.

Pecatello, L.S. and DiPietro, L. (1993). Physical activity in older adults: An overview of health benefits. *Sports Medicine* 15, 353-364.

Rogers, M.A. and Evans, W.J. (1993). Changes in skeletal muscle with aging: Effects of exercise training. *Exercise and Sport Sciences Reviews* 21, 65-102.

Rose, D.J. (2003). *Fallproof! A comprehensive balance and mobility training program*. Champaign, IL: Human Kinetics.

Seals, D.R. et al (1994). Exercise and aging: Autonomic control of the circulation. *Medicine and Science in Sports and Exercise* 26(5), 568-576.

Shephard, R.J. (1997). *Aging, physical activity and health*. Champaign, IL: Human Kinetics.

Short, K.R. and Nair, K.S. (2001). Does aging adversely affect muscle mitochondrial function? *Exercise and Sport Sciences Reviews* 29(3), 118-123.

AGONIST   *See under* DRUG; MUSCLE ACTION.

AGRANULOCYTES   *See under* LEUKOCYTES.

AIDS   The acquired immune deficiency syndrome. It is a severe depletion of critical cells of the human immune system (CD4-bearing T-cells) in the presence of major complication such as opportunistic infection or cancer. AIDS became known in the USA in 1981 and was subsequently attributed to the human immunodeficiency virus (HIV). Only when the infected status of basketball star "Magic" Johnson became known in the early 1990s did numerous sporting and medical groups begin to consider the consequences of HIV and athletics.

Transmission of HIV is thought to be via three routes: exchange of body fluids such as during intimate sexual contact, blood inoculation, and from an infected mother to her fetus. Not all HIV infected mothers transmit the virus to their babies; in the USA between 70 and 85% escape infection.

It is thought that exercise is a safe and beneficial activity for the HIV-infected person. Severely immuno-compromised individuals can expect no increase in CD4 count with exercise. Although exercise may not significantly slow the progression of HIV and the subsequent onset of AIDS, it does not appear to exacerbate HIV. Resistance training may be important in preventing the wasting process associated with AIDS. In fully developed AIDS, the capacity to exercise may be compromised by deterioration in cardiorespiratory and neuromuscular function.

Athletic competition poses no reasonable risk of HIV transmission among competitors and associated personnel. In sports where significant blood exposure can occur, the risk of HIV transmission is so low as not to warrant major changes in policy to accommodate athletes who may be HIV infected.

The use of highly active antiretroviral therapy (HAART) has served to significantly decrease the mortality of HIV-infected persons, but it is associated with a number of adverse effects (e.g. fatigue, nausea, pain, anxiety and depression). Exercise may have a positive impact on these adverse effects.

See also IMMUNITY.

Chronology

•1991 • Earvin 'Magic' Johnson of the Los Angeles Lakers tested positive for HIV and said that he would retire from playing basketball. He did play in the All-Star Game later in the 1991-92 season, and won the most valuable player award in the West's 153-113 victory. He also played for the USA basketball team in the 1992 Olympic Games that summer, winning a gold medal. A return to the National Baseball Association (NBA) in 1992 was cut short after a few players feared on-court transmission of HIV. However, Johnson returned to the NBA with the Los Angeles Lakers in 1996 and finished the season averaging 14.6 points per game. (His career average was 19.5 point per game.) After the playoff loss to Houston in the first round, Johnson announced that he was going back into retirement.

• 1993 • Former Wimbledon tennis champion Arthur Ashe died at age 49 of AIDS contracted from a blood transfusion.

• 1994 • President Bill Clinton's government temporarily relaxed government restrictions by granting a ten-day waiver to allow HIV-infected athletes from other nations to enter the USA to participate in the Gay Games. The first Gay Games was founded in 1982 by Tom Waddell, a homosexual physician who competed in the decathlon at the Olympic Games. About 1,300 athletes competed in 16 events. There were 16,000 athletes in the 1998 Gay Games. Waddell died of AIDS, aged 49, in 1987. Before his death Waddell wrote a book with Dick Schaap entitled *Gay Olympian: The Life and Death of Dr. Tom Waddell*.

Bibliography

Birk, T.J. (1996). HIV and exercise. *Exercise Immunology Review* 2, 84-95.

Calabrese, L.H. and LaPerriere, A. (1993). Human immunodeficiency virus infection. *Sports Medicine* 15(1), 6-13.

Ciccolo, J.T., Jowers, E.M. and Bartholomew, J.B. (2004). The benefits of exercise training for quality of life in HIV/AIDS in the Post-HAART era. *Sports Medicine* 34(8), 487-499.

Grinspoon, S. et al. (2000). Effects of testosterone and progressive resistance training in eugonadal men with AIDS wasting. A randomized, controlled trial. *Annals of Internal Medicine* 133(5), 348-355.

Sankaran, G., Volkwein, K.A.E. and Bonsall, D.R. (1999, eds). *HIV/AIDS in sport. Impact, issues and challenges*. Champaign, IL: Human Kinetics.

Shephard, R.J. (1998). Exercise, immune function and HIV infection. *Journal of Sports Medicine and Physical Fitness* 38(2), 101-110.

AIR POLLUTION   The presence of gases or aerosols in the atmosphere at levels considered detrimental to the quality, or life supporting capacity, of the environment. Air pollutants may be of human origin (especially emissions from combustive sources such as car engines) or of natural origin (such as volcanic eruptions).

A distinction can be made between primary and secondary pollutants. **Primary pollutants** (e.g. carbon monoxide, nitrogen oxides and particulates) exert physiological influence directly from the source of pollution. **Secondary pollutants** (e.g. aerosols, ozone and peroxyacetyl nitrate) are formed from the interactions of primary pollutants with other compounds, ultraviolet light or with each other. Nitrogen oxides can combine with hydrocarbons and oxygen in the presence of sunlight to form **photochemical smog** and ozone. There is also the presence of sulfur dioxide and particulate emissions associated with diesel engines. Hydrocarbons, carbon monoxide and particulates result from the incomplete combustion of fuel.

'**Greenhouse gases**' like water vapor, methane, nitrous oxides and carbon dioxide in the atmosphere keep the earth's average surface temperature close to a hospitable 60 degrees Fahrenheit (16 degrees Celsius). Without the 'greenhouse effect,' the earth would be a frozen globe of about 5 degrees Fahrenheit (-15 degrees Celsius) and most life would cease. There appears to be a small global warming trend; global temperatures have risen 0.6 degrees C since the 1860s. There is concern that this may be associated with degradation of air quality, an increase in weather-related deaths, and a possible increase in infectious diseases. There is debate, however, as to whether or not the burning of fossil fuels is responsible for this global warming. A report by the Intergovernmental Panel on Climate Change (2001) did not show that human activities were responsible for global warming. The main greenhouse gas is water vapor. Carbon dioxide is a minor greenhouse gas, is essential for the growth of all plants, and should not be considered a pollutant (Gray, 2002).

Almost half of the carbon monoxide, hydrocarbons and nitrogen oxides given off by the burning of fossil fuels are emitted by gasoline and diesel engines. **Carbon monoxide** is a gas formed mainly from the incomplete combustion of fossil fuels and other carbonaceous materials such as tobacco. Tobacco smoke contains 4% carbon monoxide. Smoking 15 to 25 cigarettes a day increases carbon monoxide hemoglobin level to over 6%. Side-stream smoke from the tip of a cigarette contains more carbon monoxide than the smoke that is directly inhaled. Carbon monoxide pollution is a problem for athletes, because hemoglobin has a strong affinity for carbon monoxide. The affinity of carbon monoxide for hemoglobin is 230 times that of oxygen. By competing with oxygen for hemoglobin, carbon monoxide decreases the oxygen-carrying capacity of the blood. When carbon monoxide joins with hemoglobin, carboxyhemoglobin is formed. When blood carboxyhemoglobin is increased, maximal oxygen uptake is decreased and cognitive performance measures (such as attention) also decline.

Particulates include a wide range of solid and liquid particles in air. Larger particles (5 to 10 microns) are filtered in the nose, and are deposited in the nasopharyngeal region, causing an inflammatory response. Particles of 3 to 5 microns enter the tracheobronchial region, stimulating bronchospasm, bronchial congestion and bronchitis. Particles of 0.5 to 3 microns reach the alveoli. The shift from nose to mouth breathing during exercise increases the amount of particulates reaching the alveoli. In urban areas, motor vehicles may contribute over 90% of black smoke and as much as 70% of fine particulates (PM10; less than 10 microns in diameter). Epidemiological research in the USA suggests that particulate matter may exacerbate respiratory ill-health. PM10 exposure is associated with the premature death of people who already have heart and lung disease, especially the elderly.

Volatile organic compounds, mainly hydrocarbons, are emitted into the atmosphere as a result of evaporation from fuel tanks and carburetors during refueling and delivery. Emissions of volatile organic compounds have been decreased as a result of improvement in technology.

The inhalation of various air pollutants is much higher during exercise, due to the significant increase in ventilatory rate that accompanies breathing through the nose and mouth. A combination of exercise and air pollutants causes a significant increase in bronchoconstriction and airflow obstruction when compared to the same exposure at rest.

In the higher stratosphere, **ozone** (triatomic oxygen, O_3) is beneficial as a barrier against harmful radiation, but at ground level it is an air pollutant. Most inhaled ozone is absorbed by mucous membranes in the respiratory tract. Ozone can exacerbate allergic responses and preferentially increases the production and stimulation of inflammatory cells. The epithelial cells lining the respiratory tract are particularly susceptible to damage from ozone. Individual responses differ widely but those with respiratory disease, and/or those who exercise regularly, are particularly susceptible to decreases in lung function that is associated with ozone exposure. Ozone causes an increase in breathing rate and a decrease in tidal volume for a given workload. Significant impairment of exercise performance has been observed at 0.18 parts per million (ppm) of ozone, a pollution level reached for one hour or more on about 180 days per year in the Los Angeles basin. California's topography (physical shape of the land) and its warm, sunny climate are ideal for trapping and forming pollutants. Most California cities are built on plains or in valleys surrounded by mountains. These areas are natural bowls that trap air pollution and prevent the air from circulation. On some days, temperature inversions (where the air closer to the ground becomes cooler than the air above) act as lids which trap air pollutants close to the ground. This prevents the upper, cleaner air from mixing with the lower, polluted air; it also prevents the dispersion of pollutants. In the 1980s, Los Angeles was the most polluted area in the USA with levels of ozone peaking at 0.36 ppm and more than a hundred days exceeding the standard of 0.12 ppm. Ozone levels peak during mid-afternoon. If the 1984 Olympic Games in Los Angeles had been carried out during a time of significantly high pollution levels, then endurance performance would have been affected. Little is known about the effects of air pollutants on sprint or power-type field events. The processes accounting for decreased maximum exercise performance upon significant ozone exposure are not clearly understood. It is possible that subjective respiratory discomfort (associated with increased perceived exertion) is the main factor accounting for decreased exercise performance. The combination of heat and ozone exposure has been shown to accentuate ozone-induced effects, but it is not known why this is so.

Like ozone, **peroxyacetyl nitrate** is formed by photochemical reaction and is a common constituent of smog. Peroxyacetyl nitrate serves as a stable storage form of nitrogen oxides, allowing these highly reactive compounds to be transported in the colder, higher regions of the earth's atmosphere. The nitrogen oxides are released in the warmer, lower regions of the atmosphere. Eye irritation has been reported at concentrations of Peroxyacetyl nitrate as low as 0.24 ppm. Peroxyacetyl nitrate levels of more than 0.5 ppm have been recorded in Los Angeles. There is a lack of research on the effects of peroxyacetyl nitrate during exercise.

Sulfur dioxide is a toxic, irritating, water-soluble gas. Sulfur dioxide pollution is the direct result of burning fuels that contain sulfur. It is a highly water-soluble gas that is normally absorbed in the upper airway during nasal breathing. During heavy exercise, breathing through the mouth is the predominant mode of breathing, thus much larger amounts of sulfur dioxide are delivered to the lower airway. At present ambient levels, it is unlikely that sulfur dioxide will affect athletic performance. An exception is the exercising asthmatic experiencing significant changes in airway resistance even at concentrations as low as 0.5 ppm. Sulfur dioxide also exacerbates lung diseases and breathing problems in asthmatics. Sensitivity is enhanced by cold and/or dry air.

Nitrogen dioxide is a soluble gas that can be absorbed by the mucus of the nasopharyngeal cavity, where it converts to nitrous acid and nitric acid. Nitrogen dioxide levels of 0.4 ppm do not affect physical performance during submaximal exercise, except for mild irritation of the upper-respiratory tract and impairment of mucociliary activity in bronchial tubes. Nitrogen dioxide levels of 0.34 ppm have been recorded in Los Angeles.

An **aerosol** is a suspension of liquid or solid particles in air or gas. Sulfate aerosols arise from ammonia combining with sulfuric acid to form ammonium sulfate and ammonium bisulfate. These aerosols have little effect on pulmonary function of normal people or asthmatics during exercise. Nitrate aerosols, including ammonium nitrate, also have no significant effect on pulmonary function during exercise. Sulfuric acid aerosols do have significant effects on pulmonary function during submaximal exercise.

Epidemiological studies suggest that allergic diseases, such as hay fever, have become more common over the last 50 years. Air pollution is not implicated directly, but there is evidence that air pollutants can alter airway reactivity in allergic individuals.

Chronology

•1943 • The first episodes of smog occurred in Los Angeles.

•1947 • The Air Pollution Control Act was established in California.

•1963 • The Federal Clean Air Act was passed and was the first law established to set strict air quality standards based primarily on health rather than economic considerations. The two main purposes of this act were: to limit the amount of smog by decreasing the concentration of six major pollutants in the air; and to regulate the emission of hazardous toxic air pollutants, such as benzene from chemical plants.

•1994 • In the context of decreasing air pollution, the US Department of Transportation's three-year National Bicycling and Walking Study identified strategies for doubling the percentage of total trips made by bicycling and walking, and identified scenarios for increasing bicycle trips by 3 to 5 times the current levels.

•2002 • Landmark legislation (AB 1493) to combat climate change was signed in California. The bill requires the California Air Resources Board to develop and adopt regulations that decrease greenhouse gases emitted by passenger vehicles and light-duty trucks.

Bibliography

Adams, W.C. (1987). Effects of ozone exposure at ambient air pollution episode levels on exercise performance. *Sports Medicine* 4, 395-424.

Armstrong, L.E. (2000). *Performing in extreme environments*. Champaign, IL: Human Kinetics.

California Air Resources Board. Http://www.arb.ca.gov

Folinsbee, L.J. and Raven, P.B. (1984). Exercise and air pollution. *Journal of Sports Sciences* 2, 57-75.

Gray, V. (2002). *The greenhouse delusion. A critique of "Climate Change 2001."* Brentwood, UK: Multi-science.

Jenkins, S. and Hay, D. (1996). Air pollution, health and exercise: A review. *Energy and Environment* 7(1), 51-56.

Lahohm, H., Rozendaal, S. and Thoenes, D. (2001). *Man-made global warming: Unraveling a dogma.* Brentwood, UK: Multi-science.

McDonough, P. and Moffatt, R.J. (1999). Smoking-induced elevations in blood carboxyhemoglobin levels. Effect on maximal oxygen uptake. *Sports Medicine* 27(5), 275-283.

Pierson, W.E. (1989). Impact of air pollutants on athletic performance. *Allergy Proceedings* 10(3), 209-14.

ALACTACID SYSTEM   *See under* ANAEROBIC ENERGY SYSTEMS.

ALANINE A three-carbon, glucogenic (glycogenic) amino acid. It can be synthesized in the body from pyruvate and glutamate. The production of alanine increases in exercising muscles. Alanine also serves to transport ammonia to the liver via the glucose-alanine cycle.

See GLUCOSE-ALANINE CYCLE.

ALBINISM   An inherited condition in which decreased pigment causes abnormal development of the optic nerve. It is often found with nystagmus and refractive errors, and may be associated with sensitivity to light.

ALBUMIN A simple protein found in many plant and animal tissues. It functions in osmolality and transport.

ALCOHOL   i) A class of organic compounds that contains the hydroxyl (OH) group. ii) A general term often applied to **ethanol** (ethyl alcohol), the alcohol resulting from the alcoholic fermentation of glucose. It is the main alcohol in alcoholic beverages. It is the drug most commonly abused by both athletes and non-athletes. Although it is a drug, it can also be classified as a nutrient, because it provides energy. The net caloric yield of one gram of alcohol (pure 200 proof) is 7 kcal. Contrary to popular belief, most of the calories in beer come from alcohol. With a single drink, the blood alcohol level usually peaks about 45 minutes after ingestion. Intensive mental concentration, lowered body temperature or physical exertion tends to slow the rate of alcohol absorption into the blood, as does a full stomach. The rate of metabolism of ethanol is increased by fructose. People differ substantially in their reactions to alcohol. Proof is the strength of ethanol; one degree of proof is equal to 0.5% of ethanol by volume.

Moderate drinking can be defined as the level of drinking that poses a low risk of alcohol-related problems, both for the drinkers and for others. It is difficult to provide a quantitative definition of moderate drinking, because alcohol can have different effects on different individuals. Based on differences between the sexes in terms of both weight and metabolism, the federal government in the USA defines moderation as no more than one drink per day for women (and persons over 65 years of age) and no more than two drinks per day for men. About 60% of Americans are occasional to moderate drinkers; less than 8% are heavy drinkers. About 35% of Americans abstain from alcohol. According to the National Institute on Alcohol Abuse and Alcoholism, men are at risk if they have more than 14 drinks per week or more than 4 drinks per occasion; and women are at risk if they have more than 7 drinks per week or more than 3 drinks per occasion. One of the objectives of *Healthy People 2010* in the USA is to decrease the number of college students who engage in heavy drinking of alcoholic beverages.

About 3 to 10% of alcohol is excreted unchanged via breath, urine or sweat. Some alcohol is metabolized in the cells lining the stomach. The majority of alcohol is metabolized by the liver at a rate of 8 to 10 g per hour (less than the amount in one glass of wine). At low doses, alcohol is broken down to acetaldehyde and hydrogen ions in a reaction catalyzed by alcohol dehydrogenase with NAD^+ being reduced to NADH. Excess hydrogen ions may combine with fatty acids to form triglycerides or with pyruvate to form lactate. The NADH that is produced in the alcohol dehydrogenase reaction inhibits gluconeogenesis, which in turn causes a decrease in blood glucose. Acetaldehyde is broken down to acetyl CoA, with NAD^+ being reduced to NADH. The acetate is liberated into the blood stream and metabolized in other tissues, mainly in cardiac muscle and skeletal muscle. It can replace free fatty acids in the energy metabolism of these tissues, but it is of minor importance as an energy substrate in skeletal muscle during exercise. Alcohol suppresses vasopressin release, which can lead to decreased blood pressure and dehydration. The dehydration caused by alcohol is associated with a worsening of aerobic performance. Aerobic energy production is decreased because of a slowing of the Krebs cycle. There is an increase in the NADH to NAD^+ ratio, which leads to an increase in the lactate to pyruvate ratio. The resulting hyperlactacidemia (excess of lactic acid in the blood) may be a factor in the poor aerobic performance after alcohol ingestion.

When a person drinks heavily, and there are higher concentrations of alcohol in the liver, the **alcohol dehydrogenase enzyme system** cannot cope. Therefore, another enzyme system, the **microsomal ethanol oxidizing system**, is used to metabolize alcohol. Instead of yielding ATP molecules from the first step of ethanol metabolism via formation of NADH, the microsomal ethanol oxidizing system increases the rate of ethanol metabolism and uses up ATP as NADPH converts to NADP. This partly explains why alcoholics do not gain as much weight as might be expected.

According to the American College of Sports Medicine, alcohol does not possess an ergogenic effect. Acute ingestion of alcohol can be detrimental to reaction time, hand-eye coordination, accuracy, balance and coordination. It may also have a detrimental effect on strength, power and speed. Temperature regulation may be impaired during prolonged exercise in a cold environment.

The diuretic action of alcohol is via inhibition of vasopressin secretion. The degree of diuresis is proportional to the amount of alcohol consumed. There appears to be no difference in recovery from dehydration whether the rehydration beverage is alcohol free or contains up to 2% alcohol, but drinks

containing 4% tend to delay the recovery process. The diuretic effect of alcohol is substantially blunted when alcohol is consumed by individuals who are in a state of hypohydration induced by exercising in the heat.

Alcohol is classified as a depressant drug, even though small doses may elicit a transitory stimulant effect upon ingestion, possibly via excitation of the sympathetic nervous system or disinhibition of the reticular activating system. This may account for the paradoxical agitation and anxiety experienced by some individual upon alcohol absorption. In larger doses, the depressant effect on the central nervous system becomes more apparent. Although there is no known receptor for alcohol, specific regions of the central nervous system appear to show selective sensitivity to alcohol; namely, the reticular ascending system and certain structures in the cerebral cortex. Alcohol blocks the release of the neurotransmitter acetylcholine and disrupts its synthesis. As a result, transmission in the cholinergic pathways of the central nervous system will be lowered. The disruption of acetylcholine synthesis and release accounts for the depressant effects of alcohol on the reticular activating system (the activity of which represents the level of physiological arousal) and the cerebral cortex. The lowering of arousal decreases the individual's ability to attend to specific stimuli and also decreases awareness of stressful information. Alcohol in small quantities may be used to decrease anxiety or tremor prior to competition. It might therefore be useful to target sportsmen such as archers.

Social drinking in moderation during the day(s) prior to an event does not appear to influence physical performance. Excessive intake the evening prior to competition, however, may be detrimental to performance the following morning. Alcohol hangover is caused by the toxicity of alcohol, dehydration, and the toxic effects of the congeners (impurities) such as sulfides and histamines found in alcoholic beverages. The athlete will suffer a lack of motivation to perform maximally because of the associated depressed mood state, headache and hypersensitivity to environmental stimuli.

Athletes should not consume excessive amounts

of alcohol during the recovery period, since it is likely to interfere with their ability to follow guidelines for post-exercise eating.

Alcohol may trigger exercise-induced anaphylaxis and asthma, and it can interact in a harmful way with other types of drugs such as antihistamines and analgesics. Up to a third of people with asthma complain that wine (more so than beer or spirits) will exacerbate their asthma. This is likely due to the effect of sulfites, which are used as preservatives. Histamine within alcoholic beverages may cause allergic reactions. There is generally more histamine in red than white wines. Allergic reactions to alcoholic beverages are uncommon, but non-allergic adverse reactions such as irritant reactions are more common. Anaphylaxis has been described in patients with severe reactions to proteins within grapes, yeast, hops, barley and wheat. The body constantly produces small amounts of alcohol itself. Over-ripe fruit can ferment, resulting in sufficient alcohol to trigger anaphylaxis. Alcohol can exacerbate symptoms in patients with urticaria. Some people, especially those of Asian background, experience intense facial flushing after having even small amounts of alcohol. Alcohol consumption may also trigger stronger-than-normal reactions to everyday allergens such as house dust mites. Alcohol is one of the predisposing factors thought to be important in non-allergic, non-infective rhinitis (an inflammatory condition of the nasal mucosa). Alcohol dilates blood vessels, including those in the nose, causing the nasal and sinus passages to swell.

Alcohol makes the lung liable to injury and infection by producing a decrease in alveolar levels of glutathione, an antioxidant, as well as inhibiting the response to bacterial infection. Drinking alcohol increases the risk of a common gene mutation in smokers developing lung cancer.

There is a positive association between an alcohol intake of 40 g of ethanol per day (3 or more drinks) and increased blood pressure.

Acute or chronic overuse of alcohol has a number of adverse effects including cirrhosis of the liver, which is characterized in the early stages by enlargement of the liver due to fatty change with mild fibrosis. **Alcoholism** is a primary, chronic disease with genetic, psychological, social and environmental factors influencing its development and manifestations. It is often progressive and fatal. It is characterized by impaired control over drinking, preoccupation with alcohol, use of alcohol despite adverse consequences, and distortions in thinking (most notably denial).

Women who drink while pregnant are also more likely to have a miscarriage, a still birth or a low birth-weight baby. The fetal brain and other organs begin to develop around the third week of pregnancy and are vulnerable to damage in these early weeks. There is increasing evidence that heavy alcohol use by the male can also have some effect on pregnancy and the health of the baby. Heavy alcohol use by males can lower the level of the male hormone testosterone, leading to low sperm counts and, occasionally, to infertility.

For the World Anti-Doping Agency Prohibited List 2005, the international federations for gymnastics, roller sports, triathlon and wrestling requested that alcohol be removed as a substance prohibited in their sport. Six federations agreed to a harmonized threshold of 0.1 g/L of alcohol in blood, and three federations required a specific threshold.

See also FETAL ALCOHOL SYNDROME; FRENCH PARADOX; NICOTINE; SLEEP-WAKE CYCLE.

Bibliography

American College of Sports Medicine (1982). Position statement on the use of alcohol in sports. *Medicine and Science in Sports and Exercise* 14(6), ix-xi.

Burke, L.M., Kiens, B. and Ivy, J.L. (2004). Carbohydrates and fat for training and recovery. *Journal of Sports Sciences* 22, 15-30.

Kerr, J.S. and Hindmarch, I. (1991). Alcohol, cognitive function and psychomotor performance. *Reviews on Environmental Health* 9(2), 117-122.

O'Brien, C.P. (1993). Alcohol and sport. Impact of social drinking on recreational and competitive sports performance. *Sports Medicine* 15(2), 71-77.

Shirreffs, S.M. and Maughan, R.J. (1997). Systemic circulation and fluid balance. *Journal of Applied Physiology* 83(4), 1152-1158.

Stainback, R.D. (1997). *Alcohol and sport*. Champaign, IL: Human Kinetics.

Wardlaw, G.M. (1999). *Perspectives in nutrition.* 4ᵗʰ ed. Boston, MA: WCB McGraw-Hill.

Williams, M.H. (1992). Alcohol and sport performance. *Gatorade Sports Science Exchange* 4(40).

World Anti-Doping Agency. Http://www.wada-ama.org

ALDOSTERONE   One of the mineralocorticoids. A hormone secreted by the cortex of the adrenal glands that brings about sodium and water reabsorption, and potassium excretion, by the kidneys. It is controlled by plasma potassium concentration and by the hormones renin and angiotensin. It is stimulated by low blood pressure and plasma volume, elevated potassium and sympathetic activity to the kidney. It is increased by exercise.

See also ANGIOTENSIN-CONVERTING ENZYMES INHIBITORS; PROGESTERONE.

ALIMENTARY CANAL   Enteric canal. The gut. A tube concerned with the digestion and absorption of food.

ALKALEMIA   A decreased concentration of hydrogen ions in the blood.

See also ALKALOSIS.

ALKALINE RESERVE   The buffering capacity of the blood.

ALKALOIDS   A group of nitrogen-containing compounds found in certain plants. Examples are cocaine and nicotine.

ALKALOSIS   A decreased concentration of hydrogen ions in both blood and other body fluids. **Respiratory alkalosis** may be caused by hyperventilation and a decrease of carbon dioxide in body fluids. This occurs during conditions of altitude, hypoxia and anxiety. **Metabolic alkalosis** is caused by: excessive ingestion of base such as sodium bicarbonate; constipation; excess aldosterone; or a large loss of acids, such as when there is vomiting of acidic gastric juice.

See also ACID-BASE BALANCE; ALKALEMIA.

ALLELE   *See under* GENE.

ALLERGY   A harmful (or at least irritant) response in which the immune system is implicated in the mediation of symptoms. An **allergen** is a substance that produces allergy. A number of substances are implicated in the etiology of allergic disease, including pollen, house dust, bee venom and exercise. The term 'allergy' is also used loosely to describe 'sensitivity' to environmental irritants, even when the role of the immune system is far less clear. This 'loose' usage is often applied to reactions following exposure to air pollution in addition to many other ill-defined 'sensitivities' such as non-allergic, asthmatic-type responses (e.g. exercise-induced bronchoconstriction).

The most common allergies involve antibodies of the IgE class. Allergies occur in some people who are genetically predisposed to produce more than the usual amount of IgE when they are exposed to allergens. **Atopy** refers to the largely genetic predisposition for developing an IgE-mediated response to common environmental allergens. It is the strongest identifiable predisposing factor for developing asthma.

An **allergic reaction** involves the release of histamine and other mediators of anaphylaxis. **Anaphylaxis** is a type of hypersensitivity to antigens, such as allergens, in which IgE antibodies attach to mast cells and basophils. Histamine, leukotrienes and other mediators cause the smooth muscle contraction (responsible for wheezing and gastrointestinal symptoms) and vasodilation that characterize anaphylaxis. Vasodilation and leaking of plasma into the tissues causes urticaria and angioedema and results in a decrease in effective plasma volume, which is the major cause of shock. Fluid escapes into the alveoli of the lungs and may produce pulmonary edema. Obstructive angioedema of the upper airway may also occur. Arrhythmias and cardiogenic shock may develop if the reaction is prolonged. It may result in circulatory shock and asphyxia. Anaphylactic shock triggers abrupt and widespread dilation of peripheral blood vessels. Anaphylaxis can be aggravated or even triggered by exercise.

Hyperventilation is common among people with allergies, although it is not known which is the cause and which is the effect. It is known that low levels of carbon dioxide in the blood will alter the activity of mast cells, causing them to release histamine and, in turn, can produce various allergic symptoms.

Food allergies involve allergic reaction to food proteins. The most common food allergens are found in milk, eggs, tree nuts, peanuts, soy, wheat, fish and other seafood. **Food intolerance** involves clinical gastrointestinal reactions in which the mechanism is not immunologic, or is not known. Milk intolerance is sometimes caused by an intestinal disaccharidase deficiency and is expressed by gastrointestinal symptoms. Monosodium glutamate can produce systemic symptoms that are not caused by IgE antibodies.

See also RHINITIS; URTICARIA.

Bibliography

Jenkins, S. and Hay, D. (1996). Air pollution, health and exercise: A review. *Energy and Environment* 7(1), 51-56.

ALLOMETRIC SCALING A mathematical procedure concerned with the relationship between a body size variable (X) such as stature and a physiological variable (Y) such as muscular strength. It can be expressed as $Y = a(X^b)$, where a is the proportionality coefficient and b is the scaling factor. A logarithmic transformation makes the relationship easier to visualize and it also facilitates inter-subject comparisons: $\text{Log} Y = \log a + b (\log X)$.

Bibliography

Rowland, T.W. (1996). *Developmental exercise physiology*. Champaign, IL: Human Kinetics.

ALL OR NONE LAW *See under* MUSCLE; NEURON.

ALLOSTERIC *See under* ENZYME.
ALPHA ADRENERGIC RECEPTORS *See under* AUTONOMIC NERVOUS SYSTEM.

ALPHA KETO-GLUTARIC ACID One of the intermediates in the Krebs cycle. It is also a product of the deamination of glutamic acid.

ALPHA-LIPOIC ACID *See* LIPOIC ACID.

ALPHA MOTOR NEURONS *See under* MUSCLE SPINDLE; NEURONS.

ALTERED STATE OF CONSCIOUSNESS A state of consciousness that is different from a normal awake state of consciousness. Altered states of consciousness occur under many conditions, including: in a flow state, while staring at a particular object, during great muscular effort, when arousal is extremely high or low, in conditions of fatigue, when intoxicated by certain drugs, during sexual intercourse, during pain and during hypnosis. An altered state of consciousness associated with long distance running, 'runner's high,' is thought to be associated with endorphins.

Weston (1986) suggests that altered states of consciousness occur at five different stages: "no sensory selection" (when a person is not concentrating on anything in particular); "normal sensory selection" (when doing routine work or leisure activities); "augmented sensory selection" (when concentrating on a complicated or interesting task); "hypersensory selection" (when concentrating on a single stimulus); and "total sensory selection" (an extension of the previous stage such that the person is unaware of anything except the stimulus).

See also PEAK EXPERIENCES.

Bibliography

Weston, P.G.W. (1986). Hypnosis - Some states of altered consciousness and their application in sport. In: MacGregor, J.A. and Moncur, J.A. (eds). *Sport and Medicine*. pp148-157. London: E. and F.N. Spon.

ALTITUDE The vertical distance above ground (sea) level. Medium altitude is considered as between 1,829 and 3,048 m. Above 3,048 m is considered to be high altitude. One per cent of the world's population resides above 3,300 m. The highest mountain is Mount Everest with a peak of 8,850 m.

There are changes in environmental and physiological variables with altitude. Total barometric pressure decreases with increasing altitude. Dry ambient air at both sea level and altitude contains 20.9% oxygen, so the partial pressure of oxygen decreases in direct proportion to the decrease in barometric pressure with altitude (it is equal to 0.209 multiplied by total barometric pressure). **Altitude hypoxia** refers to the decrease in partial pressure of oxygen with increasing altitude.

Altitude exposure may lead to significant weight loss because of an initial loss of water and subsequent loss of fat and muscle mass due to malnutrition. Weight losses of 3% in 8 days at 4,300 m and up to 15% after 3 months at 5,300 to 8,000 m have been reported, suggesting that this weight loss is a function of both absolute altitude and the duration of the exposure. It is thought that non-water weight loss can be avoided at altitudes of up to 5,000 m, if an adequate energy intake is maintained. Factors related to weight loss during longer exposures at higher altitudes are primary anorexia, lack of comfort and palatable food, detraining, and possibly the direct effects of hypoxia on protein metabolism. Proper acclimatization and maintenance of a high and varied nutrient intake should minimize weight losses.

Laboratory tests with simulated altitude have found a decrease in maximal oxygen uptake at altitudes as low as 1,219 m. Maximal oxygen uptake decreases about 2% for every 300 m above 1,500 m. The loss of maximal aerobic capacity is not usually improved by acclimatization. There is an increase in endurance capacity for submaximal exercise. This may possibly be explained by a decrease in ammonia accumulation at high altitude that may decrease the perception of fatigue and thus enable the athlete to work longer.

The alveolar partial pressure of oxygen averages 25 mmHg at the summit of Everest (8,850 m). For an acclimatized individual, this decreases maximal oxygen uptake by 70% to about 15 ml/O_2/kg. An unacclimatized individual loses consciousness within 30 seconds at this altitude.

The decrease in air density with altitude can have a beneficial effect on the flight of projectiles and sprinting performance. At the 1968 Olympic Games in Mexico City (2,300 m above sea level) air density was about 23% less than at sea level. Performances in sprint events were about 1.7% better than would be expected if the events had taken place at sea level.

Bob Beamon's long jump record (8.91 meters), that was achieved at altitude and with a maximum allowable following wind of 2 m/s in the 1968 Olympics, was broken by Mike Powell (8.95 meters) in 1991. The decreased air resistance at Mexico City assisted the setting of a record in the 800 m, but performance was progressively worse for races lasting longer than about two minutes. Athletes who resided permanently at high altitude performed well not only in Mexico City, but also in endurance events held at sea level. These facts led to the question of whether altitude training might have a beneficial effect on subsequent sea level performance.

Altitude acclimatization involves physiological responses that improve tolerance to the decrease in the partial pressure of oxygen with altitude. Short-term acclimatization occurs within three months to a year. The most important immediate response to altitude hypoxia is hyperventilation caused by the decreased arterial partial pressure of oxygen. Chemoreceptors in the aortic arch and carotid sinuses are stimulated by a significant decrease in arterial partial pressure of oxygen. The response from the respiratory center is to increase alveolar ventilation, causing alveolar partial pressure of oxygen to increase toward ambient partial pressure of oxygen. This facilitates oxygen transport in the lungs. In the early stages of acclimatization, the decrease in arterial partial pressure of oxygen is partially offset by an increase in submaximal cardiac output (maximal cardiac output is unchanged or slightly lower). This is due to an increase in submaximal heart rate (stroke volume is unchanged or slightly lowered). It is because of this short-term acclimatization to altitude that climbers are able to ascend and briefly survive on Mount Everest, where pressures are less than one-third of normal barometric pressure. In the longer term, submaximal cardiac output is lowered due to decreased stroke volume. Both maximal heart rate and cardiac output are lowered.

The kidneys respond to the respiratory alkalosis (caused by hyperventilation) by excreting base (alkali). The buffer (alkaline) reserve is decreased, thus lowering both the blood-buffering capacity for acid and the threshold for accumulation of acidic metabolic by-products. The oxygen-carrying capacity of the blood is increased. This is due firstly to a decrease in plasma volume causing an increase in hematocrit and hemoglobin, and secondly to erythrocythemia. The affinity for hemoglobin is decreased, probably due to an increase in the concentration of 2,3 diphosphoglycerate in red blood cells, thus facilitating oxygen uptake by the tissues. There may be an increase in the concentration of capillaries in skeletal muscle and an increase in myoglobin. There is an increase in both the number of mitochondria and the concentration of enzymes required for aerobic energy production. Carbohydrate metabolism is dramatically altered at altitude, with fat being the preferred fuel for exercise. It is possible that the preference for fat utilization may be a consequence of decreased muscle glycogen storage, which is affected by both diet and dehydration.

Acclimatization at one particular altitude does not extend to full acclimatization at a higher altitude. Maximal oxygen uptake is lowered by about 2% for every 300 m above 1,500 m. Full acclimatization to medium altitude takes about two weeks. For high altitude, it is a very slow process: sea-level subjects residing at high altitude may suffer a decrease in work capacity as great as 50% after one year. The effects of acclimatization last only about three weeks on return to sea level. Acclimatization stops and physical wellness deteriorates above 5,200 m.

On ascent to high altitude, lactate production at a given submaximal exercise load is increased when compared to the same load at sea level. After acclimatization, paradoxically, there is a decreased lactate response to the same exercise load in the absence of increased oxygen uptake or regional blood flow. Proposed explanations for this 'lactate paradox' include decreased output of glucose-mobilizing epinephrine during chronic altitude exposure and inhibition of glycolytic-pathway activation due to a decrease in intracellular ADP during chronic altitude exposure.

With regard to the differences in lactate accumulation during exercise that have been reported to occur between lowlanders and highlanders, both groups either being acclimatized

or not, these do not seem to be based upon fundamentally different metabolic features. Instead they seem merely to reflect points along the same continuum of phenotypic adaptations of which the location depends on the time spent at high altitude.

Two major experiments that have elucidated the factors determining acclimatization and tolerance to extreme altitude (over 7,000 m) were the American Medical Research Expedition to Everest and the low-pressure chamber simulation, Operation Everest II. Extreme hyperventilation is one of the most important responses to extreme altitude; it allows the climber to maintain an alveolar partial pressure of oxygen that keeps the arterial partial pressure of oxygen above dangerously low levels. There is evidence of residual impairment of the central nervous system after ascents to extreme altitude. Seasonal changes in pressure probably affect climbing performance near the summit of Mount Everest. Supplementary oxygen always improves exercise tolerance at extreme altitudes, and rescue oxygen should be available on climbing expeditions to 8,000 m peaks.

Mountain sickness is an illness that occurs if altitude acclimatization is inadequate. **Acute mountain sickness** is a condition affecting previously healthy individuals who ascend rapidly to high altitude. The symptoms include headache, nausea, vomiting, irritability and insomnia. Acute mountain sickness is classified as benign or malignant. At altitudes of 2,500 to 5,000 m, about 20 to 90% of persons not acclimatized to high altitude will experience mild symptoms of acute mountain sickness. In the Mount Everest region, about 50% of trekkers who ascend above 4,000 m over 5 days develop acute mountain sickness. Acute mountain sickness can be avoided buy limiting ascent to 300 m per day with a day of rest every 3rd day. Sleep at night should take place at least 460 m lower than the altitude climbed during the day. The altitude where each night is spent should be no more than 300 m above the altitude of the previous night, and two nights should be spent at the same altitude every 3 days. Descent should be undertaken if symptoms of acute mountain sickness occur. There is evidence to support the use of acetazolamide for the prophylaxis of acute mountain sickness. It may also decrease muscle loss and assist exercise performance. **Acetazolamide** is a carbonic acid anhydrase inhibitor that probably acts as a respiratory stimulant. It has been shown to decrease arterial partial pressure of carbon dioxide thus mimicking respiratory acclimatization. Acute mountain sickness can lead to a malignant form, **chronic mountain sickness** (high-altitude pulmonary edema; cerebral edema), or mixed forms of these two. Symptoms of these edema conditions include mental and physical fatigue, headaches and dizziness. Cerebral edema is probably the result of cerebral vasodilation and elevated capillary hydrostatic pressure. Chronic mountain sickness affects residents of high altitude and consists of extreme polycythemia.

See also under HEADACHE.

Bibliography

Armstong, L.E. (2000). *Performing in extreme environments.* Champaign, IL: Human Kinetics.

Bradwell, A.R., Dykes, P.W. and Coote, J.H. (1987). Effect of acetazolamide on exercise at altitude. *Sports Medicine* 4, 157-163.

Kayser, B. (1994). Nutrition and energetics of exercise at altitude. *Sports Medicine* 17(5), 309-323.

Kayser, B. (1996). Lactate during exercise at high altitude. *European Journal of Applied Physiology and Occupational Physiology* 74(3), 195-205.

McArdle, W.D., Katch, F.I. and Katch, V.I. (2004). *Exercise physiology: Energy, nutrition and human performance.* 5th ed. Philadelphia, PA: Lippincott, Williams & Wilkins.

Milledge, J.S. (1998). High altitude. In: Harries, M., Williams, C., Stanish, W.D. and Micheli, L.J. (eds). *Oxford textbook of sports medicine.* p255-269. New York: Oxford Medical Publications.

Reeves, J.T. et al (1992). Oxygen transport during exercise at altitude and the lactate paradox: Lessons from Operator Everest II and Pikes Peak. *Exercise and Sport Sciences Reviews* 20, 275-296.

West, J.B. (1993). Acclimatization and tolerance to extreme altitude. *Journal of Wilderness Medicine* 4(1), 17-26.

ALTITUDE TRAINING A form of training based on the premise that the physiological stress of hypoxia, in addition to training stress, will compound the training adaptations the athletes acquire and thus enhance performance. Athletes tend to choose altitudes of 2,743 to 3,658 m for altitude training. There is no doubt that altitude training benefits subsequent performance at altitude, but training at altitude provides no more benefit to sea-level performance than equivalent training at sea level. There are certain altitude acclimatization adaptations that should increase aerobic capacity and endurance performance on return to sea level. Oxygen delivery should be improved at sea level after altitude training, as altitude acclimatization increases hematocrit and hemoglobin. If, however, these effects are due to dehydration, and if blood viscosity is increased, then it is unlikely that performance would improve. Research evidence suggests that increased oxygen carrying capacity of the blood would be offset by the altitude-related decrease in maximal heart rate and maximal stroke volume. For some athletes, a worsening of maximal oxygen uptake upon return to sea level may be explained simply by detraining due to the quality of their training sessions suffering at high altitude.

Since the late 1980s, endurance athletes have followed the strategy of 'live high, train low' using devices such as the Colorado Mountain Room, which is a hypoxic apartment produced by a company called Colorado Altitude Training. It is a negative-feedback system, which features a molecular sieve that safely decreases oxygen levels until the desired altitude is reached, a carbon dioxide scrubber that eliminates excess carbon dioxide, oxygen sensors, and a control panel. The premise is that sea level maximal oxygen uptake and endurance performance can be improved by, in effect, living at a high altitude (2,000 to 3,000 m) and training simultaneously at a low altitude (i.e. lower than 1,000 m). Athletes typically 'live and sleep high' in the hypoxic apartment for 8 to 18 hours a day, but complete their training at, or near, sea level. There is equivocal evidence that using a hypoxic apartment in this manner produces beneficial changes in serum erythropoietin levels, reticulocyte count and red blood cell mass that in turn may lead to improvements in post-altitude endurance performance. Improvements in performance would not likely exceed 2 to 3%.

Bibliography

Armstrong, L.E. (2000). *Performing in extreme environments*. Champaign, IL: Human Kinetics.

Berglund, B. (1992). High-altitude training. Aspects of hematological adaptation. *Sports Medicine* 14(5), 289-303.

Ratzin Jackson, C.G. and Sharkey, B.J. (1988). Altitude, training and human performance. *Sports Medicine* 6(5), 279-284.

Sutton, J.R. (1993). Exercise training at high altitude: Does it improve endurance performance at sea level? *Gatorade Sports Science Exchange* 6(4).

Wilber, R.L. (2001). Current trends in altitude training. *Sports Medicine* 31(4), 249-265.

Wilber, R.L. (2004). *Altitude training and athletic performance*. Champaign, IL: Human Kinetics.

Wolski, L.A., McKenzie, D.C. and Wenger, H.A. (1996). Altitude training for improvements in sea level performance. Is there scientific evidence of benefit? *Sports Medicine* 22(4), 251-263.

ALVEOLAR-ARTERIAL PARTIAL PRESSURE OF OXYGEN DIFFERENCE The difference between the ideal alveolar partial pressure of oxygen and the mean arterial partial pressure of oxygen. It is considered to be an index of pulmonary inefficiency with respect to oxygen exchange. It may increase substantially during strenuous exercise, by about threefold in untrained individuals.

ALVEOLAR PRESSURE The pressure within the alveoli. Alveolar pressure determines whether air flows into or out of the lungs. When alveolar pressure is negative, as is the case during inspiration, air flows into the lungs. When alveolar pressure is positive, as is the case during expiration, air flows out of the lungs.

ALVEOLAR VENTILATION The volume of fresh air introduced into the gas-exchanging regions of the lung per minute. Alveolar ventilation is pulmonary ventilation minus dead space ventilation. **Diffusion capacity** is the rate of oxygen transfer from alveolar air to blood and combination with hemoglobin. The magnitude of diffusion capacity is determined by the alveolar-capillary surface available for gas exchange, the oxygen-carrying capacity of the blood and the pulmonary capillary blood volume. Normally the diffusion capacity of oxygen increases by 40 to 100% from rest to exercise. Increased diffusion capacity is the combined result of increased tidal volume (which opens partially-collapsed alveoli and exposes more alveolar surface to inspired gas), increased pulmonary blood flow (which opens previously collapsed capillaries and increases capillary volume and surface for diffusion) and changes in red blood cell flow pattern (so the regional distribution of red blood cells and among capillaries becomes more uniform). Diffusion limitation develops when blood crosses and leaves the pulmonary capillary bed without fully equilibrating with alveolar partial pressure of oxygen resulting in a low arterial partial pressure of oxygen and a high alveolar-arterial partial pressure of oxygen difference.

Deeper breathing (i.e. higher tidal volume) provides more effective alveolar ventilation than a similar pulmonary ventilation achieved through an increased respiratory frequency.

See also VENTILATION-TO-PERFUSION RATIO.

ALVEOLI *See under* LUNG.

ALZHEIMER'S DISEASE It is a slow, progressive disease, which starts with mild memory problems and ends with severe, fatal brain damage. It is the most common form of dementia. There is no medical treatment to cure or stop the progression of Alzheimer's disease. Up to 10% of all people 65 years of age and older have Alzheimer's disease; and up to 50% of all people 85 years of age and older have Alzheimer's disease. Three genes have been identified that cause rare, inherited forms of the disease that tend to occur before the age of 65 years. Up to 4 million Americans suffer from Alzheimer's disease.

Amyloid plaques and neurofibrillary tangles are considered hallmarks of Alzheimer's disease. **Amyloid plaques** are clumps of protein fragments that accumulate outside of cells. **Neurofibrillary tangles** are clumps of altered proteins inside cells. It is not known exactly what role plaques and tangles play in the disease process. However, amyloid can make cell membranes leak choline, and thus decrease production of acetylcholine in cells.

Alzheimer's disease is more common among individuals who have sustained a severe head injury (accompanied by loss of consciousness) during their lives.

The concept of cognitive reserve suggests that innate intelligence or aspects of life experience like educational or occupational attainments may supply reserve, in the form of a set of skills or repertoires that allows some people to cope with progressing Alzheimer's disease pathology better than others. There is epidemiological evidence that lifestyle characterized by engagement in leisure activities of intellectual and social nature is associated with slower cognitive decline in healthy elderly and may decrease the risk of incident dementia.

Bibliography

Alzheimer's Disease Education & Referral Center. Http://www.alzheimers.org.

Scarmeas, N. and Stern, Y. (2003). Cognitive reserve and lifestyle. *Journal of Clinical and Experimental Neuropsychology* 25(5), 625-633.

AMATEURISM This implies engaging in an activity simply for 'love of the game' with a code of 'fair play,' but without extrinsic rewards such as money being sought. It has been regarded as the antithesis of professionalism and commercialism.

Four different perspectives on amateurism have been identified in the sociology of sport literature. Firstly, amateurism can be regarded as a way of excluding the lower classes. In the nineteenth century, the rules and practices of sport were based on social class. For example, mechanics, artisans and laborers were disqualified from rowing. The argument was that men in such groups would have a physical advantage in sport due to the nature of their work. The ruling classes thus declared that such men were professionals and ineligible for amateur competition.

Secondly, amateurism can be regarded as an exploitative ideology. For example, the National Collegiate Athletics Association (NCAA) in America actively promotes an amateur ideology even though it functions as a cartel that completely controls the mass commercial entertainment industry that collegiate sport has become. The collegiate athletes, however, receive very low salaries relative to professional athletes. There were 4.9 million students in NCAA institutions in 2001. Of these, about 111,600 students had some form of athletic aid. For all three NCAA divisions, fewer than 23,000 had full scholarships (room, food and full tuition). The term 'student-athlete' was apparently crafted and mandated for use in the 1950s by the NCAA's executive director, Walter Byers, in order to avoid use of terms such as 'employee' or 'worker.'

Thirdly, amateurism can be regarded as an anachronism in that the original concept of amateurism simply does not apply in contemporary international sport. Hypocrisy and cheating, rather than fair play and honesty, arises because sports organizations cling unrealistically to the amateur ideal.

Fourthly, amateurism can be regarded as a worthy ideal. The hypocrisy surrounding it is not a fault of the ideal but a consequence of corruption in sport. It can be argued that elite amateur sport has moved beyond the amateur ideal to become corporate sport. At the grass roots level, however, amateur sport thrives.

See also under CHARACTER BUILDING; COMMERCIALISM; INTRINSIC MOTIVATION.

Chronology

•594 AD • Legislating for Athens, Solon laid down maxima for athletic prizes: 500 drachmae for Olympic victors and 100 drachmae for victors in the Olympic and Isthmian Games, respectively. Solon said, "…we do not look at the mere prizes which are handed out. They are tokens of victory and a way to recognize the victors, and getting kicked is a small price to pay for those who seek fame through pain." (Lucian, *Anacharsis*, 9-14) Gardiner (1910) described it as an attempt to encourage athletics among the people and perhaps to counteract the growing love of chariot racing among the aristocracy.

•1808 • At Newmarket in England, Captain Robert Barclay Allardice, a Scotsman, walked one mile in each of 1,000 successive hours. In the first week his average time was 14 minutes, 54 seconds; in the last week it was 21 minutes 4 seconds. More than 10,000 people were attracted to the event and Barclay won substantial prize money. Pedestrianism was a popular spectator sport in the eighteenth and nineteenth centuries. The first famous pedestrian was Foster Powell, who, for a wager of one hundred guineas, walked from London to York, and back (about 396 miles in 6 days). Huge crowds were willing to pay entrance fees to watch walking events. In 1796, Barclay covered 110 miles in 19 hours, 27 minutes in a muddy park. In 1801, he wagered a thousand guineas that he could walk 90 miles in 12 hours but reputedly caught a cold and lost. Then he increased the stake to 2,000 guineas, but lost again. Finally he got odds that would pay him 5,000 guineas if he won – which he did with an hour to spare. In 1813, Walter Thom published *Pedestrianism, or An Account of the Performances of Celebrated Pedestrians during the Last and Present Century: With a Full Narrative of Captain Barclay's Public and Private Matches, and an Essay on Training.* Barclay had a profound impact on athletics generally and his training methods, involving purging and sweating, and the eating of meat, were widely used throughout much of the century. He was also sponsor and trainer of Tom Cribb, the bare-knuckle fighter. He died in 1854 of paralysis after being kicked by a horse.

•1846 • In England, there was a dispute following a Manchester crew's victory in a rowing competition. Two of the crew were artisans and alleged to be unacceptable entrants on the basis that "they were not men of any property" (i.e. they were not 'gentlemen').

•1862 • In America, James Creighton was probably the first professional baseball player when reportedly paid a lump sum by the Excelsiors from Brooklyn. He died a few days after rupturing his bladder from swinging forcefully at a pitch.

•1866 • The New York Athletic Club was formed. Its purpose was to promote amateur competition in track and field in the New York area, based on the English model.

•1869 • A year following the establishment of two categories of membership by the National Association of Base Ball Players, amateur and professional, the Cincinnati Red Stockings suddenly appeared as the first openly all-professional baseball team. There was only one starter who was actually from Cincinnati; most of the others were imported from New York. The Red Stockings were not the first team of paid players. Their rival club in Cincinnati, the Buckeyes, had been playing their players steady wages.

•1871 • With the National Association of Base Ball Players being in disarray because of the battle between professionals and amateurs, nine clubs, including the Red Stockings, who were now representing Boston, but was still managed by Harry Wright, founded the National Association of Professional Base Ball Players. In response, a number of clubs formed the National Association of Amateur Base Ball Players, but it disbanded after a dispute concerning whether or not admission charges should be made.

•1879 • In the regulations for the Henley Regatta - staged on the River Thames in England - mechanics, artisans and laborers were not considered eligible for the status of amateur rowers and were therefore excluded.

•1879 • The National Association of Amateur Athletes of America (NAAAA) was founded to preserve the concept of amateurism and regulate competition.

•1888 • Fifteen of the more prominent track and field clubs joined together to form the Amateur Athletic Union (AAU) of the United States. Its purpose was to deal with the problems of professionalization and gambling in track and field and to organize national amateur championships in that sport.

•1892 • Former Yale All-America guard, and prize fighter, William (Pudge) Heffelfinger became the first known professional football player when the Allegheny Athletic Association paid him $500 to play a single game against the Pittsburgh Athletic Club. Heffelfinger scored a touchdown to win the game for Allegheny.

•1893 • The Pittsburgh Athletic Club signed one of its players (probably halfback Grant Dilbert) to the first known professional football contract in 1893. Three years later, the Allegheny Athletic Association team fielded the first completely professional team for its abbreviated two-game schedule.

•1895 • John Brallier became the first football player to openly turn professional, accepting $10 and expenses to play for the Latrobe YMCA against the Jeannette Athletic Club.

•1895 • Seven Midwest university presidents met in Chicago to discuss the regulation and control of intercollegiate athletics. Under the leadership of James H. Smart, president of Purdue University, this meeting led to the development of the Intercollegiate Conference of Faculty Representatives, also known as the Big Ten Conference. The presidents' first known action "restricted eligibility for athletics to bona-fide, full-time students who were not delinquent in their studies."

•1895 • In England, rugby union split into two distinct codes, amateur and professional. The

to the northern counties of England, became known as rugby league.

•1905 • In football, 18 players were killed and 159 were seriously injured. The brutality of the sport caused some universities, e.g. Columbia, to drop the sport. President Theodore Roosevelt's son was injured while playing football and he called two White House meetings to deal with violence in football. He put enough pressure on the college presidents to take the necessary steps for reform. The conference led to the development of a safer game. It also led to the formation of the Intercollegiate Athletic Association of the United States (IAAUS) that was officially constituted in 1906. It changed its name to the National Collegiate Athletic

Association (NCAA) in 1910.

•1912 • At the Olympic Games, Jim Thorp won the modern pentathlon, heptathlon and decathlon, but was stripped of his medals after it was discovered that he had played for a minor league baseball team in 1909 and 1910, and was thus classified as a professional athlete. Thorp was the first Native American to compete in the Olympics and to play football. In 1999 the US Government declared, "Jim Thorpe is the athlete of the century." Years after his death, his daughter was successful in persuading the International Olympic Committee (IOC) to restore his status as an Olympic champion.

•1920 • The American Professional Football Association was founded, with the first president being Jim Thorpe. In 1922, it officially changed its name to the National Football League (NFL).

•1929 • The Carnegie Foundation released the results of a study that stated physical education had been used to turn colleges and universities in giant athletic agencies.

•1932 • Paavo Nurmi of Finland was disqualified from competing, because it was determined that he had claimed travel expenses to fund his journey to a German meeting and was thus a professional athlete. Nurmi became known for his scientific approach to training and performance; after finishing 2nd in 5,000 meters at the 1920 Olympic Games he ran with a stop watch to pace himself better. He won 9 gold medals at the Olympic Games, in distances from 1,500 meters to 20,000 meters, including 5 at the 1924 Olympic Games.

•1946 • The National Collegiate Athletic Association (NCAA) held a "Conference on Conferences" for the purpose of determining "Principles for the Conduct of Intercollegiate Athletics." A code was adopted in 1948 and two years later seven schools were cited for noncompliance.

•1951 • Members of the City College of New York (CCNY) men's basketball team admitted that they took money from gamblers to 'fix' the point spread, i.e. win by a lesser amount of points than they had to. Two of the players served brief jail sentences. The New York District Attorney's office showed that between 1947 and 1951, 86 games had been fixed in 23 cities in 17 states by 32 players from seven colleges. The New York City Board of Higher Education, when investigating the CCNY program, found that the high school records of 14 players had been tampered with to make them eligible for admission.

•1957 • Having three years earlier established a "Committee on Infractions," the NCAA hired its first full-time investigator.

•1973 • The National Collegiate Athletic Association (NCAA) approved of a reorganization into three divisions based on the size of the institution and its athletic facilities, and/or the scope of its intercollegiate athletic program and/or the financial aid provided for its student-athletes.

•1974 • The International Olympic Committee (IOC) passed an amendment to its amateur code that permitted reimbursement for loss of salary, lifted restrictions on the length of time an athlete can spend away from home for training and competition, and legitimized the sponsorship of athletes by organizations such as national governing bodies, private businesses and corporations.

•1983 • The National Collegiate Athletic Association (NCAA) passed rules (Proposition 48) that set minimum standards for a first-year athlete to be eligible to play on Division I teams. Student-athletes were required to have a minimum SAT score of 700, or an ACT score of 17, and a minimum GPA of 2.0 in at least 11 courses in core classes.

•1985 • The International Amateur Athletic Federation (IAAF) created trust funds for athletes.

•1991 • The National Collegiate Athletic Association (NCAA) made several reforms including that athletes entering their fourth year must have completed at least 50% of their degree requirements.

•2002 • The National Collegiate Athletic Association (NCAA) approved new academic standards, which took effect in August 2003, that would allow student-athletes with an SAT score as low as 400 (the lowest score possible) to qualify for admittance to college, if they have earned a high school grade-point average of 3.55 or higher. Under the 'sliding scale' of the new system, the minimum score for a student-athlete with a 3.0 was lowered to 620. A student-athlete with a 2.6 GPA would need a 780. The number of high-school core courses required by student-athletes to participate in sports as a freshman was raised from 13 to 14 and the requirement of a 2.0 grade-point average in core courses was maintained. Student-athletes would not be eligible unless they had completed: 40% of their graduation requirements with a GPA of at least 1.8 by the end of their second year (up from 25%); 60% of requirements with a GPA of 2.0 by the end of their third year (up from 50% and 1.8); and 80% with a GPA of 2.0 by the end of their fourth year (up from 75% and 1.9). Other requirements included that student-athletes must pass 24 semester hours before entering their second academic year and maintain at least 18 hours each academic year and six hours per term. The NCAA argued that the standards corrected inequities in existing eligibility policies and furthermore were designed to improve graduation rates.

•2003 • Vanderbilt University, a small, but prestigious, private school with around 6,300 undergraduates, merged its athletic department with recreational activities for students under the new Office of Student Athletics, Recreation and Wellness. The goal was to integrate student athletics into the mainstream of the university. The chancellor of the university did away with the job of athletic director, offering the former athletic director a job as special assistant to the chancellor for athletic/academic reform.

Bibliography

Coakley, J. (2004). *Sports in society. Issues and controversies.* 8th ed. Boston, MA: McGraw-Hill.

Eitzen, D.S. (1989). The sociology of amateur sport: An overview. *International Review for the Sociology of Sport* 24(2), 95-106.

AMBYLOPIA 'Lazy eye.' Suppression of the image of one eye, usually because of that eye having a significantly poorer acuity or being turned in/out. Children with ambylopia can have some functional field loss or absent depth perception.

AMENORRHEA **Primary amenorrhea** can be defined as the absence of menstruation by the age of 16 years in a girl with secondary sex characteristics; **secondary amenorrhea** is the absence of three or more consecutive menstrual cycles after menarche; and **oligomenorrhea** is defined as fewer than eight menses per year (Harmon, 2002). Amenorrhea is 20 times more frequent in athletic women than in nonexercising women.

The very low body mass that frequently accompanies exercise-related menstrual irregularities has led some authors to develop a hypothesis that a critical percentage of body fat is essential to trigger normal menstruation. The weight of evidence suggests amenorrhea is not caused solely by low body-weight (or body fat).

A negative energy balance appears to be the primary factor affecting gonadotrophin-releasing hormone (GnRH) suppression in athletes engaged in sports that emphasize low body weight or leanness. Suppression of hypothalamic pulsatile release of GnRH, which normally occurs every 60 to 90 minutes, limits secretion of luteinizing hormone from the pituitary gland and, to a lesser extent follicle-stimulating hormone, which, in turn, limits ovarian stimulation and estradiol production. A prolonged follicular phase, or the absence of a critical luteinizing hormone or estradiol surge mid-cycle, results in the mild or intermittent suppression of menstrual cycles in athletes whose sports emphasize low body weight. Very low levels of luteinizing hormone result in delayed menarche or amenorrhea. Amenorrheic athletes display low plasma glucose concentrations, low insulin, low insulin-like growth factor 1 (IGF-1) / IGF binding protein-1, low leptin, low triiodothyronine, and low resting metabolic rates; as well as elevated growth hormone, and mildly elevated cortisol. All these abnormalities are signs of chronic energy deficiency.

The 'energy drain' theory does not explain reproductive dysfunction in all athletic disciplines. In sports that emphasize strength, the endocrine profile of athletes is characterized by mildly elevated levels of luteinizing hormone, elevated ratios of luteinizing hormone to follicle-stimulating hormone and mild hyperandrogenism rather than the hypoestrogenism observed in athletes engaged in sports requiring low body weight. It is not known whether the hormone profile of these women is genetically determined or secondary to activation of the adrenal axis.

There is no convincing evidence that exercise training delays menarche. There is evidence that some form of sport-specific selection occurs in gymnastics, such that late maturation contributes to a girl's decision to continue participating in the sport. It is not clear why menarche and breast development are predominantly affected by starting exercise training at a young age, whereas the onset or completion of the growth of adrenal steroid-induced pubic and axillary hair are not delayed.

The menstrual function of 66 competitors in the 1964 Olympic Games was found to be quite normal, even though 7.7% were amenorrheic and a 19 year-old had not yet menstruated (Zaharieva, 1965). By the 1970s, when more women did intense exercise training, reports of menstrual irregularities became more common. Surveys of recreational and elite distance runners show a great variability in the prevalence of secondary amenorrhea, between 1 and 44%. Menstrual cycle alterations are likely to occur after very demanding training, which causes an increased secretion of anti-reproductive hormones. These hormones can inhibit the normal pulsatile secretion pattern of the gonadotrophins. Abrupt initiation of a high volume of aerobic training can disrupt the menstrual cycle in some women. It is possible, however, that these women may be more susceptible to menstrual dysfunction than others. It may therefore not be exercise itself, but rather some aspect of athletic training (such as nutritional inadequacy), which is responsible for the observed disruption. Athletic women may become amenorrheic if reproductive immaturity, emotional stress and undernutrition co-exist with increasing exercise loads. There is an association between athletic amenorrhea and eating disorders.

The dietary issues of the female athlete with athletic menstrual dysfunction are similar to those of her eumenorrheic counterpart. The most common nutrition issues in female athletes are poor energy intake and/or poor food selection, which can lead to poor intake of protein, carbohydrate and essential fatty acids. The most common micronutrients to be low are the bone-building nutrients (especially calcium), the B vitamins, iron and zinc. Iron and zinc are typically low in the diets of female athletes if meat products are avoided.

Women with amenorrhea experience decreased lipid mobilization and increased carbohydrate metabolism, while women with normal cycles experience the opposite effect.

See under EATING DISORDERS; MENSTRUAL CYCLE.

Bibliography

Constantino, N.W. (1994). Clinical consequences of athletic amenorrhea. *Sports Medicine* 17(4), 213-223.

De Crée, C. (1998). Sex steroid metabolism and menstrual irregularities in the exercising female. A review. *Sports Medicine* 25(6), 369-406.

De Crée, C., Vermeulen, A. and Ostyn, M. (1991). Are high-performance young women athletes doomed to become low-performance old wives? A reconsideration of the increased risk of osteoporosis in amenorrheic women. *Journal of Sports Medicine and Physical Fitness* 31(1), 108-14.

De Souza, M.J. and Metzger, D.A. (1991). Reproductive dysfunction in amenorrheic athletes and anorexic patients: A review. *Medicine and Science in Sports and Exercise* 23(9), 995-1007.

Harmon, K.G. (2002). Evaluating and treating exercise-related menstrual irregularities. *The Physician and Sportsmedicine* 30(3), 29-35.

Keizer, H.A. and Rogol, A.D. (1990). Physical exercise and menstrual cycle alterations: What are the mechanisms? *Sports Medicine* 10(4), 218-235.

Loucks, A.B. (2004). Energy balance and body composition in sports and exercise. *Journal of Sports Sciences* 22, 1-14.

Manore, M.M. (2002). Dietary recommendations and athletic menstrual dysfunction. *Sports Medicine* 32(14), 887-901.

O'Donnell, E. and De Souza, M.J. (2004). The cardiovascular effects of chronic hypoestrogenism in amenorrheic athletes: A critical review. *Sports Medicine* 34(9), 601-627.

Warren, M.P. and Perlroth, N.E. (2001). Hormones and sport. The effects of intense exercise on the female reproductive system. *Journal of Endocrinology* 170, 3-11.

West, R.V. (1998). The female athlete. The triad of disordered eating, amenorrhea and osteoporosis. *Sports Medicine* 26(2), 63-71.

Zaharieva, E. (1965). Survey of sportswomen at the Tokyo Olympics. Journal of Sports Medicine and Physical Fitness 5, 215-219.

AMIDE BOND   A bond in which the hydroxyl (-OH) group of carboxylic acid is replaced by an amino (NH_2) group.

AMINATION   The addition of an amino (NH_2) group to an organic compound to produce an amine.

AMINES   Compounds, derived from ammonia, in which at least one hydrogen atoms is replaced by hydrocarbon groups.

AMINO ACIDS   Simple nitrogenous compounds that are the building blocks of peptides and proteins. Alpha-amino acids are the only kinds of amino acids in proteins. The **alpha** refers to the central carbon, onto which four different groups are attached. Amino acids (except for proline) uniformly consist of a central carbon atom chemically bonded to one hydrogen, one carboxylic acid group (-COOH), one amino ($-NH_2$), and one side group unique to each amino acid (R). To form a peptide bond, the carboxyl group of one amino group bonds to the amino group of another amino acid, releasing water in the process.

Amino acids may be classified as glucogenic (glycogenic) or ketogenic according to the destination of their carbon skeletons during degradation. If the skeleton, or part of it, is changed into a compound that may lead to the production of glucose, the amino acid is said to be **glucogenic**. If the compound is one that could lead to the formation of ketone bodies, the amino acid is said to be **ketogenic**. These amino acids would lead to the synthesis of fats, ketone bodies and sterols.

Of the known amino acids, eight (ten for children) cannot be synthesized by the body and must therefore be obtained from the diet. These eight (ten) so-called **essential amino acids** are valine, leucine, phenylalanine, tryptophan, lysine, isoleucine, methionine and threonine (for children, also arginine and histidine). Some adults can synthesize histidine, but for other adults histidine is an essential amino acid. The following are **nonesssential amino acids**: glycine, alanine, aspartic acid, glutamic acid, serine, cysteine (and cystine), tyrosine, arginine, ornithine, proline, hydroxyproline, glutamine and asparagine. There is controversy, however, as to whether or not arginine is an essential amino acid. It is believed that arginine can become essential during conditions of illness or severe physiological stress. Glutamine can become essential after trauma or during periods of critical illness that increase the body's need for it. Tyrosine and cysteine/cystine are both considered **conditional essential amino acids**, in that they can only be synthesized from methionine and phenylalanine, respectively, once needs for methionine and phenylalanine are met. People with phenylketonuria (PKU) lack sufficient amounts of an enzyme that converts phenylalanine to tyrosine, so tyrosine becomes an essential amino acid.

Most amino acids can exist in more than one form (same chemical formula but different spatial configurations of atoms). The amino acids, except for glycine, present in protein molecules are all of the L (laevorotatory) form.

Four of the amino acids - glutamate, aspartate, alanine and glutamine - are present in cells at much higher concentration than the other sixteen and have major metabolic functions in addition to their roles in proteins.

The **amino acid pool** refers to the **free amino acids** present mainly in the cytosol and circulating blood. Amino acids may join the pool during either the digestion/absorption of protein-rich foods or the degradation of body proteins. Free amino acids are used for fuel or for incorporation into protein. About 80% of the free amino acid pool is located in skeletal muscle. Free amino acids are mainly concerned with energy production through oxidation of **branched-chain amino acids** (leucine, isoleucine and valine) and the use of alanine in gluconeogenesis. Branched-chain amino acids are catabolized mainly in skeletal muscle, where the carbon skeletons provide an oxidizable source of substrate and where their nitrogen residues participate in alanine formation. Catabolism of valine and leucine to glutamine produces 16 molecules of ATP. However, the rate of amino acid oxidation during exercise is low and increases to a maximum of only 15% of the ATP used during prolonged (greater than one hour) exercise.

Leucine is an essential, ketogenic, 6-carbon, amino acid. It is abundant in globulins and albumins. The degradation of leucine takes place mainly in skeletal muscle. Leucine has a higher oxidation rate than the other branched-chain amino acids. It stimulates protein synthesis in muscle and is involved in the release of glucogenic (glycogenic) precursors, such as alanine, from muscle. During exhaustive aerobic exercise, there are decreases in leucine level and glycogen stores in skeletal muscle. Consumption of branched-chain amino acids (30-35% leucine) before or during endurance exercise may prevent, or decrease, the net rate of protein degradation. It may improve both mental and physical performance, and may also have a sparing effect on muscle glycogen degradation and depletion of muscle glycogen stores. Caution must be paid when interpreting the limited number of studies in this area, because in many studies leucine has been used as part of a mixture of branched-chain amino acids.

Endurance training may enable a larger amount of energy to be derived from amino acids. Like alanine, glutamine is synthesized in muscle tissue and is a major means for removing excess amino groups from the muscle, delivering the amino group to the kidney for excretion as ammonia. Due to its role as an energy substrate in the immune system, it has been argued that decreased levels of glutamine might impair the function of the immune system.

Advertisements for dietary supplements often contain performance claims that cannot be substantiated by published research findings or are based on inappropriate extrapolations from research findings or are simply the physiological functions of the particular substance in the body. Arginine and ornithine have been included in dietary supplements and are frequently promoted as 'growth hormone releasers.' Scientific evidence does not support the claim that these supplements have an effect on the secretion of growth hormone.

Tryptophan has been promoted as a growth hormone releaser. Detrimental effects of large doses of tryptophan include inhibition of gluconeogenesis and urea metabolism, both of which are important for athletic performance. Following an epidemic of eosinophilia-myalgia syndrome, the Food and Drug Administration (FDA) in America banned sales of tryptophan in supplement form in 1990. Although it has been claimed that the tryptophan was contaminated, it is possible that L-tryptophan itself was the cause.

The FDA actually classifies amino acids as "not generally recommended as safe," and thus should not be sold as over-the-counter supplements. In purified form, however, tryptophan can be used to fortify protein products.

Some sellers of amino acid supplements claim that only a small proportion of the amino acids from food is absorbed. This is a false claim because normally about 95 to 99% of protein from animal sources, and about 90% of protein from vegetable sources, is absorbed and used by the body. It has also been claimed that free amino acids are absorbed more rapidly than those broken down from food. There is research evidence to support this, but there is no evidence that faster absorption has greater benefits.

Bibliography

Burke, L.M. and Read, R.S.D. (1993). Dietary supplements in sport. *Sports Medicine* 15(1), 43-56.

Grunewald, K.K. and Bailey, R.S. (1993). Commercially marketed supplements for bodybuilding athletes. *Sports Medicine* 15(2), 90-103.

Hood, D.A. and Terjung, R.L. (1990). Amino acid metabolism during exercise and following endurance training. *Sports Medicine* 9(1), 23-25.

Kreider, R.B., Miriel, V. and Bertun, E. (1993). Amino acid supplementation and exercise performance. Analysis of the proposed ergogenic value. *Sports Medicine* 16(3), 190-209.

Mero, A. (1999). Leucine supplementation and intensive training. *Sports Medicine* 27(6), 347-358.

Viru, A. (1987). Mobilization of structural proteins during exercise. *Sports Medicine* 4, 95-128.

AMINO ACID DEGRADATION Breaking down of an amino acid into its amino group and carbon skeletons so that the parts may be used to synthesize other molecules, oxidized to provide energy or converted into molecules that can be excreted. It is stimulated when: i) protein foods are eaten in excess of what is required for repair and replacement of tissue; ii) a low-carbohydrate diet is followed and the carbon skeletons of amino acids are used to resupply the Krebs cycle with carbohydrate intermediates; and iii) insufficient energy is derived from the diet with the result that amino acids from body proteins are oxidized for fuel.

With few exceptions, the first step in amino acid degradation is the removal of the amino group. This usually occurs by transamination. **Transamination** involves the transfer of an amino group (NH_2) from an amino acid to an alpha keto acid, producing a new amino acid and a new alpha keto acid. Transamination involves enzymes called transaminases or aminotransferases, using Vitamin B_6 as a coenzyme. Most transaminases require alpha-ketoglutarate to accept the amino group. Transamination enables the body to use ammonia and synthesize the nonessential amino acids. The liver is the major site of transamination for most amino acids except for the branched-chain amino acids, which are transaminated in peripheral tissues such as skeletal muscle. Transamination occurs *in vivo* for all twenty primary amino acids except lysine and threonine.

If there is no demand for the amino group to form

other amino acids or for nitrogen to be used in the synthesis of nonprotein nitrogenous molecules, the amino group may be transferred to alpha-ketoglutarate, forming glutamate. Glutamate can undergo **oxidative deamination** by glutamate dehydrogenase, using NAD^+ as a coenzyme. Glutamate dehydrogenase is stimulated by low ATP and/or low GTP. The resulting ammonium ion will be converted to urea and excreted.

Following deamination, the remaining carbon skeleton can enter the Krebs cycle when the carbons have been incorporated into one of seven molecules: pyruvate, aceytl CoA, acetoacetyl CoA, alpha ketoglutarate, succinyl CoA, fumarate or oxaloacetate. All seven molecules may lead to complete oxidation through the Krebs cycle and the respiratory chain. Alternatively, the carbons from the Krebs cycle intermediates, alpha ketoglutarate, succinyl CoA and fumarate may exit the Krebs cycle when they have been converted to oxaloacetate. In this case, the carbons become involved in gluconeogenesis. Another alternative is conversion of the carbons to acetyl CoA and diversion from the Krebs cycle to form triglycerides, sterols such as cholesterol or ketone bodies. These conversions take place mainly in the liver.

AMMONIA   An alkaline gas that is soluble in water. During intense exercise, the primary source of ammonia is adenosine monophosphate (AMP) deamination; ammonium is produced as a by-product of the AMP deaminase-catalyzed reaction of the purine nucleotide cycle in which AMP is converted to inosine monophosphate (IMP). This reaction is stimulated during acidic conditions. As the ammonium is toxic to the cell, it is removed into the circulation for metabolism by the liver, excreted by the kidney, or lost through sweat.

During steady state exercise, ammonia is formed mainly from the deamination of amino acids that are oxidized in the catabolic pathways. The ammonia released from skeletal muscles undergoes reduction, by the transfer of the amine group from amino acids (mainly glutamate) to pyruvate to form alanine. Alanine is then released into the circulation where it can be taken up by the liver and metabolized.

See also UREA CYCLE.

Bibliography
Yuan, Y. and Chan, K.M. (2000). A review of the literature on the application of blood ammonia measurement in sports science. *Research Quarterly for Exercise and Sport* 71(2), 145-151.

AMP   *See* ADENOSINE MONOPHOSPHATE.

AMPHETAMINE   A class of drugs that includes amphetamine itself and the homologous substances methylamphetamine, dimethylamphetamine, benzyl-amphetamine and other substances known as 'masked amphetamines,' which are metabolized to amphetamine in the body. 'Speed' is an injectable methamphetamine used by drug addicts.

Amphetamine acts as a stimulant by releasing presynaptic dopamine. These neurons cause an increase in cardiac output, metabolic rate, blood pressure, blood glucose level, arousal, alertness and concentration. Amphetamine is also an appetite suppressant, but can lead to depression and dependence. Amphetamines were used clinically in the 1930s for treating nasal congestions, narcolepsy and obesity, and were first used by athletes as an ergogenic aid in the 1960s. The research evidence suggests that amphetamines can improve the performance of fatigued individuals, but not for individuals who are non-fatigued, alert and motivated. Amphetamines may increase time to exhaustion by masking the physiological response to fatigue, but this can lead to heat stroke and cardiac failure.

Ecstasy is a drug that is manufactured from amphetamine so as to diminish the drug's stimulant effects and increase its hallucinogenic effects. Its use has been widespread in the dance club culture that has grown since the 1990s. The most common form of ecstasy (**3, 4-methylenedioxy-methamphet-amine**; MDMA) is derived from methamphetamine by the addition of another methyl group. This additional methyl group confers increased lipophilicity to MDMA, leading to its rapid entry into the brain. MDMA acts as an indirect sympathomimetic, stimulating release and inhibiting re-uptake of epinephrine, norepinephrine and dopamine. Similar to other stimulants, it may cause tachycardia, elevated blood pressure, increased energy, anorexia and increased concentration. It has some hallucinogenic properties at high doses. MDMA has been linked with a number of deaths worldwide. Deaths result from hyperthermia, hyponatremia or cerebral edema. In 1985, the Drug Enforcement Administration (DEA) declared it a Schedule I drug.

Methcathinone has properties like those of methamphetamine and cocaine. **Methylphenidate** (Ritalin) is related to the amphetamines, but is a relatively mild CNS stimulant that is effective in the treatment of narcolepsy and attention-deficit hyperactivity disorder.

See also STIMULANTS.

Chronology

●1887 ● The first amphetamine was synthesized by a German pharmacologist, L. Edeleano, but it was not until 1910 that amphetamines were tested in laboratory animals.

●1932 ● Benzedrine (amphetamine) inhalers became available as a nonprescription medication across the USA. In sport, amphetamine became the stimulant of choice over strychnine. It was available over-the-counter until 1949.

●1960 ● Danish cyclist Kurt Jensen died during the 100 km road race at the Olympic Games. It was regarded at the time that, leading up to his death, Jensen was taking (supposedly on doctor's orders) a mixture of drugs that included amphetamine. Jensen was the first Olympian to die from drugs.

●1967 ● 29-year-old British cyclist Tommy Simpson died on his way up a 6,000 foot mountain during the 13th stage of the 2,974 mile Tour de France. From the start of the Tour 15 days before, he had cycled 1,684 miles at an average speed of 22 mph and had been allowed only one rest day. His last mumbled words were "Put me back on my bike." On the road to the mountain, Simpson grabbed a drink from a spectator: it was neat cognac. The cause of death, however, was amphetamine overdose.

●1971 ● In the USA, all potent amphetamine-like compounds in nasal inhalers were withdrawn from the market.

Bibliography

Divadeenam, K. (2002). Stimulants. Http://www.emedicine.com

Doyon, S. (2001). The many faces of ecstasy. *Current opinions in pediatrics* 13(2), 170-176.

Schwenck, T.L. (1997). Psychoactive drugs and athletic performance. *The Physician and Sportsmedicine* 25(1), 32-46.

AMPHIBIAN REFLEX   A postural reflex that emerges 4 to 6 months after birth and persists throughout life. It is essential for crawling, walking and running.

AMPUTATIONS *See under* LIMB DEFICIENCIES.

AMYLIN   A peptide hormone which, like insulin, is secreted by the beta cells of the pancreas. It is believed that amylin complements insulin by antagonizing aspects of insulin action. Amylin stimulates glycogenolysis and lactate production in muscle. In conjunction with epinephrine, it can therefore support the Cori cycle and hepatic gluconeogenesis.

AMYOTROPHIC LATERAL SCLEROSIS   Lou Gehrig's disease. Motor neurone disease. A fatal neuromuscular disease characterized by progressive muscle weakness resulting in paralysis. It is characterized by both upper and lower motor neuron damage. Symptoms of upper motor neuron damage include spasticity, fasciculations and clonus. Symptoms of lower motor neuron damage include muscle weakness and atrophy. The disease does not affect all muscles. Bowl and bladder control remains intact, as does sexual function. Most patients first notice muscle weakness in either the arms or the legs (32% in the arms and 36% in the legs). This is called **limb-onset amyotrophic lateral sclerosis**. When patients have difficulty speaking as their first symptom, it is called **bulbar amyotrophic lateral sclerosis**, because it involves the corticobulbar area of the brainstem.

Some people with amyotrophic lateral sclerosis experience apparent emotional instability, with spells of uncontrolled laughter or crying. It is now thought that this 'emotional instability,' **pseudobulbar affect**, arises from the loss of motor neurons in the top part of the brain that normally moderate the activity of the bulbar motor neurons in the brainstem. The problem is not, therefore, in the bulbar neurons themselves.

The incidence of amyotrophic lateral sclerosis is

about 2 per 100,000; and the prevalence is about 11 per 100,000. Men are much more likely to get the disease than women. Older people are more likely to get it than younger people. The average age of onset is 55 years, and 80% of cases begin between the ages of 40 to 70 years.

A common cause of death among patients with amyotrophic lateral sclerosis is respiratory failure or cardiac arrhythmias due to insufficient oxygen. Another common cause of death is respiratory infection such as pneumonia. The risk of respiratory infections increases as weakened diaphragm and chest muscles make it more difficult to clear the lungs. 50% of patients die within 18 months of diagnosis. Only 20% survive 5 years and 10% live longer than 10 years. There are rare cases where the disease progression plateaus or stops. Patients who go on a ventilator may live for many years.

The cause of the disease is not known, but one of the many possible causes could be oxidative stress from free radical production. Overabundance of glutamate in the nervous system has also been implicated.

At least 10% of cases are hereditary. It is inherited as an autosomal dominant trait. 20% of familial amyotrophic lateral sclerosis cases have a specific gene defect in the superoxide dismutase gene (SOD1 gene on chromosome 21). Other mutated genes that can lead to amyotrophic lateral sclerosis have been noted on chromosomes 2, 9, 15, 18 and on the X chromosome. 90% of all cases have no familial link (sporadic amyotrophic lateral sclerosis). A third type, Guamian, is related to the high incidence of amyotrophic lateral sclerosis on the island nation of Guam, where people eat bats that feed on cycad seeds. As bat consumption has decreased, so too has the incidence of amyotrophic lateral sclerosis.

There is no cure for the disease, but riluzole (Rilutek) is a drug that helps slow the progression of the disease, by acting as a glutamate inhibitor.

Exercise does not slow down the wasting of muscles due to amyotrophic lateral sclerosis. Heavy exercise should be avoided, but light exercise such as walking, swimming and stretching can help maintain strength in the muscles that are not yet affected by the disease. When muscle atrophy becomes severe, the only recommended exercise is stretching to preserve flexibility.

Chronology

●1939 ● At the age of 38, Lou Gehrig of the New York Yankees was diagnosed with amyotrophic lateral sclerosis. The previous year, Gehrig's batting average dropped below 0.3 for the first time since 1925. He managed only four hits in the first eight games of the 1939 season. He died in 1941.

●1942 ● A movie called *The Pride of the Yankees* was made about the life of Lou Gehrig. The movie was produced by Sam Goldwyn, featured several of Gehrig's real-life teammates (including Babe Ruth) playing themselves and included newsreel footage of Gehrig's farewell speech.

Bibliography

ALS Association. Http://www.alsa.org

Muscular Dystrophy Association. Http://www.mdausa.org

Les Turner ALS Foundation, Ltd. Http://www.lesturnerals.org

ANABOLIC STEROIDS   Drugs that have an anabolic function similar to that of testosterone, but without as much of the androgenic effects of testosterone. Chemical alterations of testosterone are made in an attempt to alter the anabolic-to-androgenic ratio in order to decrease the androgenic effects or to make the substance orally active. Removal of the methyl group at C10, for example, produces nandrolone (19-nortestosterone), which exhibits more anabolic than androgenic activity. A '**dirty steroid**' is one that has a low anabolic-androgenic ratio, e.g. Depo-testadiol (testosterone cypionate) (1:1). A '**clean steroid**' is one that has a high anabolic-to-androgenic ratio, e.g. Anavar (oxandrolone) (13:1).

Although classed as banned substances by the World Anti-Doping Association (WADA), anabolic steroids are used as ergogenic aids in sport. The American College of Sports Medicine (ACSM) has stated that the use of anabolic steroids during training, with a proper diet, may enhance lean body mass and muscular strength. Anabolic steroids have been found to exert a trophic (size-increasing) effect on skeletal and cardiac muscle fibers in subjects with low circulating levels of testosterone, such as pre-pubertal males and females. The widespread use of anabolic steroids in male athletes to increase their physical performances poses the question of whether these compounds are active in the presence of normal circulating levels of testosterone. The results of most animal studies indicate that anabolic steroids are ineffective in this situation. On the other hand, the results of the experiments performed in humans have been equivocal. According to the review of data on athletes by Hartgens and Kuipers (2004) strength gains can be 5 to 20% of the initial strength and increments of 2 to 5 kg bodyweight, which may be attributed to an increase of the lean body mass, have been observed. A decrease of fat mass does not seem to occur. The effectiveness of anabolic steroids thus remains a controversial issue.

The process by which anabolic steroids may affect the growth of muscle fibers is not fully understood. One theory is that the steroids work by stimulating receptor molecules in muscle fibers that activate specific genes to produce proteins. Anabolic steroids are believed to diffuse into the cellular cytosol and bind to the androgen receptor. The newly formed receptor-steroid complex migrates to the nucleus, interacts with the DNA and initiates transcription. The production of RNA is then increased, causing an increased rate of protein synthesis. An alternative theory is that the effects of anabolic steroids are indirect and related to certain effects of the drugs that enable the athlete to train harder. These effects include task-oriented addiction, euphoric states, increased tolerance of fatigue and increased aggressiveness.

Anabolic steroids may have an anti-catabolic effect that manifests itself by cross binding with glucocorticoid receptors, interfering with post-exercise glucocorticoid catabolic activity.

Rapid tolerance to anabolic steroids occurs in muscle tissue as the body attempts to maintain homeostasis through processes such as increased levels of cortisol in the blood. 'Stacking' involves the use of two or more different anabolic steroids at the same time. Many athletes take 10 to 100 times the recommended dosage. Injectable steroids are generally more potent than oral steroids, mainly due to the delivery route. Examples of oral anabolic steroids are: oxymetholone (Anadrol-50),

oxandrolone (Oxandrin) and stanazolol (Winstrol V). Examples of injected anabolic steroids are nandrolone (Durabolin), phenpropionate (Nandobolic) and nadrolone (Deca-Durabolin).

The main adverse effects of short- and long-term abuse of anabolic steroids reported by male athletes are: an increase in sexual drive; the occurrence of acne vulgaris; increased body hair; and aggressive behavior. A triad may exist between anabolic steroid use, weight training and behavioral change (including dependence). It is also possible that changes frequently attributed to anabolic steroids may also reflect changes resulting from the concurrent use of other substances, including alcohol, and from diet. Dependence or withdrawal effects (such as depression) seem to occur only in a small number of anabolic steroids users. Scientific data may underestimate the actual adverse effects of anabolic steroids, because of the relatively low doses administered in those studies compared to those used by many illicit users.

Administration of anabolic steroids will disturb the regular endogenous production of testosterone and gonadotrophins that may persist for months after drug withdrawal. The hypothalamus signals the pituitary gland to produce less luteinizing hormone and follicle-stimulating hormone. These decreased hormone levels result in decreased sperm production and testicular size. The effect is variable, but often involves an enhanced sex drive early in the course of steroid use and then a decrease to normal, or below normal, as the drugs are continued. Some anabolic steroid users take human chorionic gonadotrophin to counteract testicular atrophy and/or diminished sex drive. Oral steroids generally have more serious side effects compared to injectable steroids, with a far greater incidence of liver, kidney, cardiovascular and immune system problems being reported. In studies of athletes, evidence of liver damage has not been found. Anti-estrogens such as tamoxifen may be taken to prevent gynecomastia, which occurs when androgens are converted to estrogens. Anabolic steroids are converted into female sex hormones (estradiol and estrone) by the enzyme aromatase, antagonistic action to estrogens and a competitive antagonism to the glucocorticoid receptors. Adolescents taking anabolic steroids may experience premature epiphyseal closure of the long bones resulting in short stature. Anabolic steroids stimulate erythropoietin synthesis and red blood cell production as well as bone formation, but counteract bone breakdown. Anabolic steroids do not increase aerobic power or capacity.

Risk factors for cardiovascular disease may be worsened, e.g. blood pressure may be elevated. The effects on the cardiovascular system are proposed to be mediated by the occurrence of atherosclerosis (due to unfavorable influence of anabolic steroids on serum lipids and lipoproteins), thrombosis, vasospasm or direct injury to vessel walls, or may be ascribed to a combination of the different mechanisms.

Increased frequency and intensity of training sessions may explain the increased incidence of connective tissue injuries, such as rupture of the *biceps brachii* tendon, associated with steroid abuse. This is due to dysplasia of collagen fibers that decreases the tensile strength of tendons. The combination of anabolic steroids with other drugs, restrictive diets and dehydrating practices may potentiate the health risks associated with weight training and steroid use.

Other side effects of anabolic steroids include: water retention in tissue, sterility, yellowing of the eyes and skin, thickened skin and striae distensae. Additional side effects in women are male-pattern baldness, hirsutism, deepening of the voice, smaller breast size, enlargement of the clitoris, menstrual irregularities and fetal damage. Women appear to suffer more permanent side effects than men from anabolic steroids. The deepening of the female voice and the growth of body hair are generally irreversible after anabolic steroids are discontinued.

In 1993, the doping class of 'anabolic steroids' was changed to 'anabolic agents' to encompass the increasing use of beta-2 adrenoceptor agonists (such as clenbuterol) that produce anabolic effects even though they are not steroids.

The World Anti-Doping Agency (WADA) makes a distinction between exogenous and endogenous anabolic agents. Examples of **exogenous anabolic agents** are androstadienone, gestrinone, methandienone, nandrolone and stanazolol. Examples of **endogenous anabolic agents** are androstenediol, androstenedione, dehydroepiand-rosterone (DHEA), dehydrotestosterone and testosterone.

Tetrahydrogestrinone (**THG**) is a designer steroid, and exogenous anabolic agent, used by elite athletes. THG was created by modifying two other known steroids: trenbolone and gestrinone. Gestrinone is a commercialized treatment for the condition of endometriosis. The modifications made THG undetectable in doping tests.

On the basis that athletes tend to rely on unscientific information about anabolic steroids, Millar (1994) suggested that there is a case for the medical management of anabolic steroid use in sport.

See also ANDROSTENEDIONE; DEHYDRO-EPIANDROSTERONE, TESTOSTERONE.

Chronology

•1960 • John Ziegler, a physician, began giving methandrostenolone (Dianabol), an anabolic steroid manufactured by Ciba Pharmaceutical Co. (Basel, Switzerland) to three US weightlifters, who then made substantial improvements in muscle mass and strength. All three became national champions, and two of them (Bill March and Lou Riecke) set world records.

•1968 • Arnold Swartzenegger used anabolic steroids when he arrived in the USA at the age of 20. "I took them under a doctor's supervision once a year, six or weight weeks before competition," he told *Playboy* magazine in 1988. He had taken Dianabol at the age of 17 years in Germany.

•1968 • Tom Waddell, a US decathlete, told the *New York Times* that he estimated a third of the men on the US track-and-field team were using anabolic steroids at the pre-Olympic training camp held at Lake Tahoe.

•1972 • Unofficial tests for anabolic steroids were undertaken at the Olympic Games.

•1975 • The International Olympic Committee (IOC) banned anabolic steroids.

•1976 • About 250 positive dope tests were recorded at the Olympic Games in Montreal. It was the first Olympics at which athletes were tested for anabolic steroids and 8 athletes were banned. When Shirley Babashoff, a member of the US Women's Swimming Team, accused her Eastern German rivals of using anabolic steroids because of their big muscles and deep voices, an official from the East German team replied: "They came to swim, not sing." (Guttman, 1976, p146)

•1981 • US discus thrower Ben Plunknett was stripped of his world record and placed on suspension by the International Amateur Athletics Federation (IAAF) when he tested positive for anabolic steroids. Plunknett was the first person to lose a world record because of steroid use.

•1982 • Santa Monica bodybuilder Dan Duchaine published *The Underground Steroid Handbook*.

•1983 • In an exposé on the activities of Robert Kerr, author of *The Practical use of Anabolic Steroids With Athletes*, the *Los Angeles Times* wrote, "The controversial sports medicine specialist estimates that he has 4,000 patients, among them Olympic athletes from 19 countries as well as professional football, baseball, and basketball players."

•1986 • In the USA, the Food and Drug Administration (FDA) ruled that methandro-stenalone (Dianabol) and methandriol could no longer be manufactured, because of a lack of proof of medical need.

•1987 • Dan Duchaine was indicted for being part of a conspiracy to sell anabolic steroids, smuggling and tax fraud. Duchaine died in 2000, aged 47 years, of kidney failure.

•1988 • In the USA, the Anti-Drug Abuse Act made it illegal to dispense steroids for non-medical purposes.

•1988 • Ben Johnson of Canada was disqualified from victory in the 100 meters final at the Olympic Games after testing positive for an anabolic steroid. Ben Johnson had run the 100 meters in a world record of 9.79 seconds. Just prior to the Games, Johnson was administered stanazolol. Johnson had began using steroids six years earlier and was told by his coach Charlie Francis that he could not hope to become a world-class sprinter without steroids. Francis was banned for life by Athletics Canada in 1989.

•1990 • In the USA, Congress voted into law the Anabolic Steroids Control Act, which meant that even first-time users could be sent to prison.

•1996 • In baseball, Ken Caminiti won the National League Most Valuable Player Award. Caminiti turned to anabolic steroids, after tearing his rotator cuff, as a way of being able to play through the pain in the second half of the season. Caminiti used steroids so heavily that by the end of the season his testicles shrank and retracted. Doctors found that his body had virtually stopped producing its own testosterone and that his level of the hormone had fallen to 20% of normal. Due to his body's continuing inability to make the hormone in sufficient quantity, he was legally prescribed weekly shots of testosterone. In 2001, eight days after his release by the Atlanta Braves, Caminiti, who also suffered from

alcoholism, was arrested in a crack house and found guilty of cocaine possession. In 2004, Caminiti died of "acute intoxication due to the combined effects of cocaine and opiates," according to tissue and toxicology tests. A month before his death, he violated his probation by testing positive for cocaine and was sentenced to 180 days in jail. His lawyer said after his death that Caminiti had hoped eventually to mentor young players about avoiding the mistakes he made.

•1998 • Florence Griffith-Joyner ("Flo-Jo") of the USA, who set a world-record record in the 200 meters at the 1988 Olympic Games, died at the age of 38. It was widely suspected that the apparent heart attack was a result of drug abuse. "The first heart seizure of Griffith Joyner in 1996 was already symptomatic of the abuse of anabolic steroids." (Werner Franke, quoted in *The Times*, 23.9.98). Between 1987 and 1988, when her husband Al Joyner (the 1984 Olympic triple jump gold medallist) became her coach, her physique underwent a remarkable change that she attributed to intensive weight training. In 1988, her 100 meters time of 10.49 in the US Olympic trials knocked 0.27 second off the world records. The following year she retired. In 1989 Darrell Robinson, a former US 400-metres champion, alleged that Flo-Jo had bought human growth hormone from him, in preparation for the 1988 athletics season. Flo-Jo denied the allegation, but never sued Robinson.

•1990 • In the USA, the Anabolic Steroids Control Act placed these drugs into Schedule III of the Controlled Substances Act. This act requires anyone who distributes or disperses anabolic steroids to be registered with the Drug Enforcement Administration (DEA).

•1996 • In the UK, an amendment to the Misuse of Drugs Act reclassified anabolic steroids as Class C schedule drugs. It became an offence to supply, or possess these drugs with intent to supply, but it did not make it an offence to possess or use them personally.

•2003 • The United States Anti-Doping Agency (USADA) received notice from a popular track coach that several athletes were using an undetectable steroid. He sent a sample of the undetectable steroid and claimed that the source of this drug, tetrahydrogestrinone (THG) was BALCO, a nutritional company located in California. A number of elite athletes, including baseball star Barry Bonds were linked with BALCO and subsequently made testimonies in legal proceedings. A test for THG was developed at the Olympic Analytic Laboratory in Los Angeles. It was later revealed that the sample of THG (in a syringe) was sent to the USADA by Trevor Graham, coach of Justin Gatlin, the Olympic 100 m champion. THG may be based on a drug, norbeloethone, which was developed in 1966 by a pharmaceutical company, Wyeth, but never marketed. It was developed as a way of treating underweight and unusual shortness. THG is thought to be one of hundreds, or even thousands, of 'forgotten steroids.'

•2003 • Four players from the Oakland Raiders in the National Football League tested positive for THG.

•2004 • Triple Olympic champion, Marion Jones, and 100 meters world record holder, Tim Montgomery were among 27 athletes named in a federal investigator's memo as having received THG from BALCO Laboratories, according to the *San Jose Mercury News*.

•2004 • Greg Anderson, nutritional adviser of Barry Bonds, was one of four men charged in a 42-count indictment alleging they ran a steroid-distribution ring that provided drugs to dozens of athletes in the NFL, major league baseball, and track and field. Bonds denied steroid use.

Bibliography

American College of Sports Medicine (1987). Position stand on the use of anabolic androgenic steroids in Sports. *Medicine and Science in Sports and Exercise* 19(5), 534-9.

Bahrke, M.S., Yesalis, C.E. and Wright, J.E. (1990). Psychological and behavioral effects of endogenous testosterone levels and anabolic-androgenic steroids among males. *Sports Medicine* 10(5), 303-337.

Bahrke, M.S. and Yesalis, C.E. (1994). Weight training. A potential confounding factor in examining the psychological and behavioural effects of anabolic-androgenic steroids. *Sports Medicine* 18(5), 309-318.

Celotti, F. and Negri-Cesi, P. (1992). Anabolic steroids: A review of their effects on the muscles, of their possible mechanisms of action and of their use in athletics. *Journal of Steroid Biochemistry and Molecular Biology* 43(5), 469-77

Cowan, D. (1998). Drug abuse. In: Harries, M., Williams, C., Stanish, W.D. and Micheli, L.J. (eds). *Oxford textbook of sports medicine.* pp339-354. Oxford: Oxford University Press.

Denham, B.E. (1997). Sports Illustrated, the 'war on drugs,' and the Anabolic Steroid Control Act of 1990: A study in agenda building and political timing. *Journal of Sport and Social issues* 21(3), 260-273.

Hartgens, F. and Kuipers, H. (2004). Effects of androgenic-anabolic steroids in athletes. *Sports Medicine* 34(8), 513-554.

Laseter, J.T and Russell, J.A. (1991). Anabolic steroid-induced tendon pathology: A review of the literature. *Medicine and Science in Sports and Exercise* 23(1), 1-3.

Miller, A.P. (1994). Licit steroid use – Hope for the future? *British Journal of Sports Medicine* 28, 79-83.

Mottram, D.R. (1999). Banned drugs in sport. Does the International Olympic Committee (IOC) list need updating? *Sports Medicine* 27(1), 1-10.

Todd, J. and Todd, T. (2001). Significant events in the history of drug testing and the Olympic movement 1960-1999. In: Wilson, W. and Derse, E. (eds). *Doping in elite sport. The politics of drugs in the Olympic movement.* pp65-128. Champaign, IL: Human Kinetics.

Williams, M.H. (1998). *The ergogenics edge.* Champaign, IL: Human Kinetics.

Yesalis, C.E. (2000, ed). *Anabolic steroids in sport and exercise.* 2nd ed. Champaign, IL: Human Kinetics.

Yesalis, C. and Cowart, V. (1998). *The steroids game.* Champaign, IL: Human Kinetics.

ANABOLISM The synthesis in the body of complex molecules from simpler ones.

ANAEROBIC 'Without oxygen.' *See* ANAEROBIC ENERGY SYSTEMS.

ANAEROBIC CAPACITY The maximal amount of ATP resynthesized via anaerobic metabolism during a specific mode of short-duration maximal exercise.

Measures of anaerobic capacity have included oxygen debt, maximal blood lactate and oxygen deficit. The oxygen debt is not a valid measure of anaerobic capacity, since its magnitude is probably influenced by factors other than those directly involved in anaerobic metabolism. Although it is not fully understood, the excess post-exercise oxygen consumption (EPOC) after exercise may be due to a loosening of the linkage between oxidation and phosphorylation. This may be caused by: elevated tissue temperatures, changes in ionic concentrations of intracellular and extracellular fluids, and changes in metabolite and hormone levels. These changes continue during recovery and thus serve to increase oxygen consumption immediately after exercise.

The utility of maximal blood lactate as an estimate of anaerobic (lactic) capacity is controversial. In the post-exercise period, a large proportion of lactate may be metabolized before equilibrium in lactate between muscle and blood has been achieved. In such a case, maximal blood lactate cannot provide an accurate quantitative estimate of lactic capacity.

The oxygen deficit is thought by some researchers to be the only valid measure of anaerobic capacity. It is the oxygen equivalent of the total energy used during exercise that did not come from aerobic energy processes after the start of exercise. It is based on a number of assumptions, one of which is that the oxygen demand at high exercise intensities can be estimated via the linear extrapolation of the relationship between submaximal oxygen uptake and workload. The validity of this assumption is tenuous.

Anaerobic work capacity is the total amount of work performed during an exhaustive work bout that is of sufficient duration to maximize the anaerobic ATP yield (given that this ATP yield exceeds that from oxidative metabolism). Estimates of anaerobic work capacity are dependent on several factors and can only (at best) reflect anaerobic capacity.

See also under GROWTH.

Bibliography

Green, S. and Dawson, B. (1993). Measurement of anaerobic capacities in humans. Definitions, limitations and unsolved problems. *Sports Medicine* 15(5), 312-327.

Stainsby, W.N. and Brooks, G.A. (1990). Control of lactic acid metabolism in contracting muscles and during exercise. *Exercise and Sport Sciences Reviews* 18, 29-63.

ANAEROBIC ENERGY SYSTEMS These systems resynthesize ATP without using oxygen. There are two anaerobic energy systems: alactacid and lactacid.

See CREATINE PHOSPHATE; GLYCOLYSIS.

ANAEROBIC POWER The maximum amount of anaerobic energy that can be produced per unit of time. Performance tests of anaerobic power include the **Wingate test** that involves 30 seconds of maximal-effort exercise on either an arm crank or bicycle ergometer. Peak power output (the highest mechanical power generated during any 3 to 5 second period of the test) is assumed to represent anaerobic power.

Bibliography

Bouchard, C. et al. (1991). Testing anaerobic power and capacity. In: MacDougall, J.D., Wenger, H.A. and Green, H.J. (eds). *Physiological testing of the high performance athlete.* 2nd ed. pp175-221. Champaign, IL: Human Kinetics.

Inbar, O. Bar-Or, O and Skinner, J.S. (1996). *The Wingate Anaerobic Test.* Champaign, IL: Human Kinetics.

Vanderwalle, H., Peres, G. and Monod, H. (1987). Standard anaerobic exercise tests. *Sports Medicine* 4, 268-269.

ANAEROBIC THRESHOLD *See under* LACTATE THRESHOLD.

ANALGESIC *See under* OPIATE; PAIN.

ANAPHYLAXIS *See under* ALLERGY; ASTHMA.

ANASTOMOSIS Direct intercommunication of the branches of two or more veins or arteries without any intervening network of capillary vessels.

ANATOMICAL LANDMARKS Standard anatomical landmarks include: acromiale, acropodion, cervicale, dactylion, epigastrale, gluteale, gnathion, iliocristale, iliospinale, mesosternale, metacarpale radiale, metacarpale ulnare, orbitale, pternion, radiale, sphyrion, stylion, tragion, trochanterion, tibiale mediale, tibiale laterale, vertex, sphyrion fibulare, metatarsale tibiale, metatarsale fibulare, omphalion, suprasternale, symphysion and thelion.

ANATOMICAL POSITION Anatomical standing position. A standard position used in anthropometric description. It is a standing position with head and eyes directed forward, upper limbs hanging by the sides with the palms forward, thumbs pointing away from the sides, fingers pointing directly downward, feet together and toes pointing directly forward. The **fundamental position** is a standard position that involves an erect posture with the feet slightly separated and parallel, with the arms hanging easily at the sides with the palms facing the body. The fundamental position is the position usually accepted as the point of reference for analyzing all the movements of the body's segments, except those of the forearm, hand and fingers; whereas the anatomical position is usually accepted as the point of reference for the movements of the forearm, hand and fingers.

ANATOMICAL SNUFF BOX A depression on the back of the back of the hand, when the thumb is extended and abducted, which is so named because it could be used as place to hold tobacco for snorting. The tendons of the *extensor pollicis brevis* and *abductor pollicis brevis* make the lateral border of the anatomical snuff box; the medial border is formed by the tendon of the *extensor pollicis longus*. Situated deeply in this space is the radial artery (and its pulse), covered by the radial vein. Two of the carpal bones (scaphoid and trapezium) and the styloid process of the radius can be palpated within the snuff box.

ANATOMY The science of structure of the body. **Functional anatomy** is the study of the body components needed to achieve a human movement or function.
See also KINESIOLOGY.

Chronology

●285 AD ● Herophilus, of the great medical school in Alexandria, emphasized the importance of exercise and wrote commentaries on the works of Hippocrates. The work of Herophilus was described by later scholars such as Galen.

●1510 ● Leonardo da Vinci attempted to publish a textbook of anatomy and physiology that he had collaborated on with Marcantonio della Torre, a young Paduan lecturer in medicine. During the Renaissance, there were major advancements in art and literature and revolution in science. Some of the great artists, such as Michelangelo, studied the human form very closely. The anatomical drawings by Leonardo da Vinci were arguably the most artistic of the Renaissance. The artists started to dissect human bodies. During the Middle Ages, beliefs about physiology were always based on Galen and there was frequent confusion due to misunderstanding of his work. Leonardo was the first to question the views of Galen.

●1543 ● Andreas Vesalius, the 'father of modern anatomy,' published his *De Humani Corporis Fabrica* in Basle. He dissected human bodies and based his work on observations rather than relying on the authority of Galen. His work was thus not accepted by many of the traditional scholars of the time.

Bibliography

Behnkne, R.S. (2001). *Kinetic anatomy*. Champaign, IL: Human Kinetics.

Enoka, R.M. (2002). *Neuromechanics of human movement*. 3rd ed. Champaign, IL: Human Kinetics.

Hamilton, N. and Luttgens, K. (2002). *Kinesiology. Scientific basis of human motion*. 10th ed. Madison, WI: Brown & Benchmark.

Rasch, P.J. (1989). *Kinesiology and applied anatomy*. 7th ed. Philadelphia, PA: Lea & Febiger.

Seeley, R., Stephens, T. and Tate, P. (2000). *Anatomy and physiology*. 5th ed. Boston, MA: McGraw-Hill.

Stone, R.J. and Stone, J.A. (1997). *Atlas of skeletal muscles*. 3rd ed. Boston, MA: McGraw-Hill.

Thompson, C.W. and Floyd, R.T. (2004). *Manual of structural kinesiology*. 15th ed. St Louis: Mosby-Year Book, Inc.

Watkins, J. (1999). *Structure and function of the musculoskeletal system*. Champaign, IL: Human Kinetics.

Wirhed, R. (1984). *Athletic ability and the anatomy of motion*. 2nd ed. London: Wolfe Medical.

ANDROGEN A substance with male sex hormone activity, concerned with the development and maintenance of many male sexual characteristics.
See TESTOSTERONE.

ANDROGEN SUPPLEMENTS Androgen prohormone supplements. Most studies indicate that some androgen supplements in sufficient doses do convert to more active substances such as testosterone. At the same time, however, increases in estrogen subfractions can be measured. The net effect is no increase in protein synthesis, muscle or strength.

Cholesterol converts to pregnenolone in the delta-5 pathway. Pregnenolone converts to 17-hydroxypregnenolone in the delta-5 pathway or it converts to progesterone. 17-hydroxypregnenolone converts to dehydroepiandrosterone (DHEA) in the delta-5 pathway or it converts to 17-hydroxyprogesterone. DHEA converts to 5-androstenediol in the delta-5 pathway or to androstenedione. Androstenedione converts to testosterone in the delta-4 pathway, or it converts to estrone or it interconverts with 4-androstenediol. Testosterone converts to dihydrotestosterone in the delta-4 pathway, or it converts to estradiol, or interconverts to 4-androstenediol.

The closer a hormone's precursor is to the end product, the more pronounced the conversion to the final hormone product should be. For example, DHEA should convert to testosterone more abundantly than its precursors, and androstenedione more abundantly than DHEA, because it is closer to the final product in the synthetic pathway.

Dehydroepiandrosterone (DHEA) and its sulfated ester, **dehydroepiandrosterone-sulfate** (DHEAS), represent the most abundant adrenal steroids in the circulation. DHEA (also known as prasterone) and DHEAS interconvert. DHEAS therefore serves as a major precursor to DHEA. DHEA is a weak androgen, but it can be converted to the stronger androgens, testosterone and dihydrotestosterone, in tissues. Decline in DHEA levels with aging has been associated with increased deposits of intra-abdominal fat. DHEA and/or androstenedione supplements do not seem to have a positive effect on hormone profiles and increases fat-free mass during resistance training. DHEA levels are high at birth, but fall during childhood before rising sharply during puberty and peaking during young adulthood. There is no empirical evidence that DHEA or DHEAS have any ergogenic effects. Adverse effects of these supplements include irreversible virilization in women. DHEA supplements were first marketed in 1985, as a weight-loss aid, but were banned by the Federal Drug Agency (FDA) in the USA because they lacked safety and effectiveness reviews. The ban ended with the passage of the Dietary Supplement Health and Education Act in 1994. The sale and distribution of DHEA for therapeutic purposes was banned by the FDA in 1996 until its safety and value could be reviewed. Manufacturers then began selling it as a nutritional aid rather than a therapeutic drug. DHEA is on the World Anti-Doping Agency (WADA) list of banned substances.

Androstenedione is an intermediate or precursor hormone between DHEA and testosterone that is normally produced by the adrenal glands and the gonads. It assists the liver in the synthesis of other biologically active steroid hormones, such as testosterone. It can also convert into estrogen. Classed as a dietary supplement by the FDA, it has been commercially manufactured and sold in the USA since 1996. It is on the WADA list of banned substances, and certain other sporting organizations (e.g. National Football League) in America, but not others (e.g. Major League Baseball).

There is no empirical evidence for any effect of androstenedione on serum levels of testosterone or for any effect on muscle strength or body composition. Androstenedione ingestion is likely to cause individuals to test positive for steroid use, because it increases urinary concentrations of androsterone, etiocholanolone and both compounds' hydroxylated derivatives: 5 alpha and 5 beta-androstan-3, 17 beta-diols; testosterone; and epitestosterone.

While androstenedione is converted directly to testosterone, 19-norandrostenedione converts to nortestosterone (also known as **nandrolone**) and does not undergo significant 5-alpha reduction to dihydrotestosterone. The main urinary excretion products are noretiocholanolone and norandrosterone, the same urinary compounds that characterize nandrolone use. The use of 19-norandrostenedione at dosages from 10 micrograms to 75 mg/day can elevate the concentration of urinary markers for nandrolone enough to cause an athlete to test positive for the prohormone.

Chronology

•1988 • The International Olympic Committee (IOC) recorded 304 positive tests in accredited laboratories for nandrolone.

•1998 • Baseball batter Mark McGwire of St. Louis Cardinals admitted to using androstenedione, which is not banned by Major League Baseball. McGwire broke the major league home run record. In his career of only 12 full seasons, McGwire hit 583 home runs.

•1998 • Mark Richardson and Dougie Walker were both cleared by UK Athletics when research indicated that some legal dietary supplements can contain enough nandrolone to produce positive results.

•1999 • A representative from La Fédération Internationale de Natation (FINA) told the Court of Arbitration for Sport (CAS) in Lausanne that the Irish swimmer Michelle de Bruin (née Smith) took the banned substance androstenedione between 10 and 12 hours before drug testers called at her home in 1998 to take a urine sample that would prove to contain a lethal dose of alcohol - she added what was believed to have been whisky to her urine sample in order to spoil the test result. The CAS judged that de Bruin deserved the four-year ban that had been imposed on her, but she continued to protest her innocence.

•1999 • Linford Christie, 39-years old, the 1992 Olympic 100 meters champion, was tested positive for nandrolone. The result of 200 nanograms per milliliter of urine is 100 times the permitted level of two nanograms per milliliter and far higher than recent positive tests such as Czech tennis player Peter Korda (50 to 100 nanograms), British sprinter Dougie Walker (10 to 12 nanograms) and French footballer Antoine Sibierski (2.1 nanograms). Walker was cleared of doping charges. A UK Athletics disciplinary committee said that the metabolites of nandrolone found in his urine sample could have come from the banned substance nandrolone itself or two other substances that were not banned: 19-norandrostenedione or 19-norandrostenediol. Walker was unable to explain why 19-norandrosterone, a nandrolone metabolite, was detected in his system, but suspected food supplements from a company whose products he endorsed. Wilhelm Scheanzer, head of the Institute of Biochemistry in Germany where Christie was tested positive was quoted in the *News of the World* as saying, "I would say it is not possible for the body to produce this amount of nandrolone naturally. Nor would it show at this level through eating vegetables or meat which have been contaminated with steroids." Christie was later cleared by UK Athletics of committing any doping offence.

•2004 • British tennis player, Greg Rusedski tested positive for nandrolone, but was later cleared of a doping offence. It is possible that the body may naturally create a form of nandrolone, especially if that person has eaten large quantities of meat contaminated with the substance. In 2003, seven players on the Association of Tennis Professionals (ATP) tour were cleared of failing tests for nandrolone after the ATP admitted its own trainers were to blame, having unwittingly handed out banned substances in supplements. The tests of the 7 players who were cleared by the ATP all showed the presence of metabolites 19-norandrostenedione or 19-norandrostenediol in roughly the same quantities. Rusedski's positive test came in July 2003, two months after the ATP said it had stopped its trainers from providing supplements. The World Anti-Doping Agency (WADA) called into question the ATP's investigation, and launched its own inquiry into how so many samples showed elevated levels of nandrolone.

Bibliography

Armsey, T.D. and Green, G.A. (1997). Nutrition supplements: Science vs. hype. *The Physician and Sportsmedicine* 25(6), 76-92.

Corrigan, B. (2002). DHEA and sport. *Clinical Journal of Sports Medicine* 12(4), 236-241.

Earnest, C.P. (2001). Dietary androgen 'supplements.' Separating substance from hype. *The Physician and Sportsmedicine* 29(5), 63-79.

Kreider, R.B. (1999). Dietary supplements and the promotion of muscle growth with resistance exercise. *Sports Medicine* 27(2), 97-110.

World Anti-Doping Agency. Http://www.wada-ama.org

ANDROSTENEDIONE   See under ANDROGEN SUPPLEMENTS.

ANEMIA   Any condition in which the number of red blood cells and/or the amount of hemoglobin is less than normal. It is characterized by a decreased oxygen-carrying ability of the blood, tiredness, shortness of breath and headache.

Sports anemia is a condition in which there is an increased destruction of red blood cells and a decrease in hemoglobin levels as a result of exercise. A distinction can be made between short-term sports anemia and long-term sports anemia. The distinction is couched in terms of whether the observed changes in iron status are due to iron deficiency or the effects of exercise. **Short-term sports anemia** is not a true anemia. It is a 'dilutional pseudoanemia,' because iron deficiency is not the cause of limited red blood cell production. It is an early adaptation to endurance exercise. It is thought that the initial drop in hemoglobin can be accounted for by an increase in plasma volume that is accompanied by an unequal increase in red blood cell mass. Red blood cell destruction also contributes to the decrease in hemoglobin. Red blood cells are vulnerable to oxidative damage, because of their continuous exposure to oxygen and their high concentrations of polyunsaturated fatty acids and heme iron. If red blood cell destruction does not exceed the rate of red blood cell production, then no detrimental effect to athletic performance should occur. An increased rate of red blood cell turnover may actually be advantageous, because young cells are more efficient in transporting oxygen. It is not clear whether or not short-term sports anemia is detrimental to performance.

Endurance athletes can have **long-term sports anemia**, which may be underpinned by iron deficiency. Iron storage parameters such as serum ferritin may not be true indicators of iron status in athletes. Estimates of iron loss in endurance athletes may therefore be exaggerated.

Accelerated destruction and turnover of red blood cells because of mechanical trauma, compounded by an adaptational increase in the red blood cell mass seems to be the most convincing of the various explanations of the compromised hematological status of some endurance trained athletes. Weight (1993) concluded that sports anemia as a unique entity does not exist and that the suboptimal red cell indices and negative iron status observed in athletes occur independently of each other. Although some athletes experience a 'frank anemia,' it develops for the same reason as the clinical entity in the non-athletic population and is therefore not related to exercise, per se.

Hemolysis involves the destruction of red blood cells with the release of hemoglobin into the surrounding fluid. **Footstrike hemolysis** can cause true anemia in athletes, especially elite distance-runners. **Hemolytic anemia** is caused by the rupture or hemolysis of an excessive number of erythrocytes. This can occur in sickle cell anemia. Red blood cell removal is normally an extravascular process that does not involve hemolysis. **Haptoglobin** (a plasma protein) delivers hemoglobin to the liver, where the iron is salvaged. The plasma content of haptoglobin can be depleted if sufficient numbers of red blood cells are destroyed. When haptoglobin is depleted, the hemoglobin released from damaged red blood cells spills into the urine, coloring it red-to-brown (hemoglobinuria).

Other types of anemia include pernicious anemia, aplastic anemia, renal anemia, hemorrhagic anemia, megaloblastic anemia and sickle cell anemia. **Pernicious anemia** results from lack of vitamin B_{12} absorption. It is pernicious (deadly) because of the associated nerve degeneration that can result in eventual paralysis and death. **Aplastic anemia** is

caused by a defect in bone marrow. This leads to deficiency of red and white blood cells. **Renal anemia** is associated with a decreased production of erythropoietin due to a pathological state of the kidneys. **Hemorrhagic anemia** is caused by rapid loss of blood. **Megaloblastic anemia** occurs when megaloblasts replace red blood cells and may occur as a result of cellular deficiency of either folate or vitamin B_{12}. When red blood cell precursors in the bone marrow cannot form new DNA, they cannot divide normally but they continue to grow and become large, fragile, immature cells called megaloblasts. Megaloblasts mature into macrocytes, abnormally large red blood cells with short life span.

Sickle cell anemia is a hereditary human disease in which normal hemoglobin molecules are genetically altered; the hemoglobin contains one substituted amino acid due to a mutation in DNA. The gene encoding the beta chain of the hemoglobin molecule, located on chromosome 11, can be mutated in a variety of ways that result in different types of sickle cell disease. Sickle cell disease affects more than 50,000 Americans, with the highest frequency in people of African descent. The hemoglobin content of the blood is only about half the normal amount. The red blood cells are fewer in number and of an abnormal sickle shape. Exercise causes symptoms such as dizziness, breathing difficulties and increased pulse rate.

Sickle cell trait is a disease that is not as severe as sickle cell anemia. The individual receives an abnormal hemoglobin gene from only one parent. Sickle cell trait is present in 8% of African Americans, but is usually covert and benign. Research evidence suggests that patients with sickle cell trait have an exercise capacity that is probably normal or near normal. There is controversy as to whether sickle cell trait increases the risk of exercise-induced death. Between 1970 and 1993, more than 30 cases of collapse associated with sickle cell trait were reported. However, in cases of sudden death, it has been secondary to rhabdomyolysis occurring in sickle cell trait athletes performing at intense exertion under hot conditions, too soon after arriving at altitude. Maximal exercise, especially in heat or at altitude, can evoke a life-threatening syndrome of sickling, metabolic acidosis, collapse, acute renal failure, hyperkalemia and fulminant (sudden-onset) rhabdomyolysis. Athletes with sickle cell trait should adhere to the guidelines for fluid replacement and acclimatization to hot conditions and altitude.

Bibliography

Eichner, E.R. (1988). 'Sports anemia:' Poor terminology for a real phenomenon. *Gatorade Sports Science Exchange* 1(6).

Eichner, E.R. (1993). Sickle cell trait, heroic exercise and fatal collapse. *The Physician and Sportsmedicine* 21(7), 51-64.

Höberman, J. (1997). *Darwin's athletes. How sport has damaged Black America and preserved the myth of race.* Boston, MA: Houghton Mifflin Company.

Shaskey, D.J. and Green, G.A. (2000). Sports hematology. *Sports Medicine* 29(1), 27-38.

Smith, J.A. (1995). Exercise, training and red blood cell turnover. *Sports Medicine* 19(1), 9-31.

Weight, L.M. (1993). Sports anemia. Does it exist? *Sports Medicine* 16(1), 1-4.

ANENCEPHALY   *See under* BRAIN.

ANEURYSM   A localized swelling or dilation of a vein, an artery or the heart, due to weakening of the vessel wall by disease, injury or an abnormality present at birth. Aneurysms may occur in any blood vessel in the body, but the most common place is the abdomen below the renal arteries. The aneurysm may continue to grow larger until it ruptures. In the USA, aneurysm rupture affects about 15,000 people per year. An aorta is considered aneurismal when it grows more than 50% over its normal size. A normal aorta below the renal arteries measures about 2.3 cm in diameter in men and 1.9 cm in diameter in women, but varies with age and body size. Aneurysms are four times more common in men than women and occur most often after 55 years of age. A **pseudoaneurysm** is not a true aneurysm, but rather a collection of extravascular blood (clotted, free-flowing or both).

See also VASCULAR FRAGILITY.

ANGINA PECTORIS   Pain in the chest caused by partial occlusion of a coronary artery that is thought to be associated with inadequate blood supply to the myocardium. The pain usually lasts one to three minutes. One theory to explain angina pectoris is that metabolites within an ischemic segment of the heart muscle stimulate myocardial pain receptors. Exercise training results in a higher angina threshold.

See NITRATES.

ANGIOEDEMA   Subcutaneous edema that is of sudden onset and recurrent. It usually disappears within 24 hours and is seen mainly in young women, especially as an allergic reaction. Hereditary angioedema is a form of angioedema inherited as an autosomal dominant trait.

ANGIOGENESIS   *See under* CAPILLARIES.

ANGIOMA   A localized vascular lesion of the skin and subcutaneous tissue that results from overgrowth or blood or lymph. Now known as hemangioma or lymphangioma.

ANGIOTENSIN   A class of peptides that bring about vasoconstriction. The **renin-angiotensin-aldosterone** pathway is a mechanism for the control of blood pressure. Sympathetic stimulation, renal artery hypotension and decreased sodium delivery to the distal tubules stimulate the release of renin by the kidney. **Renin** is an enzyme that acts upon a circulating substrate, angiotensinogen, which undergoes proteolytic cleavage to form the **angiotensin** I, which is converted to angiotensin II by angiotensin-converting enzyme (ACE); **angiotensin II** stimulates the cortex of the adrenal glands to secrete aldosterone.

See also under NEUROTRANSMITTER.

ANGIOTENSIN-CONVERTING   ENZYME ACE. An enzyme that is present on the inner surface of blood vessels in many parts of the body, especially in the lungs. It catalyzes the conversion of angiotensin I to angiotensin II.

A decrease in ACE activity reverses the decline in physical performance due to peripheral muscle factors in those with congestive heart failure and may halt or slow the decline in muscle strength in elderly women.

In humans, the ACE gene is found in one of two forms: D-allele (deletion) and I-allele (insertion). The I-allele is due to the presence of a 287 base pair DNA fragment that the D-allele is missing. Montgomerie et al. (1998) carried out research with 78 British Army recruits, before and after 11 weeks of boot camp. Before training, the recruits with two copies of the I-allele and those with two copies of the D-allele had identical results when their muscles were tested. After training the recruits with two I alleles were able to curl a barbell for 11 times as long as those with two D-alleles. These recruits had lower levels of ACE in their blood. It is believed that the I-allele is responsible for production of lower levels of ACE in plasma and tissues. The I allele is found more frequently in elite 5000 m runners, high-altitude mountaineers and elite rowers than in the general population, but athletes with two D-alleles are more common among swimmers and 200 m runners. The I-allele is associated with lower ACE activity and superior endurance performance; this may be related to increased muscle efficiency. For high-altitude mountaineers, the increased muscle efficiency may conserve fat-free mass. The D-allele is associated with training-related strength gain and improved power, secondary to increased ACE and angiotensin II.

Bibliography

Gayagay, G. et al. (1998). Elite endurance athletes and the ACE I allele – the role of genes in athletic performance. *Human Genetics* 103, 48-50.

Jones, A., Montgomerie, H.E. and Woods, D.R. (2002). Human performance: A role for the ACE genotype. *Exercise and Sport Sciences Reviews* 30(4), 184-190.

Jones, A. and Woods, D.R. (2003). Skeletal muscle RAS and exercise performance. *International Journal of Biochemistry and Cell Biology* 35(6), 855-866.

Montgomery, H.E. et al. (1998). Human gene for physical performance. *Nature* 393, 221-222.

Woods, D.R. and Montgomerie, H.E. (2001). Angiotensin-converting enzyme and genetics at high altitude. *High Altitude Medicine and Biology* 2(2), 201-210.

ANGIOTENSIN-CONVERTING ENZYMES INHIBITORS ACE inhibitors. Drugs used to treat high blood pressure, e.g. Enalapril, Captopril. ACE inhibitors block the formation of angiotensin II, a potent vasconstrictor. This promotes vasodilation and decreases the liberation of aldosterone. ACE inhibitors are also effective in the treatment of heart failure and renal insufficiency secondary to diabetes. ACE inhibitors do not affect aerobic capacity.

ANGLE The ratio of the arc to the radius of the arc. The **radian** is a unit of angular measure. It is equal to the angle subtended at the center of a circle by an arc that is of equal length to the radius. There are 2π radians in a circle; one radian is equal to 57.29578 degrees.

Absolute angle is the angle of inclination of a body segment. It describes the orientation of the segment in space. The most commonly used convention for calculating absolute angles is to place a coordinate system at the distal end point of the segment. The angle using this convention is measured in a counter-clockwise direction from the right horizontal. **Relative angle** is the angle between the longitudinal axes of two segments. An **angle-angle diagram** plots a relative angle, such as that between two adjacent body segments against the absolute angle of a body segment (i.e. the angle relative to a reference in the surroundings). Comparative analysis of cyclical activities (such as running) can be facilitated by angle-angle diagrams, because the start and finish of an event are located at about the same point on the diagram.

See ANGULAR DISPLACEMENT.

ANGULAR ACCELERATION The time rate of change of angular velocity, either in angular speed or in direction of the axis. The average angular acceleration is equal to the final angular velocity minus the initial angular velocity divided by the time taken. The units are radians per second per second (rad/s^2). The US Customary units are revolutions per second per second or degrees per second per second.

See also MOMENT OF INERTIA.

ANGULAR DISPLACEMENT The change in angular position; it is the angle through which a body is rotated about an axis. Angular displacement is a vector quantity, which means that it expresses both magnitude and direction.

ANGULAR IMPULSE   A change in angular momentum equal to the product of torque and the time interval over which the torque acts. When an angular impulse acts on a system, the result is a change in the total angular momentum of the system. In the discus, for example, the aim is to maximize the angular impulse exerted on the discus before release in order to maximize its momentum and the ultimate horizontal displacement following release.

ANGULAR MOMENTUM   The angular analogue of linear momentum. It is calculated by multiplying the angular velocity by the moment of inertia. The Standard International unit is the kilogram meter-squared per second ($kg.m^2/s$).

The **law of conservation of angular momentum** states that the angular momentum of a system remains the same in the absence of external forces (i.e. forces from outside the system). Conservation of angular momentum is evident in activities such as diving where the body is isolated, and in situations where external resistive torque/force is negligible, such as sprint ice-skating. Once a diver leaves the board, the only external force acting on him is gravity. Gravity acts through the center of gravity of the body, which serves as the location of the axis of rotation during free flight. The gravitational force does not have any perpendicular distance from the axis of rotation and thus can produce neither torque nor angular impulse. Assuming air resistance is negligible, there is no change in the diver's angular momentum until he lands or collides with another object (even though gravity is accelerating the diver's center of gravity linearly downward).

Because of the law of conservation of momentum, angular momentum may be transferred from one body (or body part) to another as the total angular momentum remains unchanged. An example is the sequence of segmental rotations that occur in throwing and kicking actions. In a throwing action, the initial angular momentum generated by application of torque to the leg and trunk segments

is transferred to the much lighter upper arm. The decrease in moment of inertia between the trunk and the arm produces an increase in the angular velocity of the upper arm.

In sports such as diving, **zero momentum rotations** are initiated in mid air when the total body angular momentum is zero. A skilful diver can rotate 180 degrees or more in the air with zero angular momentum, because in a piked position there is a large discrepancy between the radii of gyration for the upper and lower extremities with respect to the longitudinal axes of these two major body segments. In accordance with the conservation of angular momentum, if a part of the body rotates one way, the remainder of the body rotates with equal and opposite angular momentum.

When an airborne skateboarder thrusts his arms out wide, the moment of inertia of his upper body is increased. Throwing his outspread arms in one direction creates a torque through the body that can twist his legs (and the skateboard) up to 180 degrees in the opposite direction. In this, 'frontside 180,' the two rotations cancel each other out and thus the skater's total angular momentum remains zero.

Angular momentum can also be transferred or converted to linear momentum (or vice versa). For example, the angular momentum of the hammer becomes linear momentum when it is released.

See also ENERGY; FORCE; POWER; SUMMATION OF VELOCITY PRINCIPLE; WORK.

ANGULAR MOTION   Motion that is not linear. If the axis of rotation is fixed, all particles in the body travel in a circular motion. If the axis of rotation is not fixed, the motion is a combination of translation and rotation. In biomechanics, the motion of many limb segments is assumed to occur about fixed axes, even though the joint centers are not actually fixed. The Standard International (SI) unit is the radian. The US customary unit is the degree.

The angular analogue of Newton's first law is that a rotating body will continue in a state of uniform angular motion unless acted on by an external torque. The angular analogue of Newton's second law is that an external torque will produce an angular acceleration of a body that is proportional and in the direction of the torque, and inversely proportional to the moment of inertia of the body. Torque is the product of moment of inertia and angular acceleration. The angular analogue of Newton's third law is that for every torque exerted by one body on another body, there is an equal and opposite torque exerted by the one body on the other. A long jumper swings her legs forward and upward in preparation for landing. To counteract this lower-body torque, the remainder of the body moves forward and downward, producing a torque equal and opposite to the lower-body torque. The torques and counter-torques are equal and opposite, but the angular velocity of these two body portions is different because the moments of inertia are different. See also under POWER; WORK.

ANGULAR VELOCITY   The rate of change of angular displacement with respect to time. The Standard International units are radians per second (rad/s). The US Customary units are revolutions/min or degrees/sec.

Assuming constant angular velocity, an object (such as a ball) moving at the end of a long radius (such as an arm-club lever) will have a greater linear velocity than one moved at the end of a short radius. Thus it is an advantage for an athlete to use as long a lever as possible to impart linear velocity to an object if the long lever length does not significantly compromise angular velocity. Assuming constant linear velocity, shortening the radius will increase the angular velocity and lengthening it will decrease the angular velocity. For any given angular velocity, the linear velocity is proportional to the radius. If the radius doubles, the linear velocity also doubles. For any given linear velocity, the angular velocity is inversely proportional to the radius.

See also SUMMATION OF VELOCITY PRINCIPLE.

ANIONS   *See* NEGATIVE IONS.

ANKLE EQUINUS   A structural limitation of dorsal flexion with less than 10 degrees available from the neutral position.

ANKLE JOINT   A joint complex that involves the tibiotalar, fibulotalar and distal tibiofibular joints. The **tibiotalar joint** is a diarthrotic hinge joint. The proximal articulating surface is concave and is the inferior portion of the tibia (medial malleolus). The distal articulating surface is convex and is the medial portion of the talus. The **fibulotalar joint** is an amphiarthrosis. The proximal articulating surface is the inferior medial fibula; the distal articulation is the superior lateral side of the talus. The **distal tibiofibular joint** is an amphiarthrosis that is formed by the distal ends of the medial fibula and lateral tibia. The distal syndesmotic ligaments prevent separation of the distal tibia and fibula and help transmit force through the distal fibula on weight bearing.

Medial anatomic structures are: the posterior tibial tendon, the *flexor digitorum longus* muscle, the neurovascular bundle and the *flexor hallucis longus* muscle. Lateral anatomic structures are: the tendons of the *peroneus brevis* and *peroneus longus* muscles and the sural nerve. Anterior anatomic structures are: the anterior tibial tendon, the *extensor hallucis longus* muscle, the neurovascular bundle, the *extensor digitorum longus* muscle and the *peroneus tertius* muscle. Posterior anatomic structures are: the Achilles tendon and the os trigonum (Stieda's process).

The movement at the ankle joint is primarily dorsal/plantar flexion, with minor components of inversion/eversion and adduction/abduction.

See FOOT; SUBTALAR JOINT.

ANKLE JOINT, INJURIES   The posterior-process fracture (Shepherd's fracture) typically occurs when a woman in high heels catches the heel during stairway-descent and sustains a plantar-flexion sprain, fracturing the posterolateral (Stieda's) process of the talus or dislodging the os trigonum. An avulsion fracture of the anterior process of the calcaneus is caused by inversion and plantar flexion.

See also FRACTURES.

ANKLE LIGAMENTS   The ligaments of the ankle may be grouped into three complexes: lateral, medial and interosseus. The **lateral complex**

involves the anterior talofibular ligament, calcaneofibular ligament and posterior talofibular ligament. The **medial complex** involves four bands (three superficial and one deep) of the deltoid ligament. The **interosseus complex** (syndesmosis) involves the anterior and posterior tibiofibular ligaments and interosseus membrane.

Sprains are the most common injuries to the ankle, and consist of either partial or complete tears. About 70% of ankle sprains occur at the lateral complex, of which the anterior talofibular ligament is the weakest and the most frequently injured. They occur from inversion, when the foot is in a plantar flexed and supinated position. Being vertical and under tensile stress, the anterior talofibular ligament is usually damaged first. If the stress continues, it tears completely. Tear of the calcaneofibular ligament may ensue in 20% of cases. The strongest ligament of the lateral complex (the posterior talofibular ligament) is rarely involved. The mechanism of injury is often landing from a jump or a sudden change of direction. Inversion sprains are the most common of all sports injuries, occurring especially in sports such as basketball, volleyball and soccer. One of the risk factors is pes cavus. With a rotational sprain, resulting from cutting across a plantar flexed, inverted foot, not only the lateral complex but also the interosseus complex may be involved. As a consequence, the neck of the fibula may be fractured (Maisonneuve fracture). Isolated tear of the calcaneofibular ligament is rare, but may occur when inversion is combined with dorsal flexion.

Injuries to the medial complex are rare (less than 10% of ankle sprains) because it is much stronger than the lateral complex. The medial complex may be injured when an athlete suffers an eversion injury, usually associated with external rotation of the leg while the foot is fixed. With larger eversion forces, medial complex injuries or medial malleolus fractures extend through the interosseus membrane and a Maisonneuve fracture may result. If the ligament complex is stronger than the bone, an avulsion fracture of the medial malleolus may occur. Another injury associated with eversion is a syndesmosis (interosseus complex) sprain ('**high ankle sprain**;' **distal tibiofibular diastasis**);

there is a partial tear of the anterior tibiofibular ligament.

Forces generated by excessive dorsal flexion result in the talus being jammed into the mortise, since the anterior part of the talus is wider than the posterior part. This may result in separation of the syndesmosis in addition to an osteochondral fracture of the talus.

Proprioceptive exercises have been found to protect the ankle joint from re-injury.

Bibliography

Osborne, M.D. and Rizzo Jr, T.D. (2003). Prevention and treatment of ankle sprain in athletes. *Sports Medicine* 33(15), 1145-1150.

ANKLE TAPING Prophylactic taping can effectively decrease excessive ankle inversion before exercise, but the restraint may be lost during exercise. Semi-rigid ankle orthotics can substitute for taping. Since taping and rigid/semi-rigid devices interfere with normal movement, however, there is concern that they might actually be a risk factor for injury. In this respect, taping is less of a concern because it interferes least with normal movements. In comparison to low-top shoes, high-top shoes are more effective in restricting mechanically imposed ankle inversion range of movement. Low-top shoes, however, also limit mechanically imposed ankle inversion stress with the ankle in the position in which ankle injury occurs most frequently. A superior mechanical restriction of ankle range of movement, however, does not necessarily imply a superior preventive effect.

According to Robbins and Waked (1998), sense of foot position in humans is precise when barefoot, but is distorted by athletic footwear. This may account for the high frequency of ankle sprains in athletes wearing shoes. The development of footwear to retain maximal tactile sensitivity, and thus sense of foot position, should therefore be developed.

See also RUNNING INJURIES.

Bibliography

Robbins, S. and Waked, E. (1998). Factors associated with ankle injuries. Preventive measures. *Sports Medicine* 25(1), 63-72.

Verhagen, E.A., van der Beek, A.J. and van Mechelen, W. (2001). The effect of tape, braces and shoes on ankle range of motion. *Sports Medicine* 31(9), 667-677.

ANKYLOSING SPONDYLITIS   *See under* ARTHRITIS.

ANNULAR   Shaped like a ring.

ANOREXIA   Lack or loss of appetite. *See* EATING DISORDERS.

ANOREXIA ATHLETICA   *See under* EATING DISORDERS.

ANOREXIA NERVOSA   A life-threatening eating disorder that is characterized by: resistance to maintain body weight, at or above, a minimally normal weight for age and height; intense fear of weight gain or being 'fat,' even though underweight; distorted perception of body weight or shape; undue influence of weight or body shape on self-evaluation; denial of the seriousness of low body weight; and amenorrhea.

Warning signs of anorexia nervosa include: dramatic weight loss; preoccupation with weight, food, calories, fat grams and dieting; refusal to eat certain foods, progressing to restrictions against whole categories of food; frequent comments about feeling 'fat' or overweight despite weight loss; anxiety about gaining weight or being 'fat;' denial of hunger; development of food rituals, such as eating foods in certain orders; consistent excuses to avoid mealtimes or situations involving food; excessive, rigid exercise regimen; withdrawal from usual friends and activities; and behaviors and attitudes indicating that weight loss, dieting, and control of food are becoming primary concerns.

Health consequences of anorexia nervosa include abnormally slow heart rate and low blood pressure; osteoporosis; muscle loss and weakness; severe dehydration, which can result in kidney failure; fainting, fatigue and overall weakness; dry hair and skin; and growth of a downy layer of hair called **lanugo** all over the body, including the face, in an effort to keep the body warm.

0.5 to 1% of American women suffer from anorexia nervosa. It typically appears in early to mid-adolescence. 90 to 95% of anorexia nervosa sufferers are girls and women. 5 to 20% of individuals with anorexia nervosa will die from the disorder.

Risk factors for anorexia nervosa include: high parental education and income, early feeding problems, low self-esteem, high neuroticism, maternal overprotection, and eating disorders among family members.

Epling et al. (1983) suggested that dieting and exercising initiate the anorexic cycle and that as many as 75% of anorexia nervosa cases are exercise induced. Strenuous exercise tends to suppress appetite, which serves to decrease the value of food reinforcement. As a result, food intake decreases and bodyweight is lost. As bodyweight decreases, there is increased motivation for more exercise. The problem with this line of reasoning is that not all persons with anorexia engage in exercise and it cannot explain bulimia nervosa.

In males, emotional and mental characteristics associated with anorexia nervosa include: intense fear of becoming fat or gaining weight; depression; social isolation; strong need to be in control; rigid, inflexible ('all-or-nothing') thinking; decreased interest in sex or fear around sex; possible conflict over gender identity or sexual orientation; difficulty expressing feeling; perfectionism; and belief that others are overreacting to his low weight or caloric restriction. Males with anorexia see themselves, and are seen by others, as more feminine than other men, both in attitudes and behavior. In general, males with anorexia appear to identify more closely with their mothers than their fathers.

Chronology

•1994 • On 26 July, five days after her 22nd birthday, Olympic-hopeful gymnast Christy Henrich died of multiple organ failure after five years of starving herself. Her weight of 61 lb was an improvement upon her 47 lb that she weighed on 4 July. For two years she had been in and out of various hospitals. In 1988 Henrich, who trained with Julissa Gomez at Al Fong's gym, was 10th at the Senior Nationals and missed the Olympic team by 118 thousandths of a point. This left her devastated. At a meet in Budapest during 1988, a US judge told Henrich that she would have to lose weight if she wanted to make the Olympic team. At that time she weighted 90 pounds. Upon returning to the States, her mother recalls the first words out of Christy's mouth: she was fat and she would have to lose weight; that was the only way she would reach her dreams. Henrich resorted to anorexia and bulimia as a way to control her weight. In 1989, she placed 2nd in the nationals and was 4th in the world. But, as Joan Ryan explained in *Little Girls in Pretty Boxes*, "The medals hanging from the walls of her home, the newspaper clippings, the national rankings, the fourth-place finish at the 1989 World Championships – they were no match for her own certainty that she was a failure. She carried the failure in the curve of her thighs, the soft skin under her chin, anywhere she couldn't see bone." Nancy Marshall, a 1972 Olympic gymnast, who also suffered from an eating disorder during her competitive career said, "If you have trusting parents, an ambitious coach and a gymnast like Christy, who is a textbook perfectionist, highly intense, and driven – then you have a time bomb."

Bibliography

National Eating Disorders Association. Http://www.NationalEatingDisorders.org

Epling, W.F., Pierce, W.D. and Stefan, L. (1983). A theory of activity based anorexia. *International Journal of Eating Disorders* 3, 27-46.

Fichter, M.M. and Daser, C. (1987). Symptomatology, psychosexual development and gender identity in 42 anorexic males. *Psychological Medicine* 17, 409-418.

Noden, M. (1994). Dying to win. *Sports Illustrated*, 8 August, 52-60.

Ryan, J. (1995). *Little girls in pretty boxes*. New York: Doubleday.

ANOREXIANTS A group of drugs that include sympathomimetic amines (e.g. amphetamines), serotonin agonists (e.g. flenfluramine) and monoamine oxidase inhibitors (e.g. sibutramine).

ANOXIA *See under* HYPOXIA.

ANTAGONIST *See under* DRUG; MUSCLE ACTION.

ANTERIOR Ventral. It refers to the front surface of the body.

ANTERIOR CRUCIATE LIGAMENT *See under* KNEE LIGAMENTS.

ANTERIOR INTEROSSEUS SYNDROME The anterior interosseus branch of the median nerve can be compressed by the fibrous edge of the *flexor digitorum superficialis* muscle or the deep head of the *pronator teres* muscle, as a result of overuse or external compression. Anterior interosseus syndrome may afflict tennis players who wear over-tight, counter-force braces. Possible causes include: anatomic variations in vessels, muscle origins or nerves, as well as space-occupying lumps such as ganglia. *See* PERIPHERAL NERVE INJURIES.

ANTERIOR PLANE Sagittal plane. The plane that runs parallel to the vertical plane and divides the body into right and left halves.

ANTERIOR SUPERIOR ILIAC SPINE Blunt bony projection on the anterior border of the ilium, forming the anterior end of the iliac crest.

ANTEVERSION *See under* FEMORAL NECK.

ANTHROPOMETRY Measurement of the structure of the human body. It can be subdivided into five classes: lengths (including stature), diameters, girths (circumferences), skinfolds and weights (e.g. body weight).

See also KINANTHROPOMETRY; KINESI-OLOGY.

Chronology

•1654 • A thesis entitled *Anthropometria* by Johann Sigismund Elsholtz, a German physician, was issued in Padua. Elsholtz invented the use of the term 'anthropometry.'

•1861 • Edward Hitchcock supervised the first significant college program in physical education at Amherst College. Hitchcock had been appointed as "Professor of Hygiene and Physical Education" in 1859 and at the same time was first officially recognized college director of physical education in the USA. He was probably also the first person in physical education to take anthropometric measurements. He recorded the age, weight, height, finger reach, chest girth, lung capacity and strength of each student five times during their college course.

•1869 • Archibald MacLaren's *A System of Physical Education* was published. MacLaren had become widely recognized as an authority on the scientific study of physical education and a pioneer in anthropometry.

•1879 • Dudley A. Sargent was appointed as Harvard's first assistant professor of physical training and as director of its new Hemenway Gymnasium. Upon entrance, all Harvard freshmen were given an examination that included anthropometric measurements and strength tests. Sargent developed a series of strength test items using a dynamometer that William T. Brigham, a Harvard graduate, had first brought over from Paris eight years earlier. Brigham was the first to become interested in anthropometry when he was crossing the Pacific on a ship with a number of Chinese.

•1885 • In America, the Association for the Advancement of Physical Education (AAPE) was founded after William G. Anderson convened about sixty individuals who were interested in promoting the field of physical education. The following year it became the American Association for the Advancement of Physical Education (AAAPE). In 1903, it became known as the American Association of Physical Education Association (AAPE). The AAPE created the Committee of Anthropometry and Vital Statistics at its first meeting. A major concern was the lack of standardization in measurement, e.g. Edward Hitchcock and Dudley Sargent had both developed their own protocol that that they felt was superior.

•1888 • A student of Dudley A. Sargent at Harvard, George W. Fritz, designed and made the first multiple camera and automatic labeling device for Sargent to photography students in his physical examination at the Hemenway Gymnasium.

•1896 • Jay Seaver's *Anthropometry and Physical Examinations* described the measurements that Edward Hitchcock had performed at Amherst, the 1877 study of American school children by Henry P. Bowditch, George W. Peckham's study of the growth of school children in Milwaukee from 1880-1883, and William T. Porter's 1892-1893 study of the children in the public schools of St. Louis.

•1898 • In Belgium, a commission composed of professionals from medicine and gymnastics was appointed to consider the merits of the Belgian and Swedish systems of gymnastics. It recommended that the schools adopt the more scientific Swedish system. Other recommendations included periodical physical examinations and anthropometric measurements.

•1898 • Dudley A. Sargent standardized his strength tests for large-scale intercollegiate competition. However, intense rivalry led to so many violations of the rules, fake records, and juggling of the instruments that Sargent felt it had lost its special value.

•1911 • Abram Flexner's influential study of medical education found that the medical degree was very superficial in the USA as compared with medical degrees in Europe. Consequently, medical training in the USA was improved. Ever since the *Flexner Report*, medical schools have devoted the first two years of study to the basic sciences - chemistry, physiology and pathology - as the foundation for later clinical training. The tougher four-year curriculum plus internship and postgraduate work made the relatively unrenumerative position of physical education director unattractive to medically qualified professionals. One of the consequences of this was a decrease in the popularity of anthropometric measurements on freshmen in US universities.

•1965 • The International Committee on Physical Fitness Research was founded. One of its aims was to standardize tests in physical fitness.

ANTIBODY   *See* IMMUNOGLOBULIN.

ANTICIPATION   Predicting a response before it occurs. It can help overcome the limitations of reaction time. Expert tennis players can return hard tennis serves, because they learn to perceive their opponents' preparatory movements prior to the actual hitting of the ball.

Inexperienced soccer players tend to focus more frequently on the ball and players passing the ball, whereas experienced players tend to focus on the positions and movements of other players.

Novice goalkeepers spend more time fixating on the kicker's trunk, arms and hip areas, and less time on the head, non-kicking foot and ball.

See also EXPERTISE; PERCEPTION; TIMING ACCURACY.

Bibliography

Abernethy, B. (1991). Visual search strategies and decision making in sport. *International Journal of Sport Psychology* 22, 189-210.

Savelsbergh, G.J.P. et al. (2002). Visual search, anticipation and expertise in soccer goal keepers. *Journal of Sports Sciences* 20, 279-287.

Williams, A.M., Davids, K., Burwitz, L. and Williams, J.G. (1994). Visual search strategies in experienced and inexperienced soccer players. *Research Quarterly for Exercise and Sport* 65, 127-135.

ANTI-DIURETIC HORMONE   ADH. *See* VASOPRESSIN.

ANTIGEN   *See under* IMMUNITY.

ANTIHISTAMINES   Drugs that antagonize the action of histamine and are used to treat certain allergic conditions such as hay fever. The latest antihistamine medications, unlike earlier ones, do not have sedative side effects. Single oral administrations of non-sedative antihistamines seem to have no effect on exercise performance or tolerance in asymptomatic individuals. The effects of antihistamine treatment on exercise are not clearly understood. There is growing evidence, however, that pre-treatment with antihistamines may prevent or attenuate some exercise-induced, histamine-mediated disorders such as urticaria, pruritus (itching), anaphylaxis and gastrointestinal bleeding.

Bibliography
Montgomery, L.C. and Deuster, P.A. (1993). Effects of antihistamine medications on exercise performance. Implications for sports people. *Sports Medicine* 15(3), 179-195.

ANTIOXIDANT   An agent that prevents or inhibits oxidation of a substance by combining with oxygen.
    See FREE RADICALS; NUTRITION; VITAMIN C; VITAMIN E.

ANTI-SOCIAL PERSONALITY DISORDER   A mental disorder with the following diagnostic criteria: (A) There is a pervasive pattern of disregard for and violation of the rights of others occurring since age 15 years, as indicated by 3 (or more) of the following: (i) failure to conform to social norms with respect to lawful behavior as indicated by repeatedly performing acts that are grounds for arrest; (ii) deceitfulness, as indicated by repeated lying, use of aliases, or conning others for personal profit or pleasure; (iii) impulsivity or failure to plan ahead; (iv) irritability and aggressiveness, as indicated by repeated physical fights or assaults; (v) reckless disregard for safety of self or others; (vi) consistent irresponsibility, as indicated by repeated failure to sustain consistent work behavior or honor financial obligations; (vii) lack of remorse, as indicated by being indifferent to or rationalizing having hurt, mistreated, or stolen from another. (B) The individual is at least 18 years of age. (C) There is evidence of Conduct Disorder with onset before age of 15 years. (D) The occurrence of antisocial behavior is not exclusively during the course of Schizophrenia or a Manic Episode.

Bibliography
American Psychiatric Association. (1994). *Diagnostic and statistical manual of mental disorders*. 4th ed. Washington, DC: American Psychiatric Association.

ANXIETY   A condition in which there is a certain degree and pattern of high arousal in combination with unpleasant emotion, such as fear and/or negative images and thoughts such as worry. Anxiety may be associated with fear of failure, lack of readiness to perform and concerns about social evaluation by others. Athletes who derive their self-esteem primarily from experiencing success in sport may be more likely to experience fear of failure.
    Anxiety can be assessed using psychophysiological measures of arousal in combination with self-report inventories of emotions and cognitions. In everyday life, anxiety tends to be used as synonymous with stress. In psychology, stress is a separate but related construct.
    Spielberger (1966) distinguished between **state anxiety** (the degree of anxiety an individual experiences at a given point in time) and **trait anxiety** (an enduring personality characteristic relating to both the frequency and intensity of an individual's state anxiety). Based on the theories of McGrath and Spielberger, Martens (1977) proposed an explanation of anxiety in sport that involved a distinction between an "objective competitive situation" and a "subjective competitive situation." An **"objective competitive situation"** is defined as a situation in which all the following three factors are present: a standard of excellence, the presence of an evaluator who is aware of the standard and comparison of the performance outcome against the standard. The **"subjective competitive situation"** refers to an individual's cognitive appraisal of a particular objective competitive situation and determines whether a pre-competition state anxiety response will occur. The evaluation of the state anxiety response (successful or unsuccessful) is also considered to be a factor in

determining appraisals of future subjective competitive situations. It is hypothesized that individuals with high trait anxiety manifest greater increases in state anxiety than individuals who are rated as low trait anxious, when the situation is perceived as threatening. This prediction has been supported by research using questionnaire ratings of anxiety such as the Sport Competition Anxiety Test (SCAT) and Competitive State Anxiety Inventory-2 (CSAI-2). CSAI-2 is based on a multi-dimensional theory of state anxiety, which differentiates between cognitive state anxiety (worry; negative thoughts and images) and somatic state anxiety (perceived arousal).

Multidimensional Anxiety theory predicts that cognitive and somatic anxiety will differentially influence athletic performance. It predicts a strong, negative linear relationship between cognitive state anxiety and performance; and a less strong, inverted-U relationship between somatic anxiety and performance. The detrimental effect of anxiety on performance may be due to cognitive state anxiety, which causes less attention to be devoted to task relevant information and impairs a person's ability to discriminate between relevant and irrelevant information. CSAI-2 also includes a self-confidence subscale. Self-confidence is negatively related to cognitive state anxiety, but on the same continuum. Research using CSAI-2 has suggested that the influence of performance on subsequent anxiety may be greater than the influence of pre-competitive anxiety on subsequent performance. The **Matching Hypothesis** states that an anxiety-management technique should be matched to a particular anxiety problem, i.e. somatic anxiety should be dealt with using physical relaxation (e.g. progressive relaxation); and cognitive anxiety should be dealt with mental relaxation (e.g. autogenic training). The research evidence to support this hypothesis is equivocal.

While Multidimensional theory makes no specific predictions about the combined effects of cognitive and somatic anxiety, the **Cusp Catastrophe model** predicts that cognitive anxiety is not always detrimental to performance. It suggests that at low levels of cognitive anxiety, changes in physiological arousal should lead to small and continuous changes in performance. However, at high levels of cognitive anxiety, changes in physiological arousal may lead to small changes in performance when physiological arousal is either low or high, but may lead to large changes in performance when physiological arousal is at intermediate levels. At low levels of physiological arousal, cognitive anxiety has a positive linear relationship with performance. At high levels of physiological arousal, however, cognitive anxiety has a negative relationship with performance. It also follows that performers can experience both cognitive anxiety and self-confidence at the same time. Cognitive anxiety may decrease attentional resources available for performing the task at hand, but they may also motivate increased cognitive and physical efforts to perform that task. Cohen et al. (2002) argue that the inclusion of physiological arousal at the expense of somatic anxiety is a critical error in the conceptualization of the Cusp Catastrophe theory.

According to Hanin (1989), individual athletes tend to perform best when their own pre-competition anxiety level is within a relatively narrow range or zone. When pre-competition anxiety is either higher or lower than this zone, performance deteriorates. This relation appears to be described by an inverted-U curve. There are considerable inter-individual differences in the optimal anxiety level of athletes. Hanin's **Zone of Functioning (ZOF) theory** predicts that a large percentage of athletes perform best when anxiety is high or low rather than moderate. Inter-individual variability in the optimal zone of anxiety exists for every sport and different levels of expertise. Many athletes appear to perform best when experiencing high levels of anxiety. Subsequently any interventions that act to calm an athlete down may actually have a detrimental effect on athletic performance. Hanin (1997) extended the Individualized ZOF concept beyond anxiety to show how ZOF uses a variety of emotions.

Smith's (1986) model of anxiety postulates that both the intensity and duration of cognitive and somatic anxiety are influenced by the objective competitive sport situation, the sport-specific trait anxiety of the person and the person's psychological defenses for coping with anxiety-provoking competitive situations. The above factors influence state anxiety through their impact on the following processes: appraisal of situational demands; appraisal of resources to deal with the immediate situation; appraisal of the nature and likelihood of potential consequences if the demands are not met; and the personal meanings attached to the consequences.

See also DEPRESSANTS; DEPRESSION; EMOTION; MOOD STATE; PSYCHO-DYNAMICS; QUALITY OF LIFE; SELF-EFFICACY.

Bibliography

Burton, D. (1988). Do anxious swimmers swim slower? Reexamining the elusive anxiety-performance relationship. *Journal of Sport and Exercise Psychology* 10, 45-61.

Burton, D. and Naylor, S. (1997). Is anxiety really facilitative? Reaction to the myth that cognitive anxiety always impairs performance. *Journal of Applied Sport Psychology* 9, 295-303.

Cohen, A., Pargman, D. and Tenenbaum, G. (2003). Critical elaboration and empirical investigation of the Cusp Catastrope model: A lesson for practitioners. *Journal of Applied Sport Psychology* 15, 144-159.

Eysenck, M. (1983). Anxiety and individual differences. In: Hockey, R. (ed). *Stress and Fatigue in Human Performance*. pp273-298. Chichester, England: John Wiley and Sons.

Eysenck, M.W. and Calvo, M. (1992). Anxiety and performance: The Processing Efficiency theory. *Cognition and Emotion* 6, 409-434.

Fazey, J. and Hardy, L. (1988). The inverted-U hypothesis: A catastrophe for sport psychology? *British Association of Sports Sciences Monograph* No. 1. Leeds: National Coaching Foundation.

Feltz, D.L. (1988). Self confidence and sports performance. *Exercise and Sport Sciences Reviews* 16, 423-458.

Hanin, Y.L. (1989). Interpersonal and intragroup anxiety in sports. In: Hackfort, D. and Spielberger, C.D. (eds). *Anxiety in sports: An international perspective*. pp19-28. New York: Hemisphere Publishing.

Hanin, Y.L. (1997). Emotions and athletic performance: Individual zones of optimal functioning model. *European Yearbook of Sport Psychology* 1, 29-72.

Hanin, Y.L. (2000, ed). *Emotions in sport*. Champaign, IL: Human Kinetics.

Hardy, L. (1996). Testing the predictions of the Cusp Catastrophe model of anxiety and performance. *The Sports Psychologist* 10, 140-156.

Hardy, L. and Parfitt, G. (1991). A catastrophic model of anxiety and performance. *British Journal of Psychology* 82, 163-178.

Jones, G. (1995). Competitive anxiety in sport. Biddle, S.J.H. (ed). *European perspectives on exercise and sport psychology*. pp128-153. Champaign, IL: Human Kinetics.

Martens, R. (1977). *Sport Competition Anxiety Test*. Champaign, IL: Human Kinetics.

Martens, R., Vealey, R.S. and Burton, D. (1990). *Competitive anxiety in sport*. Champaign, IL: Human Kinetics.

Maynard, I.W., Smith, M.J. and Warwick-Evans, L. (1995). The effects of a cognitive intervention strategy on competitive state anxiety and performance in semiprofessional soccer players. *The Sport Psychologist* 9, 51-64.

Raglin, J.S. (1992). Anxiety and sport performance. *Exercise and Sport Sciences Reviews* 20, 243-74.

Smith, R.E. (1996). Performance anxiety, cognitive interference, and concentration enhancement strategies in sports. In Sarason, I.G, Pierce, G.R. and Sarason, B.R. (eds). *Cognitive interference: Theories, methods and findings*. pp261-284. Hillsdale, NJ: Erlbaum.

Spielberger, C.D. (1966, ed). *Anxiety and behavior*. New York: Academic Press.

ANXIETY DISORDERS   The broad diagnostic category that includes panic attacks, panic disorders, phobias, obsessive-compulsive disorders and other conditions of excessive worry and unease. More than 19 million Americans suffer from anxiety disorders. People with anxiety disorders are at higher risk for developing comorbid depression.

A **panic attack** is a discrete period of intense fear or discomfort, in which at least four of the following symptoms develop abruptly and reach a peak within 10 minutes: palpitations, pounding heart or accelerated heart rate, sweating, trembling or shaking, sensations of shortness of breath or smothering, feeling of choking, chest pain or discomfort, nausea or abdominal distress, feeling dizzy, unsteady, lightheaded or faint; feelings of unreality or being detached from oneself, fear of losing control or going crazy, fear of dying, paresthesias (numbness or tingling sensations), and chills or hot flushes. Panic attacks usually occur in the aftermath of stress, prolonged emotion, specific worries or frightening experiences. **Panic disorder** is the recurrence of unexpected panic attacks.

Phobias are intense, persistent and unreasonable fears in relation to specific objects that cause avoidance behaviors.

Post-traumatic stress disorder is an anxiety disorder that may be triggered by rape, accidents and military combat, for example. About 30% of men and women who have spent time in war zones experience post-traumatic stress disorder. One million war veterans developed it after serving in Vietnam. Many people with post-traumatic stress disorder have recurrent flashbacks of the trauma in the form of memories, nightmares or frightening thoughts, especially when they are exposed to events or objects reminiscent of the trauma. More than 5 million Americans experience post-traumatic stress disorder during the course of a year, tending to have abnormal levels of stress hormones. For example, cortisone levels are lower than normal; epinephrine and norepinephrine levels are higher than normal. Corticotropin releasing factor levels seem to be elevated in people with post-traumatic stress disorder and this may explain their tendency to be easily startled.

Obsessive-compulsive disorder is an anxiety disorder in which a person has recurrent and unwanted ideas or impulses (**obsessions**) and an urge or compulsion to do something to relieve the discomfort caused by the obsession. The obsessive thoughts range from the idea of losing control, to themes surrounding religion or keeping things or parts of one's body clean all the time. **Compulsions** are behaviors that help decrease the anxiety surrounding the obsessions. The most common compulsions are washing and checking behaviors. Most people (90%) who have obsessive-compulsive disorder have both obsessions and compulsions. The thoughts and behaviors a person with obsessive-compulsive disorder has are senseless, repetitive, distressing and sometimes harmful, but they are also difficult to overcome. Children are not necessarily aware that their obsessions or compulsions are excessive behaviors. Obsessive-compulsive disorder is indicated by four (or more) of the following: (i) is

occupied with details, rules, lists, order, organization or schedules to the extent that the major point of the activity is lost; (ii) shows perfectionism that interferes with task completion (e.g. is unable to complete a project because his or her own overly strict standards are not met); (iii) is excessively devoted to work and productivity to the exclusion of leisure activities and friendship (not accounted by obvious economic necessity); (iv) is overcon-scientious, scrupulous and inflexible about matters of morality, ethics or values (not accounted for by cultural or religious identification); (v) is unable to discard worn-out or worthless objects even when they have no sentimental value; (vi) is reluctant to delegate tasks or to work with others unless they submit to exactly his or her way of doing things; (vii) adopts a miserly spending style toward both self and others; (viii) money is viewed as something to be hoarded for future catastrophes; and (ix) shows rigidity and stubbornness.

Bibliography

American Psychiatric Association. (1994). *Diagnostic and statistical manual of mental disorders*. 4th ed. Washington, DC: American Psychiatric Association.

National Center for Post-Traumatic Stress Disorder. Http://www.ncptsd.org

AORTA   The main artery of the human body. It leaves the left ventricle of the heart to supply arterial blood to the many arteries that branch off it. The aortic arch is a loop in the aorta found a short distance from where it leaves the heart.

See also ANEURYSM.

APATITE   A complex mineral consisting of calcium fluoride phosphate or calcium chloride phosphate.

APERT'S SYNDROME   A relatively uncommon craniofacial condition (occurring with a frequency of 1 in 160,000 live births) that is associated with craniofacial and digital developmental failure with craniosynostosis (early closing of one or more of the sutures of the infant's head) and syndactyly, midface hypoplasia and often hydrocephalus. It is caused by a single gene alteration of fibroblast growth factor. It is indicated by a flat head appearance, microcephalus, defective formation of facial bones, bulging eyes, and malformed hands and feet. Mental retardation is sometimes present. The malformed hands and feet necessitate adapted physical activity.

Bibliography

World Craniofacial Foundation. Http://www.worldcf.org

APOLIPOPROTEIN *See under* CHOLESTEROL.

APONEUROSIS A flattened or ribbon-shaped tendon, which joins muscles to bone, cartilage, ligament or other connective tissue.

APOPHYSEAL JOINTS Synovial joints between adjacent vertebrae, connected at the superior and inferior facets located on the laminae.

APOPHYSIS A growth area at the point of a tendon insertion; it is a cartilaginous structure near the end of a long bone. The apophysis is subjected primarily to tensile forces, whereas the epiphysis is subjected mainly to compressive forces. Apophyseal injuries occur at sites where major muscle tendons apply traction (tension) to soft bone. It is not clear whether intensively trained young athletes are at greater risk of injury than children engaged in free play activities.

APOPHYSITIS Irritation or inflammation of an apophysis. Traction (tensile) apophysitis can occur at a number of locations: the medial epicondyle of the elbow (Little Leaguer's elbow), the tibial tubercle (Osgood Schlatter's disease), the superior pole of the patella (quadriceps tendon injury), the inferior pole of the patella (Sinding-Larsen-Johansson syndrome), the calcaneus (Sever's disease), the ischial tuberosity (origin of the *semimembranosus*, *semitendinosus* and long head of *biceps femoris*), the navicular (accessory navicular syndrome), the base of 5th metatarsal (Iselin's disease) and other sites.

See also AVULSION FRACTURE; ILIAC CREST APOPHYSITIS; OLECRANON OSTEO-CHONDROSIS.

APOPTOSIS Programmed cell death. It is a type of cell death that differs morphologically and biochemically from necrosis, although both appear to occur after exercise. In normal tissues, it provides a physiologic way to eliminate terminally differentiated, damaged or genetically altered cells, thus facilitating tissue remodeling after cell injury. Apoptosis is an important defensive barrier that inhibits carcinogenesis by eliminating mutant cells. Accelerated apoptosis has been documented to occur in a variety of disease states, such as AIDS and Alzheimer's disease, as well in the aging heart. Free radicals are intermediate messengers in several apoptosis signaling pathways. Administration of antioxidants inhibits apoptosis. Phaneuf and Leeuwenburgh (2001) speculate that exercise-induced apoptosis is a normal regulatory process that serves to remove certain damaged cells without a pronounced inflammatory response, thus ensuring optimal body function.

Bibliography

Phaneuf, S. and Leeuwenburgh, C. (2001). Apoptosis and exercise. *Medicine and Science in Sports and Exercise* 33(3), 393-396.

APPENDIX Vermiform appendix. A narrow vestigial process projecting from the cecum of the large intestine that is in the lower part of the abdomen of some mammals (including humans). **Appendicitis** is inflammation of the appendix. It may be acute or chronic. Rupture of an appendix can lead to feces and bacteria being sprayed over abdominal contents, causing peritonitis. If the appendix becomes obstructed (e.g. with hardened fecal material) venous circulation may be compromised leading to an increase in bacterial growth and pus. Chronic appendicitis may involve gangrene, rupture into the bowels, and peritonitis.

APPETITE The psychological desire to eat. Some drugs (e.g. amphetamines) decrease appetite; other drugs (e.g. antihistamines) increase appetite.

See also ANOREXIA; HUNGER; SATIETY.

APRAXIA *See* DEVELOPMENTAL COORDIN-ATION DISORDER.

ARACHIDONIC ACID An important mediator of the acute inflammatory process. It is the product of the interaction between enzymes supplied by leukocytes and phospholipids derived from the membranes of destroyed cells.

ARACHNOID *See under* HEAD.

ARCHIMEDES' PRINCIPLE The force of buoyancy is equal to the weight of the displaced fluid. *See under* BODY COMPOSITION.

ARCH SYSTEMS *See under* FOOT.

ARCUATE LIGAMENT *See under* KNEE LIGAMENTS; ULNAR NERVE.

AREA It is a two-dimensional measure of length. The Standard International unit is square-metres (m^2). 1 ft^2 is equal to 0.0929 m^2.

ARGININE A glucogenic (glycogenic), six carbon amino acid. It has a role in many protein structures, in the production of creatine, and in the urea cycle. Arginine is the precursor molecule for nitric oxide. *See under* GROWTH HORMONE.

ARM *See under* SKELETON.

ARNOLD-CHIARI MALFORMATION A condition in which the cerebellum protrudes into the spinal canal. **Arnold-Chiari I type malformation** usually causes symptoms in young adults and is often associated with syringomyelia. **Arnold-Chiari II type malformation** is a congenital defect of the hindbrain in which the posterior cerebellum herniates downward, displacing the medulla into the cervical spinal canal and obstructing the normal flow of cerebral spinal fluid. It is associated with myelomeningocele and hydrocephalus, which usually are apparent at birth. Myelomeningocele usually causes paralysis of the legs and, less commonly, the arms. If left untreated, hydrocephalus can cause mental impairment.

Symptoms of progressive brain impairment may include dizziness, an impaired ability to coordinate movement, double vision, and involuntary, rapid, downward eye movements. Most patients who have surgery experience a decrease in their symptoms.

Bibliography

March of Dimes Birth Defects Foundation. Http://marchofdimes.com

The National Institute of Neurological Disorders and Stroke. Http://www.ninds.nih.gov

AROUSAL A physiological construct that is most often defined as the state of general activation in the body that varies on a continuum of deep sleep to intense excitement. The reticular formation is involved in arousal. Arousal can be measured by electroencephalography and by other physiological measures such as heart rate.

There is conceptual confusion in some of the sport psychology literature between arousal and anxiety. One way of resolving such confusion is to assume that arousal is a construct based on physiological variables, while anxiety also involves self-report of cognitions and emotions.

Until recently, sport psychologists have assumed that the relationship between arousal and performance in sport is best described by an inverted-U (parabolic) relationship in which there is an optimal level of arousal for performance. Before and after the optimal point, performance drops off in a smooth manner. This relationship originates from the experimental work of Yerkes and Dodson (1908) that involved mice learning a choice discrimination task under weak, moderate and strong arousal. Shock was used to manipulate arousal. Performance was measured as the number of trials needed for the mice to select the brighter of two compartments. Task difficulty was manipulated by altering the difference in brightness between the two compartments. Learning was best under moderate stimulus levels and demonstrated the inverted-U relationship between arousal and performance. On more difficult tasks, the decrease in performance under increasing arousal conditions occurred earlier than it did for less difficult tasks.

One theory to explain the inverted-U relationship between arousal and performance as applied to humans concerns the narrowing of attention as arousal increases. This results in the filtering out of irrelevant cues (as arousal increases to the optimal point) and then relevant cues (as arousal increases beyond the optimal point).

It is now thought inappropriate to instruct athletes to raise or lower their physiological arousal without considering the quantity and quality of arousal-related cognitions.

Until recently, it has generally been assumed that arousal is unidimensional. In other words, functions such as heart rate and brain waves reflect the same underlying mechanism. There is evidence, however, that the variables used to measure arousal are not highly correlated, function independently and show different patterns corresponding to different emotional states. It is now thought that there may be more than one arousal system operating within the brain, and that emotions are not simply generalized arousal plus situation-specific cognitions about that arousal.

See ATTENTION; EMOTION.

Bibliography

Gould, D. and Udry, E. (1994). Psychological skills for enhancing performance: Arousal regulation strategies. *Medicine and Science in Sports and Exercise* 26(4), 478-485.

Neiss, R. (1988). Reconceptualizing arousal: Psychobiological states in motor performance. *Psychological Bulletin* 103(3), 345-366.

ARRHYTHMIAS *See* CARDIAC ARRYTHMIAS.

ARTERIAL DISSECTION A tear in the lining of an artery. A **cerebral arterial dissection** occurs when such a tear occurs in the carotid or vertebral arteries, the major arteries to the brain. The flow of blood in between the layers of the torn blood vessel may cause the artery to narrow and even close off entirely.

ARTERIAL ENDOFIBROSIS A disease that usually affects the external iliac artery in highly trained athletes. Since the early 1980s, an increasing incidence of iliac arterial stenosis has been reported in competition cyclists as well as many other male and female athletes.

Approximately 1 in 5 top-level cyclists will develop sports-related flow limitations in the iliac arteries.

These flow limitations may be caused by a vascular lumen narrowing due to endofibrotic thickening of the intima and/or by kinking of the vessels. In some athletes, extreme vessel length contributes to this kinking. Endofibrotic thickening is a result of repetitive vessel damage due to hemodynamic and mechanical stress. Athlerosclerotic intimal thickening is rarely encountered in these young athletes. This type of sports-related flow limitation shows no relationship with the classical risk factors for atherosclerosis, such as smoking, hypercholesterolemia or family predisposition for arterial diseases. If an athlete reports typical claudication-like complaints in a leg at maximal effort, which disappear quickly at rest, approximately 2 out of the 3 will have a flow limitation in the iliac artery. Conservative treatment consists of diminishing or even completely stopping the provocative sports activity. If conservative treatment is insufficient or deemed unacceptable, surgical treatment might be considered. In the early stages, when kinking has not yet led to intimal thickening or excessive lengthening, simple surgical release of the iliac artery is effective. For patients with excessive vessel length or extensive endofibrotic thickening, a vascular reconstruction may be necessary.

Bibliography

Abraham, P., Saumet, J.L. and Chevalier, J.M. (1997). External iliac artery endofibrosis in athletes. *Sports Medicine* 24(4), 221-226.

Abraham, P. et al. (1997). Lower extremity arterial disease in sports. *American Journal of Sports Medicine* 25(4), 581-584.

Abraham, P. et al. (2004). Past, present and future of arterial endofibrosis in athletes: A point of view. *Sports Medicine* 34(7), 419-425.

Arko, F.R. and Olcott, C. (2003). Arterial and venous injuries in athletes. Findings and their effect on diagnosis and treatment. *The Physician and Sportsmedicine* 31(4), 41-48.

Bender, M.H.M. et al. (2004). Sports-related flow limitations in the iliac arteries in endurance athletes: Etiology, diagnosis, treatment and future developments. *Sports Medicine* 34(7), 427-442.

Paraf, F. et al. (2000). External iliac artery endofibrosis of the cyclist. *Annals of Pathology* 20(3), 232-234.

Scavee, V. et al. (2003). External iliac artery endofibrosis: A new possible predisposing factor. *Journal of Vascular Surgery* 38(1), 1809-1810.

ARTERIAL-MIXED VENOUS OXYGEN CONTENT DIFFERENCE The difference in the oxygen content of the arterial and venous blood. It increases linearly with increases in exercise intensity. It also increases slightly with training. Possible mechanisms to explain the latter effect include a rightward shift of the oxyhemoglobin-dissociation curve, adaptations in mitochondria, increased myoglobin and/or increased muscle capillary density. Increased muscle capillary density leads to a shorter diffusion distance from capillaries to cells.

ARTERIAL PRESSURE *See under* BLOOD PRESSURE.

ARTERIAL STIFFNESS *See under* COMPLI-ANCE; PULSE PRESSURE; VENOUS COMPLIANCE.

ARTERIOLES Small blood vessels that connect capillaries to arteries. Arterioles possess properties similar to arteries but in addition can be surrounded circumferentially by layers of smooth muscle fibers that enable vasoconstriction and vasodilation.

ARTERIOSCLEROSIS A term which refers to the many conditions in which the arteries become thickened, hard and less elastic. *See under* CARDIOVASCULAR DISEASE.

ARTERY A tube that carries blood away from the heart to the arterioles, which in turn lead to capillaries. Arteries have limited ability to be distended (stretched) and to increase their vascular volume. This property is termed compliance. **Metarterioles** are short vessels that connect arterioles with the venules, creating a shortcut through the capillary bed. *See* AORTA.

ARTHRALGIA Pain in a joint.

ARTHRITIS Any condition associated with inflammation of a joint. More than 100 disorders have been identified that may lead to arthritis. The most common types of arthritis are osteoarthritis, fibromyalgia syndrome, rheumatoid arthritis, gout and ankylosing spondylitis.

Osteoarthritis is a heterogeneous group of conditions that lead to joint symptoms and signs associated with defective articular cartilage and changes to the underlying bone and joint margins. The term 'osteoarthritis' is also used to cover joint pain that appears to have a mechanical basis in the absence of clinical or radiographic evidence of cartilage loss. Symptoms of osteoarthritis usually include brief joint stiffness upon awakening, and joint pain or tenderness following use of the affected joints. The joints most commonly affected are the hips, spine and the thumb bases of the distal interphalangeal joints of the hand. **Primary osteoarthritis** occurs in the absence of any known predisposing factor, or etiology. It occurs most frequently in women and diabetics. **Secondary osteoarthritis** is the result of some underlying pre-existing condition or disorder. Four main categories of causes of secondary osteoarthritis are metabolic disorders, anatomic derangements (e.g. genu varus/genu valgus), major trauma (or surgery to a joint after trauma) and inflammatory disease (e.g. rheumatoid arthritis). In the USA, the prevalence of osteoarthritis is approximately 1 in 13 (20 million people). By the age of 40 years, almost everyone has some osteoarthritic changes in weight-bearing joints (e.g. hip and knee joints).

Osteoarthritis can be prevented only by decreasing or eliminating its risk factors, the most important of which are excess mechanical stresses brought about by anatomical or functional defects. These defects can be corrected by decreasing occupational or sports hazards and avoiding large or abrupt forces. The onset of osteoarthritis appears to depend on the frequency, intensity and duration of physical activity. There is some evidence that previous injury predisposes an athlete to osteoarthritis later in life.

Aerobic training may benefit osteoarthritis patients because of increases in aerobic capacity, muscle strength, pain tolerance, positive mood and increased social activity.

Fibromyalgia syndrome is a condition with generalized muscular pain, fatigue and poor sleep. It is not a true form of arthritis and does not cause deformity of the joints.

Rheumatoid arthritis is an autoimmune disease with unknown cause that affects more than 2.1 million people in the USA. It is a chronic inflammatory condition that affects joints, connective tissue, muscles and other tissues throughout the body. As inflammation spreads through a joint, articular cartilage is destroyed, cysts form in adjacent bone, scar tissue is formed, and the joint capsule becomes thickened. As a consequence, joint mobility is impaired. It is more common in women than in men, and usually begins between the ages of 20 and 30 years or 45 and 55 years. The average age of onset of **juvenile rheumatoid arthritis** is 6 years, with two peaks of incidence occurring between ages 2 and 4 years and between ages 8 and 11 years. It affects five times as many girls as boys. The knee is involved more often than other joints, causing a slight limp as the child walks. The characteristic swelling gives the appearance of knock-knees. Rheumatoid arthritis in children may be systemic (**Still's disease**), affecting the whole body, or peripheral, affecting only the joints. Still's disease is characterized by high fever and evanescent (transient) salmon-colored rash. **Adult-onset Still's disease** is also systemic and is a form of **polyarthritis** (inflammation of several joints). The cause of Still's disease is unknown.

In spite of enlargement of the liver and spleen, pericarditis and other side effects, rheumatoid arthritis is rarely fatal. It does cause severe disability in about 25% of the cases and mild to moderate disability in 30%. The purposes of movement for the child with rheumatoid arthritis are relief of pain and spasm, prevention of flexion contractures and other deformities, maintenance of normal range-of-motion for each joint and maintenance of strength (especially in the extensor muscles).

Gout is a metabolic disease resulting from a defect in the metabolism of purines. Crystal deposits of the sodium salt of uric acid accumulate in the joint. 95% of victims are middle-aged men. The first metatarsophalangeal joint is the most frequently affected joint. Factors leading to increased levels of uric acid and then gout include excessive alcohol intake, high blood pressure, kidney disease, obesity and certain drugs.

Ankylosing spondylitis is a relatively rare condition occurring mostly in males in their late teens or early twenties. It starts as an inflammation of the sacro-iliac joint.

There are many different kinds of drugs used to treat arthritis. Anti-inflammatory drugs generally work by slowing the body's production of prostaglandins. In the USA, the Federal Drug Agency (FDA) has approved three non-steroidal anti-inflammatory drugs for over-the-counter marketing: ibuprofen (e.g. Advil), naproxen sodium (Aleve) and Ketoprofen (e.g. Actron). A new type of NSAID, cyclooxygenase-2 inhibitors (COX-2 inhibitors), helps suppress arthritis with less stomach irritation. Remicade is a class of drug known as biologic response modifiers which block the action of tumor necrosis factor, believed to play a role in joint inflammation and damage.

The following activities are contraindicated for individuals with arthritis: all jumping, hopping and leaping activities; activities in which falls might be frequent; contact sports; diving; horseback riding; and sitting for long periods. Swimming is highly recommended, especially strokes such as the front crawl that emphasize extension. *See also* CHONDROMALACIA.

Bibliography

American College of Rheumatology. Http://www.rheumatology.org

Arthritis Foundation. Http://www.arthritis.org

Gordon, N.F. (1993). *Arthritis: Your complete exercise guide*. The Cooper Clinic and Research Institute Fitness Series. Champaign, IL: Human Kinetics.

Ike, R.W., Lampan, R.M. and Castor, C.W. (1989). Arthritis and aerobic exercise. *The Physician and Sportsmedicine* 17(2), 128-137.

International Stills Disease Foundation. Http://www.stillsdisease.org

Millar, A.L. (2003). *Action plan for arthritis: ACSM Action Plan for Health series*. Champaign, IL: Human Kinetics.

Panush, R.S. and Brown, D.G.(1987). Exercise and arthritis. *Sports Medicine* 4, 54-64.

Panush, R.S. and Inzinna, J.D. (1994). Recreational activities and degenerative joint disease. *Sports Medicine* 17(1), 1-5.

Petrella, R.J. (2000). Is exercise effective treatment for osteoarthritis of the knee? *British Journal of Sports Medicine* 34(5), 326-331.

Saxon, L., Finch, C. and Bass, S. (1999). Sports participation, sports injuries and osteoarthritis. Implications for prevention. *Sports Medicine* 28(2), 123-135.

ARTHROGRYPOSIS   Arthrogryposis multi-complex congenital. It involves the presence of multiple joint contractures at birth, and typically affects the hands, wrists, elbows, shoulders, hips, knees and feet. It is relatively rare, occurring in about 1 in 3,000 births. Each year in the USA about 500 infants are born with arthrogryposis. It is a nonprogressive disease and the severity varies widely, with some persons in wheelchairs and others only minimally affected. Persons with arthrogryposis may excel in track activities in a motorized chair. People with arthrogryposis have restricted range of motion, thus emphasis should be placed on exercises and activities that increase flexibility. Swimming encourages development of flexibility and also serves to strengthen weak muscle around joints.

Bibliography

Avenues: A National Support Group for Arthrogryposis Multicomplex Congenital.

Http://www.sonnet.com/avenues/pamplet.html

Winnick, J.P. (2000, ed). *Adapted physical education and sport*. 3rd ed. Champaign, IL: Human Kinetics.

ARTHROPATHY   Any disease of the joints.

ARTHROPLASTY   Reconstructing a joint through surgery.

ARTICULATION   *See* JOINT.

ASCORBIC ACID   *See* VITAMIN C.

ASOMATOGNOSIA   Failure to recognize parts of one's own body.

ASPARAGINE   A nonessential, glucogenic (glycogenic), four-carbon amino acid that is an amide of aspartate, another amino acid. If asparagine is degraded for energy, the enzyme asparaginase catalyses its conversion to aspartate, which is transaminated to oxaloacetate in a vitamin B_6-dependent reaction. Oxaloacetate either combines with acetyl CoA and enters the Krebs cycle, or is converted to phosphoenolpyruvate (PEP) and proceeds in gluconeogenesis.

ASPARTAME   A sugar substitute made from phenylalanine and aspartic acid that is found in 'diet' beverages and used as a non-nutritive sweetener.

ASPARTATE   A nonessential, glucogenic (glyco-genic), four-carbon, amino acid. It is sometimes referred to as aspartic acid. Aspartate is involved in the malate-aspartate shuttle in glycolysis. Aspartate is the donor of one of the nitrogens in urea. Three of aspartate's carbons, and one nitrogen, are incorporated into the pyrimidine ring of the pyrimidine bases cytosine, thymine and uracil. These bases are involved in protein synthesis. The degradation of aspartate by transamination to oxaloacetate permits its carbon skeleton to enter the Krebs cycle. In this process alpha ketoglutarate is converted to glutamate, which undergoes oxidative deamination (catalyzed by glutamate dehydro-genase), yielding an ammonium ion and reforming alpha ketoglutarate. The carbons of aspartate can also enter the Krebs cycle via fumarate from the urea cycle.

ASPARTIC ACID   *See* ASPARTATE.

ASPERGER'S SYNDROME   A type of pervasive developmental disorder characterized by severe and sustained impairment in social interaction, coupled with stereotypies, obsessions and compulsions, which seriously impacts function. Asperger's syndrome is much more common than autism, and appears to have a somewhat later onset than autistic disorder. Unlike autistic disorder, there are no clinically significant delays in language, cognitive function, self-help skills, adaptive behaviors (except for social interaction) or curiosity about the environment.

The diagnostic criteria used by the American Psychiatric Association are: (A) Qualitative impairment in social interaction, as manifested by at least two of the following: marked impairment in the use of multiple nonverbal behaviors such as eye-to-eye gaze, facial expression, body postures and gestures to regulate social interaction; failure to develop peer relationships appropriate to developmental level; and a lack of spontaneous seeking to share enjoyment, interests or achievements with other people; and a lack of social or emotional reciprocity. (B) Restricted repetitive and stereotyped patterns of behavior, interests and activities, as manifested by at least one of the following: encompassing preoccupation with one or more stereotyped and restricted patterns of interest that is abnormal either in intensity or focus; apparently inflexible adherence to specific, nonfunctional routines or rituals; stereotyped and repetitive motor mannerisms (e.g. hand or finger flapping or twisting, or complex whole-body movements); and persistent preoccupation with parts of objects. (C) The disturbance causes clinically significant impairment in social, occupational or other important areas of functioning. (D) There is no clinically significant general delay in language. (E) There is no clinically significant delay in cognitive development or in the development of age-appropriate self-help skills, adaptive behavior (other than in social interaction) and curiosity about the environment in childhood. (F) Criteria are not met for another specific Pervasive Developmental Disorder of Schizophrenia.

The major diagnostic criterion for delay in language is inability to use single words by age 2 years and to speak in phrases by age 3 years. While many individuals with autism have mental retardation, a person with Asperger's syndrome possesses an average to above average intelligence. Therefore, Asperger's syndrome should not be referred to as 'high-functioning autism.'

People with Asperger's syndrome love winning and praise, but find losing and criticism hard to take.

Bad behavior often results from an inability to communicate their frustrations and anxieties. Some talk incessantly on a topic of interest only to themselves without knowing the listener's lack of interest. They often appear to talk 'at' rather than 'to' people, giving information rather than holding proper conversations.

Bibliography

American Psychiatric Association (1994). *Diagnostic and Statistical Manual of Mental Disorders*. 4th ed. Washington, DC: American Psychiatric Association.

Asperger Syndrome Coalition of the USA. Http://www.asperger.org

ASPHYXIA   Impairment of ventilatory exchange of oxygen and carbon dioxide; combined with hypercapnia and hypoxia or anoxia. Traumatic asphyxia results from direct, massive trauma to the thorax.

ASPIRIN   Acetyl salicylic acid. It is a drug that is commonly used as an analgesic (pain-relief) agent, antipyretic agent (to decrease elevated body temperature), anti-inflammatory agent and anti-coagulant. At low dosages, it inhibits the formation of thromboxane A_2, decreasing platelet aggregation and platelet plug formation. Thromboxane A_2 is formed from a phospholipid, arachidonic acid, located in the membrane of platelets. At high dosages, however, aspirin decreases formation of prostacyclin, which actually increases the likelihood of clot formation. There is evidence that a single daily dose of about 325 mg of aspirin can have a highly protective effect against acute myocardial infarction in men with unstable angina pectoris and a significant decrease in mortality. There do not seem to be adverse effects associated with taking aspirin and engaging in exercise. Some individuals, however, are allergic to aspirin and it could lead to anaphylaxis.

There is no evidence of an overall increase in the risk of congenital malformations through use of aspirin during the first trimester of pregnancy. There may, however, be an association between aspirin exposure during the first trimester and an increased risk of **gastroschisis**, which is a defect in the abdominal wall resulting from rupture of the amniotic membrane that envelopes the embryo.

See also EPHEDRINE; NON-STEROIDAL ANTI-INFLAMMATORY DRUGS.

Bibliography

De Meersman, R.E. (1990). Aspirin and exercise as a prophylaxis for heart disease: Is it safe? *Sports Medicine* 9(2), 71-75.

Kozer, E. et al. (2002). Aspirin consumption during the first trimester of pregnancy and congenital anomalies: A meta-analysis. *American Journal of Obstetrics and Gynecology* 187(6), 1623-1630.

ASSERTIVENESS   *See under* COMMUNICA-TION.

ASSIMILATION   *See under* COGNITIVE DEVELOPMENT.

ASTEREOGNOSIA   A state in which a person is unable to recognize objects by touch.

ASTHMA   A disease characterized by an increased responsiveness of the trachea and bronchi to various stimuli. Symptoms include constriction of the respiratory passages, impaired breathing, wheezing, coughing, urticaria and anaphylaxis. **Cough-type asthma** is characterized by a chronic, non-productive cough that is exacerbated by exercise and upper respiratory tract infections. About 30 to 50% of patients suffering cough-type asthma may progress to '**classical asthma**' with wheezing.

The classical mechanism triggering an asthma attack is coupling of an antigen to immunoglobulin-E antibodies on the surface of sensitized mast cells, leading to the release of various biochemical mediators causing airway smooth muscle constriction. The antigen-antibody interaction may also stimulate vagal neural reflexes directly to cause bronchoconstriction.

Asthma is characterized by the presence of increased numbers of eosinophils, neutrophils, lymphocytes and plasma cells in the bronchial tissues, bronchial secretions and mucus. Physical stimuli, such as cooling and cold air exposure, may directly stimulate the release of chemical mediators.

Other triggers of asthma include air pollution, allergy, drugs, cigarette smoke, emotion, exercise, infection and stress. Regardless of the triggers of asthma, the repeated cycles of inflammation in the lungs with injury to the pulmonary tissues followed by repair may produce long-term structural changes ('remodeling') of the airways. Prolonged bronchospasm leads to secondary mucosal edema and mucus accumulation.

During an acute asthmatic attack, lung units distal to the constricted bronchi are hypoventilated, and regions of low ventilation-perfusion ratio develop. Patients typically hyperventilate initially, maintaining a normal partial pressure of oxygen in arteries, while partial pressure of carbon dioxide decreases. As the attack worsens, the distribution of ventilation-perfusion becomes more abnormal, and partial pressure of oxygen in the arteries declines despite persistent hyperventilation. People with asthma adapt to hyperventilation. If their asthma disappears perman-ently, then an increased rate of breathing will cause serious problems unless it is corrected, because increased hyperventilation makes the carbon dioxide levels fall.

In the USA, the prevalence of asthma is approximately 1 in 15 (17.4 million) people. Asthma affects up to 25% of children in Western urban environmental settings. During childhood and adolescence, asthmatic individuals seem to have physical activity levels comparable with those of the normal pediatric population. However, differences in physical activity levels may develop during the time of maturation from adolescence into adulthood.

Although most asthmatics tend to develop exercise-induced bronchoconstriction, sport and exercise are now accepted as valuable in the management of asthma. About 80% of people with asthma have symptoms triggered by exercise. Symptoms of exercise-induced asthma include coughing, wheezing, chest tightness, and difficulty in breathing that is triggered by exercise. Symptoms usually begin after exercise and worsen about fifteen minutes after exercise stops. If exercise is attempted within three hours, the symptoms are less severe. Team sports, involving intermittent exercise, such as football, are less likely to cause asthma symptoms than continuous exercise. Since it is likely that exercise-induced asthma is related to physical stimuli directly causing mast cell degranulation, prophylactic use of an inhaled bronchodilator or a mast cell-stabilizing drug, such as cromolyn sodium, before exercise, commonly prevents attacks.

Approximately 10 to 15 million Americans are scuba divers. Conditions present during scuba diving may provoke airway obstruction in asthmatic patients. Theoretically, asthmatic patients may face a greater than normal risk of pulmonary barotrauma from lung overdistention on ascent through the water. However, it has been found that asthmatic patients with normal airway function at rest, and with little airway reactivity in response to exercise or cold air inhalation, have a risk of pulmonary barotrauma similar to that of nonasthmatic individuals. People with asthma can participate in parachute jumping or skydiving if their asthma is completely controlled, and if neither cold air nor exercise is a trigger.

A number of drugs have been developed to control asthma. Inhaled corticosteroids are the most effective anti-inflammatory treatment available for persistent asthma. These drugs function by suppressing the generation of cytokines, recruitment of eosinophils, and release of inflammatory mediators. Side effects include cough, dysphonia (a disorder of oral speech) and oral thrush. All of these side effects can be greatly decreased by the use of a spacer and mouth washing after treatments. A **spacer** device attached to an inhaler decreases the amount of oropharangeal deposition and drug swallowed. It is used with pressurized metered inhalers. It is possible that inhaled corticosteroids may have a dose-dependent adverse effect on linear growth in some children. Both cromolyn sodium and nedocromil have anti-inflammatory effects by blockading chloride channels and the modulation of mast cell mediator release and eosinophil recruitment. Both of these drugs can be used in exercise-induced bronchospasm and in mild, persistent asthma. The two leukotriene-modifying drugs currently available are Zafirlukast and Zileuton. Their role in asthma treatment has not been firmly established. Zileuton is a 5-lipoxygenase inhibitor. Zafirlukast is a leukotriene receptor antagonist. Oral

corticosteroids can be useful in short courses for speeding resolution of asthma exacerbations. Like inhaled corticosteroids, these drugs function by suppressing the generation of cytokines, recruitment of eosinophils, and release of inflammatory mediators. The side effects of long-term corticosteroid use include: pituitary-hypothalamic axis suppression; osteoporosis; growth suppression; dermal thinning; hypertension; diabetes; cataracts; muscle weakness; and Cushing's syndrome. Short-acting beta$_2$ agonists are the medications of choice in treating asthma exacerbations and exercise-induced bronchospasm. The regularly scheduled, daily use of these drugs is not recommended. Side effects include tachycardia, skeletal muscle tremor, hypokalemia, increased lactic acid and headache. Beta$_2$ selective agents are preferred due to decreased potential for excessive cardiac stimulation. Long-acting beta$_2$ agonists function to relax the bronchial smooth muscle via the stimulation of beta$_2$ receptors. These medications have a duration of at least 12 hours. Side effects include tachycardia, skeletal muscle tremor and hypokalemia. Theophylline, the most common methylxanthine, causes mild to moderate bronchodilation. There is some evidence that theophylline may also have a mild anti-inflammatory component. Side effects include insomnia, gastric upset, and aggravation of gastric ulcers or reflux.

There is no evidence to suggest that non-asthmatics can benefit from taking anti-asthma medication as an ergogenic aid. It thus seems that anti-asthmatic drugs merely allow the asthmatic to overcome respiratory disadvantage. There is insufficient evidence to recommend the use of room air ionizers to decrease symptoms in patients with chronic asthma.

See also EXERCISE-INDUCED BRONCHO-CONSTRICTION; LEUKOCYTES.

Chronology

•1972 • Rick De Mont, who a year later was to become the first swimmer to break the four-minute barrier in the 400m freestyle, became the first swimmer to be stripped of an Olympic gold medal when he tested positive for ephedrine. This was included in the 16-year old's asthma medication, which he declared on his medical form. American team doctors had failed to notify De

Mont that the drug was banned.

Bibliography

Blackhall, K., Appleton, S. and Cates, C.J. (2003). Ionizers for chronic asthma. *Cochrane Database Systems Reviews* 3: CD002986.

Cummiskey, J. (2001). Exercise-induced asthma: An overview. *American Journal of Medical Science* 322(4), 200-203.

Fireman, P. (2003). Understanding asthma pathophysiology. *Allergy and Asthma Proceedings* 24(2), 79-83.

Koehle, M. et al. (2003). Asthma and recreational SCUBA diving: A systematic review. *Sports Medicine* 33(2), 109-116.

Langdeau, J.B. and Boulet, L.P. (2001). Prevalence and mechanisms of development of asthma and airway hyperresponsiveness in athletes. *Sports Medicine* 31(8), 601-616.

Morton, A.R. and Fitch, K.D. (1992). Asthmatic drugs and competitive sport: An update. *Sports Medicine* 14(4), 228-242.

Mottram, D.R. (1999). Banned drugs in sport. Does the International Olympic Committee (IOC) list need updating? *Sports Medicine* 27(1), 1-10.

National Asthma Campaign. Http://www.asthma.org.uk

Neuman, T.S. et al. (1994). Asthma and diving. *Annals of Allergy* 73(4), 344-350.

O'Connell, E.J. et al. (1991). Cough-type asthma: A review. *Annals of Allergy* 66(4), 278-282; 285.

Storms, W.W. (2003). Review of exercise-induced asthma. *Medicine and Science in Sports and Exercise* 35(9), 1464-1470.

Welsh, L., Roberts, R.G.D. and Kemp, J.G. (2004). Fitness and physical activity in children with asthma. *Sports Medicine* 34(13), 861-870.

ASTIGMATISM   A cylindrical curvature of the cornea that prevents light rays from focusing properly on the retina. As a consequence, both near and far objects may appear blurry. It often occurs in combination with myopia and hyperopia.

ASTRAGALUS   *See* TALUS.

ASYMMETRICAL TONIC NECK REFLEX   A primitive reflex that is rare in the newborn infant, but persists through to the age of 3 to 4 months. It is elicited as a result of turning the head to one side. As the head is turned, the arm and leg on the same side will extend while the opposite limbs assume an acute flexed posture. It helps to break up flexor- and extensor-pattern dominance so that each side of the body can function separately.

When a baby is born it can only focus its eyes at about 8 inches. Outside of this range, the baby can see movement and shadow, but it cannot focus. Through the asymmetrical tonic neck reflex, the baby slowly extends the vision from near point fixation to distance, and is therefore vital for eye-hand coordination training.

Failure of this reflex to become integrated prevents learning to roll from supine to prone and vice versa, because the extended arm gets in the way. It interferes with limb movement, which, in turn, impairs the development of normal hand-eye coordination. An associated problem is loss of visual fixation. It prevents independent flexion of the limb to bring it toward the midline, such as during feeding. Children and adults with severe cerebral palsy often exhibit a persistent asymmetrical tonic neck reflex. A degree of asymmetrical tonic neck reflex is normal in all children and adults.

See also SYMMETRIC TONIC NECK REFLEX.

ASYSTOLE   Absence of contractions of the heart.

ATAXIA   A symptom of coordination difficulties that can be associated with infections, injuries, other diseases, or degenerative changes in the central nervous system. In cerebral palsy, stroke and traumatic brain injury, the ataxia is of cerebellar-vestibular origin. Ataxia is diagnosed only in people who can walk unaided. When persons can maintain balance with eyes open, but not closed, ataxia is usually the diagnosis. To compensate for extreme unsteadiness of gait, the arms are typically overactive in balance-saving movements. Falls are frequent.

Ataxia is also used to denote a group of specific degenerative diseases of the nervous system called the hereditary and sporadic ataxias. **Hereditary ataxia** is degenerative and the severity depends on the type of ataxia. A number of genes for hereditary ataxias have been identified, the first of which was called the **spinocerebellar ataxia type I**. It is inherited as an autosomal dominant trait. The various abnormal genes that cause ataxia have in common that they make abnormal proteins that affect nerve cells, primarily in the cerebellum (and in other parts of the brain) and the spinal cord. **Sporadic ataxia** can be either 'pure cerebellar,' where only the cerebellum is involved, or **olivopontocerebellar ataxia**.

Friedreich's ataxia is an inherited condition in which there is progressive degeneration of the sensory nerves of the limbs and trunk, which results in diminished kinesthetic input. Inheritance is autosomal recessive. It first occurs between the ages of 5 and 15 years, and is often associated with diabetes or heart disease. The primary indicators are ataxia, clumsiness and lack of agility. The majority of persons have heart problems, such as heart murmur. Diabetes develops in 10 to 40% of persons. Visual abnormalities include nystagmus and poor visual tracking. Many associated defects, such as diminished fine motor control and tremor of the upper extremities, may also develop and affect sport performance.

Bibliography

National Ataxia Foundation. Http://www.ataxia.org

National Organization for Rare Disorders. Http://www.rarediseases.org

Sherill, C. (2004). *Adapted physical activity, recreation and sport. Cross disciplinary and lifespan.* 6th ed. Boston, MA: McGraw-Hill.

ATENOLOL *See under* BETA-BLOCKERS.

ATHEROSCLEROSIS *See under* CARDIO-VASCULAR DISEASE.

ATHETOSIS An involuntary overflow disorder that is characterized by constant, unpredictable and purposeless movement caused by fluctuating muscle tone that is sometimes hypertonic and sometimes hypotonic. Damage to the basal ganglia in the cerebral white matter is the primary cause of athetosis. It is the second most common type of motor disorder after spasticity.

Constant movement is most troublesome to the head and upper extremities, thus there are difficulties with facial expression, eating and speaking. The head is usually drawn back, but may roll unpredictably from side to side with tongue protrusion and drooling. Lack of head control causes problems of visual pursuit and focus that impair ability to read and perform hand-eye accuracy tasks. Constant movement of the fingers and wrist render handwriting and fine muscle coordination almost impossible.

There are many types of athetosis, such as dystonia (with fluctuating muscle tone), mixed with spasticity (in which muscle tone is most hypertonic), mixed with floppy baby syndrome (in which muscle tone is primarily hypotonic), and mixed with ataxia. Changes from one type to another sometimes occur with age, particularly from floppy baby to dystonic children.

Chorea and athetosis can occur together (choreoathetosis). The disease that most often produces choreoathetosis is Huntington's disease.

Most persons with athetosis are quadriplegic. Many persons with athetosis use wheelchairs, but some have enough motor control to walk. Their gait is typically unsteady or staggering, with short steps taken in order to maintain balance. They walk with trunk and shoulder girdle leaning backward, reinforcing extensor muscle tone, to prevent collapsing. The hips and knees tend to be hyperextended, with lumbar lordosis, and the feet in dorsal flexion, pronation and eversion. Persons with such gait can compete in track athletics, but wear knee and elbow pads and gloves.

ATHLETE'S FOOT Tinea pedis. A very common infection of the feet caused by mold-like fungi (dermatophytes). It is contagious and is spread by direct contact, or contact with shoes, stockings, and shower or pool surfaces. Risk factors include poor hygiene, closed footwear, prolonged wetness of the feet (such as from sweating during exercise) and minor skin or nail injuries. The infection can be controlled by application of over-the-counter anti-fungal powders or creams, such as those containing miconazole and clotrimazole.

ATHLETE'S HEART *See under* CARDIAC HYPERTROPHY.

ATHLETIC IDENTITY *See under* SELF CONCEPT.

ATHLETIC PUBALGIA   *See under* HERNIA.

ATHLETIC TRAINING   An allied-health profession that specializes in: prevention of athletic injuries; recognition, evaluation and assessment of athletic injuries; the immediate care of athletic injuries; and treatment, rehabilitation and reconditioning of athletic injuries. In cooperation with physicians and other allied-health personnel, the athletic trainer functions as an integrated member of the athletic healthcare team in secondary schools, colleges and universities, sports medicine clinics, professional sports programs, industrial settings and other health-care environments.

See also SPORTS PHYSIOTHERAPY.

Chronology

•1914 • *Athletic Training* was published by Michael C. Murphy, the athletic trainer and coach of football and track at Yale and then the University of Pennsylvania.

•1917 • *The Trainer's Bible* was published by Samuel E. Bilik, former trainer at the University of Illinois.

•1921 • *Training for Sports* was published by Walter Camp, Yale's famous football coach.

•1931 • *Training, Conditioning, and the Care of Injuries* was published by Walter E. Meanwell, a physician and former basketball coach at the University of Wisconsin, and Knute Rockne, the legendary Notre Dame football coach.

•1938 • *Athletic Injuries: Prevention, Diagnosis and Treatment* was published by Augustus Thorndike, Jr, Harvard's team physician. It was regarded as the authoritative work on the subject until Don H. O'Donoghue's Treatment of Injuries to Athletes was published in 1962.

•1938 • The National Athletic Training Association (NATA) was formed. It ceased to exist after 1944, but reformed in 1950. It has a current membership of about 23,000 and is the professional organization to which most athletic trainers belong.

•1967 • The American Medical Association (AMA) first recognized the role of the athletic trainer as an important part of the health care of the athlete.

•1969 • The first National Athletic Trainer's Association (NATA) certification examination took place.

•1980 • A resolution was passed by the National Athletic Trainers Association (NATA) board of directors that all existing NATA-approved programs become academic major or major equivalents in athletic training by 1990 or sooner.

Bibliography

Anderson, M.K., Hall, S.J. and Martin, M. (2004). *Foundations of athletic training: Prevention, assessment and management*. 3rd ed. Philadelphia, PA: Lippincott, Williams and Wilkins.

Arnheim, D.D. and Prentice, W.E. (2002). *Essentials of athletic training*. 5th ed. Boston, MA: McGraw-Hill.

Berryman, J.W. (1995). *Out of many, one: A history of the American College of Sports Medicine*. Champaign, IL: Human Kinetics.

Hillman, S.K. (2000). *Introduction to athletic training*. Champaign, IL: Human Kinetics.

National Athletic Trainers' Association. Http://www.nata.org

Schenck, R. (2002, ed). *Athletic training and sports medicine*. 2nd ed. Rosemount, IL: American Academy of Orthopedic Surgeons.

ATHLETICISM   *See under* CHARACTER BUILDING.

ATLANTO-AXIAL JOINT   Articulation of the atlas (the first cervical vertebra) with the axis (the second cervical vertebra). There are four distinct joints, one of which is a pivot joint. Movement involves rotation of the atlas (and hence the cranium) upon the axis.

Approximately 10 to 30% of youth with Down syndrome have **atlanto-axial joint instability**. Instability indicates that the ligaments and muscles surrounding the joint are lax and that the vertebrae can slip out of alignment easily. Almost all are asymptomatic. The cause is not fully understood. Symptomatic atlanto-axial joint instability results from subluxation (excessive slippage) that is severe enough to injure the spinal cord, or from dislocation at the atlanto-axial joint. The neurologic manifestations of symptomatic atlanto-axial joint instability include easy fatigability, difficulties in walking, abnormal gait, neck pain, limited neck mobility, torticollis, incoordination and clumsiness, sensory deficits, spasticity and hyper-reflexia. In rare cases, symptoms may progress to paraplegia, hemiplegia, quadriplegia, or death.

Since 1983, Special Olympics has required a physician's statement, based on x-ray analysis, that indicates absence of atlanto-axial joint instability in persons with Down syndrome as a prerequisite for unrestricted participation in Special Olympics. Forceful flexion or extension of the neck, which occurs in gymnastics, swimming and other sporting events, may dislocate the atlas, causing damage to the spinal cord. Eleven years after its original position statement, which supported the use of x-ray testing for atlanto-axial joint instability, the American Academy of Pediatrics (AAP) stated that uncertainty exists concerning the value of cervical spine x-rays in screening for possible catastrophic neck injury in athletes with Down syndrome. Pueschel (1998) opposed the revised AAP statement, arguing that the x-ray may not be ideal, but it is the best screening available. Pueschel's arguments are: i) symptomatic atlanto-axial joint instability (that may occur in up to 1 to 2% of all children with Down syndrome) is a serious disorder, which justifies the work and expense required to detect it; ii) while it isn't known if asymptomatic atlanto-axial joint instability turns into symptomatic atlanto-axial joint instability, it hasn't been disproven; iii) the lack of reports of spinal cord injury from any activity associated with Special Olympics may mean either that such an injury is a rare occurrence or that the Special Olympics's precautionary measures are effective at preventing such injuries; iv) if one waits for significant neurologic signs to appear, spinal cord damage may have already occurred – by waiting, an individual at risk with no symptoms will not be detected; and v) lateral neck x-rays may also detect the less common but more serious atlanto-occipital instability, or degenerative changes in the cervical spine.

Nonachondroplasia dwarfism is also associated with atlanto-axial instability.

Bibliography

American Academy of Pediatrics Committee on Sports Medicine and Fitness (1995). Atlantoaxial instability in Down syndrome: Subject review. *Pediatrics* 96(1), 151-154.

Pueschel, S. (1998). Should children with Down syndrome be screened for atlanto-axial instability? *Archives of Pediatric and Adolescent Medicine* 152(2), 123-125.

ATLANTO-OCCIPITAL FUSION   Occipitaliza-tion of the atlas. It is a fusion of the atlas to the occipital bone. One of the most common skeletal abnormalities of the upper cervical spine, the onset of symptoms is usually in the third or fourth decade

of life but younger patients are usually asymptomatic. Symptoms include torticollis. Trauma may be a precipitating factor in at least 50% of reported symptomatic cases.

ATLAS   The first cervical vertebra. *See under* ATLANTO-AXIAL JOINT.

ATOM   A unit of matter consisting of a single nucleus with one or more electrons in orbit around that nucleus.

ATOMIC NUMBER   *See under* ELEMENT.

ATOMIC WEIGHT   *See under* MOLE.

ATOPY   *See under* ALLERGY.

ATP   *See* ADENOSINE TRIPHOSPHATE.

ATRESIA   Congenital absence or closure of a normal body opening or tubular structure. Tricuspid atresia is the absence of tricuspid orifice; circulation being made possible by the atrial septal defect (shunt is from left atrium to right atrium).

ATRIAL FIBRILLATION   A cardiac arrhythmia that is common in older adults. When the atria are fibrillating, impulses arrive from the atrial muscle at the atrioventricular node rapidly but also irregularly. The **internodal pathways** conduct the impulse from the sinus node to the atrioventricular node. The **atrioventricular node** is where the impulse from the atria is delayed before passing into the ventricles. The **atrioventricular bundle** conducts the impulse from the atria into the ventricles.

Atrial fibrillation is characterized by a rapid, irregular heart rate and the absence of a properly timed atrial contraction, resulting in a decline of cardiac output (as much as 20% in those with relatively normal ventricles). About 70% of people who have atrial fibrillation are between 65 and 85 years old, and most suffer from hypertension, ischemic heart disease, congestive heart failure or other underlying conditions such as pulmonary disease. In patients with cardiac disease, cardiac output may decline by up to 40%. Atrial fibrillation may compromise ability to perform physical activity. Patients with atrial fibrillation are at increased risk of developing atrial thrombus that may embolize to organs including the brain.

Bibliography

Reiss, R.A. (1999). Managing atrial fibrillation in active patients and athletes. *The Physician and Sportsmedicine*, 27(3), 73-83.

ATRIAL NATRIURETIC PEPTIDE

Atrial natriuretic hormone. Atrial natriuretic factor. A fluid-regulating hormone that is secreted by certain cells of the atria in the heart when they are stretched by the effects of elevated blood pressure. It is secreted during hyperhydration or increased venous return. It has two target organs: the kidney and the adrenal cortex. In the kidney, it inhibits sodium reabsorption and renin release. In the adrenal cortex, it inhibits the secretion of aldosterone. It thus has diuretic and natriuretic (salt-excreting) effects.

There is evidence that atrial natriuretic peptide is elevated during and immediately following exercise. The predominant stimuli for the release of atrial natriuretic peptide during exercise appear to be increases in atrial pressures and atrial distension. Elevations in plasma atrial natriuretic peptide may in part by responsible for the increase in urine flow reported when exercise is performed at low or moderate intensities.

Atrial natriuretic peptide also has vascular effects that may be important in buffering or moderating the blood pressure response to exercise.

Bibliography

Freund, B.J., Wade, C.E. and Claybaugh, J.R. (1988). The effects of exercise on atrial natriuretic factor release mechanisms and implications for fluid homeostasis. *Sports Medicine* 6(6), 364-377.

ATRIAL REFLEX

Bainbridge reflex. A reflex initiated by an increase in venous return and blood congestion in the atria. Stretching of the atrial walls produces an increase in heart rate and force, by directly stimulating the sinoatrial node and by stimulating baroreceptors in the atria, which trigger reflexive adjustments that result in increased sympathetic stimulation of the heart.

ATRIUM

One of the chambers of the heart; there is one on each side of the heart. It receives blood from the veins and pumps it into the ventricle. *See also under* LUNGS.

ATROPHY

Decrease in size of cells and tissue. *See* MUSCLE ATROPHY.

ATTENTION

The selection of information from the perceptual system. It depends on both sensory input and past experience. Information processing models of the attentional process hypothesize that at some stage a 'bottleneck' or selective filter occurs in order to restrict the amount of information that can be attended to at a particular moment in time. Attention is often defined in terms of whether or not there is interference between two tasks that a person is performing simultaneously. Information processing models assume that the capacity to process information is limited and that performance will be adversely affected if capacity is overtaxed by task requirements (capacity changes as task requirements change).

Attention is often considered as synonymous with conscious control. It is widely believed that many highly learned sports skills become automatic in the sense that they are executed without much attention. On the other hand, in the early stages of learning a skill there would seem to be a need for more conscious attention. Automaticity occurs when a person performs a skill or engages in an information-processing activity without demands on attention capacity. Logan (1998) regards automaticity as an acquired skill that should be viewed as a continuum of varying degrees of automaticity. Rather than study attention as a process, sport psychologists have tended to study attention as a personality variable called attentional style.

See AROUSAL; MOTOR LEARNING; NICOTINE.

Bibliography

Landers, D.M. (1982). Arousal, attention and skilled

performance: Further considerations. *Quest* 33, 271-283.

Logan, G.D. (1998). What is learned during automatization? II Obligatory encoding of spatial location. *Journal of Experimental Psychology: Human Perception and Performance* 24, 1720-1736.

ATTENTIONAL STYLE   The characteristic manner in which a person attends to the environment. Nideffer's (1976) two-dimensional model of the direction (internal-external) and width (broad-narrow) of attention has been extensively used by sport psychologists. A self-report inventory called the "Test of Attentional and Interpersonal Style" (TAIS) includes six attentional style subscales: Broad-External (the ability to effectively integrate many external stimuli simultaneously), External Overload (the tendency to become confused and overloaded with external stimuli), Broad-Internal (the ability to effectively integrate several ideas at one time), Internal Overload (the tendency to become overloaded by internal stimuli), Narrow Focus (the ability to effectively narrow attention where appropriate) and Reduced Focus (chronically narrowed attention). A strong correlation has been found between the 'overload' subscales of TAIS and trait anxiety.

In a study of tennis players, Van Schoyck and Grasha (1981) found that a tennis-specific version of TAIS was more valid than the TAIS. It was found that the direction of attention was not a strong factor. The results suggested instead that the 6 attentional scales of the TAIS could be collapsed into two scales reflecting Wachtel's (1967) concepts of "scan" and "focus." Scan refers to the allocation of attention to many aspects of the stimulus field, including both external stimuli and internal processes. It can be broad or narrow. Focus refers to the degree to which a person can bring various factors to bear on each other and can use them simultaneously to construct a more complete and balanced picture of his internal or external world. Similar results have been obtained from studies of basketball players, cricketers and fencers. The factors under focus seem to relate to the subjective experience of an inability to concentrate. Anxiety would seem to have a negative effect on an individual's ability to integrate stimuli and may be associated with increased scanning, where the person continually shifts from one input cue to another.

The main technique in Nideffer's Attentional Control Training is "**centering**," which involves progressive relaxation and breathing exercises. It also involves use of the TAIS. Techniques to stay centered include: use of verbal or kinesthetic cues to focus concentration or re-trigger lost concentration; mental rehearsal of successful performance immediately after a failure; use of biofeedback to show the effects of thoughts and imagery on the body; training to improve attentional focus, such as focusing on a single thought for as long as possible; and associating concentration with pre-performance routines or rituals.

A distinction has been made between "association" and "dissociation" with respect to marathon running. An **associative strategy** involves a narrow-internal attentional focus and a monitoring of bodily sensations. It contrasts with a **dissociative style** that is characterized by distraction, such as focus on external objects or task-irrelevant thoughts like recounting events from daily life. Although there is equivocal evidence as to which attentional style is more effective, there is some evidence that association may be related to faster performance, and that dissociation relates to lower perceived exertion and possibly greater endurance. Association may allow runners to continue performing despite painful sensory input and may lead to increased risk of injury; dissociation does not appear to increase the risk of injury.

See INJURY; PAIN; PERCEIVED EXERTION; RUNNING.

Bibliography

Masters, K.S. and Ogles, B.M. (1998). Associative and dissociative cognitive strategies in exercise and running: 20 years later on, what do we know? *The Sport Psychologist* 12(3), 253-270.

Morgan, W.P. and Pollock, M.L. (1977). Psychologic characterization of the elite distance runner. *Annals of the New York Academy of Sciences* 301, 382-403.

Nideffer, R.M. (1976). Test of Attentional and Interpersonal style. *Journal of Personality and Social Psychology* 34, 394-404.

Nideffer, R.M. (1990). Use of the Test of Attentional and Interpersonal Style (TAIS) in sport. *The Sport Psychologist* 4(3), 285-300.

Nideffer, R.M. and Sagal, M-S (1998). Concentration and attention control training. In Williams, J.M. (ed). *Applied sport psychology: Personal growth to peak performance.* 3rd ed. pp296-315. Mountain View, CA: Mayfield.

Schmid, A. and Peper, E. (1998). Strategies for training concentration. In Williams, J.M. (ed). *Applied sport psychology: Personal growth to peak performance.* 3rd ed. pp316-328. Mountain View, CA: Mayfield.

Summers, J.J. and Ford, S.K. (1990). The Test of Attentional and Interpersonal Style: An evaluation. *International Journal of Sport Psychology* 21(2), 102-111.

Van Schoyck, S.R. and Grasha, A.F. (1981). Attentional style variations and athletic ability: The advantages of a sports-specific test. *Journal of Sport Psychology* 3, 141-165.

Wachtel, P.L. (1967). Conception of broad and narrow attention. *Psychological Bulletin* 68, 417-429.

ATTENTION-DEFICIT HYPERACTIVITY DISORDER

ADHD. A persistent pattern of inattention and/or hyperactivity-impulsivity that is more frequent and severe than that typically observed in individuals at a comparable level of development. Some symptoms of ADHD must have been present before the age of 7 years. Three ADHD subtypes are recognized by the American Psychiatric Association (1994): ADHD, combined type; ADHD, predominantly inattention type; and ADHD, predominantly hyperactivity-impulsivity type. Approximately one-third of people with ADHD do not have the hyperactive component.

ADHD is not recognized by Individuals with Disabilities Education Act (IDEA), thus is not eligible for special education services, except in conjunction with disabilities specified in the IDEA. Children who do not qualify for services under IDEA can receive help under an earlier law, the National Rehabilitation Act, Section 504, which defines disabilities more broadly.

Inattention is characterized by the inability to sustain attention to a task, respond to a task, abide by rules or follow instructions at the same level as others of the same age. **Hyperactivity-impulsivity** (disinhibition) encompasses behaviors such as fidgeting, the inability to remain seated, blurting out answers before hearing the whole question, and talking excessively. Some children manifest the core symptoms of inattention, distractibility and impulsivity, but they do not exhibit hyperactive behavior (in some cases they are actually hypoactive).

Attention-deficit disorder, with or without hyperactivity, is estimated to affect 1 to 10% of all children. It is at least 2 or 3 times more common in boys than in girls. If one person in a family is diagnosed with ADHH, there is a 25 to 35% probability that any other family member also has ADHD (compared to a 4 to 6% probability for a person in the general population). It often continues into adolescence and adulthood. Approximately 50 to 70% of children with ADHD will continue to have significant problems with ADHD symptoms and behaviors as adults.

The etiology of ADHD is neurological with evidence implicating chemical and/or structural differences in the frontal lobes, basal ganglia, reticular activating system and brain stem, as well as the major neurotransmitter systems. In persons with ADHD, the number and density of dopamine transporters and dopamine transporter binding sites are increased by up to 70%. The following central nervous system (CNS) stimulants seem to be the most effective in treating the symptoms of ADHD in both children and adults: methylphenidate (Ritalin), dextro-amphetamine (Dexedrine or Dextrostat) and pemoline (Cylert). These drugs inhibit the dopamine transporter, increasing the time that dopamine has to bind to its receptors on other neurons, and improve attention, coordination and balance.

The right prefrontal cortex and basal ganglia (caudate nucleus and globus pallidus) are significantly smaller than normal in children with ADHD. The right prefrontal cortex is involved in editing one's behavior, resisting distractions and developing an awareness of self and time. The caudate nucleus and the globus pallidus help to switch off automatic responses, in order to allow more careful deliberation by the cortex and to coordinate neurological input among various regions of the cortex. The vermis region of the cerebellum is also smaller in ADHD children. In people with ADHD, the brain areas that control attention use less glucose, indicating they are less active. It appears from this research that a lower level of activity in some parts of the brain may cause inattention. These differences may be inherited, or caused by disease or trauma. Mutations in several genes that are normally very active in the prefrontal cortex and basal ganglia might play a role. Non-genetic factors that have been linked to ADHD include premature birth, maternal alcohol and tobacco use, exposure to high levels of lead in early childhood and brain injuries (especially those that involve the prefrontal cortex).

Before the age of 6 years, most children speak out loud to themselves frequently, reminding themselves how to perform a particular task or trying to cope with a problem. Internalization of self-directed speech is delayed in boys with ADHD. Barkley (1998) argues that inattention, hyperactivity and impulsivity of children with ADHD are caused by their failure to be guided by internal instructions and by their inability to curb their own inappropriate behaviors. Children with ADHD who take stimulant medication, such as Ritalin, are not only are less impulsive, restless and distractible, but are also better able to hold important information in mind, to be more productive academically, and to have more internalized speech and better self-control. As a result, they tend to be liked better by other children and to experience less punishment for their actions, which improves their self-image.

Many children born with fetal alcohol syndrome show much of the same inattention and/or hyperactivity-impulsivity as children with ADHD. It is also thought that abuse of drugs such as cocaine may lead to ADHD.

The following conditions can mimic ADHD: underachievement at school due to a learning disability; attention lapses caused by petit mal seizures; a middle ear infection that causes an intermittent hearing problem; and disruptive or unresponsive behavior due to anxiety or depression. 20 to 30% of patients with ADHD have a learning disability. Nearly 50% of children with ADHD (mostly boys) tend to have oppositional defiant disorder. At some point, many children with ADHD experience other emotional disorders. A very small proportion of people with ADHD have Tourette's syndrome.

Hyperactive children frequently have problems both with motor coordination and in team activities. Comorbidity may exist between ADHD and developmental coordination disorder. Sensory integration dysfunction may mimic or co-exist with ADHD.

ADHD is a controversial problem in sport, because participants with this disorder often require banned stimulant medication during competition. Treatment of ADHD athletes with methylphenidate (Ritalin) may be suitable, because a cessation of therapy 24 hours before competition is usually adequate for drug clearance and avoidance of a positive result from drug testing. *See also* SENSORY INTEGRATION DISORDER.

Bibliography

Alexander, J.L. (1990). Hyperactive children: Which sports have the right stuff. *The Physician and Sportsmedicine* 18(4), 105-108.

American Psychiatric Association (1994). *Diagnostic and Statistical Manual of Mental Disorders.* 4th ed. Washington, DC: American Psychiatric Association.

Barkley, R.A. (1998). Attention-deficit hyperactivity disorder. *Scientific American* 279 (3) (September), 66-71.

Berk, L.E. (1994). Why children talk to themselves. *Scientific American* 271(5) (November), 78-83.

Children and Adults with Attention-Deficit/Hyperactivity Disorder. Http://www.chadd.org

Corrigan, B. (2003). Attention-deficit hyperactivity disorder in sport: A review. *International Journal of Sports Medicine* 24(7), 535-540.

Harvey, W.J. and Reid, G. (2003). Attention-deficit/hyperactivity disorder: A review of research on movement skill performance and physical fitness. *Adapted Physical Activity Quarterly* 20(1), 1-25.

Hickey, G. and Fricker, P. (1999). Attention deficit hyperactivity disorder, CNS stimulants and sport. *Sports Medicine* 27(1), 11-21.

Mottram, D.R. (1999). Banned drugs in sport. Does the International Olympic Committee (IOC) list need updating? *Sports Medicine* 27(1), 1-10.

National Attention Deficit Disorder Association. Http://www.add.org

ATTENUATE   To weaken, dilute or diminish.

ATTRIBUTION THEORY   A theory of

motivation that is concerned with common sense explanations of behavior and the effect of such explanations on future behavior. Heider (1958) argued that people make inferences, from their own and other people's behavior, as to whether that behavior is caused by environmental or personal forces. Weiner (1974, 1979) modified Heider's theory and used it in educational psychology. It has been found that attributions are part of everyday psychology, being emitted more frequently when an outcome is unexpected and when a specific goal is not achieved. Sport psychologists have used Weiner's theory extensively, primarily in research that compares the attributions of winners and losers.

Fundamental attribution error is the tendency, in explaining other people's behavior, to overestimate personality factors and underestimate the influence of the situation. In a study of 34 male and female swimmers who had just participated in an important national competition, Wolfson (1997) found that swimmers perceived themselves as more affected than others by both internal and external factors. Sande, Goethals and Radloff (1988) have suggested that actor-observer differences might emanate from people's views that they are more complex and multi-faceted than others. People believe that more factors, both internal and external, will affect them than other people. This is likely to be due to a combination of motivational and information processing effects.

People tend to give internal attributions to positive outcomes and external attributions to negative events. This phenomenon is called the '**self-serving bias**' and seems to be concerned with maintaining self-esteem. There is evidence to suggest that self-serving attributions are more extreme in the context of larger-sized teams and for attribution measures focused on the team rather than on the individual. Ability seems to exhibit the greatest self-serving attribution effects.

A similar phenomenon to 'self-serving bias' is '**basking in reflected glory**.' Being a sports fan may serve functions of self-presentation or image management (Cialdini et al, 1976). Persons in need of enhancing their public image may accomplish this by associating themselves with successful athletes and athletic teams. They may benefit from athletic success, vicariously, by 'basking in reflected glory.' In support of the theory, it has been found on American university campuses that the apparel of the home team was more popular after the football team's victories than after losses. It has also been found that students talk about their winning team as "us" and their losing team as "them." Snyder et al. (1983) used the expression '**cutting off reflected failure**' to refer to how individuals avoid the negative evaluations that arise from being associated with a negatively valued other, in order to protect self-image and self-esteem.

Laboratory animals that have previously received unpleasant experiences, about which they could do nothing, are found to be less ready to undertake action when in a stimulus situation that requires a relatively simple response in order to avoid an unpleasant experience. This phenomenon has been called '**learned helplessness**,' because the animals do little to help themselves. It seems to be a similar phenomenon to that of people, typically suffering from depression, who believe that they have no control over bad events. Learned helplessness in people is found to be more likely when attributions are internal, stable and general. Learned helplessness may be a factor in dropout and burnout from sport. '**Negative self-fulfilling prophecies**' are psychological barriers that lead to a vicious circle of expectation of failure leading to actual failure with the result that self-confidence is lowered and expectancy of future failure increased. Ultimately learned helplessness may result. Self-confidence is associated with '**positive self-fulfilling prophecy**,' i.e. that expecting something to happen actually helps to make it happen.

Research in sport has shown that performance satisfaction is one of the best predictors of emotion and that attributions play a role. The athlete who believes his success to be the result of external factors, such as good luck, will experience less pride and satisfaction than will the athlete who attributes the success to internal factors, such as ability. Similarly, greater shame and dissatisfaction are experienced when failure is attributed to internal factors than when loss is believed to have resulted from external factors. There is a greater expectancy of success when the athlete perceives positive outcomes to be the result of stable factors, such as high personal ability, rather than unstable factors, such as luck. Before competition, females tend to perceive their personal ability much lower than their male counterparts, and consequently they have lower expectations of success. Before 10 years of age, children are unable to distinguish between the relative contribution of personal effort and ability to their success or failure.

Attributional retraining is a technique in which individuals are taught to change undermining attributions to more facilitative ones. It focuses on the importance of effort, rather than less controllable attributions such as luck or task difficulty.

Bibliography

Biddle, S.(1993). Attribution research and sport psychology. In Singer, R.N., Murphey, M. and Tennant, L.K. (eds). *Handbook on research on sport psychology*. pp437-464. New York: MacMillan.

Cialdini, R.B. et al. (1976). Basking in reflected glory: Three (football) field studies. *Journal of Personality and Social Psychology* 34, 366-375.

Cialdini, R.B. and Richards, K.D. (1980). Two indirect tactics of image management: Basking and blasting. *Journal of Personality and Social Psychology* 39, 406-415.

Heider, F. (1958). *The psychology of interpersonal relations*. New York: John Wiley & Sons.

Leith, L.M. (1989). Causal attribution and sport behavior: Implications for practitioners. *Journal of Sport Behavior* 12(4), 213-225.

McAuley, E. and Duncan, T.E. (1989). Causal attributions and affective reactions to disconfirming outcomes in motor performances. *Journal of Sport and Exercise Psychology* 11, 187-200.

Miserandino, M. (1998). Attributional retraining as a method of improving athletic performance. *Journal of Sport Behavior* 21(3), 286-297.

Mullen, B. and Riordan, C.A. (1988). Self-serving attributions for performance in naturalistic settings: A meta-analytic review. *Journal of Applied Social Psychology* 18(1), 3-22.

Rejeski, W.J. and Brawley, L.R. (1983). Attribution theory in sport: Current status and new perspectives. *Journal of Sport Psychology* 5, 77-97.

Sande, G.N., Goethals, G.R. and Radloff, C.E. (1988). Perceiving one's own traits and others': A multifaceted self. *Journal of Personality and Social Psychology* 54, 13-20.

Snyder, C.R., Higgins, R.C. and Stucky, R.J. (1983). *Excuses: Masquerades in search of grace*. New York: Wiley-Interscience.

Weiner, B. (1985). An attributional theory of achievement motivation and emotion. *Psychological Review* 92, 548-513.

Wolfson, S. (1997). Actor-observer bias and perceived sensitivity to internal and external factors in competitive swimmers. *Journal of Sport Behavior* 20(4), 477-484.

ATWATER GENERAL FACTORS *See under* ENERGY YIELD OF NUTRIENTS.

AUDIENCE EFFECTS *See under* HOME ADVANTAGE; SOCIAL FACILITATION.

AUDITORY REFLEX Any reflex caused by stimulation of the auditory (vestibulocochlear) nerve, especially momentary closure of both eyes produced by a sudden sound.

AUDITORY SYSTEM *See under* AGING.

AURICULAR HEMATOMA *See* CAULIFLOWER EAR.

AUTISTIC DISORDER Autism. A pervasive developmental disorder significantly affecting verbal and nonverbal communication and social interaction, which is generally evident before the age of 3 years, and adversely affects a child's educational performance. Other behaviors often associated with autism are engagement in repetitive activities and stereotyped movements, resistance to environmental change or change in daily routines, and unusual responses to sensory experiences. Students with autism typically evidence motor clumsiness. There is also a lack of spontaneous or imaginative play, with neither imitation of others' actions, nor initiation of pretend games. Autistic disorder does not apply if a child's educational performance is adversely affected primarily because the child has a serious emotional disturbance (Federal Register, 1992). Autism is a spectrum disorder (the symptoms and characteristics of autism can present themselves in a wide variety of combinations, from mild to severe).

According to the American Psychiatric Association, there are three diagnostic criteria for autism: (A) A total of six or more items from (1), (2), and (3), with at least two from (1), and one each from (2) and (3). (1) Qualitative impairment in social interaction, as manifested by at least two of the following: marked impairment in the use of multiple nonverbal behaviors such as eye-to-eye gaze, facial expression, body postures and gestures to regulate social interaction; failure to develop peer relationships appropriate to developmental level; a lack of spontaneous seeking to share enjoyment, interests or achievements with other people; and lack of social or emotional reciprocity. (2) Qualitative impairments in communication as manifested by at least one of the following: a delay in, or total lack of, the development of spoken language (not accompanied by an attempt to compensate through alternative modes of communication such as gesture or mime); in individuals with adequate speech, marked impairment in the ability to initiate or sustain a conversation with others; stereotyped and repetitive use of language or idiosyncratic language; and lack of varied, spontaneous make-believe play or social imitative play appropriate to developmental level. (3) Restricted repetitive and stereotyped patterns of behavior, interests and activities, as manifested by at least one of the following: encompassing preoccupation with one or more stereotyped and restricted patterns of interest that is abnormal either in intensity or focus; apparently inflexible adherence to specific, nonfunctional routines or rituals; stereotyped and repetitive motor mannerisms (e.g. hand or finger flapping or twisting, or complex whole-body movements); and persistent preoccupation with parts of objects. (B) Delays or abnormal functioning in at least one of the following areas, with onset prior to age 3 years: social interaction, language used in social communication, or symbolic /imaginative play. (C) The disturbance is no better accounted for by Rett's Disorder or Childhood Disintegrative Disorder.

Current research links autism to biological and neurological differences in the brain. In some cases, the cause appears to be genetic, but no specific gene has yet been identified. Autism also sometimes appears to be acquired and is linked to childhood diseases such as rubella, metabolic problems and brain injury. Some individuals with autism may also have other disorders that affect the functioning of the brain, such as attention-deficit hyperactivity disorder, epilepsy, mental retardation and Down syndrome; or genetic disorders such as Fragile X Syndrome, Landau-Kleffner Syndrome and Tourette's Syndrome. Approximately 25 to 30% may develop a seizure pattern at some period during life.

Determining intellectual function is difficult because people with autism tend to score low on tasks demanding verbal skills and abstract reasoning, but high on tasks requiring memory and visual-spatial or manipulative skills. About 20% of people with autism have IQs above 70; 20% have IQs between 50 and 70; and 60% have IQs below 50. The estimated 80% of people with autism who have IQs of less than 70 can profit from the same kinds of programming as people with mental retardation.

About one-third of persons with autism are able to live and work quite independently by adulthood. The other two-thirds remain severely disabled. There is evidence that partial or total recovery can result from structured early childhood intervention programs (e.g. Kaufman, 1994; Maurice, 1993). A well-known individual who recovered from autism is Raun Kaufman. Raun's parents established a private institute in Sheffield, Massachusetts in the early 1980s that continues to be a popular training center for parents of children with autism. It emphasizes a psychotherapy approach, i.e. acceptance and imitation (mirroring) of the child's autistic behaviors until she or he is ready to give them up or replace them with more age-appropriate activities. Central to this approach is the presence of an adult in a one-to-one therapeutic relationship almost every hour of the day. Much of the intervention used is dance or movement therapy.

Individuals with autism respond in unusual or bizarre ways to input from one or more sense modalities. Sometimes the children appear unaware of stimuli, but more often their responses are exaggerated. High-pitched noises, such as whistles, result in anxiety, fear and anger reactions, such as screaming, crying, or rocking with their hands over their ears. Visual stimuli such as moving objects seem to excessively stimulate some children with autism. These stimuli often cause stereotyped behaviors (stimming) like extended gazing or twirling, spinning or tapping behaviors. The extreme pleasure derived from certain visual stimuli and concurrent body response to stimming is similar to what many people feel during sexual orgasm, except that the pleasure seems to continue for hours or until the child is stopped from stimming. Stopping a child from stimming usually results in screaming.

Many children with autism appear to be functionally deaf, in that they do not seem to hear noises or speech. The only way to get their attention is through firmly taking hold of one or both shoulders. Firm pressure is better than light touch because many children are tactile defensive to light touch stimuli. Many children with autism dislike being hugged, but they do develop attachment behaviors. About 50% of children with autism do not talk. Many were using words before the onset of autism.

With help, about 50% of children with autism slowly learn to talk and use language more or less appropriately. Many use stereotyped and repetitive phrases, pronoun reversal (i.e. saying "you" instead of "I"), and **echolalia** (involuntary repetition of words spoken by others).

Eye contact is important in one-to-one interactions. Contrary to popular understanding, many children and adults with autism may make eye contact, show affection, smile and laugh, and demonstrate a variety of other emotions, although in varying degrees. Sometimes visual, motor and/or processing problems make it difficult to maintain eye contact with others. Rather than looking at other people directly, some individuals with autism use peripheral vision.

Physically guiding a person with autism through a new movement pattern has traditionally been the teaching method of choice, but comparison of verbal/visual and verbal/physical teaching models shows equivalent results. Connor's (1990) teaching suggestions for autism include: teach to the preferred modality; minimize unnecessary external stimuli; limit the amount of relevant stimuli presented at one time; limit the use of prompts (cues); and teach in a game-like environment to facilitate generalization. Research by Collier and Reid (1987) does not support limiting prompts. Reinforcement, task analysis, and physical prompting are the three keys to motor skill improvement for most persons with autism according to Reid et al. (1991). Traditional punishments, like time-outs, are seldom effective because the child with autism prefers to be alone. Therefore, the emphasis must be on reinforcers that are personally meaningful enough to motivate compliance with the teacher's requests.

Most persons with autism are eligible for Special Olympics training and competition. Persons with autism want to do the same things every day in precisely the same way; such preoccupation with repetition and routine is an advantage in sport and fitness training.

See also ASPERGER'S SYNDROME; SAVANTISM; SENSORY INTEGRATION DISORDER.

Bibliography

Autism Society of America. Http://www.autism-society.org

Center for the Study of Autism. Http://www.autism.org

Collier, D. and Reid, G. (1987). A comparison of two models designed to teach autistic children a motor task. *Adapted Physical Activity Quarterly* 4, 226-236.

Connor, F. (1990). Physical education for children with autism. *Teaching Exceptional Children* 23, 30-33.

Kaufman, B.N. (1994). *Son-rise: The miracle continues.* Tiburon, CA: H.J. Kramer.

Maurice, C. (1993). *Let me hear your voice.* New York: Alfred A. Knopf.

Reid, G., Collier, D. and Cauchon, M. (1991). Skill acquisition by children with autism: Influence of prompts. *Adapted Physical Activity Quarterly* 8, 357-366.

AUTOGENIC FACILITATION *See under* STRETCH REFLEX.

AUTOGENIC INHIBITION *See under* STRETCHING.

AUTOGENIC TRAINING A psychotherapeutic system that has been used as a relaxation technique by athletes. It involves associating a series of verbal cues and images (especially visual and kinesthetic images) with psychophysiological responses. These are practiced in a sequential order to achieve the autogenic (self-generated) response. The six steps are heaviness in the extremities, warmth in the extremities, regulation of cardiac activity, regulation of breathing, warmth in the abdominal region, and cooling of the forehead.

Bibliography

Schultz, J. and Luthe, W. (1959). *Autogenic training: A psychophysiological approach in psychotherapy*. New York: Grune and Statton.

AUTOIMMUNE DISEASE   A disease in which the immune system wrongly identifies normal body components as foreign and mounts an attack on the body. It is caused by the body producing antibodies and sensitized cytotoxic T cells that destroy its own tissues. 5% of adults in the USA are afflicted. The most common autoimmune diseases are: glomerulonephritis, Graves' disease, myasthenia gravis, rheumatoid arthritis, systemic lupus erythematosus and Type I diabetes mellitus.

AUTONOMIC DYSREFLEXIA   Hyper-reflexia. It is an exaggerated response of the nervous system to a specific trigger, such as an overfull bladder, which occurs because the brain is no longer able to control the body's response to the trigger. A reflex is initiated that causes vasoconstriction and increases blood pressure to level that may be dangerous or even fatal. For a person with an intact spinal cord, this same stimulus also sets in motion another set of reflexes that moderates the constriction of blood vessels. Autonomic dysreflexia is most often seen in people with spinal injuries higher than the fourth to sixth thoracic vertebrae (T4 to T6). In wheelchair athletics, a technique called '**boosting**' has been used as an ergogenic aid to exploit autonomic dysreflexia. A wheelchair athlete might put a nail on their chair to sit on. They do not feel it, but autonomic dysreflexia is exploited with the result that blood pressure is elevated and hormones such as epinephrine are released in order to improve performance by as much as 15%. Allegedly, some Paralympic athletes have kinked or blocked off the catheter used to drain their bladder in order to achieve autonomic dysreflexia.

AUTONOMIC NERVOUS SYSTEM   An efferent system of nerve fibers that innervates smooth muscle, cardiac muscle and glands. The most important parts of the brain involved in control of the autonomic nervous system are the hypothalamus and regions of the brain stem. The autonomic nervous system consists of the sympathetic and the parasympathetic nervous systems. The **para-sympathetic nervous system** is responsible for controlling many bodily functions under normal resting conditions. The **sympathetic nervous system** is concerned with energy expenditure and prepares the body for emergency situations (the '**fight or flight**' response). While the sympathetic and parasympathetic systems are usually antagonist to one another, there are some exceptions to this principle. During extreme fear or excitement, for example, the sympathetic system is dominant but a not-uncommon parasympathetic symptom is involuntary discharge of the bladder or bowels.

The parasympathetic nervous system involves the motor components of cranial nerves III, VII, IX and X in the brain stem and three spinal nerves in sacral segments 2 to 4. The sympathetic nervous system involves the 12 thoracic segments and the first 2 or 3 lumbar segments of the spinal cord.

Nerves of the autonomic nervous system do not go directly from the spinal cord to target glands or effectors. They make synapses with a second order of neurons in structures known as **ganglia**. **Synapses** can be categorized as either electrical or chemical, depending on how the effects of activity in one neuron (the **pre-synaptic or pre-ganglionic neuron**) are passed on to another (the **post-synaptic or post-ganglionic neuron**). If the effects of the pre-synaptic neuron are passed on directly by the flow of current, then it is an **electrical synapse**. If the effects of the pre-synaptic neuron are passed on indirectly by a neurotransmitter, then it is a **chemical synapse**. Neurotransmitters are released in minute amounts at synapses. Whether a given neurotransmitter produces an excitatory post-synaptic potential or an inhibitory post-synaptic potential in a given post-synaptic neuron, is dependent upon the ionic channels opened by the post-synaptic receptors for that neurotransmitter. A single pre-synaptic neuron contains only one neurotransmitter, but it can produce either an excitatory or inhibitory post-synaptic potential in different post-synaptic cells. Not all the pre-ganglionic fibers of the sympathetic nervous system synapse in the ganglia of the sympathetic chain; some travel to the more peripheral ganglia or to medulla of the adrenal glands.

In both the sympathetic and parasympathetic nervous systems, the neurotransmitter released from the terminals of the pre-ganglionic nerve fibers is acetylcholine. The neurotransmitter released from the post-ganglionic nerve fibers on to effector organs differs in the two divisions of the autonomic nervous system. At parasympathetic synapses, acetylcholine is the neurotransmitter. At sympathetic synapses, norepinephrine is the neurotransmitter. The effects of norepinephrine are supplemented by epinephrine. Acetylcholine is released from a small number of post-ganglionic sympathetic nerve fibers, while the adrenal medulla produces and releases epinephrine and norepinephrine. The adrenal medulla resembles a sympathetic ganglion in that it is innervated by sympathetic pre-ganglionic nerve fibers. When activated, these nerve fibres release catecholamines into the bloodstream.

A nerve fiber is said to be **cholinergic** if it secretes acetylcholine when an impulse reaches its ending (receptor). There are two types of cholinergic receptor: nicotinic and muscarinic. **Nicotinic receptors** (so named because nicotine mimics the action of acetylcholine at such receptors) are found on both sympathetic and parasympathetic post-ganglionic neurones. The stimulation of nicotinic receptors results in vasodilation of skeletal muscle blood vessels and increased sweating. **Muscarinic receptors** are present on all effectors (muscles and glands) innervated by parasympathetic post-ganglionic nerve fibers. The stimulation of muscarinic receptors results in increased heart rate, decreased vasodilation of myocardial blood vessels, increased contractility of atrial myocardium, and decreased tone of the intestinal tract lumen.

A nerve fiber is said to be **adrenergic** if it secretes epinephrine or norepinephrine when an impulse reaches its ending. There are two types of adrenergic receptor (adrenoceptor): alpha and beta. Stimulation of **alpha-adrenoceptors** results in vasoconstriction of blood vessels in the myocardium, skeletal muscle, skin and abdominal viscera; bladder sphincter contraction; pilomotor erection; and dilation of the iris. There are two types of beta-adrenergic receptor. **Beta-1 adrenergic receptors** are found in the heart, kidneys and adipose tissue. The stimulation of beta-1 receptors results in increased heart rate, increased myocardial contractility and increased lipolysis. **Beta-2 adrenergic receptors** are found in the liver, bronchi and arteries. The stimulation of beta-2 receptors results in vasodilation of myocardial blood vessels, decreased airway resistance, increased glycogenolysis in the liver and increased glycogenolysis in skeletal muscle.

Autonomic responses to exercise can be divided into three categories: metabolic (liver and muscle glycogenolysis, lipolysis and pancreatic responses), cardiovascular (inotropic and chronotropic effects on the heart, decrease in the flow of blood to the liver and gastrointestinal tract) and thermoregulatory (sweating). Heat stress is associated with sweating and an increase in skin blood flow, which occur in the absence of more widespread sympathetic responses. Widespread sympathetic responses, constituting the 'fight or flight' syndrome, are seen during vigorous sustained exercise.

See also under BLOOD PRESSURE.

Bibliography

Green, J.H. (1990). *The autonomic nervous system and exercise.* London: Chapman and Hall.

AUTOREGULATION (i) A process that maintains a generally constant physiological state in a cell or organism. (ii) The tendency of blood flow to an organ or part of the body to remain at or return to the same level despite changes in the pressure in the artery that supplies it with blood.

AUXILLARY CELLS   *See under* LEUKOCYTES.

AV NODE   *See under* HEART BLOCK.

AVOGADRO'S NUMBER   *See under* MOLE.

AVULSION FRACTURE   An indirect injury that occurs when a force applied to a tendon or ligament is transferred to its bony attachment site, with the result that a piece of bone is pulled away from the attachment site. Avulsion fractures are more common than tendinous ruptures in skeletally immature athletes, as the physis is the weakest link. Common avulsion fractures in children involve the following muscles (and their attachments): the forearm flexors (medial epicondyle of the humerus), *sartorius* muscle (anterior superior iliac spine), *rectus femoris* muscle (anterior inferior iliac spine), *iliopsoas* (lesser trochanter of femur), abdominal muscles (iliac crest) and hamstrings (ischial tuberosity); also the patellar tendon (tibial tuberosity) and Achilles tendon (calcaneus).

Avulsions of the *sartorius* muscle (anterior superior iliac spine) are relatively common, due to sudden contractions of the *sartorius*, and can be bilateral. The mechanism in 75% of cases is a sudden pull on the *sartorius* while running with the hip in extension and knee in flexion, but it can also result from kicking. Anterior inferior iliac spine avulsions are also seen with kicking and running, but occur less frequently (partly because of earlier fusion).

Avulsions of the iliac crest can occur, rarely, due to forceful contractions of numerous muscle attachments (most commonly the gluteals, *transversus abdominis* and the abdominal obliques), but may also follow direct injury. They typically follow rapid changes in direction at speed, and due to their late fusion, can be seen up until 25 years of age.

Avulsions of the ischial tuberosity are possibly the most common adolescent injury of the hip. They are frequently the result of explosive athletic events and sudden, forceful contraction of the hamstrings with the hip in flexion and the knee in extension, and also when doing the splits in gymnastics. The lesser trochanter apophysis is rarely avulsed. Avulsions of the greater trochanter can result from sudden abduction normally produced by 'cutting' motions.

AWARENESS   *See* ATTENTION; BODY AWARENESS; CONSCIOUSNESS; DIRECTIONAL AWARENESS; TEMPORAL AWARENESS.

AXILLARY NERVE   The last nerve to issue from the posterior spinal cord before it becomes the radial nerve. It supplies the *deltoid* muscle and *teres minor* muscle, and may be injured as a result of anterior shoulder dislocation.
See also under PERIPHERAL NERVE; THROMBOSIS.

AXILLARY VEIN   Subclavian vein. *See under* THROMBOSIS.

AXIS   i) The second cervical vertebra, which is involved in the atlanto-axial joint.
ii) The axis of rotation.

AXON   Nerve fiber. *See under* NEURON.

AXONOPATHY   A disorder disrupting the normal functions of the axons.

AXONOTMESIS   Axonal degeneration with maintenance of the epineurium, perineurium and endoneurium. It is characterized by a complete loss of motor, sensory and sympathetic function along the distribution of the injured nerve. Muscle atrophy occurs and reflexes may be lost.

B

BABINSKI REFLEX   Plantar grasp reflex. Foot grasp reflex. A primitive reflex that is present at birth and persists through the first year of life. It is elicited by applying slight pressure to the outer margin of the sole of the foot. As a result, the toes of the foot flex and adduct as if to grasp. This reflex enhances body awareness and strengthens the foot muscles. It is due to incomplete myelination of the nervous system. Failure of this reflex to integrate properly interferes with balance in walking and standing. It is often seen in conjunction with the positive supporting reflex (increased extensor tone that results in toe walking).

It is an important neurological test for spinal cord damage because it gives an easily detectable abnormal response if the spinal cord has been injured. If there is damage to the lateral corticospinal tract, there will be extension and abduction of the toes instead.

BABKIN REFLEX   *See* PALMAR MANDIBULAR REFLEX.

BACTERIA   A group of single-cell micro-organisms, some of which produce poisonous substances called toxins that lead to ill health in humans. They contain only one chromosome and lack many organelles found in human cells.

BAINBRIDGE REFLEX   *See* ATRIAL REFLEX.

BAKER'S CYST   *See* POPLITEAL CYST.

BALANCE   i) An instrument that is used in weighing. ii) A condition of partial or complete equilibrium or adjustment. iii) A term that refers to the control processes that maintain body parts in the specific alignments necessary to achieve different kinds of mobility and stability. Postural control involves keeping or returning the body's center of mass over its base of support. Balance in young children is heavily influenced by vision, whereas adults rely more on tactile and kinesthetic input. Sensory systems (vestibular, kinesthetic, tactile and visual) interact with environmental variables to enable balance. **Static balance** involves maintaining one's equilibrium while the center of gravity remains stationary. Activities that include static balance include balancing on one foot. **Dynamic balance** involves maintaining one's equilibrium as the center of gravity shifts. Activities that require dynamic balance include walking along a narrow beam. There is low correlation between different tests of static and dynamic balance. A test of vestibular function is to seat a person on a stool and spin them rapidly. 20 seconds of spinning normally results in 9 to 11 seconds of nystagmus (rapid eye movements), an automatic midbrain response. A longer or shorter duration of nystagmus indicates a lack of vestibular integration. No dizziness or discomfort, or the opposite (including nausea), indicates the presence of vestibular problems also. Spinning is contraindicated when individuals are seizure-prone, or have inner ear or upper-respiratory infections.

See also under AGING.

Bibliography

Cook, G. (2003). *Athletic body in balance*. Champaign, IL: Human Kinetics.

BALL AND SOCKET JOINT   Enarthrosis. *See under* JOINT.

BALLISTIC MOVEMENT   *See under* MOTOR UNIT; MOVEMENT.

BARBITURATES   *See under* DEPRESSANTS.

BARORECEPTORS   Nerve endings found mainly in the walls of the carotid sinuses and the aortic arch. They are sensitive to stretch, and thus to changes in blood pressure. They send nerve impulses to the medulla of the brain, which helps regulate blood pressure.

BAROREFLEX   Baroreceptor reflex. Venous pooling leads to a decrease in central venous pressure that leads to a decrease in mean arterial pressure, which in turn leads to decreased blood flow to the brain. The decrease in arterial blood pressure is detected by arterial baroreceptors, which trigger an increase in sympathetic activity and a decrease in parasympathetic activity. This brings about increases in heart rate, myocardial contractility and vascular resistance. The Valsalva maneuver is a simple test of the baroreceptor reflex.

BAROSINUSITIS Inflammation of one or more of the paranasal sinuses. Inflammation is caused by a pressure gradient, almost always negative, between the sinus cavity and the surrounding ambient atmosphere. Consider an aircraft pilot making a descent. Ambient pressure increases and pressure cannot equalize across the nasal cavity to the sinus because of blockage at the ostium. Air volume decreases in the sinus cavity and a negative pressure is created.

Bibliography

Thiringer,   J.K.   (2002).   Barosinusitis. Http://www.emedicine.com

BAROTRAUMA Tissue injury caused by changing pressure.
    See under HYPERBARIC PHYSIOLOGY.

BARREL CHEST   Increased anterior-posterior chest diameter caused by increased functional residual capacity due to air trapping from small airway collapse. It is frequently seen in patients with chronic obstructive diseases such as chronic bronchitis and emphysema. In persons with severe, chronic asthma who become permanently hyperventilated because of their inability to exhale properly, the excess air retained in the lungs tends to expand the anterior-posterior dimensions. It is also seen in kyphosis. Barrel chest is normal for infants and preschool children.

BARTON'S FRACTURE   *See under* ELBOW FRACTURES.

BASAL GANGLIA   *See under* BRAIN.

BASAL METABOLIC RATE   *See under* ENERGY EXPENDITURE.

BASE   (i) Alkali. A substance that dissociates, providing negative ions and accepting positive ions (protons). A **basic solution** is one in which the concentration of hydrogen ions is less than the concentration of hydroxide ions. (ii) Single-ring (pryrimidine) or double-ring (purine) component of a nucleic acid.

BASEBALL FINGER   *See* MALLET FINGER.

BASE PAIR   A pair of nitrogenous bases, most commonly one purine and one pyrimidine, held together by hydrogen bonds in a double-stranded region of a nucleic acid molecule.

BASOPHILS   *See under* LEUKOCYTES.

B CELLS   *See under* LEUKOCYTES.

BED REST   *See under* IMMOBILIZATION.

BEE POLLEN A mixture of bee saliva, plant nectar and the pollen of flowering plants. It is used by athletes as an ergogenic aid and is taken in the form of tablets or loose powder. It contains over 50% carbohydrate. There is no evidence that bee pollen has an ergogenic effect. It can cause allergic reactions and anaphylaxis.

BEHAVIOR   Any act of a person or animal. Overt behavior is observable. Covert behavior is non-observable.

BEHAVIORAL INTERVENTIONS Interventions that are based on behaviorism.

BEHAVIORISM   The school of thought that regards psychology as the study of behavior and denies the importance of mental processes in the explanation of behavior. Behavior is seen as acquired, maintained and modified as a function of environmental causes. In the 'ABC Model of Behavioral Analysis,' 'A' refers to antecedent conditions (what precedes the person's behavior), 'B' refers to the person's overt behavior and 'C' refers to the consequences of the person's behavior.

See also CLASSICAL CONDITIONING; OPERANT CONDITIONING.

BENDING   A force that includes all the changes that occur with compression, tension and shear. Bending of a structure occurs when forces produce equal and opposite moment actions about a section of that structure. Tensile stresses and strains act on one side of the neutral axis, and compressive stresses and strains act on the other side; there are no stresses and strains along the neutral axis. The magnitude of the stresses is proportional to their distance from the neutral axis of the bone. The farther the stresses are from the neutral axis, the higher their magnitude.

Forces acting perpendicular to the long axis of a beam (e.g. a long bone) create bending. The concave (inner) surface of the bone experiences compressive stress; the convex (outer) surface of the bone is subjected to tensile stress. The maximum stresses occur at the surface of bone, with lower stresses developed away from the surface towards the midline (neutral axis) of the bone. The bone resists the bending moment created by external forces. **Bending moment** is a quantitative measure of the tendency of a force to bend a structure. It is calculated as the product of the applied force and the perpendicular distance from the point of force application to the axis. The Standard International unit is the newton meter (N.m). The US Customary unit is foot pound force (ft.lbf).

Fractures from three-point bending and four-point bending are both common, especially in long bones. **Three-point bending** occurs when three parallel forces acting on a structure produce two equal moments, each being the product of one of the two peripheral forces and its perpendicular distance from the axis of rotation (the point at which the middle force is applied). If loading continues to the yield point, the structure, if homogeneous, symmetrical and with no structural or tissue defects, will break at the point of application of the middle

force. A **'boot-top' fracture** occurs when one bending moment acts on the proximal tibia as a skier falls forward over the top of the ski boot, while an equal moment, produced by the fixed foot and the ski, acts on the distal tibia. As the proximal tibia is bent forward, tensile stresses and strains act on the posterior side of the bone, and compressive stresses and strains act on the anterior side. The tibia and fibula fracture at the top of the boot. **Four-point bending** occurs when two force couples acting on a structure produce two equal but opposite moments. Because the magnitude of the bending moment is the same throughout the area between the two force couples, the structure breaks at its weakest point.

BENNETT'S FRACTURE   *See under* METACAR-PALS, FRACTURES.

BENZODIAZEPINES   *See under* DEPRES-SANTS.

BETA-ADRENERGIC AGONISTS   Beta-2 agonists. Drugs that are used for the treatment of asthma, but which have also been described as 'partitioning agents' because beta-2 agonists such as clenbuterol (administered orally) have an anabolic effect, increasing muscle hypertrophy and decreasing fat deposition.

For the World Anti-Doping Agency Prohibited List 2005, all beta-2-agonists were prohibited in- and out-of-competition. All beta-2-agonists including their D- and L- isomers are prohibited except "formoterol, salbutamol, salmeterol, and terbutaline permitted by inhalation only to prevent and/or treat asthma and exercise induced asthma/bronchoconstriction." Medical notification under the Therapeutic Use Exemption (TUE) standard is required. When a urinary concentration of salbutamol above 1000 ng/mL is found, the athlete has the responsibility to prove that this results from a therapeutic use of inhaled salbutamol.

See CLENBUTEROL.

Bibliography

World Anti-Doping Agency Prohibited List. Http://www.wada-ama.org

BETA-ADRENERGIC BLOCKERS   *See* BETA BLOCKERS.

BETA-ADRENERGIC RECEPTORS   *See under* AUTONOMIC NERVOUS SYSTEM.

BETA-BLOCKERS   Beta-adrenergic blockers. Drugs used clinically to treat high blood pressure, in addition to angina pectoris, arrhythmias, anxiety and migraine headaches. Beta-blockers decrease blood pressure by inhibiting the secretion of renin and by antagonizing (preventing the stimulation of) beta-adrenergic receptors.

The **water-soluble beta-blockers**, such as atenolol, do not affect the central nervous system. The **lipid-soluble beta-blockers**, such as propranolol, may act via the central nervous system. There is evidence that lipid-soluble beta-blockers can have a beneficial effect on anxiety and essential tremor. These drugs have been used in target sports, such as archery, which require steadiness. **Non-selective beta blockers**, such as propanolol, have the same potency for beta-1 and beta-2 receptors. [Cardio-]**Selective beta blockers**, such as atenonol, have a greater affinity for beta-1 than beta-2 receptors. Selective beta-blockers without intrinsic sympathomimetic activity (e.g. atenolol) lead to the greatest decrease in exercise-induced blood pressure and heart rate increases. **Nebivolol** is a highly selective, long-acting beta-blocker with vasodilating properties, which acts in part via the endothelial L-arginine/nitric oxide pathway. In contrast to atenolol, nebivolol does not decrease maximal and endurance exercise capacity, and does not increase perceived exertion significantly.

Beta-blocker therapy is contraindicated for patients who receive insulin therapy for diabetes mellitus, because beta-blockers may depress the response of the sympathetic nervous system to, and warning signs of, hypoglycemia. Warning signs of hypoglycemia include nervousness and tachycardia.

Beta-blockers are prohibited in competition only by the international federations of certain sports (e.g. diving and synchronized sports). The international federations of certain other sports (e.g. archery, shooting) also prohibit beta-blockers out of competition.

Chronology

•1984 • Beta-blockers were used by most competitors in the Olympic modern pentathlon.

•1985 • Beta-blockers were added to the International Olympic Committee (IOC)'s list of prohibited classes of substances.

Bibliography

Head, A. (1999). Exercise metabolism and beta-blocker therapy. An update. *Sports Medicine* 27(2), 81-96.

Lenz, T.L., Lenz, N.J. and Faulkner, M.A. (2004). Potential interactions between exercise and drug therapy. *Sports Medicine* 34(5), 293-306.

Todd, J. and Todd, T. (2001). Significant events in the history of drug testing and the Olympic movement 1960-1999. In: Wilson, W. and Derse, E. (eds). *Doping in elite sport. The politics of drugs in the Olympic movement*. pp65-128. Champaign, IL: Human Kinetics.

Van Baak, M.A. (1988). Beta-adrenoceptor blockade and exercise. An update. *Sports Medicine* 4, 209-225.

Van Bortel, L.M. and van Baak, M.A. (1992). Exercise tolerance with nebivolol and atenolol. *Cardiovascular Drugs and Therapy* 6(3), 239-247.

Wagner, J.C. (1991). Enhancement of athletic performance with drugs. An overview. *Sports Medicine* 12(4), 250-265.

World Anti-Doping Agency. Http://www.wada-ama.org

BETA-HYDROXY-BETA-METHYLBUTYRATE   HMB. It is a metabolite of leucine. About 2 to 10% of leucine oxidation proceeds to HMB. Small amounts are produced endogenously, but it is also found in catfish, citrus fruits and breast milk. It has been used as a nutritional supplement, after claims that high levels decrease protein catabolism, thereby creating a net anabolic effect. In trained individuals and elite power athletes, HMB intake does not appear to enhance lean body mass or strength.

Bibliography

Armsey, T.D. and Green, G.A. (1997). Nutrition supplements: Science vs. hype. *The Physician and Sportsmedicine* 25(6), 76-92.

Maughan, R.J., King, D.S. and Lea, T. (2004). Dietary supplements. *Journal of Sports Sciences* 22, 95-113.

Slater, G.J. and Jenkins, D. (2000). Beta-hydroxy-beta-methylbutyrate (HMB) supplementation and the promotion of muscle growth and strength. *Sports Medicine* 30(2), 105-116.

BETA-LIPOPROTEINS Low-density lipoproteins (LDL). *See under* CHOLESTEROL.

BETA LIPOTROPHIN   *See under* ENDOR-PHINS.

BETA OXIDATION *See under* FATTY ACIDS.

BIACROMIAL-TO-BICRISTAL RATIO   A measure of proportionality where **biacromial width** is the distance between the left and right acromion processes, and **bicristal width** is the distance between the left and right iliocristales.

BIARTICULAR MUSCLE *See under* MUSCLE, MULTI-JOINT.

BICARBONATE BUFFER   *See under* BUFFERING.

BICARBONATE ION An ion that combines with a hydrogen ion, neutralizing it.

BICEPS BRACHII REFLEX With the elbow flexed and the forearm supinated, the tendon of the *biceps brachii* is pressed down with a thumb or forefinger in the middle of the cubital fossa and the thumb or forefinger is then tapped with a reflex hammer. This stretches the *biceps brachii* muscle and it should respond by reflexively flexing.

BICEPS TENDON INJURY The origin of the long head of the biceps tendon is closely associated with the rotator cuff tendons and the glenoid labrum. The tendon rides over the top of the humerus and enters the joint capsule before exiting through the bicipital groove. Working with the rotator cuff, the long head of the *biceps brachii* imparts a downward force during overhead activities to enhance the stability of the glenohumeral joint.

Inflammation of the distal biceps tendon's synovial sheath is an overuse syndrome resulting from friction across the bicipital tuberosity during repetitive elbow hyperextension or vigorous flexion and supination (especially in throwing sports).

Rupture of the distal biceps tendon is usually an acute injury, as a result of sudden and vigorous extension force while flexing the *biceps brachii* muscle. The overloaded tendon is avulsed from the bicipital tuberosity. It is associated with abuse of anabolic steroids, especially in bodybuilding.

BICYCLE ERGOMETER   A stationary bicycle used as an ergometer. The most commonly used types of bicycle ergometers are based on either mechanical braking or electrical braking.

Mechanically-braking devices allow resistance to pedaling to be varied by use of a braking device on a moving flywheel attached to the pedals. Because the work rate is related to the pedal frequency or speed of the flywheel, a particular work rate is achieved only if the subject cycles within a very narrow range of speed. Electrically-braking cycle ergometers use a magnetic field to produce a resistance to pedaling that can be made to vary with the flywheel speed.

See OXYGEN UPTAKE, MEASUREMENT OF; TREADMILL.

Chronology
•1896 • French medical student E. Bouny developed the first bicycle ergometer. He installed a mechanical brake directly at the wheel of a jacked-up bicycle frame.

BIGOREXIA   *See* BODY DYSMORPHIC DISORDER.

BILATERAL TRANSFER   *See under* MOTOR LEARNING, TRANSFER OF.

BILE A yellow-green material that contains water, bile salts and acids, pigments, cholesterol, phospholipids and electrolytes. It is secreted by the liver, stored in the gall bladder and released into the small intestine where it promotes the breakdown and absorption of lipids.

BILIRUBIN   A yellow bile pigment found as sodium bilirubinate (soluble), or as an insoluble calcium salt in gallstones, formed from hemoglobin during normal and abnormal destruction of erythrocytes by the reticuloendothelial system.

BINGE EATING DISORDER Compulsive overeating. A type of eating disorder not otherwise specified. It is characterized by frequent episodes of eating large quantities of food in short periods of time, feeling out of control over eating behavior, feeling ashamed or disgusted by the behavior. It occurs in approximately 1 to 5% of the general population (60% female, 40% male).

Binge eating disorder is often associated with symptoms of depression. Other health consequences of binge-eating disorder include high blood pressure, high cholesterol levels, heart disease, diabetes mellitus and gall bladder disease.

In males, binge eating is often triggered by uncomfortable feelings such as anger, anxiety or shame; and may be used as a means of relieving tension, or to 'numb' feelings. Emotional and mental characteristics of binge eating disorder in males include: feelings of disgust, guilt or depression during and after overeating; rigid, inflexible thinking; strong need to be in control; difficulty expressing feelings; perfectionism; working hard to please others; and social isolation, depression, moodiness and irritability.

Bibliography

National Eating Disorders Association. Http://www.NationalEatingDisorders.org

BIOAVAILABILITY The degree to which the amount of an ingested nutrient is absorbed and is available to the body. *See* ENERGY YIELD OF NUTRIENTS.

BIOCHEMICAL PATHWAY A diagram showing the order in which intermediate molecules are produced in the synthesis or degradation of a metabolite in a cell.

BIOCHEMISTRY The study of chemical processes in living organisms. Biochemistry and physiology are inextricably linked. In making a distinction between biochemistry and physiology, however, it can be said that biochemistry usually refers to the study of events at sub-cellular and molecular level (rather than cellular level). *See* METABOLISM.

Bibliography

Houston, M.E (2001). *Biochemistry primer for exercise science.* 2nd ed. Champaign, IL: Human Kinetics.

Mathews, C.K., Van Holde, K.E. and Ahern, K. (2000). *Biochemistry.* 3rd ed. San Francisco, CA: Benjamin/Cummings.

Maughan, R., Gleeson, M. and Greenhaff, P.L. (1997). *Biochemistry of exercise and training.* Oxford: Oxford University Press.

Stenesh, J. (1989). *Dictionary of biochemistry and molecular biology.* 2nd ed. New York: John Wiley and Sons.

Stryer, L, Berg, J. and Tymoczko, J. (2002). *Biochemistry.* 5th ed. New York: W.H. Freeman.

Viru, A-M. and Viru, M. (2001). *Biochemical monitoring of sport training.* Champaign, IL: Human Kinetics.

BIOELECTRICAL IMPEDANCE *See under* BODY COMPOSITION.

BIOFEEDBACK A technique used to teach voluntary control of physiological responses that are under control of the autonomic nervous system. Electronic devices are used to detect and amplify responses such as heart rate or muscle tension, giving visual or auditory feedback to the subject. The biofeedback equipment provides information that is not usually available to consciousness. The subject develops cognitive strategies to increase or decrease the signal. The theoretical basis of biofeedback is poorly understood, but the constructs of closed-loop control and feedback have often been invoked, as has operant conditioning. Biofeedback has been used for relaxation training.

Bibliography

Blumenstein, B., Bar-Eli, M. and Tenenbaum, G. (2002, eds). *Brain and body in sport and exercise: Biofeedback applications in performance enhancement.* Chichester, UK: John Wiley & Sons.

Liebermann, D.G. et al. (2002). Advances in the application of information technology to sport performance. *Journal of Sports Sciences* 20(10), 755-769.

Petruzzello, S.J., Landers, D.M., Salazar, W. (1991). Biofeedback and sport/exercise performance: Applications and limitations. *Behavior Therapy* 22(3), 379-392.

Sandweiss, J.M. and Wolf, S.L. (1985, eds). *Biofeed-back and sports science*. New York: Plenum Press.

Zaichkowsky, L.D. and Fuchs, C.Z. (1988). Biofeedback applications in exercise and athletic performance. *Exercise and Sport Sciences Reviews* 16, 381-422.

BIOLOGICAL RHYTHM   A sequence of events, which, in a steady state, repeat themselves in time with the same order and same interval. Biological functions exhibit cycles of activity with a characteristic period, thus providing an internal clock ('body clock') that is important for the precise timing of physiological processes and for prediction of external events. The suprachiasmatic nucleus cells of the hypothalamus are thought to be one of the loci of the internal clock.

Many biological functions have circadian (about 24-hour) rhythms that can be represented by a sine wave. Examples include heart rate, body (core) temperature, sleep-wake cycle, metabolic rate, total water content, electrolyte content and flexibility. The female menstrual cycle has a circalunar (about 28-day) cycle. Normally biological rhythms become synchronized with the zeitgebers (time givers) of light-dark cycle illumination and social signals. Light is thought to act as a zeitgeber via the transmission of photic information along the retinohypothalamic tract (a neural pathway connecting the retinae of the eyes with the suprachiasmatic nucleus). Even without exposure to the solar light-dark cycle or to other zeitgebers, such as rest-activity patterns and the timing of meals, humans still maintain a circadian rhythm that varies between 23.5 and 28 hours. The tendency of the internal clock to run slow with a period greater than 24 hours explains why people tend to go to bed later and sleep later on weekends and during holidays. This resistance to change is normally beneficial, since it means that the body clock does not adjust inappropriately if a person gets up for a snack in the middle of the night, for example. A corollary of this, however, is that night-shift workers suffer from the body clock's slow adjustment to a change in habits.

It is difficult to correlate changes in biological rhythms with performance. It is generally found that the correlation is not strong, but there are wide individual differences. Optimal time of day for exercise is determined not only by biological rhythms, but also by factors such as the intensity of exercise and environmental conditions. In general, athletic performance improves as the day proceeds, with the peak occurring during the middle to late afternoon. In hot climates, this is often partly due to a more favorable ambient temperature. Athletic performance that has a greater dependence on cognitive skills may peak earlier in the day than performance that has a greater dependence on motor skills involving large muscle groups. Rather than being independent rhythms, performance rhythms may fluctuate with arousal, which tends to be lowest early in the morning, increases during the day and shows a slight decrease in the middle afternoon.

Post-prandial low ('post-lunch dip') is a period of decreased alertness that occurs between 1 and 4 pm. Work performance decreases, there is a tendency to nod off and the risk of accidents increases. It is exacerbated by a large, heavy lunch. However, it will occur whether or not lunch is eaten.

Biological rhythms should not be confused with '**Biorhythms**,' which is a theory lacking in scientific foundation. It involves attempts to predict times for optimal performance based on the phasing of three independent cycles, which are purported to exist in each individual (a physical cycle of 23 days, an emotional cycle of 28 days and an intellectual cycle of 33 days).

See also JET LAG.

Bibliography

Atkinson, G. and Reilly, T. (1996). Circadian variation in sports performance. *Sports Medicine* 21(4), 292-312.

Hines, T.M. (1998). Comprehensive review of Biorhythm Theory. *Psychological Reports* 83, 19-64.

Munnings, F. (1991). Exercise: Is any time prime time? *The Physician and Sportsmedicine* 19(5), 101-104.

Reilly, T., Atkinson, G. and Waterhouse, J. (1997). *Biological rhythms and exercise*. Oxford: Oxford University Press.

Winget, C.M., DeRoshia, C.W., Holley, D.C. (1985). Circadian rhythms and athletic performance. *Medicine and Science in Sports and Exercise* 17(5), 498-516.

BIOMECHANICS   The study of the structure and function of biological systems by means of the methods of mechanics. **Mechanics** is a branch of science that deals with forces and the effects of forces, specifically the motion and deformation of matter. It includes the study of rigid bodies, solid deformable bodies and fluids. **Statics** is the branch of mechanics that is concerned with the description and analysis of a body (or body part) that is completely stationary or moving at a constant velocity. It is concerned with forces that tend to cause motion. **Dynamics** is concerned with a body (or body parts) undergoing acceleration.

Direct dynamics involves mechanical analysis of a system that starts with force and determines movement. **Inverse dynamics** involves mechanical analysis of a system that starts with movement and determines force. It involves the calculation of kinetic variables for joints and body segments from segmental anthropometric and kinematic data. It is usually supplemented, where necessary by measurement of external forces acting on the subject (such as from a force plate).

Quantitative biomechanics involves a numeric description or evaluation of movement based on data collected during performance of the movement. **Qualitative biomechanics** involves a non-numeric description or evaluation of movement based on direct observation.

Sport biomechanics is mainly concerned with determination of optimal techniques for performance in sport, the design of sports equipment, and investigation of the stresses placed upon the body during performance. *See also* KINESIOLOGY.

Chronology

•350 BC • In *Parts of Animals, Movement of Animals, and Progression of Animals*, Aristotle described the actions of muscles and subjected them to geometrical analysis.

•1633 • The Italian astronomer Galileo Galilei was convicted of heresy by the Inquisition and forced to repudiate Copernican theory (i.e. the sun, rather than the earth, is at the center of the solar system). Included in Galileo's unpublished treatise *De Animaliam Motibus* (The Movement of Animals) were studies of human jumping biomechanics, gait analysis of horses and insects, and the study of human suspension in liquid. He also studied the strength of biomaterials such as bone.

•1680 • In *De Motu Animalium*, Italian scientist Giovanni A. Borelli applied an understanding of mechanics and physical principles developed by Galileo to the interpretation of all muscular action.

•1867 • Guillaume B.A. Duchennes published his *Physiology of Motion* for which he used electrophysiological methods to analyze human movements in both normal and diseased subjects.

•1935 • Arthur Steindler's textbook *Human Body Under Normal and Pathological Conditions* offered the first formal presentation of basic information on the application of mechanics to the internal structures of the human body. It also made reference to Newton's laws.

•1966 • The first laboratory for biomechanics research was developed by Richard Nelson at Pennsylvania State University.

•1970 • The first meeting in North America for physical education researchers in biomechanics was held at Indiana University.

•1973 • The International Society of Biomechanics was founded at the 4th International Seminar on Biomechanics at Pennsylvania State University.

•1977 • The US Olympic Committee developed a program of biomechanical services for amateur athletes.

Bibliography

Adrian, M.J. and Cooper, J.M. (1995). *Biomechanics of human movement*. 2nd ed. Dubuque, IA: WCB Benchmark.

Alexander, R.M. (1992). *The human machine*. London: Natural History Museum Publications.

Bartlett, R. (1997). *Introduction to sports biomechanics*. London: E & FN Spon.

Bartlett, R. (1998). *Sports biomechanics: Reducing injury and improving performance*. New York: E & FN Spon.

Bell, F. (1998). *Principles of mechanics and biomechanics*. Cheltenham, UK: Stanley Thornes.

Bloomfield, J., Ackland, T.R., and Elliott, B.C. (1994). *Applied anatomy and biomechanics in sport*. Melbourne: Blackwell Scientific Publications.

Carr, G. (2004). *Sport mechanics for coaches*. 2nd ed. Champaign, IL: Human Kinetics.

Enoka, R.M. (2002). *Neuromechanics of human movement*. 3rd ed. Champaign, IL: Human Kinetics.

Hall, S.J. (2003). *Basic biomechanics*. 4th ed. Boston, MA: WCB McGraw-Hill.

Hamill, J. and Knutzen, K.M. (2003). *Biomechanical basis of human movement*. 2nd ed. Philadelphia, PA: Lippincott Williams & Wilkins.

Hay, J.G. (1993). *The biomechanics of sports techniques*. 4th ed. Englewood Cliffs, New Jersey: Prentice Hall.

Knudson, D.V. and Morrison, C.S. (2002). *Qualitative analysis of human movement*. 2nd ed. Champaign, IL: Human Kinetics.

Kreighbaum, E. and Barthels, K.M. (1996). *Biomechanics: A qualitative approach*. 4th ed. Needham Heights, MA: Allyn and Bacon.

Le Veau, B.F. (1992). *Williams and Lissner's biomechanics of human motion*. 3rd ed. Philadelphia, PA: W.B. Saunders.

Levangie, P.K. and Norkin, C.C. (2001). *Joint structure and function: A comprehensive analysis*. 3rd ed. Philadelphia, PA: F.A. Davis Company.

McGinnis, P. (1999). *Biomechanics of sport and exercise*. Champaign, IL: Human Kinetics.

Nigg, B.M. and Herzog, W. (1999, eds). *Biomechanics of the musculoskeletal system*. Chichester, UK: John Wiley.

Nigg, B.M., MacIntosh, B.R. and Mester, J. (2000, eds). *Biomechanics and biology of movement*. Champaign, IL: Human Kinetics.

Nordin, M. and Frankel, V.H. (2001). *Basic biomechanics of the musculoskeletal system*. 3rd ed. Philadelphia, PA: Lippincott Williams & Wilkins.

Robertson, D.G.E. et al. (2004). *Research methods in biomechanics*. Champaign, IL: Human Kinetics.

Stergiou, N. (2004, ed). *Innovative analyses of human movement. Analytical tools for human movement research*. Champaign, IL: Human Kinetics.

Vaughan, C.L. (1989, ed). *Biomechanics of sport*. Boca Raton, FL: CRC Press.

Wilkerson, J.D. (1997). Biomechanics. In: Massengale, J.D. and Swanson, R.A. (eds.). *The history of exercise and sport science*. pp321-366. Champaign, IL: Human Kinetics.

Winter, D.A. (1990). *Biomechanics and motor control of human movement*. 2nd ed. New York: John Wiley and Sons.

Zatsiorsky, V.M. (2000, eds). *Biomechanics in sport. Performance enhancement and injury prevention. Vol. IX of the Encyclopedia of Sports Medicine*. Oxford: Blackwell Science.

Zatsiorsky, V.M. (2002). *Kinetics of human motion*. Champaign, IL: Human Kinetics.

BIOSYNTHESIS   Anabolism. *See under* METABOLISM.

BIOTIN   A water-soluble B-vitamin that exists in many foods, either in its free form or bound to a protein. It is important as a coenzyme in carboxylation reactions, during which it carries an activated carbon dioxide molecule (in a carboxyl group) from one active site to another on a carboxylase. Biotin-dependent enzymes are found in the cytosol and mitochrondria. Biotin is needed for the synthesis and degradation of fatty acids, gluconeogenesis and protein degradation. Only D-biotin is biologically active as a coenzyme. Biotin is synthesized by intestinal microflora and absorbed, but not enough is obtained to meet dietary requirements for the vitamin.

Egg yolk, liver and yeast are rich sources of biotin. The adequate intake level for biotin assumes that current average intake of biotin are meeting the dietary requirement.

Bibliography

Oregon State University. The Linus Pauling Institute. Micronutrient Information Center. Http://lpi.oregonstate.edu/infocenter

BIPOLAR DISORDER   Manic depression. It involves an alternating pattern of emotional highs (mania) and lows (depression). Signs and symptoms of mania include: feelings of euphoria, extreme optimism and inflated self-esteem; rapid speech, racing thoughts, agitation and increased physical activity; poor judgment and recklessness; difficulty sleeping; tendency to be easily distracted; inability to concentrate; and extreme irritability. Signs and symptoms of the depression phase include: persistent feelings of sadness, anxiety, guilt or hopelessness; disturbances in sleep and appetite; fatigue and loss of interest in daily activities; difficulty in concentrating; recurring thoughts of suicide; and depression. **Bipolar I disorder** is characterized by one or more manic episodes or mixed episodes (symptoms of both a mania and a depression occurring nearly every day for at least one week) and one or more major depressive episodes. It is the most extreme form of the illness and is marked by extreme manic episodes. **Bipolar II disorder** is characterized by one or more depressive episodes, accompanied by at least one hypomanic episode. **Hypomanic episodes** have symptoms similar to manic episodes, but are less severe and must be clearly different from a person's non-depressed mood. **Cyclothymic disorder** is characterized by chronic fluctuating moods involving periods of hypomania and depression. The periods of both depressive and hypomanic symptoms are shorter, less severe and do not occur with regularity as experienced with bipolar I and II. **Bipolar disorder not otherwise specified** is a form of the illness that does not fit into one of the above definitions. In the USA, bipolar disorder affects more than 2 million adults, or about 1% of the population aged 18 years or older. It often begins in adolescence or early adulthood, and may persist for life. 80 to 90% of people suffering from bipolar disorder have relatives with some form of depression. Lithium is effective in controlling mania.

Bibliography

American Psychiatric Association (1994). *Diagnostic and statistical manual of mental disorders*. 4th ed. Washington, DC: American Psychiatric Association.

BIRTH DEFECTS *See* TERATOGENS.

BIRTH ORDER Firstborn children are more likely to be high achievers and more likely to be more active than later-born children.

BLACK EYE *See* PERIORBITAL HEMATOMA.

BLACK HEEL *See* TALON NOIR.

BLADDER A hollow muscular storage organ that is found behind the pubic symphysis (under the midline of the abdominal quadrants) and is a reservoir for urine produced by the kidneys. Because it is in a well-protected area, the bladder is rarely injured in sport. However, a blunt force to the lower abdominal region may injure the bladder that is distended by urine. '**Runner's bladder**' is hematuria associated with contusion of the bladder as a result of long-distance running. Running with an empty bladder increases the risk of gross hematuria, because no fluid cushion exists between the posterior wall and the base of the bladder.
See under MICTURITION.

BLIND Blindness and visual impairment are largely

problems of old age. Visual impairment may be congenital or adventitious (diagnosed at age of 2 or 3 years, or later). Approximately half a million persons in the USA are legally blind. In the USA, it is defined as a visual acuity of 20/200 or less in the better eye with the best correction, i.e. what a person with perfect vision sees form a distance of 200 feet, a person who is legally blind sees from a distance of 20 feet or less. Most blindness in school-age persons is attributed to birth defects, such as congenital cataracts or retinopathy of prematurity. Under federal legislation in the USA, **visual impairment** is defined as impairment in vision, which, even with correction, adversely affects a child's educational performance. The term includes both partial sight and blindness.

Impairment of the visual field, the area viewed by one or both eyes at a time, is associated with any one of, or combination of the following symptoms: peripheral field loss (less than 170 to 180 degree of sight from side to side or top to bottom), central field loss (unable to see what is straight ahead), scotomas ('holes' or 'blind spots' scattered throughout the visual field), field cuts (unable to see pieces or an entire half of the visual field in each eye) and islands of vision (visual field is decreased to only small areas in one or both eyes).

Cortical visual impairment is due to damage to the visual cortex of the brain or the visual pathways, which results in the brain not adequately receiving or interpreting visual information. Children with cortical visual impairment often also have cerebral palsy, seizure disorder and developmental delays as a result of damage to the brain. They may exhibit inattention to visual stimuli, preference for touch over vision when exploring objects, and difficulty visually discriminating objects that are placed close together or in front of a visually complex background.

Postural deviations may result from holding their heads in certain positions to maximize vision. A slow shuffling gait characterizes many persons who are blind.

Mastery of motor milestones for blind infants is in a different order from that of sighted infants, with milestones requiring vision being delayed most.

Stereotypies are common in persons with visual impairment; '**blindisms**' are habits such as hand waving or finger flicking. Due primarily to sedentary lifestyles, persons with visual impairment have lower fitness than sighted persons. As a result of the overprotection experienced by many persons who are blind, and the consequent lack of opportunity to free explore their environment, fearfulness and dependence may be a characteristic of persons with visual impairment. Boundaries for various games should be marked by a change in floor or ground surfaces that can be perceived by the soles of the feet. Braille can be used on swimming pool walls to designate the changing water depths.

See also CATARACTS; GLAUCOMA; RETINA.

Chronology

•1838 • The first physical activity program for students who are blind was begun at the Perkins School for pupils with visual disabilities in Boston. Its director, Samuel G. Howe, advocated the health benefits of physical activity that involved outdoor recreation.

•1946 • Goalball was invented by Hanz Lorenzen of Austria and Sett Reindle of Germany, as a way to rehabilitate post-World War II veterans who were blind. The sport is now played in more than a hundred countries. Each team tries to roll the ball, which contains a bell, across the opponents goal while the other team tries to stop them. Goalball can be used in mainstream physical education, with sighted peers participating on equal terms with those who are visually impaired. All team members are required to wear a blindfold.

•1976 • The US Association for Blind Athletes (USABA) was created to provide competitive opportunities for legally blind athletes. USABA members compete against athletes with and without visual disabilities. It covers Alpine and Nordic skiing, goalball, judo, powerlifting, swimming, tandem cycling, track and field, and wrestling. The first national championship was held in 1977.

•1976 • Goalball was introduced as a medal event at the Paralympic Games in Toronto after its success as a demonstration event at the 1972 Paralympic Games in Heidelberg.

•1976 • James Mastro became the first blind athlete to be placed on an Olympic team. He was alternate to the US Olympic wrestling team. He didn't compete in the Olympic Games that year, but he later won a bronze medal in the 1996 Paralympic Games. Mastro was the first person with a visual impairment to earn a PhD in physical education in the USA. He studied adapted and developmental physical education at Texas Woman's University.

•1981 • The International Blind Sport Association (IBSA) was founded in Paris.

•1994 • The US Association of Blind Athletes (USABA) began a nationwide public service campaign utilizing elite blind athletes as peer leaders with schools and community organizations.

•2000 • Marla Runyan, a former Paralympian, became the first legally blind American to compete in the Olympic Games, finishing 8th in the Women's 1,500 m run. As a teenager, she was diagnosed with Stargardt disease, a condition that can cause visual impairment and even blindness in teenagers and young adults.

Bibliography

International Blind Sports Association. Http://www.ibsa.es/eng.

Runyan, M. and Jenkins, S. (2001). *No finish line: My life as I see it*. New York: G.P. Putnam's Sons.

Winnick, J.P. (2000, ed). *Adapted physical education and sport*. 3rd ed. Champaign, IL: Human Kinetics.

BLINKING   Regular and full opening and closing of the eye cleans and refreshes the front of the eye while providing nutrients and dissolved oxygen for the tissues of the cornea. The eyeball is kept moist by tears secreted by the lacrimal apparatus, together with the mucous and oily secretions of the other secretory organs and cells of the lids and conjunctiva. The secretion produces the pre-corneal film, which consists of an inner layer of mucus, a middle layer of lacrimal secretion, and an outer oily film that decreases the rate of evaporation of the underlying watery layer. It includes lyozyme, an enzyme that has dissolves the outer coats of many bacteria.

A distinction can be made between spontaneous and reflex blinking. **Spontaneous blinking** occurs regularly without stimuli at a rate that depends on a number of factors including visual acuity and environmental conditions. It remains fairly constant for a given individual, and is determined by the 'blinking center' in the globus pallidus of the caudate nucleus. **Reflex blinking** occurs in response to various stimuli, such as bright lights, approaching noises, touch, and loud noises.

The average blink rate is once every 3 to 6

seconds, but individuals with dry eyes tend to blink considerably less. Looking at computer screens for long periods of time can dry out the eyes. Cathode-ray tube monitors are worse than TFT (thin film technology) monitors, as the former give out static which dry out the eyes. Air conditioning and central heating also tend to dry out eyes. Cosmetics can cause dry eyes, especially oily make-up removers that may destabilize the tear film.

Tear supplements include Viscotears from Ciba Vision, which is a viscous gel. It is most effective when it is used as a course of treatment applied three to four times per day for up to 28 days.

Bibliography
All About Vision. Http://www.allaboutvision.com

D & J Brower Opticians. Http://www.brower.co.uk

BLISTER An injury caused by skin being rubbed against a hard or rough surface. The heat that is generated causes the epidermis to separate from the dermis and fluid accumulates in the dermal layer. Blisters occur most commonly on the palms and soles from repeated friction. They appear as tender vesicles filled with clear fluid or blood, or, if ruptured, as erosions with remnants of the epidermal roof. When possible, the epidermal roof should be left intact to serve as a natural barrier against infection. Blisters larger than a centimeter in diameter should be drained by puncturing the skin with a sterile needle or scalpel to prevent further expansion from peripheral pressure. Once drained, the blister can be covered with a membrane dressing such as DuoDerm® to protect against additional friction. Lubricating the skin or applying powders such as Zeasorb® may help to decrease friction and subsequent blisters.

Bibliography
Basler, R.S., Hunzeker, C.M. and Garcia, M.A. (2004). Athletic skin injuries. Combating pressure and friction. *The Physician and Sportsmedicine* 32(5). Http://www.physsportmed.com

BLOOD The fluid circulated by the heart and blood vessels. It is a liquid connective tissue. All blood cells begin as stem cells the bone marrow before differentiating and maturing into corpuscles. Blood transports substances to and from tissues. It is composed of plasma and corpuscles. **Plasma** contains water (90%), proteins (7%) and other substances (3%). Proteins are albumen (55%), globulin (41%) and fibrinogen (4%). Other substances include glucose and urea. **Corpuscles** are red blood cells (4.5 to 5.5 million/mm^3), white blood cells (6 to 10 thousand/mm^3) and platelets (150 to 400 thousand/mm^3).

See LEUKOCYTES; PLATELETS; RED BLOOD CELLS.

BLOODBORNE PATHOGENS Pathogenic microorganisms that can potentially cause disease. They may be present in human blood and other bodily fluids including semen, vaginal secretions, cerebrospinal fluid, synovial fluid and any other fluid contaminated with blood. The two most significant bloodborne pathogens are hepatitis B virus and HIV.

BLOOD-BRAIN BARRIER A physical barrier that exists between the blood and cerebrospinal fluid, which is the interstitial fluid in the central nervous system.

BLOOD CLOTTING The conversion of blood from liquid- to jelly-form when blood vessels are injured, thus preventing the escape of blood. **Fibrinogen** (also known as factor I) is a soluble protein of the globulin class that is found in blood plasma. Elevated levels of fibrinogen have been shown to correlate with myocardial infarction and stroke, probably as a result of enhanced blood viscosity and increased thrombogenicity.

During the clotting process, fibrinogen is converted into an insoluble protein called **fibrin** by the proteolysis of the enzyme thrombin. **Prothrombin** is a pro-enzyme of thrombin.

The breakdown of fibrin clots is referred to as **fibrinolysis** or **fibrinolytic activity**. The term **coagulation (fibrinolytic) potential** reflects an increased potential for coagulation, while coagulation per se may or may not be occurring. Fibrinolysis is the lysis of inappropriate or excessive blood clot, which may or may not be occurring when the enzymes that stimulate fibrinolysis are activated. Enhanced fibrinolytic activity could potentially decrease the risk of clots and hence coronary heart disease. An inhibition of fibrinolysis increases the risk of arterial thrombosis. High visceral abdominal obesity is directly related to decreased fibrinolytic activity.

It seems that exercise of moderate intensity is followed by activation of blood fibrinolysis without concomitant hypercoagulability, while exercise of high intensity is associated with concurrent activation of blood coagulation and fibrinolysis. Moderate exercise may be the most appropriate way known to lower plasma fibrinogen concentrations. Fibrinolytic activity associated with exercise appears to be mediated via beta-adrenoceptor stimulation, augmenting vascular endothelial release of plasminogen activator. There is evidence that exhaustive exercise is associated with a raising of blood fibrinogen, particularly in the 20% of the population who inherit a gene that gives them higher levels of fibrinogen when leading a normal life. Chronic aerobic exercise training may decrease coagulation potential and increase fibrinolytic potential in both healthy individuals and cardiovascular disease patients.

Bibliography

El-Sayed, M.S., Ali, Z.E-S. and Ahmadizad, S. (2004). Exercise and training effects on blood hemostasis in health and disease: An update. *Sports Medicine* 34(3), 181-200.

Ernst, E. (1993). Regular exercise reduces fibrinogen levels: A review of longitudinal studies. *British Journal of Sports Medicine* 27(3), 175-176.

Womack, C.J., Nagelkirk, P.R. and Coughlin, A.M. (2003). Exercise-induced changes in coagulation and fibrinolysis in healthy populations and patients with cardiovascular disease. *Sports Medicine* 33(11), 795-807.

BLOOD CORPUSCLE *See under* BLOOD.

BLOOD DONATION After donating 450 mL of whole blood, plasma volume falls 7 to 13%, then recovers within 24 to 48 hours. The hemoglobin level decreases 10 to 20 g/L. With an adequate iron supply, hemoglobin returns to baseline after 3 to 4 weeks. Blood donation is contraindicated for endurance athletes who will soon be competing.

Bibliography

Schnirring, L. (2001). Donating blood. What active people need to know. *The Physician and Sportsmedicine*. 29(6), 11-15.

BLOOD DOPING An ergogenic aid that has been used to increase performance in events involving the aerobic energy systems. It is also known as induced erythrocythemia, red blood cell reinfusion or 'blood boosting.' Some studies have reported maximal oxygen uptake increases of 10 to 15%. Oxygen uptake during submaximal exercise is unchanged.

The American College of Sports Medicine (1987) stated that the use of blood doping as an ergogenic aid for athletic competition is unethical and unjustifiable, but that autologous red blood cell infusion (i.e. the athlete's own blood) is an acceptable procedure to induce erythrocythemia in clinically controlled conditions for the purpose of legitimate scientific inquiry. Blood doping was first used as an experimental procedure to investigate oxygen transport during acute hypoxia.

Blood doping involves blood being taken from the athlete and the erythrocytes removed for frozen storage with the plasma being immediately reinfused. The blood is usually withdrawn in lots of about half a liter over a period of 3 to 8 weeks. A problem with early research was that American Red Cross blood donation regulations specified that refrigerated blood must be used within 21 days; it takes about 8 weeks for the body to replace naturally the erythrocytes lost following withdrawal. The erythrocytes that have been separated from the plasma are preserved via glycerol freezing, allowing preservation for up to three years. If homologous transfusion (donated blood) is going to be given, then storage is not necessary. The individual continues training to full aerobic capacity during the following 4 to 8 weeks. Reinfusion is usually done 1 to 7 days prior to the athletic event. At the time of autologous reinfusion, the frozen erythrocytes are thawed and reconstituted with a physiologic saline solution. Intravenous infusion takes place over a period of 1 to 2 hours. The major effect of blood doping is related to the increase in total erythrocyte mass and hemoglobin, which can be as great as 20%; the transient increase in blood volume and cardiac output following reinfusion is too short lived to be of any real importance. This enables an increased transport of oxygen, and therefore a potentially greater reserve of blood that can be diverted to non-exercising tissues to improve thermoregulation. The increased red cell mass also improves lactate buffering.

Blood doping may have the opposite effect to that intended. A large infusion of erythrocytes could increase blood viscosity, causing a decrease in cardiac output and a decrease in the amount of oxygen carried to the working muscle. One quart of blood will not lead to excessive viscosity, but has been associated with improved performance. There is also a detraining effect produced by the repeated venesection required to obtain an adequate amount of stored blood for autologous reinfusion. *See also* ERYTHROPOIETIN.

Chronology

•1972 • Rumors circulated during the Olympic Games in Munich that Finnish athlete Lasse Viren used blood doping. Viren, however, is said to have attributed his 5000 m and 10,000 m victories to a diet that included reindeer milk.

•1984 • After the Olympic Games, the US Olympic Committee revealed that seven members (four medallists) of its 24-member Olympic cycling team had received blood transfusions prior to competition. A year later 'blood doping' was banned by the International Olympic Committee (IOC).

Bibliography

American College of Sports Medicine (1987). Position stand on blood doping as an ergogenic aid. *Medicine and Science in Sports and Exercise* 19, 540-542.

Jones, M. and Tunstall-Pedoe, D.S. (1989). Blood doping - A literature review. *British Journal of Sports Medicine* 23(2), 84-8.

Sawaka, M.N., Joyner, M.J. et al. (1996). American College of Sports Medicine position stand. The use of blood doping as an ergogenic aid. *Medicine and Science in Sports and Exercise* 28(6), i-viii.

BLOOD FLOW *See under* BLOOD PRESSURE; BLOOD VISCOSITY.

BLOOD GLUCOSE *See under* GLUCOSE.

BLOOD GROUPS Blood types. About 200 different blood group substances have been identified and placed within 19 known blood group systems. The most commonly encountered blood group system is the **AB0 (Landsteiner) system**. According to the AB0 blood grouping system, there are four different kinds of blood types: A, B, AB, or 0 (null). With **blood group A**, there are A antigens on the surface of the red blood cells and B antibodies in the blood plasma. With **blood group B**, there are B antigens on the surface of the red blood cells and A antibodies in the blood plasma. With **blood group AB**, there are both A and B antigens on the surface of the red blood cells and no A or B antibodies at all in the blood plasma. With **blood group 0**, there are neither A or B antigens on the surface of the red blood cells, but both A and B antibodies in the blood plasma.

Blood transfusions should be done with exactly matched blood. When red blood cells carrying one or both antigens are exposed to the corresponding antibodies, they agglutinate, i.e. they clump together. The agglutinated red cells can clog blood vessels and stop the circulation of the blood to various parts of the body. The agglutinated red blood cells also crack and their contents leak out into the body. The red blood cells contain hemoglobin, which becomes toxic when outside the cell. This can have fatal consequences for the patient.

People usually have antibodies against those red cell antigens that they lack. Transfused blood must not contain red blood cells that the recipient's antibodies can clump. People with blood group 0 are called **"universal donors"** and people with blood group AB are called **"universal receivers."**

For a blood transfusion to be successful, it is also necessary for Rh blood groups to be compatibile between the donor blood and the patient blood. There are a number of Rh antigens (the most common one is designated D), and all produce red blood cells that are '**Rh positive.**' About 15% of the population have no Rh antigens and are thus '**Rh-negative.**' A person with Rh-negative blood does not have Rh antibodies naturally in the blood plasma (as one can have A or B antibodies, for instance). But a person with Rh-negative blood can develop Rh antibodies in the blood plasma if he or she receives blood from a person with Rh-positive blood, whose Rh antigens can trigger the production of Rh antibodies. A person with Rh-positive blood can receive blood from a person with Rh-negative blood without any problems. **Maternal-fetal incompatibility** of the Rh blood groups in humans may result in a disease called **erythroblastosis fetalis** or **hemolytic disease of the newborn**, which may be so severe as to kill the fetus or the newborn infant. During birth, there is often a leakage of the baby's red blood cells into the mother's circulation. If the baby is Rh-positive (having inherited the trait from its father) and the mother is Rh-negative, these red cells will cause her to develop antibodies against the Rh antigen. The antibodies, usually of the IgG class, do not cause any problems for that child, but can cross the placenta and attack the red blood cells of a subsequent Rh-positive fetus. This destroys the red cells and results in anemia and jaundice.

Bibliography

National Blood Service. Http://www.blood.co.uk

BLOOD LACTATE   *See under* LACTIC ACID.

BLOOD LIPIDS   *See under* LIPIDS.

BLOOD PLASMA   It is the fluid in which blood corpuscles float.
   See BLOOD VOLUME.

BLOOD PRESSURE   This is the pressure of the blood on the walls of the arteries. **Blood flow** is the result of a difference in pressure between two points in the circulation. This difference in pressure is a pressure gradient. The amount of blood entering the arterial system from the left ventricle is determined by the cardiac output. The amount of blood leaving through the arterioles is determined by the peripheral resistance. If it can be assumed that central venous pressure is zero, then mean arterial pressure is the product of cardiac output and systemic vascular resistance. It can also be described as the sum of diastolic arterial pressure and one third of the pulse pressure.

   Systolic blood pressure is the highest pressure recorded at the brachial (arm) artery when the left ventricle of the heart pumps blood into the aorta. **Diastolic blood pressure** is the lowest pressure recorded when the heart relaxes. Blood pressure is expressed as two numbers: systolic pressure/ diastolic pressure. Normal blood pressure is equal to 120/80 millimeters of mercury (mm Hg).

   Blood pressure may be measured directly by using a catheter. More commonly, it is measured indirectly using a sphygmomanometer. Arterial blood pressures measured from within peripheral arteries exaggerate systolic blood pressures, but provide representative mean and diastolic pressures of the central arterial circulation. Manual and automated sphygmomanometry are the best non-invasive indirect methods of blood pressure measurement to estimate ascending aortic systolic pressures. Both methods, however, significantly underestimate diastolic pressures at rest and during exercise. The error in diastolic pressure measurement increases as exercise intensity increases. Ascending aorta pressures should ideally be used as a gold standard or criterion method for blood pressure measurement during exercise and instrument/method validation.

   Blood pressure is much lower in the pulmonary circulation than the systemic (body) circulation. In both circulations, when the blood passes from the arteries to the arterioles, there is a sharp drop in both systolic and diastolic blood pressure. There is a further fall as the blood goes from the arterioles to the capillaries. There are successive falls in pressure as blood returns to the heart from the capillaries to the venules, to the veins, and to the heart.

   With the body supine or prone, the pressure in the arteries of the head and feet are about equal to that at (and applied by) the heart. Although the pressure intensity introduced at the heart must be transmitted without loss to the head and the feet, the net result is that the pressure at the head is lower than at heart level, and that at the feet is considerably higher. The increased blood pressure gradient from head to feet can cause edema (swelling) in the legs.

   During exercise of moderate intensity, systolic

pressure rises about 35% but diastolic pressure barely changes. During exercise of high intensity, systolic exercise may rise even higher and diastolic pressure may increase about 35%. When exercise involves very forceful muscular contractions and breath holding, both systolic and diastolic pressures may increase more than two or threefold. This may cause the Valsalva maneuver.

Endurance training tends to cause a decrease in both systolic and diastolic blood pressure at rest and during submaximal exercise. The decrease is greater for systolic pressure, but is unlikely to be greater than 5 to 10 mm Hg.

See also DOUBLE PRODUCT; GROWTH; HYPERTENSION; HYPOTENSION; PRESSOR RESPONSE; VALSALVA MANEUVER.

Bibliography

Griffin, S.E., Robergs, R.A. and Heyward, W.H. (1997). Blood pressure measurement during exercise: A review. *Medicine and Science in Sports and Exercise* 29(1), 149-159.

BLOOD SERUM The fluid that separates from clotted blood. *See under* BLOOD.

BLOOD SUGAR Blood glucose.

BLOOD VESSEL *See* ARTERIES; ARTERIOLES; CAPILLARIES; VEINS; VENULES.

BLOOD VESSEL COMPLIANCE The ability of a vessel to distend with increasing transmural pressure (inside minus outside pressure across the wall). It is an important function of large arteries and veins. At lower pressures, the compliance of a vein is about 20 times greater than an artery. Thus veins can accommodate a large change in blood volume with only a small change in pressure. At higher volumes and pressures, venous compliance becomes similar to arterial compliance. Hence veins can be used as arterial by-pass grafts.

With respect to the respiratory system, compliance refers to the distensibility of the respiratory system; it is the volume change produced by a change in the distending pressure.

An increased stiffness of the aorta and large arteries leads to an increase in pulse pressure through a decrease in arterial compliance and effects on wave reflection. Strength training results in stiffer arteries. When arteries are stiff, the pressure wave gets reflected more readily from the periphery of the circulation and the combination of the outgoing wave and the reflected wave results in a sharper pressure waveform, and hence a wider pulse pressure. There is evidence that increased stiffness of the arteries is associated with aging, hypertension and coronary heart disease. Wide pulse pressure may be a risk factor for heart disease and stroke. Thus weightlifting may be harmful to the cardiovascular system.

A number of dietary and lifestyle interventions have been shown to modify large artery behavior. These include aerobic exercise training and consumption of omega-3 fatty acids.

Bibliography

Bertovic, D.A. et al. (1999). Muscular strength training is associated with low arterial compliance and high pulse pressure. *Hypertension* 33, 1385-1391.

Dart, A.M. and Kingwell, B.A. (2001). Pulse pressure: A review of mechanisms and clinical relevance. *Journal of the American College of Cardiology* 37(4), 975-984.

Duprez, D.A. et al. (2001). Small and large artery elasticity indices in peripheral arterial occlusive disease (PAOD). *Vascular Medicine* 6, 211-214.

O'Rourke, M.F. et al. (2002). Clinical applications of arterial stiffness: Definitions and reference values. *American Journal of Hypertension* 15, 426-444.

BLOOD VISCOSITY A measure of the internal friction of blood as it flows through the vascular system. Blood viscosity is conventionally determined at the physiological temperature of 37 degrees Celsius. Blood is more viscous than water, because there is greater friction between adjacent layers in the flowing blood than in water.

The main determinants of whole blood viscosity are: plasma viscosity; hematocrit; shear stress and shear rate; the deformability and aggregation of red blood cells; fibrinogen concentration; and temperature.

Blood is a non-Newtonian fluid, meaning that the ratio of shear stress to shear rate alters depending on the speed of flow. Relatively greater force is required to move the blood slowly than to move it fast. Blood is able to remain fluid even at a very high hematocrit value. This is mainly due to the flexibility of red blood cells and their ability to shape and reshape easily. The comparatively low blood viscosity at a high shear rate is partly due to the deformability of red blood cells.

Plasma viscosity increases with increasing protein concentration, but different proteins will have different effects on plasma viscosity depending on the shape and size of the protein. The increase in viscosity with increasing hematocrit increases as the shear rate (flow rate) decreases. At low shear rate, an increase in red blood cell concentration promotes red blood cell aggregation, which increases effective cell volume and blood viscosity. At high shear rate, an increase in red cell concentration promotes deformation of red blood cells, which decreases effective cell volume and hence compensates for the increase in viscosity.

An increase or decrease in temperature elevates blood viscosity, and this temperature effect is to some extent dependent on shear rate. The increase in whole blood viscosity as a result of exercise is mainly attributed to an increase in hematocrit and plasma viscosity, whereas the deformability and aggregability of red blood cells remains unaltered. The increases in plasma viscosity and hematocrit have been ascribed to exercise-induced hemoconcentration as a result of fluid transfer from the blood to the interstitial spaces. The blood of endurance athletes is more dilute and this has been attributed to an expansion of plasma volume as a result of training.

See also ANEMIA.

Bibliography
El-Sayed, M.S. (1998). Effects of exercise and training on blood rheology. *Sports Medicine* 26(5), 281-292.

BLOOD VOLUME An increase in blood volume produces an increase in central venous pressure. If blood volume decreases (due to dehydration, for example), central venous pressure decreases along with venous pressure and end-diastolic volume. The resulting decrease in cardiac output triggers a decrease in mean arterial pressure.

BLOUNT'S DISEASE *See* TIBIA VARUS.

BODY AWARENESS *See under* SELF CONCEPT.

BODYBUILDING A sport that involves the use of weight training to develop the size, density, visual separation, symmetry and harmony of body parts. The bodybuilder needs to minimize subcutaneous fat, which may be as low as 6% in males and 10% in females. Competition involves posing on a stage in front of judges, who subjectively rate the contestants.

Bodybuilding training tends to involve 6 to 12 repetitions with short to moderate periods of rest in between sets. All top bodybuilders use 'split' systems of training, which involve the use of a few selected muscles or muscle groups in each training session. All muscles are trained over 4 days or 6 days. 'Double split' training involves 2 sessions each day, with 2 to 5 exercises being done per muscle group, and 20 to 25 sets per muscle group. For most muscle groups, two sessions per week seem to be sufficient. Bodybuilding methods aim at total overloading and depletion of energy stores. Optimal recovery time is not known. To prevent overtraining when using split routines, it is important to train all muscles that act together in one training session and, for very intensive sessions, a recovery period of about 72 hours should occur. Bodybuilding training techniques include super setting (alternating agonists and antagonists of a joint with minimal rest between exercises), compound setting (performing two different exercises for the same muscle group in an alternating fashion with little or no rest between exercises) and pre-exhaustion (fatiguing a muscle in a single joint and isolated movement prior to performing a multiple joint exercise involving the same muscle, e.g. preceding squats with leg curls to give hamstring fatigue). It is not clear what process associated with contraction failure would relate to increased protein synthesis.

The high volume of training coupled with moderate relative intensity (expressed as percentage of one-repetition maximum) appears to be optimal for overall muscle hypertrophy. There is evidence of a relative lack of individual fiber hypertrophy in bodybuilders who possess large limb growth. This has led to the suggestion that larger muscles in bodybuilders may be associated with an increase in the number of muscle fibers (i.e. hyperplasia). Bodybuilders tend to have a significantly lower proportion of fast-twitch fibers than other strength athletes and a larger number and size of slow-twitch fibers. These characteristics are similar to those found in endurance athletes. Bodybuilders have higher citrate synthase activity in type II fibers than other types of weight lifters who train with heavier loads and longer rest periods.

Relative to non-athletes or other strength-trained athletes, it seems that bodybuilders possess greater arm than leg strength.

Lambert et al. (2004) suggest that the diet for bodybuilders, during both the off-season and pre-contest phases, should be 55 to 60% carbohydrate, 25 to 30% protein, and 15 to 20% fat. In both the off-season and pre-contest phases, adequate dietary carbohydrate should be ingested (55 to 60% of total energy intake) so that training intensity can be maintained. During the off-season, the diet should be slightly hyperenergetic (15% increase in energy intake) and during the pre-contest phase it should be hypoenergetic (15% decrease in energy intake). For 6 to 12 weeks before competition, bodybuilders attempt to retain muscle mass and decrease body fat to very low levels. During the pre-contest phase, the bodybuilder should be in negative energy balance so that body fat can be oxidized. According to Lambert et al, there is evidence that a relatively high protein intake (around 30% of energy intake) will decrease loss of fat-free mass relative to a lower protein intake (15%) during energy restriction.

See also BODY DYSMORPHIA; MUSCLE GROWTH, EXERCISE-INDUCED; PROTEIN; RESISTANCE TRAINING.

Chronology

•1894 • Eugen Sandow (born in Prussia as Friederich Wilhelm Mueller) went to Chicago to pose as a Greek statue in the World Fair and to make a show called the "Sandow Trocadero Vaudevilles." He built his musculature to the same proportions as classical Greek and Roman sculpture, and was described by Dudley A. Sargent as "the most wonderful specimen of man I have ever seen." Sandow marketed photographs of himself (sometimes clad only in a leaf) and had a number of body-building manuals published in his name including *The Body Building, Or Man in the Making*, the first training book of bodybuilding. He could raise a barbell weighing about 271 lb over his head with one arm in a movement he called "The Bent Press," which involved being sideways and forwards. In London (32 St. James Street), Sandow built the first modern gymnasium. It was marketed to a rich clientele. He became the personal fitness instructor to King George V, and was one of the first to advocate a government ministry of health and compulsory physical education in schools. Sandow developed a successful mail order business. An advert in A.G. Spalding & Bros. (1909) catalog showed "Sandow's Parent Spring Grip Dumb Bells" (made in two halves connected by steel springs) that were sold with a chart of exercises by Sandow.

•1903 • Bernarr McFadden, a businessman in America, promoted an approach of physical development through weightlifting. He promoted a competition to declare, "The Most Perfectly Developed Man in the World." The 1921 winner, Angelo Sicilian, changed his name to become Charles Atlas. Atlas won in 1922, but it was not held in 1923 because McFadden knew Atlas would win. McFadden was a "weak, sickly child," who became "a complete physical wreck" at the age of 16 years. McFadden also published *Physical Culture* magazine.

Bibliography

Anderson, R. (2004). Sandow. Http://www.sandowmuseum.com

Baechle, T.R. (2000, ed). *Essentials of strength training and conditioning*. 2nd ed. Champaign, IL: Human Kinetics.

Green, J. (1986). *Fit for America. Health, fitness, sport and American society*. New York: Pantheon Books.

Lambert, C.P., Frank, L.L. and Evans, W.J. (2004). Macronutrient considerations for the sport of bodybuilding. *Sports Medicine* 34(5), 317-327.

Tesch, P.A. (1992). Training for bodybuilding. In: Komi, P.V. (ed). *Strength and power in sport*. pp370-380. Oxford: Blackwell Scientific Publications.

BODY CLOCK *See under* BIOLOGICAL RHYTHMS

BODY COMPOSITION The body can be subdivided into two components: fat and fat-free mass. The **fat-free mass**, formerly referred to as the lean body mass, is composed of all of the body's non-fat tissue, including bone, muscle, connective tissue and organs. The direct method of assessing body composition is by cadaver (fresh dead body) dissection analysis. The most common indirect methods involve body density measurement and measures of skinfold thickness. **Hydrostatic weighing** is an indirect method of determining body density. It is based on Archimedes' principle that a body's loss of weight in water equals the weight of the volume of water it displaces. To determine body density, the following steps may be taken. Firstly, body volume is computed as the difference between body weight measured in air and body weight measured under water. Secondly, a temperature correction is made for the density of water. Thirdly, body volume is calculated as the difference between body weight measured in air and that measured under water, divided by the density of water. Fourthly, body volume must be corrected for residual volume of the lungs. This can be found using the modified oxygen-dilution technique. Finally, body density is calculated as mass divided by volume.

Body density is usually converted to % body fat using the **Siri equation**: % Body fat $= (495/D) - 450$, where D is body density.

Absolute body fat is equal to body weight multiplied by % body fat. **Lean body weight** is equal to body weight multiplied by absolute body fat. The Siri equation assumes that the density of lean body material is 1.1 grams per cubic centimeter (g/cm^3) and that the density of fat is $0.9\ g/cm^3$. The single value for the density of lean tissue is problematic, however, because there are wide individual differences in the densities and proportions of fat-free components.

There are a number of other methods used to assess body composition. The trained eye has been shown to be an accurate assessor of both absolute and relative amounts of body fat. **Bioelectrical impedance** is based on the concept that the flow of electrical current through the body is facilitated through hydrated, fat-free body tissues and extracellular fluid compared to fat tissue, because of the greater electrolyte content of the fat-free

component (i.e. lowered electrical resistance). Impedance to the flow of electric current relates to the quantity of total body water, which in turn can be extrapolated to estimate free-fat mass, body density and % body fat.

24-hour creatinine excretion is a widely used biochemical marker for body muscle mass estimation and hence body composition. After a creatine-controlled diet, the total 24-hour urine is analyzed for creatinine content. A problem, though, is that no definitive creatinine equivalence for human muscle has been established. A less common method for estimating muscle mass is the use of plasma or serum creatinine values.

BODPOD® Body Composition System uses air displacement plethysmography and is based on Boyle's law that a volume of air compressed under isothermal conditions decreases in proportion to a pressure change. The subject sits in a structure composed of a front (test) and rear (reference) chamber, each of known volume, and separated by a moving diaphragm. Changes in pressure between the two chambers cause the diaphragm to oscillate, and thus reflects any change in the chamber volume. The subject takes several breaths into an air circuit to assess thoracic gas volume, which when subtracted from measured body volume yields true body volume. Body density is calculated as body mass (measured in air) divided by body volume (measured in BODPOD). The Siri equation is then used to convert body density into % body fat.

Magnetic resonance imaging (MRI) is a high-cost method in which the hydrogen nuclei of water and lipid molecules are excited by electromagnetic radiation in the presence of a magnetic field, resulting in a detectable signal, which is measured. The amount of water and lipid and their freedom of motion define the signal size, permitting discrimination between these tissues. The degree of perturbation of a body placed in an electromagnetic field depends on the quantity of conducting material (mainly electrolytes in lean body mass). **Total body electrical conductivity** is a high-cost method in which the subject lies on a stretcher and is slid into a large solenoid coil. It correlates highly with hydrostatic weighing. **Computed tomography** is a high-cost method that can give a ratio of intra-abdominal to extra-abdominal fat. **Dual-energy X-ray absorptiometry** (DEXA) allows simultaneous measurement of bone mineral, fat and non-bone lean tissue. It depends on geometric models and the assumption of constant hydration in fat-free soft tissues. **Doubly-labeled water** is a method used over 7 to 14 day periods. A form of indirect calorimetry, it measures the isotopes of hydrogen and oxygen in excreted water and carbon dioxide. The subject ingests a small quantity of two kinds of water; one labeled with the hydrogen isotope deuterium ($2H_2$) and the other labeled with an isotope of oxygen (oxygen-18). Both isotopes occur naturally and are radioactive. The body excretes oxygen-18 as part of water ($H_2^{18}O$) and carbon dioxide ($C^{18}O_2$); it excretes deuterium only as part of water (^2H_2O). The difference between the rate of deuterium loss and oxygen-18 loss is used to calculate carbon dioxide output and determine total energy expenditure. *See also* SKINFOLD FAT.

Bibliography

Barr, S.I., McCargar, L.J. and Crawford, S.M. (1994). Practical use of body composition analysis in sport. *Sports Medicine* 17(5), 277-282.

Behnke, A.R. and Wilmore, J.H. (1974). *Evaluation and regulation of body build and composition*. Englewood Cliffs, NJ: Prentice-Hall.

Bloomfield, J., Ackland, T.R., and Elliott, B.C. (1994). *Applied anatomy and biomechanics in sport*. Melbourne: Blackwell Scientific Publications.

Brodie, D.A. (1988). Techniques of measurement of body composition. *Sports Medicine* 5, 11-40 and 74-98.

Eckerson, J.M, Housh, T.J. and Johnson, G.O. (1992). The validity of visual estimation of percent body fat in lean males. *Medicine and Science in Sports and Exercise* 24, 615-618.

Eston, R.G. and Reilly, T. (1994). *Laboratory manual of tests, procedures and data for kinanthropometry and exercise physiology*. London: E. and F.N. Spon.

Heyward, V.H. and Wagner, D.R. (2004). *Applied body composition and assessment*. 2nd ed. Champaign, IL: Human Kinetics.

Roche, A.F., Heymsfield, S.B. and Lohman, T.G. (1996). *Human body composition*. Champaign, IL: Human Kinetics.

Ross, W.D. and Marfell-Jones, M.J. (1991). Kinanthropometry. In: MacDougall, J.D., Wenger, H.A. and Green, H.J. (eds).

Physiological testing of the high performance athlete. 2nd ed. pp223-308. Champaign, IL: Human Kinetics.

Weiner, J.S. and Louri, J.A. (1981). *Practical human biology*. London: Academic Press.

Wilmore, J.H. et al (1980). Further simplification of a method for determination of residual lung volume. *Medicine and Science in Sports and Exercise* 12, 216-218.

BODY DEROTATIVE REFLEXES *See* SEGMENTAL ROLLING REFLEXES.

BODY DYSMORPHIC DISORDER An excessive preoccupation with an imagined or minor defect of a localized facial feature or body part, resulting in decreased social, academic and occupational functioning. Pathologic body dissatisfaction in men was first referred to in the medical literature as **reverse anorexia nervosa** ('**bigorexia**'). Patients with body dysmorphic disorder are preoccupied with an ideal body image and view themselves as ugly or misshaped. Body dysmorphic disorder must be distinguished from eating disorders, such as anorexia nervosa, that involve a preoccupation with overall body shape and weight. About one third of men who have muscle dysmorphia also have an eating disorder, such as bingeing, or an idiosyncratic pattern, such as a focus on high-protein diets. More than half of men with muscle dysmorphia use steroids and the others are tempted. Use of nutritional supplements is almost universal in men with muscle dysmorphia.

Research using the Muscle Dysmorphia Inventory has found that elite-level body builders are significantly more likely to engage in characteristics associated with muscle dysmorphia than are elite-level power lifters.

There is debate as to whether muscle dysmorphia should be classified as a subcategory of body dysmorphic disorder. Chung (2001) argues that the historical and clinical aspects of muscle dysmorphia are more consistent with its classification as an obsessive-compulsive disorder.

Bibliography

American Psychiatric Association (1994). *Diagnostic and statistical manual of mental disorders*. 4th ed. Washington, DC: American

Psychiatric Association.

Chung, B. (2001). Muscle dysmorphia: A critical review of the proposed criteria. *Perspectives in Biological Medicine* 44(4), 565-574.

Lantz, C.D., Rhea, D.J. and Cornelius, A.E. (2002). Muscle dysmorphia in elite-level power lifters and bodybuilders: A test of differences within a conceptual model. *Journal of Strength and Conditioning Research* 16(4), 649-655.

Olivardia, R., Pope, H.G. and Hudson, J.I. (2000). Muscle dysmorphia in male weightlifters: A case-control study. *American Journal of Psychiatry* 157(8), 1291-1296.

Pope, H.G. et al. (1997). Muscle dysmorphia. An under-recognized form of body dysmorphic disorder. *Psychosomatics* 38(6), 548-557.

Pope, H.G. et al. (1999). Evolving ideals of male body image as seen through action toys. *International Journal of Eating Disorders* 26(1), 65-72.

Pope, H.G., Phillips, K.A. and Olivardia, R. (2000). *The Adonis complex: The secret crisis of male body obsession.* New York City: The Free Press.

Schnirring, L. (2000). When to suspect muscle dysmorphia. Bringing the 'Adonis complex" to light. *The Physician and Sportsmedicine* 28(12).

BODY FAT   *See under* BODY COMPOSITION.

BODY IMAGE   *See under* SELF CONCEPT.

BODY-IN-SAGITTAL PLANE RIGHTING REFLEX   *See* LANDAU REFLEX.

BODY MASS INDEX   BMI. Quetelet's index. It is the ratio of body weight (in kilograms) to height (in meters) squared. A BMI of greater than 55% of adults in the USA is classified as either overweight (body mass index = 25 to 29.9 kg/m^2) or obese (BMI greater than or equal to 30 kg/m^2). A limitation of the body mass index is that there is no way to distinguish between fat-mass and fat-free mass. *See under* OBESITY.

BODY PIERCING   A cosmetic procedure in which the skin is retracted with a hemostat, the skin is pierced with a hollow 12- to 16-gauge needle, jewelry is attached to the needle and the jewelry is threaded through the hole. Tongue piercing is a two-step procedure in which a 14-gauge or larger 'barbell' is initially placed to accommodate swelling. Piercing of the tongue has resulted in chipped teeth. A piercing can take a year or longer to heal. Medical complications from body piercing include infection and cyst formation. Some people have an allergic reaction to the metal. 1 in 10 people have a bleeding complication from piercings; and 1 in 15 will have a large scar or reaction at the site. If a nerve is pierced, nerve damage can result. In team sports, the most obvious problems are friction and shearing forces that may rip the metal out of the skin. With trauma, tongue barbells can become dislodged and cause airway obstruction or become lodged in the gastrointestinal tract. About half of navel piercings become infected, as it is an area that is prone to waistband irritation, moisture and debris collection. HIV and hepatitis B can be transmitted by non-sterile piercing practices. In a study of 874 owners/managers of piercing businesses in Australia, less than 39% correctly identified recommended sterilization procedures.

Chronology

•c. 300 AD • The Romans pierced a metal ring through the foreskin of slaves and athletes. The purpose was to prevent erections so that athletes would perform better. It was believed that any sexual activity would take away energy needed for athletic performance.

Bibliography

News Brief (1999). Body piercing and sports: An opening for trouble? *The Physician and Sportsmedicine*, 27(2), 27-33.

Oberdorfer, A. et al. (2003). Skin penetration operators' knowledge and attitudes toward infection control. *American Journal of Health Behavior* 27(2), 125-134.

Wilkinson, B. (1998). *Coping with the dangers of tattooing, body piercing and branding.* New York, NY: The Rosen Publishing Group.

BODY-RIGHTING REFLEX   A postural reflex that may not be evident until the 5th month and persists through the first year. The infant is placed supine and the head is gently turned to one side or other. The body rotates in the direction the head is turned to regain the front-facing relationship between the head and shoulders.

BODY SCHEMA   *See under* SELF CONCEPT.

BODY SIZE   The height and weight of a person. *See* BODY WEIGHT; STATURE.

BODY WEIGHT   The force exerted by gravity on a body. The Standard International (SI) unit is the newton (N). Weighing involves the determination of the body's mass by comparing its weight with that of a known mass. The most recommended type of instrument for measuring weight is weighing scales designed on the balance-arm principle with two balance arms.

See BODY MASS INDEX; GROWTH.

BODY WEIGHT REDUCTION   *See* DIETING.

BODY WEIGHT REDUCTION   (ATHLETES) 'Making weight.' Athletes may decrease bodyweight for one or more of the following reasons: to compete in a lower weight class, to improve performance or to improve aesthetic appearance. Rapid bodyweight reduction (dehydration in 12 to 96 hours) is used by athletes in weight-class sports, such as wrestling. This typically involves fluid restriction and increased exercise. This practice has been discouraged by the American College of Sports Medicine because of the following potentially harmful side effects: decreased muscular strength and power, decreased endurance performance, lower blood and plasma volumes, decreased cardiac function, decreased maximal oxygen uptake, impaired thermoregulation, decreased renal function, decreased glycogen concentration and loss of electrolytes. After rapid bodyweight loss, rehydration and re-establishment of electrolyte homeostasis may take more than 5 hours to accomplish.

The maximum rate of acceptable body mass reduction appears to be about 1% of body mass per week. Any weight loss of glycogen includes water loss. Around 60% of the weight of glycogen is actually water. A loss of body mass over a period of time exceeding a month or a total body mass loss of more than 5% may have a negative effect on vitamin and mineral status, with negative consequences for athletic performance.

Bibliography
American College of Sports Medicine (1976). Weight loss in wrestlers. *Medicine and Science in Sports and Exercise* 8, 11-13.

Brownell, K.D., Rodin, J. and Wilmore, J.H. (1992, eds). *Eating, body weight and performance in athletes: Disorders of modern society*. Philadelphia, PA: Lea and Febiger.

Fogelholm, M. (1994). Effects of bodyweight reduction on sports performance. *Sports Medicine* 18(4), 249-267.

Horswill, C.A. (1992). When wrestlers slim to win: What's a safe minimum? *The Physician and sportsmedicine* 20(9), 91-101.

Oppliger, R.A. et al. (1996). American College of Sports Medicine Position stand on weight loss in wrestlers. *Medicine and Science in Sports and Exercise* 28(6), ix-xii.

BOHR EFFECT   *See under* CARBON DIOXIDE; HEMOGLOBIN.

BOLUS   A chewed, moistened lump of food that is ready to be swallowed.

BOMB CALORIMETER   *See under* ENERGY YIELD OF NUTRIENTS.

BONE   A form of connective tissue that is comprised of fibrous tissue (mainly collagen) and bone matrix (mainly calcium phosphate). The inorganic mineral salts such as calcium phosphate give bone hardness and rigidity. The organic matrix of collagen and ground substance gives bone flexibility and resilience. **Modeling** is the formation of new bone. **Remodeling** involves resorption and (re)formation of bone.

The main bone cells are osteocytes, osteoblasts and osteoclasts. **Osteocytes** are found in lacunae (small spaces) lying in or between the lamellae. **Osteoblasts** are found on the surfaces of bone and are involved with bone deposition. **Osteoclasts** are usually found in depressions (**Howship's lacunae**) at the surfaces of bone tissue and are associated with bone resorption. It is a large multi-nucleated cell derived from blood monocytes.

Bone cells produce two types of tissue, woven bone and lamellar bone. **Woven bone** has a lower mineral content than lamellar bone and forms rapidly in periods of intensive growth such as adolescence, fracture healing or periods of rapid bone remodeling. **Lamellar bone** forms more slowly than woven bone and is more organized. It has thin layers of bone with collagen arranged in a perpendicular matrix.

Microscopically, bone is an **osteon** or **haversian system** composed of concentric layers of a mineralized matrix surrounding a central canal containing blood vessels and nerve fibers. Macroscopically, bone is composed of compact and cancellous bone. **Compact (cortical)** bone is hard and predominates in the long bones. **Cancellous (trabecular** or **spongy)** bone is generally softer than cortical bone and predominates in bones of the axial skeleton. The long axis of an osteon is approximately parallel to the major axis of stress, usually the long axis of the bone.

Bone is an **anisotropic** material; its behavior will vary according to the direction of load application. In general, bone can handle the greatest loads in the longitudinal direction and the least amount of load when applied across the surface of bone. Bone is stronger in the longitudinal direction because it has been habitually loaded in that direction. The resulting compressive forces are essential for growth and development of bone. If compressive load exceeds the stress limits of a bone, however, then a fracture will occur.

Bone remodels in response to the mechanical demands placed on it; it is laid down where needed and resorbed when not needed. **Minimal effective strain** is the threshold for a stimulus that initiates new bone formation. A load or force that exceeds this threshold, and is repeated a sufficient number of times, will cause osteoblasts to secrete osteoid and leads to the formation of new bone. The stimulus must include forces considerably greater than normally attained by habitual activity. **Wolff's law** states that the ability of bone to adapt by changing its size, shape and internal structure depends on the mechanical stresses established by the load. Hence professional tennis players have greater bone cortex thickness of the upper limb on the playing side than the non-playing side. Physical activity affects bone density and bone width, but it does not influence bone length. With aging there is a significant decrease in the amount of cancellous bone and a

decrease in the thickness of cortical bone. This leads to decreases in bone strength and stiffness. *See under* SKELETON.

BONE INJURY   *See* AVULSION; EPIPHYSITIS; FRACTURES; STRESS FRACTURES.

BONE MARROW   A connective tissue found in the interior of bones. It is the primary site of erythrocyte and leukocyte production.

BOOSTING   *See under* AUTONOMIC DYSREFLEXIA.

BORON   An element that is currently not considered to be an essential mineral for humans. Adverts for nutritional supplements have claimed that boron can exert anabolic effects on strength-trained athletes, but there is no convincing scientific evidence to support this claim.

BOTOX®   An abbreviation for 'botulinum toxin' (botulinum toxin A), which is a protein made by a bacterium called *Clostridium botulinum*, which causes botulism, a sometimes fatal form of food poisoning. BOTOX® contains a purified version of the protein, without the harmful protein. BOTOX® injection treatment is the name used for the process of injecting BOTOX® product into a patient. BOTOX® injection treatments are approved in the USA by the Food and Drug Administration (FDA) for cosmetic use, as well as the treatment of several medical conditions such as cervical dystonia and migraine.

BOTOX® Cosmetic is the most popular cosmetic procedure in the USA, being used by about 1.6 million people in the USA in 2003. BOTOX® Cosmetic also refers to the drug used for the temporary improvement in the appearance of moderate to severe glabellar lines (frown lines). These frown lines come from muscles called corrugator and/or procerus muscles. BOTOX® Cosmetic is injected directly into these muscles, before it enters the nerve endings to block the release of acetylcholine. The effects of BOTOX® Cosmetic take 3 to 5 days to appear. For most people, the effects usually last 3 to 6 months. In general, 3 or 4 treatments per year are usually needed to lessen the appearance of wrinkles. The most common side-effects following the use of BOTOX® Cosmetic for glabellar lines are headache, respiratory infections, temporary eyelid droop, nausea and influenza.

Bibliography
Botox Information. Http://www.botox-cosmetic-surgery.com

BOUNDARY LAYER   *See under* DRAG.

BOUTONNIERE DEFORMITY   *See under* PROXIMAL INTERPHALANGEAL JOINT.

BOWLER'S THUMB   Perineural fibrosis of the ulnar digital nerve. It is found in ten-pin bowlers, who constantly irritate the ulnar digital nerve of the thumb when placing it within the thumbhole of the ball. Preventative measures include enlarging the thumbhole and padding the thumb. See also PERIPHERAL NERVE INJURY.

BOXER'S FRACTURE   *See under* META-CARPALS, FRACTURES.

BOXER'S KNUCKLE   An injury, most commonly in the third metacarpophalangeal joint, which may result in bursitis over the metacarpal head, a distraction strain of the tendon of the *extensor digitorum communis* muscle, or a sprain of the intermetacarpal ligaments. It commonly occurs in boxers who have their outstretched hands bandaged before a fight, and thus the bandage is too tight when the hand is flexed to make a fist.

BOYLE'S LAW   *See under* GAS.

BRACHIAL   Of the arm.

BRACHIAL INDEX   The ratio of forearm length to arm length. Throwers and sprint swimmers tend to have above-average brachial indices. Weightlifters tend to have below-average brachial indices. *See* PROPORTIONALITY.

BRACHIALIS MUSCLE   In rock climbers, the *brachialis* muscle may be chronically overloaded because the forearms are used in a pronated, semi-flexed position. The resulting microtrauma and inflammation of the musculotendinous unit has been called climber's elbow.

BRACHIAL PLEXUS   A plexus that is formed mainly from the anterior rami of nerve roots of four cervical vertebrae and one thoracic vertebra (C5, C6, C7, C8 and T1). It passes between the anterior and middle scalene muscles of the neck, between the clavicle and first rib, under the tendon of the *pectoralis minor* muscle, and then anteriorly to the glenohumeral joint to form the radial, ulnar and median nerves.

Compression of the brachial plexus may occur within the interscalene triangle, between the clavicle and first rib, or under the tendon of the *pectoralis minor* muscle where it inserts into the coracoid process.

Anatomical variants, such as a cervical rib or fibrous bands, can constrict the plexus as it passes between the anterior and middle *scalene* muscles. A fracture malunion of the clavicle can lead to compression in the costoclavicular space.

Repetitive overhead shoulder motion in athletes, such as football quarterbacks and tennis players, can produce shoulder girdle depression that narrows the costoclavicular space. Depression of the shoulder girdle lowers the scapula and the coracoid process. This can effectively compress the brachial plexus as it passes under the tendon of *pectoralis minor*.

The plexus is susceptible to several stretch injuries. Common mechanisms include anterior glenohumeral dislocations, and the forces that drive the head and shoulder in opposite directions during a tackle or collision.

The most common cervical root or brachial plexus injury in the athlete is the '**burner**' (pinched-nerve syndrome; 'stinger;' nerve stretch). A burner is common in American footballers and it involves numbness down one upper extremity. A burner can result from one or more of the following causes: brachial plexus lesions resulting from the head being forced to one side while the opposite shoulder is depressed (most common); entrapment of the nerve root or roots in the spinal column, protruded or ruptured intervertebral disc, and a combination of nerve root and brachial plexus lesion. Boxers and weightlifters sustain burners from neck hyper-extension injuries. A direct blow to the region of Erb's point may also injure the plexus. Dislocation or subluxation of the glenohumeral joint, though not considered to be a classic mechanism for burners, can stretch the distal plexus and mimic the symptoms of a burner.

See also SUPRASCAPULAR NERVE INJURY.

BRADYCARDIA   A slow resting heart rate, usually in the range of 45 to 55 beats per minute but occasionally even lower.

Bibliography
Stamford, B. (1988). Bradycardia: Low heart rate. *The Physician and Sportsmedicine* 16(5), 180.

BRADYKININ A plasma protein that is a powerful stimulator of smooth muscle contraction, inducing hypotension, and increasing blood flow and permeability of capillaries.

See also under NEUROTRANSMITTER.

BRAIN   The part of the central nervous system enclosed within the skull. By the age of 8 years, the brain has nearly reached its mature size.

The **white matter** is comprised of all the nerve fibers. These are grouped together as tracts and given names (e.g. pyramidal and extrapyramidal). In the cerebrum, these tracts collectively are called the internal capsule. The **gray matter**, made up of concentrations of cell bodies, is the cortex or outer covering of the cerebrum and cerebellum; and nuclei with specific names like thalamus, hypothalamus and basal ganglia.

The brain can be divided into three main parts: the forebrain, the cerebellum and the brainstem. The **forebrain** consists of the cerebrum and the diencephalon. The **cerebrum** is the cerebral cortex and the internal capsule. The **cerebral cortex** is the surface of the cerebral hemispheres. It is the area

of the brain primarily concerned with higher cognitive processes that enable thought, emotion, perception, memory, language and voluntary movement. The cortex can be subdivided by function into three areas: sensory, motor and association. The **sensory cortex** receives information from the sense organs. The **motor cortex** is involved with the control of movement. The **supplementary motor area** is involved in motor planning and coordination of movements. The **association cortex** is the remainder of the cortex.

A distinction can be made between cortical and subcortical. **Cortical** refers to the functions of the cerebral cortex and the cortical tracts that carry neural impulses from one part of the brain to another, thereby enabling the integration and association of different kinds of data. **Subcortical** refers to functions of all the structures of the central nervous system except the cerebral cortex and cortical tracts. Subcortical functions include skilled movements that no longer require conscious attention and automatic movements like postural reactions and basic movement patterns that enable activities of daily living.

The **internal capsule** contains clusters of cell bodies that perform specific functions. These include the limbic system, basal ganglia and thalamus.

The **frontal lobe** is the anterior part of the cerebrum. The **parietal lobe** is immediately posterior to the frontal lobe. The **occipital lobe** is located posterior and inferior to the parietal lobe. The **temporal lobe** is located inferior to the frontal and parietal lobes on the sides of the cerebrum. The **diencephalon** consists of the thalamus and hypothalamus, each of which contains many small nuclei. The **thalamus** processes much of the sensory input that is transmitted to the cortex. It thus plays a role in the direction of attention, and it is also involved in the control of movement. The **hypothalamus** is involved in homeostasis, controlling life-sustaining functions such as motivation, thermoregulation, feeding and drinking. It is the major link between the endocrine and nervous systems.

The **brainstem** connects the forebrain and cerebellum to the spinal cord. It is the bundle of nerve tissues that extends upward from the spinal cord to the base of the cerebrum. The brain stem regulates muscle tone, postural tone and reflexes; and it is also important for many of the functions controlled by the autonomic nervous system. Its three main regions are the medulla oblongata, pons and midbrain. The **medulla oblongata** is connected to the spinal cord. The **pons** is connected to the cerebellum. The **midbrain** is connected to the forebrain. It forms a link between the pons and the cerebral hemispheres. The **red nucleus** and **substantia nigra** are located in the midbrain, and both form part of the extrapyramidal motor system. The midbrain regulates postural reactions. These include all of the automatic patterns that enable stability and mobility in activities of daily living. The midbrain also receives all of the sensory information from the eyes, which helps to explain why vision is so important to balance. Pathological muscle tone and reflexes are caused when the brain stem receives sensory information about touch, pressure or movement that is experienced by body parts and does not permit this sensory input to travel to higher levels of the brain. Also located within the brain stem is the **reticular formation** that regulates attention, arousal and wakefulness. It consists of two activating systems. The **ascending reticular activating system** extends from the medulla to the lower thalamus where it branches into the hypothalamus and thalamus regions. It then branches into the cerebral cortex. The cortex projects nerve fibers to the ascending reticular activating system, thus enables cortical activity to activate the reticular formation. The **descending reticular activating system** extends downwards from the brain stem into the spinal cord and controls motor activity.

Functionally, the brain may be divided into two systems: the limbic system and the sensorimotor system. The **limbic system** evokes motor activity related to survival behavior such as feeding (e.g. chewing). The limbic system includes the amygdala, hippocampus, fornix and cingulate gyrus of the cerebral cortex. It is concerned with emotional behavior and learning. The **sensorimotor system** is concerned with sensation and motor behavior. Neural integration of the limbic and sensorimotor

systems allows intentional control of movement. The cerebellum, basal ganglia and cerebral cortex are all involved in the control of movement. The **cerebellum**, located inferior to the forebrain and posterior to the brainstem, is important in the automatic performance of skilled movement. It is also essential for good balance, muscle tone, eye movements, and the timing of fast movements. The cerebellum contains about half the neurons in the brain. Cerebellar disorders include ataxia, dysequilibrium (balance problems with falling to the affected side), hypotonia and nystagmus. The **basal ganglia** comprise the following nuclei: caudate, putamen, globus pallidus, subthalamic nuclei and substantia nigra. The caudate and putamen nuclei are combined to form the striatum. The basal ganglia receive a major input from the cerebral cortex and send most of their output, via the thalamus, back to the cortex. The basal ganglia are concerned with motor planning in that the output neurons code for various aspects of movement, such as direction, amplitude and velocity.

There are two major systems by which signals are transmitted from the brain to the spinal cord in order to produce movement. These are known as the pyramidal system and the extrapyramidal system. Both systems send nerve fibers down the spinal cord, where they activate (directly or indirectly) alpha motor neurons or gamma motor neurons. The **pyramidal system**, thought to be involved with voluntary movement of a specific nature, involves nerve cells that lie mainly in the motor cortex (**precentral gyrus**). The **extrapyramidal system**, thought to be concerned with large and general movement patterns, involves nerve cells that lie mainly in the pre-motor cortex. Frontal lobe areas (4, 6 and 8), post-central areas (1, 2, 3 and 50) and temporal lobe area (22) are involved in the extrapyramidal system.

The brain, like the spinal cord, has a number of peripheral nerves, called **cranial nerves**. Within the brain stem are the processing centers for 10 of the 12 pairs of cranial nerves that convey information to the brain from the special senses (sight, smell etc.) and the general senses. They also control the voluntary muscles of the eyes, mouth, face, pharynx and larynx, in addition to many visceral structures.

Shape anomalies of the head due to prenatal influences are **anencephaly** (partial or complete absence of the brain), **microcephalus** (abnormally small brain), **hydrocephalus** (large head caused by increased cerebrospinal fluid in the ventricles of the brain) and **craniostenosis** (narrowed or flat cranium). In general, microcephalus is associated with severe mental retardation. It is also an indicator of specific conditions like fetal alcohol syndrome. Hydrocephalus often accompanies spina bifida. Hydrocephalus does not cause mental retardation immediately. Hydrocephalus is controlled by a surgical procedure called 'shunting,' which relieves the fluid build up in the brain by redirecting it into the abdominal area. When treatment (shunting) is ineffective, mental retardation develops slowly as increased pressure within the cranium damages the brain. *See also* ELECTROENCEPHALOGRAPHY; HEAD INJURIES.

BRASSIERE   Bra. External breast supports (brassières) decrease breast motion. Sports bras are either encapsulation- or compression-type. The **compression bra** flattens the breasts against the body. This design is thought to be more effective for females with smaller breasts (sizes A or B). The **encapsulation bra** contains moulded cups that separate and support the breasts individually. This design is thought to be more effective for females with larger breasts (sizes C or D). Most sports bras have cups that are seamless or have covered seams to avoid irritation to the nipples. Underwire must be carefully positioned so as not to place pressure on the lymph nodes under the armpit. Pregnant women are usually discouraged from wearing underwire bras, as the rigid component is thought to interfere with milk production.

The straps need to be positioned so that they lie in a direct line over the nipple of the breast. This allows for better vertical breast support, as the support of the straps can work in the direct line of force created by vertical breast movement. Fabric in the straps should be wider than the straps of a fashion bra to allow a greater area for the force to be distributed over. Cross-back sports bras have been found to be less effective in limiting vertical breast displacement when compared with a traditional backed sports bra. The bra should be a blend of at least 50% cotton and a 'breathable' material such as Lycra™ mesh to help evaporate sweat and keep odor in check. Cotton provides more comfort than synthetic materials, lesser stretch and greater support.

Schultz (2004) argues that advertisements and "iconic sports-bra moments" that circulate around Brandi Chastain's celebration of the US women's soccer victory in the 1999 World Cup, normalize ideals of femininity that are considered achievable through technologies of disciplined body management, and sexualize sports bras and the women who wear them. It doesn't escape Schultz's attention, however, that Chastain's gesture may have been motivated to market the Nike bra or Chastain herself. Several weeks before the 1999 World Cup, Chastain had appeared in *Gear* magazine naked above the waist except for soccer balls covering her breasts.

Chronology

•c. 100 AD • Women in ancient Rome supported their breasts by wearing bands around their chests or binding their breasts with a length of cloth or leather.

•1837 • Madam George introduced a "Callisthenic Corset" to avoid injuries during exercise.

•1863 • The first patent for a brassière was filed, but it was not until the 1920s that brassières began to replace corsets as the favored undergarment of women in the USA.

•1887 • At the Wimbledon tennis tournament, women competitors had to retire to the dressing rooms between matches to unhitch their bloody corsets.

•1911 • The "sports corset" was one of the first undergarments to incorporate elastic.

•1914 • The modern soft brassière was invented by socialite Mary Phelps Jacob. She and her maid sewed together two handkerchiefs and some ribbons when getting dressed for a ball. They eventually sold the patent to Warner Brothers. Brassières were not initially designed to support the breasts, but rather to cover bare breasts as fashions led to a drop in the height of corsets towards waist level.

•1977 • Hinda Miller of the USA was frustrated by the lack of comfort and support for her breasts she experienced during running in her regular brassière. With another American woman, Lisa Lindhal, Miller sewed two jock straps together to form a prototype of their first 'jog bra.' In the first year of production, 25,000 jog bras were sold and in 1996 over 41 million were sold.

•1990 • A study of female athletes undertaken by Nike's Advanced Research and Development division found that 31% reported breast-related problems. Excessive breast movement causes chafing and pain by spraining the Cooper's ligaments, and movement between the breast and bra can cause soreness and bleeding.

•1998 • The sports bra industry was worth $412 million in retail sales.

•1999 • At the Rose Bowl in Pasadena, California, over 90,000 people watched the US women's soccer team defeat China in the World Cup final. Chastain whipped off her jersey and exposed her black Nike Inner Active sports bra.

Bibliography

Page, K-A. and Steele, J.R. (1999). Breast motion and sport brassière design. Implications for future research. *Sports Medicine* 27(4), 205-211.

Schultz, J. (2004). Discipline and push-up: Female bodies, femininity, and sexuality in popular representations of sports bras. *Sociology of Sport Journal* 21, 185-205.

BREAST   The female breasts are situated on the chest wall within the superficial fascia, with the deep layer of the fascia marking the breast's posterior boundary and the superficial portion of the fascia marking the anterior boundary. There are three major structural components within female breasts: the skin, the subcutaneous tissue and the corpus mammae.

The **corpus mammae** is the functional section of the breast. It can be subdivided into the parenchyma and the stroma. The **parenchyma** is composed of ductular, lobular and alveolar structures, whereas the **stroma** is composed of connective tissue, lymphatics, fat tissue, blood vessels and nerves. Each breast consists of several lobes separated by septa (walls) of connective tissue. Each lobe consists of several lobules, which, in turn, are composed of connective tissue in which are embedded the secreting cells (alveoli) of the gland. The ducts from the various lobules unite, forming a single lactiferous (milk-carrying) duct for each lobe. The connective tissue in the stroma of the breast, '**Cooper's ligaments**,' comprises thin sheets of fibrous bands that are located within the superficial

fascia and separate the breast's lobules. Although not true ligaments, Cooper's ligaments do provide limited support to the breast region as they are attached to the deep fascia that overlays the *pectoralis* muscles. Because of the lack of internal breast support, it is possible that the skin covering the breast may also act as a support for the breast. The skin of the breast includes the nipple, areola and the general covering skin. The skin lies immediately above a layer of subcutaneous tissue.

Female breasts are affected by hormonal changes including those associated with: menstruation, pregnancy, oral contraceptives and menopause. The influx of estrogen and progesterone can increase breast size and can often make them tender. The glandular tissue of breasts decreases in size as hormone levels decrease. Each adult female breast weighs about 200 g with the left breast often being larger than the right breast. During pregnancy, the breast increases in size and weight to between 400 and 600 g, increasing to between 600 and 800 g during lactation. Exercise usually results in a large displacement of the breasts, often leading to breast pain. Therefore, female athletes are advised to wear brassières.

Contusions to the breast may produce fat necrosis or hematoma formation. This may lead to the formation of localized breast mass.

Bibliography

Page, K-A. and Steele, J.R. (1999). Breast motion and sport brassière design. Implications for future research. *Sports Medicine* 27(4), 205-211.

BREAST AUGMENTATION   Augmentation mammoplasty. A surgical procedure to enhance the size and shape of a woman's breast for one or more of the following reasons: (i) the woman feels her breast size is too small; (ii) to correct a decrease in breast volume after pregnancy; (iii) to balance a difference in breast size; and (iv) as a reconstructive technique following breast surgery.

A breast implant is a silicone shell filled with either silicone gel or saline (salt water). The use of silicone-filled implants was banned by the Food and Drug Administration (FDA), except for women participating in approved studies, because of a high incidence of both acute and long-term complications such as granulomas, skin loss and scar contracture. From 1985 to 1998, the FDA received 127,500 adverse reports on silicon breast implants and 49,661 on saline-filled implants. Saline-filled implants are now preferred. The FDA could not find conclusive evidence linking breast implants to cancer or autoimmune disease. However, it did not conclude that breast-implant surgery is safe.

Breast augmentation typically improves the individual's self image. According to the American Society of Plastic Surgeons (ASPS), approximately 200,000 women received breast implants in 2000. Low self-esteem drove 80% of those women to have the surgery. The ASPS reported that 94% of women who had their breasts enlarged in 2000 were content with the size, shape and firmness of their breasts after surgery.

In a study of 30 breast augmentation candidates and 30 physically similar women who were not interested in breast augmentation, the breast augmentation candidates rated their ideal breast size, as well as the breast size preferred by women, as significantly larger than did controls. They also reported greater investment in their appearance, greater distress about their appearance in a variety of situations, more frequent teasing about their appearance, and more frequent use of psychotherapy in the year before the operation.

Implants may be of two shapes, round implants or teardrop implants. The **round implants** are disc shaped and exhibit equal fullness in all four quadrants of the breast. The **teardrop implants** are shaped more like the breast than round implants. Teardrop implants tend to become round with the forces of healing, and also they may rotate, giving an unnatural appearance. The most common size of breast implants range from 200 to 600 cm^3. Breast implants are designed so that, as volume increases, so does diameter and projection. Women tend naturally to choose an implant volume that is in proportion with body size and breast diameter. Most plastic surgeons make an incision under the breast, because it has the advantage of having the scar hidden in the shadow of the crease under the breast.

Breast implants may be placed under or over the

pectoralis major muscle. In general, thin and small-breasted women should favor breast implants under the muscle. Advantages for placing the implants under the muscle include less interference with mammography and less rippling in the upper half of the breast. When bodybuilders pose, and forcibly contract their *pectoralis major* muscle, their implants will rise if placed behind (under) the muscle. Although an implant is more obvious in front of (over) the muscle, there is less movement with posing.

Following breast implant surgery, the body may begin to produce milk. This production may cease spontaneously or after medication is given to stop milk production.

Patients can usually resume daily activities and return to work one week after receiving breast implants. Chest muscles may feel sore for two to three weeks. According to Mele (2000), if breast implants are placed over the muscle, all exercise can be resumed 6 to 8 weeks after the surgery (assuming there are no post-operative complications). If the breast implants are placed under the muscle, which Mele does in about 95% of cases, then no exercise should be done for the first two weeks. Walking can be done after two weeks. Lower body training can be resumed after one month. Jogging and light upper body weights can be resumed after two months. Unrestricted exercise, including heavy weightlifting may be resumed after three months. Mele notes that some physicians may consider this postoperative plan to be conservative and cautious, but notes postoperative bleeding can occur even after 3 to 4 weeks in patients who start exercising too early.

Bibliography

American Society of Plastic Surgeons. Http://www.plasticsurgery.org

Chicago Plastic Surgery. Http://www.chicagoplasticsurgery.net

Loftus, J.M. Risks and complications of breast augmentation. Http://www.infoplasticsurgery.com

Mele, J.A. (2000). Exercise and breast implants. Http://www.breastimplants411.com

Sarwer, D.B. et al. (2003). Body image concerns of breast augmentation patients. *Plastic and Reconstructive Surgery* 112(1), 83-90.

BREAST FEEDING Breast milk is the optimal food for the health, growth and development of infants. Human milk contains more than 100 different oligosaccharides that vary with the duration of pregnancy, the duration of breastfeeding and the genetic make-up of the mother. For breast-fed infants, oligosaccharides serve a function similar to dietary fiber in adults, making stools easier to pass. Breast milk has been shown to decrease the incidence of respiratory infections, gastro-intestinal infections, ear infections, allergies, diarrhea and bacterial meningitis. **Bifidus factor**, one of the protective factors found in milk, fosters the growth of the bacterium *lactobacillus bifidus*, which in turn interferes with the growth of harmful bacteria in the baby's digestive system.

In terms of energy, the recommended daily allowance (RDA) for breastfeeding women is 500 kcal per day higher than the RDA for nonpregnant, nonlactating women, but this may be an overestimation of actual needs, especially for sedentary women.

In many cultures, lactating women are encouraged to drink alcohol to optimize breast milk production and infant nutrition, but scientific evidence suggests that maternal alcohol consumption may slightly decrease milk production. Some of the alcohol consumed by a lactating woman is transferred to her milk and consumed by the infant. This alcohol consumption may adversely affect the infant's sleep and gross motor development.

During the first 4 to 6 months of infancy, exclusive breastfeeding is recommended because it enables a matching of lactose concentration to the maturing gut, especially while colonic microflora and pancreatic amylase production are developing. Colonic microflora are responsible for colonic carbohydrate scavenging, converting any carbohydrate entering the colon into short-chain fatty acids. Any disturbances or inappropriate development of this microflora, such as incorrect infant formula, infection, or antibiotics, leads to colonic carbohydrate overloading and diarrhea. Caffeine can enter breast milk, and high amounts can cause the baby to become wakeful and agitated.

The **milk ejection reflex** involves the release of milk from the alveoli of the breast into the ducts, caused by a combination of neurogenic and hormonal reflexes involving the hormone oxytocin and, to a lesser extent, vasopressin. *See also* GALACTOSEMIA.

Bibliography
Insel, P., Turner, R.E. and Ross, D. (2004). *Nutrition*. 2nd ed. Sudbury, MA: Jones and Bartlett.

Menella, J. (2001). Alcohol's effect on lactation. *Alcohol Research and Health* 25(3), 230-234.

BREAST LIFT Mastopexy. A surgical procedure to raise and reshape sagging breasts by removing excess skin and repositioning the remaining tissue and nipples (at least for a time; no surgery can per-manently delay the effects of gravity). Mastopexy can also decrease the size of the areola, the darker skin surrounding the nipple. Breast implants inserted in conjunction with mastopexy can increase both the firmness and size of the breasts. Many women seek mastopexy because pregnancy and nursing have left them with stretched skin and less volume in their breasts.

Bibliography
American Society of Plastic Surgeons. Http://www.plasticsurgery.org

BREAST STROKER'S KNEE A chronic medial collateral ligament (MCL) sprain that results from repetitive stress on the MCL. During the whip kick, a valgus stress is applied to the knee when the hip is in an abducted and internally rotated position, and as the knee moves rapidly from flexion to extension in an externally rotated position. Decreasing the width of the kick helps to prevent this injury. *See also* KNEE LIGAMENTS.

BREATH-HOLD DIVING *See under* HYPER-BARIC PHYSIOLOGY.

BREATHING This involves movement of air in and out of the lungs. It is part of external respiration. The flow of air into and out of the lungs is determined by a pressure gradient between the ambient air and the air within the lung. This pressure gradient is brought about by contraction of the diaphragm and intercostal muscles in normal breathing.

Inhalation (**inspiration**) is the movement of air into the lungs. It occurs when atmospheric pressure exceeds the pressure within the alveoli. **Exhalation** (**expiration**) is the movement of air out of the lungs. This occurs when the pressure within the alveoli exceeds atmospheric pressure.

Two types of deep breathing are possible: abdominal breathing and chest breathing. **Chest breathing** at rest expands the lungs by increasing the volume in the chest cavity through elevation of the ribs. Air rushes into the lungs as a vacuum is created in the lungs. At rest, this is accomplished by the action of the intercostal muscles and the diaphragm. When chest breathing is used during exercise, muscles in the shoulder region assist in elevating the rib cage. **Abdominal (diaphrag-matic) breathing** involves moving the diaphragm downward to push the abdomen out during expiration. The diaphragm plays a greater role during inhalation. Abdominal breathing is enhanced by relaxation of the abdominal muscles during inhalation. Abdominal breathing is more economical than chest breathing, but it may seem unnatural and feel uncomfortable. Rhythmical abdominal breathing (generated by aerobic exercise) has been associated with enhanced quality of life. At rest, most people are abdominal breathers when lying down and chest breathers when standing upright. As most exercise is done in the upright position, chest breathing predominates. Cycling favors abdominal breathing, because of the belly-down posture and breathing can be coordinated with pedaling frequency.

In mammals, mechanical constraints appear to require that locomotion and breathing be synchronized. In running, humans differ from quadrupeds because they employ several phase-locked patterns (4:1, 3:1, 2:1; 1:1; 5:2; and 3:2), although a 2:1 coupling appears to be favored.

Entrainment is synchronization of limb movement and breathing frequency during rhythmical exercise, e.g. a runner always exhaling during the push-off phase. It occurs without conscious thought. Subjects who entrain naturally have a lower energy cost during exercise when they entrain, but not when they breathe randomly. When subjects are forced to breathe in specific entrainment patterns, however, rather than being allowed to breathe spontaneously, they do not exhibit any decrease in energy cost nor do they perceive any decrease in breathing effort with entrained breathing. Distance runners are thus taught to consciously control their breathing and to breathe deeply. Most experienced distance runners coordinate their breathing with their stride, inhaling for several strides, then exhaling for the same number of strides. The novice runner often breathes in a rapid, shallow manner that limits the air to the upper respiratory tract. This method is inefficient, as there is no gas exchange with the blood in the upper respiratory tract.

Most people automatically shift from nose to mouth breathing as exercise intensity increases. **Oral breathing** allows air to enter and exit much faster than **nasal breathing**, because there is less resistance to overcome. Oral breathing helps to cool the body during heat stress, because the air does not need to be warmed. Research evidence suggests that during near-maximal exercise, a breathing rate of 30 to 35 breaths per minute is most efficient. Sprinters breathe infrequently, if at all, because sprint performance is anaerobic.

A **nasal dilator** is a small strip that is placed across the bridge of the nose, and has recently been worn by many athletes including rugby players. There is no convincing evidence to support the use of nasal dilators as a physiological ergogenic aid. Because arterial saturation is already about 97 to 98% at rest and is maintained close to this level during exercise, the use of nasal dilators during exercise does not appear to be warranted. Nasal dilators have been helpful to people who suffer from nasal congestion during sleep, decreasing air resistance in the nasal cavity by 30%.

Hyperpnea refers to significantly increased breathing. **Dyspnea** refers to difficulty in breathing. During exercise, it is caused by an inability to decrease the blood partial pressure of carbon dioxide and hydrogen ions.

See also SECOND WIND; STITCH; VALSALVA'S MANEUVER.

Chronology

•1891 • Reporting on research with an elite cyclist, sports physician Philippe Tissié noted that the rider's large nostrils would facilitate the ingestion of air.

•1995 • Rugby players could be seen wearing nose clips, which had been invented for sleep apnea patients, with the aim of inhaling more air.

Bibliography

Bramble, D.M. and Carrier, D.R. (1983). Running and breathing in mammals. *Science* 219 (4582), 252-256.

Dawson, G. (1997). A review: Nasal dilators: Fact or fiction? *New Zealand Journal of Sports Medicine* 25(4), 61-63.

Höberman, J. (1992). *Mortal engines. The science of performance and the dehumanization of sport.* New York: The Free Press.

Stamford, B. (1986). A talk about breathing. *The Physician and Sportsmedicine* 14(5), 252.

Stamford, B. (1992). Tips for better breathing. *The Physician and Sportsmedicine* 20(9), 201-202.

BREATHING MUSCLES   The **diaphragm**, a muscle that inserts on itself via a central tendon, changes the volume of the thoracic and abdominal cavities by drawing the central tendon inferiorly. When the central tendon is drawn inferiorly, inspiration takes place, the volume of the thoracic cavity is increased and that of the abdominal cavity is decreased. In addition to functioning as a breathing muscle, the diaphragm assists the abdominal muscles in increasing intra-abdominal pressure. The *intercostales externi* draw the ventral part of the ribs upward, increasing the volume of the thoracic cavity for inspiration. The *scaleni* lift the first two ribs, and the *sternocleidomastoid* lifts upward on the sternum. The *levatores costarum* and the *serratus posterior superior* raise the ribs in inspiration.

The *intercostales interni* draw the ventral part of the ribs downward, decreasing the volume of the thoracic cavity for expiration. The *subcostales* and the *transversus thoracis*, which lie deep to the *intercostales interni*, also draw the ventral part of the ribs downward, decreasing the volume of the thoracic cavity for forceful expiration. The *serratus posterior inferior* pulls the ribs down, resisting the pull of the diaphragm. The *rectus abdominis* pulls downward on the lower ribs at the same time that they and other abdominal muscles compress the abdominal contents upward toward the diaphragm.

BREATHING RATE   *See* RESPIRATORY FREQUENCY.

BREATHING RESERVE   *See* VENTILATORY RESERVE.

BREATHING VALVES   *See under* OXYGEN UPTAKE, MEASUREMENT.

BRITTLENESS   The amount of strain to failure. The lower the strain to failure, the more brittle the material. A brittle material is one that has little or no plastic deformation. The breaking point of the material is near its elastic limit. Bone afflicted by osteoporosis is more brittle than normal bone. *See also under* PLASTIC BEHAVIOR; TOUGHNESS.

BRONCHI   *See under* LUNGS.

BRONCHITIS   Inflammation of the bronchial lining. It is a form of obstructive pulmonary disease. **Chronic bronchitis** is a chronic inflammation of the bronchial tubes that lasts at least three months each year for at least two consecutive years. It is characterized by inflammation and thickening of airway diameter. It can also lead to destruction of the normal tissue and fibrosis. There is a high rate of mucus secretion and the lungs are predisposed to infection. **Bronchiectasis** is inflammation and dilation of the bronchi. **Small airway disease** is an early manifestation of the same pathological processes that eventually lead to chronic bronchitis and/or emphysema. *See* CHRONIC OBSTRUCTIVE PULMONARY DISEASE.

BROWN FAT   Brown adipose tissue. It is a type of fat in which the cells contain many large mitochondria causing the fat to appear brown. These mitochondria contain large amounts of pigmented cytochromes and can produce large amounts of metabolic heat. The thermogenic property of brown fat stems from the ability of its mitochondria to perform controlled uncoupling of oxidative phosphorylation. When the uncoupling pathway is activated, the use of substrate results in the production of heat rather than ATP. Brown fat is activated by the sympathetic nervous system via stimulation of beta-adrenergic receptors. There are large amounts of brown fat in infants, but it mostly disappears by the second decade of life. Adults have only about 1% of their body weight as brown fat. Some brown fat remains in certain areas such as around the kidneys and in the posterior neck. The activity of brown fat is increased after a meal and during cold temperatures. *See under* COLD STRESS; THERMOGENESIS.

BRUISE *See* CONTUSION.

BTPS Gas volume conditioned to body temperature and ambient atmospheric pressure, and fully saturated with vapor at the individual's body temperature.

BUCCAL SMEAR TEST *See under* HEREDITY.

BUFFERING Processes that minimize changes in the concentration of hydrogen ions, thus maintaining acid-base balance. There are three types of buffering: chemical, ventilatory and renal. In response to an acid-base imbalance, chemical buffering takes place in less than a second in order to prevent drastic changes in the pH of body fluids. Ventilatory buffering occurs within minutes, and renal buffering occurs within hours or days.

Chemical buffering involves substances in body fluids that accept hydrogen ions. The most important chemical buffers are bicarbonates, phosphates and proteins (including hemoglobin). The **bicarbonate buffer** involves carbonic acid and sodium bicarbonate. The **phosphate buffer** involves phosphoric acid and sodium phosphate. It is important in intracellular fluid where there is a relatively high concentration of phosphates. **Protein buffers** are important in venous blood for buffering hydrogen ions released from the dissociation of carbonic acid. Important buffers within muscle include creatine phosphate, inorganic phosphate, protein-bound histidine residues and carnosine.

Ventilatory buffering occurs via control of ventilation. This is especially important during exercise. An increased concentration of free hydrogen ions in extracellular fluid and plasma directly stimulates the respiratory center in the brain and causes an immediate increase in alveolar ventilation. This leads to a decrease in alveolar partial pressure of carbon dioxide, and carbon dioxide is removed from the blood.

Renal buffering occurs in the kidneys and is the only way to eliminate acids other than carbonic acid. The kidneys excrete either acidic or alkaline urine in response to changes in the concentration of hydrogen ions. The renal tubules secrete greater or lesser amounts of hydrogen ions into the urine and reabsorb greater or lesser amounts of bicarbonate ions, respectively.

It does not seem that exercise training enhances the body's overall buffering capacity (alkaline reserve). *See also* CARBON DIOXIDE.

BULBAR Pertaining to the muscles of the face, mouth and throat.

BULIMIA NERVOSA An eating disorder that involves a secretive cycle of binge eating followed by purging. Binge eating is characterized by regular intake of large amounts of food accompanied by a sense of loss of control over eating behavior; regular use of inappropriate compensatory behaviors such as self-induced vomiting, laxative or diuretic abuse, fasting, and/or obsessive or compulsive exercise; and extreme concern with body weight and shape.

Bulimia nervosa affects 1 to 2% of adolescent and young adult women. Approximately 80% of bulimia nervosa patients are female. About 50% of anorectics also suffer from bulimia. Normal weight bulimia is when bulimia occurs without anorexia. Risk factors for bulimia nervosa include: childhood obesity, early onset of menarche, weight concern, perfectionism, low self-esteem, social pressure about weight/eating, family dieting, eating disorders among family members, inadequate parenting, parental discord, parental psychopathology, childhood sexual abuse and chronic illness (e.g. diabetes).

Bulimia nervosa is frequently associated with

symptoms of depression and changes in social adjustment. The recurrent binge-and-purge cycles can damage the entire digestive system and purge behaviors can lead to electrolyte and chemical imbalances in the body that affect the heart and other major organ functions. The esophagus may become inflamed and possibly rupture due to the frequent vomiting. Chronic irregular bowel movements and constipation may occur as a result of laxative abuse. Gastric rupture can result from binge eating. Up to 89% of patients with bulimia nervosa show signs of the tooth erosion usually associated with regurgitation. Loss of tissue and erosive lesions on the surface of teeth due to the effects of acid can appear as early as 6 months from the start of the problem. Teeth can become brittle, translucent, and weak. There may also be enlargement of the salivary glands, dry mouth, and reddened, dry, cracked lips.

Emotional and mental characteristics associated with bulimia nervosa in males include: intense fear of becoming fat or gaining weight; depression; social isolation; strong need to be in control; rigid, inflexible ('all-or-nothing') thinking; possible conflict over gender identity or sexual orientation; difficulty expressing feelings; and working hard to please others.

Bibliography

National Eating Disorders Association. Http://www.NationalEatingDisorders.org

BULK FLOW   Flux of a solution as a whole, including all its solutes. Bulk flow of water occurs when large masses of water move as in water through a pipe. The water is flowing in response to a water potential gradient from a region of high water potential to a region of low water potential. Water can be made to move uphill, but only if pressure is applied. The pressure raises the water potential.

BULK MODULUS   The ratio of the change in pressure acting on a volume to the fractional change in volume. Bulk modulus is a type of elastic modulus.

BUNION   A bony prominence (exostosis) of the first metatarsal head, often associated with hallux valgus. *See also* HALLUX VALGUS; TAILOR'S BUNION.

BUOYANCY   The upward force on a body that is wholly or partially immersed in a fluid. The **center of buoyancy** is the center of mass of the fluid that would occupy the space of the immersed part of a body floating in the fluid. It is the centroid of the volume of liquid displaced by a body. For a body completely submerged in a liquid, the center of buoyancy coincides with the center of volume of the body. *See* ARCHIMEDES' PRINCIPLE.

BURNER   *See under* BRACHIAL PLEXUS.

BURNOUT   It is a reaction to chronic stress, leading to a loss of motivation for an activity, to which an individual was previously committed and dedicated. Elite athletes and coaches have dropped out of sports at the peaks of their careers maintaining that they were 'burned out' and that their participation was no longer fun or rewarding. There is exhaustion, which is described as a loss of concern, energy, interest and trust. From the exhaustion comes a negative change in an individual's response to others and decreased performance. Athletes who report being burned out typically have been competing for a long time and have trained extremely hard. They have felt pressure from coaches and parents to perform at high levels. Perfectionism is a possible contributor to burnout. Entrapment is a component of burnout that occurs when individuals, especially coaches, lose their enthusiasm for the job, but feel they must stay on for a variety of reasons.

Henschen (1998) describes one potential series of events that may eventually lead to athletic burnout. First, there is a **slump**, which is an extended period of relatively low personal performance. There is no detectable performance execution problem, but the outcome is not up to normal personal standards. The athlete begins to develop a negative attitude or tries to overcompensate with more training. A vicious circle begins to develop with overtraining leading to staleness. The final outcome, when severe enough, is burnout.

Contrary to the above, Coakley (1992) has argued

that burnout in elite adolescent athletes does not have its origins in chronic stress. Instead, burnout is rooted in social processes that interfere with a young person developing desired identities apart from athletic identity and denies them the autonomy and independence that are so important in the lives of adolescents. The stress associated with burnout is a collateral product of the athlete's lack of control over conditions of his or her own participation. Internalization of this lack of control leads to the burnout symptoms noted above.

A distinction can be made between dropout and burnout. According to Schmidt and Stein (1991), while candidates for burnout perceive their alternatives as less attractive or even non-existent, dropout occurs when a person elects to switch to an activity that is equally or more attractive than the current one.

See also OVERTRAINING; SELF CONCEPT; SPORT COMMITMENT.

Bibliography

Coakley, J. (1992). Burnout among adolescent athletes: A personal failure or social problem? *Sociology of Sport Journal* 9, 271-285.

Dale, J. and Weinberg, R. (1990). Burnout in sport: A review and critique. *Journal of Applied Sport Psychology* 2, 67-83.

Henschen, K.P. (1998). Athletic staleness and burnout: Diagnosis, prevention, and treatment. In: Williams, J.M. (ed). *Applied sport psychology: Personal growth to peak performance.* 3rd ed. pp398-408. Palo Alto, CA: Mayfield Publishing Co.

Raedeke, T.D. (1997). Is athlete burnout more than just stress? A sport commitment perspective. *Journal of Sport and Exercise Psychology* 19(4), 396-417.

Schmidt, G.W. and Stein, G.L. (1991). Sport commitment. A model integrating enjoyment, dropout and burnout. *Journal of Sport and Exercise Psychology* 13, 254-265.

Smith, R.E. (1986). Toward a cognitive-affective model of athletic burnout. *Journal of Sport Psychology* 8, 36-50.

BURSAE   Fluid-filled sacs, usually located near joints, that are either permanent or acquired. **Permanent (constant) bursae** are endothelium-lined structures, found between tendon and bone or skin that facilitate smooth gliding of tendons over areas of high friction. Permanent bursae contain synovial cells that secrete collagen, proteoglycans and enzymatic proteins. These substances act as lubricants. **Acquired (adventitial) bursae** do not contain endothelial cells or synovial fluid. They develop secondary to degeneration of fibrous tissues, in areas that are subject to repeated stress such as those over bony prominences.

Bursitis is inflammation of a bursa(e) and may be caused by acute trauma, such as a direct blow; or by chronic trauma from overuse, pyrogenic infection secondary to a puncture wound and miscellaneous inflammatory processes such as gout and rheumatoid arthritis. **Septic bursitis** is sometimes related to seeding from an infection at a distant site, such as paronychia, cellulitis or forearm infection. **Nonseptic bursitis** may be caused by crystalline deposition disease (such as gout) or be related to rheumatoid arthritis, and has been associated with atopic dermatitis (a type of eczema). A **hemobursa** occurs when there is bleeding into a bursa. The usual cause of hemobursa is a direct impact such as a fall. It may also be caused by indirect injury, such as tendon rupture. Hemobursae occur frequently in sports such as volleyball, which demand repeated contact with a hard surface or object.

See also HIP JOINT, BURSITIS.

C

CADAVER DISSECTION ANALYSIS Dissection of fresh human cadavers (dead bodies). It may be performed for direct body composition. *See under* BODY COMPOSITION.

CAFFEINE A central nervous system (CNS) stimulant that has been used as an ergogenic aid for many years. It is a member of the group of chemicals called methylxanthines, which are found in over 60 species of plant. Coffee is derived from the beans of several species of coffea plants, e.g. *Coffea arabica*. Tea is made from the *Camellia sinensis* plant and its predominant methylxanthine, **theophylline**, is also a CNS stimulant. Chocolate contains small amounts of caffeine. The predominant methylxanthine in chocolate, **theobromine**, named after the cocoa tree (*Theobroma cacao*), does not bind as well into the adenosine receptors as caffeine and is virtually inert as a CNS stimulant. Adenosine generally decreases the concentration of the major neurotransmitters, including serotonin, dopamine, acetylcholine, norepinephrine and glutamate. Caffeine is an adenosine receptor antagonist and increases the concentration of these major neurotransmitters.

A brewed cup of coffee (6 oz) typically contains 60 to 100 mg of caffeine and soft drink beverages (8 oz) contain about 30 to 60 mg.

There is strong evidence that caffeine can improve performance by directly affecting the CNS. Although there are wide individual differences in response to caffeine, a dose of 80 to 200 mg leads to increased alertness, shortened reaction time, improved concentration and decreased perception of fatigue. Even small quantities of caffeine seem to have a facilitative effect on activities that require quick reaction time and rapid movements.

Caffeine causes vasoconstriction (except in the renal afferent artery), increased diuresis and naturesis, and increased gastric secretion. Due to its mild vasoconstriction and stimulant effects, caffeine is used in pain and anti-migraine medications. Most headache sufferers can consume up to 200 mg per day, but some patients with frequent headaches need to abstain from caffeine use.

Positive effects of caffeine can be obtained in a variety of exercise conditions with caffeine doses of 3 mg/kg or less. Coffee may not produce an ergogenic effect in circumstances where caffeine is effective, even though the same plasma concen-tration results. Although the research evidence is equivocal, it seems that caffeine has an ergogenic effect during exercise of greater than 30 minutes at moderate intensity (75 to 80% of maximal oxygen uptake). Costill et al. (1978) were the first to demonstrate that caffeine ingestion resulted in increased endurance. It seems that the increased endurance is a result of increased fatty acid oxidation and thus a glycogen-sparing effect. It is not clearly understood whether caffeine acts directly on adipose and peripheral vascular tissue, or indirectly via its stimulating effect on epinephrine released from the adrenal medulla. Considering the latter, it is possible that epinephrine acts as an antagonist of the adenosine receptors on adipocyte cells that usually repress lipolysis. Inhibition of adenosine receptors increases cellular levels of cyclic AMP that, in turn, activate hormone-sensitive lipases to promote lipolysis, hence releasing free fatty acids into the plasma. Increased levels of free fatty acids in the plasma then contribute to increased fatty acid oxidation, thus sparing glycogen. It is possible, however, that the sparing of muscle glycogen by caffeine may be unrelated to increased delivery of free fatty acids as a substrate. Instead, it may be due to increased neuromuscular efficiency and a subsequent decreased demand for glycogen and other fuels.

Ergogenic effects of caffeine are less apparent in individuals who are habitual users of caffeine or who consume a high-carbohydrate diet. High carbo-hydrate levels stimulate insulin release, which appears to block the effect of caffeine in raising levels of free fatty acids. Epinephrine responses to caffeine ingestion may be greater in non-users compared to habitual caffeine users.

Too much caffeine has adverse effects. **Caffeine intoxication** occurs after recent consumption of more than 250 mg. Signs include restlessness, nervousness, excitement, insomnia, muscle twitching, flushed face, diuresis, gastrointestinal disturbance, rambling flow of thought and speech, tachycardia or cardiac arrhythmia, periods of inexhaustibility, and psychomotor agitation. There is strong evidence that repeated daily administration of caffeine leads to decreased responsiveness to physiological effects (i.e. tolerance).

The most frequently reported **caffeine withdrawal** symptom is headache that is gradual in development, diffuse, throbbing and sometimes severe. Symptoms may begin 6 to 12 hours after stopping or decreasing consumption, peak in 1 to 2 days and persist for a week. Caffeine withdrawal can result from as little as a single cup of coffee per day.

About 0.5 to 4% of caffeine is excreted unchanged and can thus be detected in urine. Until January 2004, when the World Anti-Doping Agency (WADA) removed it from the list of prohibited substances, an athlete found to have a urine caffeine concentration of more than 12 mg/l was deemed to be guilty of doping. *See also* EPHEDRINE.

Chronology

•1972 • Before the Olympic Games, caffeine was classed as a drug and banned by the International Olympic Committee (IOC). It was then removed from the doping list from until the use of large amounts of caffeine was banned again before the 1984 Olympic Games.

•1997 • Daniel Komen of Kenya failed two drug tests because of excess caffeine ingested from a cola drink.

•1997 • Tests of caffeine levels in 'energy' drinks by the Ministry of Food and Fisheries in the UK found that caffeine levels were on average three times higher than levels in ordinary cola drinks with concentrations often exceeding 300 mg/l. (MAFF *Food Surveillance Information Sheet*, No 103, March 1997).

•2001 • Following the death of three healthy young people, two of whom died after mixing Red Bull with vodka, the Swedish National Food Administration issued a public warning telling people not to take Red Bull mixed with alcohol or after heavy exercise. Red Bull has 27 grams of sugar per can and about 50 mg of caffeine. Mixing energy drinks with exercise or alcohol can increase the risk of seizures, elevated heart rates and even heart attacks.

Bibliography

American Psychiatric Association. (1994). *Diagnostic and statistical manual of mental disorders*. 4th ed. Washington, DC: American Psychiatric Association.

Costill, D.L. Dalsky, G.P. and Fink, W.J. (1978). Effects of caffeine ingestion on metabolism and exercise performance. *Medicine and Science in Sports* 10, 155-158.

Dodd, S.L., Herb, R.A. and Powers, S.K. (1993). Caffeine and exercise performance: An update. *Sports Medicine* 15(1), 14-23.

Graham, T.E. and Spriet, L.L. (1996). Caffeine and exercise performance. *Gatorade Sports Science Exchange* 9(1).

Graham, T.E. et al. (1998). The metabolic and exercise endurance effects of coffee and caffeine ingestion. *Journal of Applied Physiology* 85, 883-889.

Griffiths, R.R. and Mumford, G.K. (2000). Caffeine: A drug of abuse. *American College of Neuropharmacology*. Http://www.acnp.org.

Nehling, A. and Debry, G. (1994). Caffeine and sports activity: A review. *International Journal of Sports Medicine* 15(5), 215-223.

Schwenck, T.L. (1997). Psychoactive drugs and athletic performance. *The Physician and Sportsmedicine* 25(1), 32-46.

Spriet, L.L. and Gibala, M.J. (2004). Nutritional strategies to influence adaptations to training. *Journal of Sports Sciences* 22, 127-141.

Tarnopolsky, M.A. (1993). Protein, caffeine and sports. Guidelines for active people. *The Physician and Sportsmedicine* 21(3), 137-149.

CALCANEAL BUMP *See under* ACHILLES TENDON.

CALCANEAL TENDON *See* ACHILLES TENDON.

CALCANEONAVICULAR LIGAMENT *See under* FOOT.

CALCANEUS The heel bone in humans. *See also* PLANTAR FASCIA.

CALCIFEROL *See* VITAMIN D.

CALCITONIN *See under* CALCIUM.

CALCITRIOL *See* VITAMIN D.

CALCIUM An element, which as a 'macromineral' in the human body, makes up 2% of total body weight. It is important as a structural component of bone, where 99% of it is stored. The **calcium pump** is a form of active transport, which is involved in skeletal muscle contraction. Calcium ions stored in the sarcoplasmic reticulum of muscle fibers are involved in the linkage of actin and myosin during the process of muscle contraction. It thereby controls the provision of ATP when required. The release of neurotransmitters at synapses is stimulated by the influx of calcium ions into the axon. Calcium ions in the plasma act as catalysts for blood clotting.

Parathyroid hormone is a hormone of the **parathyroid gland**, which is an endocrine gland located on the posterior aspect of the lobes of the thyroid gland. Parathyroid hormone raises the level of calcium in the blood plasma, mainly by increasing calcium absorption from bones. It is controlled by plasma calcium and is stimulated by low plasma calcium. It is increased by exercise. **Calcitonin** is a thyroid hormone involved in the metabolism of calcium in the body. Its major effect is to increase deposition of calcium and to prevent removal of mineral matter from the bones. Calcitonin decreases plasma calcium.

Athletes tend to have enhanced calcium status as assessed by bone mineral density. The exceptions to this are female athletes suffering from amenorrhea.

Milk (8 oz) contains 300 mg of calcium. Spinach (half a cup, cooked) contains 115 mg of calcium, but 16.3 servings are required to equal the absorbable calcium in 8 oz of milk. Oxalic acid is the most potent inhibitor of calcium absorption; it is found in high concentrations in spinach and rhubarb. Phytic acid is a less potent inhibitor of calcium absorption than oxalic acid. Only concentrated sources of phytic acid, such as wheat bran or dried beans, substantially decrease calcium absorption.

The use of an Adequate Intake (AI) rather than a recommended dietary allowance reflects the difficulty of estimating the intake of dietary calcium that will result in optimal accumulation and retention of calcium in the skeleton when other factors such as physical activity also interact to affect bone health. The adequate intake of calcium is 1300 mg for 9 to 18 year olds, 1000 mg for 19 to 50 year olds, and 1200 mg for adults older than 51 years of age. Only about 25% of boys and 10% of girls aged 9 to 17 years are estimated to meet the AI recommendations. Dairy foods provide 75% of the calcium in the American diet. During the most critical period for peak bone mass, however, adolescents tend to replace milk with soft drinks.

Bibliography

Food and Nutrition Board, Institute of Medicine (1997). *Dietary Reference Intakes for calcium, phosphorus, magnesium, vitamin D and fluoride.* Washington, DC: National Academy Press.

Oregon State University. The Linus Pauling Institute. Micronutrient Information Center. Http://lpi.oregonstate.edu/infocenter

Tate, C.A., Hyek, M.F. and Taffet, G.E. (1991). The role of calcium in the energetics of contracting skeletal muscle. *Sports Medicine* 12(3), 208-217.

CALCIUM-CHANNEL BLOCKERS Calcium antagonists. This is an important category of vasodilators. These drugs decrease the inflow of calcium ions into vascular smooth muscle fibers and also decrease cardiac workload by decreasing the entry of calcium ions into cardiac muscle fibers. Frequently prescribed for coronary heart disease and hypertension, calcium antagonists have been shown to lower blood pressure both in persons at rest and during exercise. They decrease vascular smooth muscle contractility and cause negative inotropic and chronotropic effects on the myocardium. Other adverse affects include bradycardia. Maximal oxygen uptake and endurance performance are not impaired following the administration of calcium antagonists. Unlike the administration of only calcium antagonists, the combination of calcium antagonists and beta-blockers has a detrimental effect on exercise performance. This detriment is significantly less than when beta blockers only are administered.

Bibliography

Kindermann, W. (1987). Calcium antagonists and exercise performance. *Sports Medicine* 4, 177-193.

CALCIUM PUMP *See under* CALCIUM;

MUSCLE CONTRACTION.

CALLUS   Tyloma. It is a thickening of the skin on the plantar aspect of the foot that occurs secondary to excessive pressure against one or more metatarsal heads. It is the skin's compensatory attempt to protect itself from chronic friction. Calluses form most commonly on weight-bearing areas of the soles of the feet and on the palms, where rackets or golf clubs rub the skin over the distal metacarpal heads. Although calluses are generally asymptomatic, they may cause discomfort when they become too thick. Calluses help to prevent injury to the dermis. Properly fitted shoes, gloves, or cushioned grips on rackets can minimize callus formation.

Bibliography

Basler, R.S., Hunzeker, C.M. and Garcia, M.A. (2004). Athletic skin injuries. Combating pressure and friction. *The Physician and Sportsmedicine* 32(5), 33-40.

CALORIC VALUE OF FOOD   *See under* ENERGY YIELD OF NUTRIENTS.

CALORIE   The quantity of heat required to raise one gram of water through one degree Celsius. Although the calorie was replaced by the joule as the main unit of heat in the metric system in 1950, the calorie is still widely used, especially in quoting the energy value of food. Physiologists use the kilocalorie (1000 calories) as a unit, but they tend to call it a 'calorie.'

CALORIMETRY   Measurement of energy consumption. **Direct calorimetry** measures the heat given off from metabolism, thus is a measure of oxygen consumption. **Indirect calorimetry** involves either closed-circuit or open-circuit spirometry.

   Closed-circuit spirometry consists of the subject inspiring via a face-mask from a container filled with oxygen. The expired air goes back to the container of oxygen via a soda-lime canister that absorbs the carbon dioxide in the expired air. Changes in the volume of oxygen in the container are recorded as oxygen is consumed.

Open-circuit spirometry consists of the subject breathing in air from the atmosphere. The flow and composition of expired air are measured to estimate oxygen consumption. For indirect calorimetry to be valid, all the energy must be generated from aerobic metabolism; ATP and creatine phosphate stores are maintained, with insignificant amino acid or protein metabolism. Although the assumptions are unlikely to be strictly true in practice, the error is usually small when the subject being measured is at rest.

   See OXYGEN UPTAKE, MEASUREMENT; STEADY STATE.

Chronology

•1777 • French scientist Antoine L. Lavoisier repeated Joseph Priestley's experiments and found that air consists of an "eminently respirable air" and an inert gas. Two years later, Lavoisier named the new gas as oxygen and his text *Traité Elementaire de Chemie* marked the modernization of chemistry.

•1782 • Antoine L. Lavoisier started collaboration with the mathematician Pierre S. LaPlace to measure the heat production of living animals using a modification of Joseph Black's (1761) device that was probably the first calorimeter and consisted of a block of ice into which was placed a substance of known mass and temperature. Lavoisier and LaPlace determined the heat produced from the amount of water produced as the substance cooled to the temperature of the ice. The animal's warmth melted the ice and the volume of water formed was measured. Knowing that 80 kcal of heat melts 1000 g of ice, this allowed the heat production to be measured. The animal chamber was surrounded by an inner jacket of ice and an outer jacket of iced water that provided perfect insulation, because it has the same temperature as the ice in the inner jacket. Lavoisier and LaPlace demonstrated later that, during exercise, oxygen is consumed and carbon dioxide is produced.

Bibliography

McClean, J.A. and Tobin, G. (1987). *Animal and human calorimetry*. Cambridge: Cambridge University Press.

c AMP   *See* CYCLIC AMP.

CANCER   A malignant tumor. **Malignant** means that the tumor is capable of progressive and unrestrained growth and/or is capable of distant spread via the lymphatic system or the circulatory system, resulting in development of secondary deposits of tumor known as **metastases**. **Benign** tumors are non-cancerous; they do not spread. There are more than 100 different types of cancers. A **carcinogen** is a physical agent or chemical reagent that causes cancer.

Cancer is the second most prevalent cause of death, after cardiovascular disease, in most Western countries. In the USA, there are more than 500,000 cancer deaths per year. The lifetime risk of developing cancer is 43.5% and 38.3% in males and females, respectively. There are about 9 million Americans alive with a history of cancer. In 2001, the most common cancers in males were prostate (198,100), lung (90,700), and colon and rectum (67,300). The most common cancers in females are breast (192,200), lung (78,800), and colon and rectum (68,100). Lung cancer mortality rates are 20 times higher in males than females. Causes of cancer include poor nutrition (33%) and tobacco use (31%).

The exact cause of cancer is unknown, but it is thought to result from acquired changes in the genetic make-up of a particular cell or group of cells that ultimately leads to failure of the normal mechanism regulating their growth.

There is strong evidence that lack of physical activity is causally related to colon cancer. It has been estimated that 12 to 14% of colon cancer could be attributed to lack of frequent involvement in vigorous physical activity. A high body mass index has been reported to be associated with an increased risk of colon cancer in sedentary men, but not in physically active men. There is evidence that a physically active occupation offers some protection against colon cancer and intestinal neoplasia. It is likely that between 3.5 and 4 hours of vigorous activity per week may be needed to optimize protection. Possible mechanisms of protection include: changes in gastro-intestinal transit time; altered immune function and prostaglandin levels; decreasing insulin and insulin-like growth factor levels; decreasing obesity; and enhancing free radical scavenger systems.

Risk of breast cancer is increased by early onset of menarche, a great number of regular ovulatory cycles, and late menopause. Exercise may protect against breast cancer by decreasing exposure to estrogens.

Physical inactivity is a significant risk factor for prostate cancer. There is evidence that exercise can decrease the risk of prostate cancer. Possible mechanisms include modulation of hormone levels, prevention of obesity, enhanced immune system and decreased oxidative stress. Exercise may also be of benefit in men undergoing treatment for prostate cancer. There is evidence that higher levels of testosterone may contribute to the development of prostate cancer. African Americans have the highest prostate cancer incidence rates in the world, and they have 15% higher levels of testosterone than other North American males. Repeated bouts of exercise may lower blood levels of testosterone, thus exposing the prostate to less testosterone.

Firm epidemiological evidence shows a significant inverse relationship between the amounts of occupational or leisure time physical activity and decrease in all-cause cancer risk. Overall susceptibility to cancer shows a 'U'-shaped relationship to body mass index. This partly reflects the adverse influences of cigarette smoking and a tall body-build for those with low body mass indices and partly reflects the adverse effect of obesity at the opposite end of the body mass index distribution. Endurance athletes are less likely to smoke, decreasing the risk of many tumors.

A Western lifestyle may increase cancer risk through alterations in the metabolism of insulin and insulin-like growth factors. Insulin increases the bioactivity of insulin growth factor-1 (IGF-1), by enhancing its synthesis and by decreasing several of its binding proteins (e.g. IGF-1 binding protein-1). Insulin and IGF-1 both stimulate anabolic processes as a function of available energy and elementary substrates (e.g. amino acids). The anabolic signals by insulin or IGF-1 can promote tumor development by inhibiting apoptosis, and by stimulating cell proliferation. Furthermore, both insulin and IGF-1 stimulate the synthesis of sex steroids, but inhibit the synthesis of sex hormone-binding globulin, a binding protein that regulates the bioavailability of circulating sex steroids to tissues. Chronic hyperinsulinemia may be a cause of cancers of the colon, pancreas and endometrium, and possibly also the breast. On the other hand, elevated plasma IGF-1 appears to be related to an increased risk of prostate cancer and breast cancer in young women.

Bibliography

American Cancer Society (2001). *Cancer facts and figures.* Atlanta: American Cancer Society.

Friedenreich, C.M. and Rohan, T.E. (1995). A review of physical activity and breast cancer. *Epidemiology* 6(3), 311-317.

Hardman, A.E. (2001). Physical activity and cancer risk. *Proceedings of the Nutritional Society* 60(1), 107-113.

Kaaks, R. and Lukanova, A. (2001). Energy balance and cancer: The role of insulin and insulin-like growth factor-I. *Proceedings of the Nutritional Society* 60(1), 91-106.

Latikka, P., Pukkala, E. and Vihko, V. (1998). Relationship between the risk of breast cancer and physical activity. *Sports Medicine* 26(3), 133-143.

Quadrilatero, J. and Hoffman-Goetz, L. (2003). Physical activity and colon cancer. A systematic review of potential mechanisms. *Journal of Sports Medicine and Physical Fitness* 43(2), 121-138.

Schneider, C.M., Dennehy, C.A. and Carter, S.D. (2003). *Exercise and cancer recovery.* Champaign, IL: Human Kinetics.

Shephard, R.J. and Shek, P.N. (1998). Associations between physical activity and susceptibility to cancer. Possible mechanisms. *Sports Medicine* 26(5), 293-315.

Slattery, M.L. (2004). Physical activity and colorectal cancer. *Sports Medicine* 34(4), 239-252.

Torti, D.C. and Matheson, G.O. (2004). Exercise and prostate cancer. *Sports Medicine* 34(6), 363-369.

CANNABINOIDS *See under* MARIJUANA.

CANTILEVER A long bar or beam fixed at only one end to a vertical support used to hold a structure such as bridge in position.

CAPACITANCE The property of being able to store an electric charge. Membrane capacitance is the capacitance of a cell membrane, as of an axon or muscle fiber. *See under* VEIN

CAPILLARIES Minute blood vessels that communicate freely with each other to form networks. Blood is delivered to the capillaries by terminal arterioles. Capillaries are the smallest diameter blood vessels and possess a wall composed of a single cell layer. Some arteriole-to-capillary junctions are surrounded by a layer of smooth muscle and regulate blood flow through a capillary bed. Such structures are termed **pre-capillary sphincters**. **Angiogenesis** is the formation of new capillaries that interconnect to form new vessels.

CAPITATE BONE Os magnum. It is the largest of the carpal bones, located in the distal row.

CAPSULITIS Inflammation of a capsule, such as that of a joint. **Adhesive capsulitis** is adhesive inflammation between the joint capsule and the peripheral articular cartilage of the shoulder, with obliteration of the subdeltoid bursa. *See under* ELBOW JOINT.

CARBOHYDRATE A class of chemical compounds composed of carbon, hydrogen and oxygen. There are three major subclasses of carbohydrates: monosaccharides, oligosaccharides and polysaccharides. **Monosaccharides** are simple sugars such as glucose and fructose. Honey contains fructose and glucose. **Sugar alcohols** (e.g. sorbitol, manitol) are derivatives of monosaccharides formed by replacing a hydrogen atom with a hydroxyl (-OH) group. **Dissaccharides** consist of two monosaccharide units. Sucrose is formed from one glucose unit and one fructose unit. Extracted from cane sugar and sugar beet, sucrose is refined to become table sugar. Maltose is a disaccharide composed of two molecules of glucose. It is a product of the enzymatic hydrolysis of starch, dextrin or glycogen. An **alpha bond** links two monosaccharides. During digestion of carbohydrates, hydrolysis can separate disaccharides into monosaccharides; the addition of a molecule of water splits the bond between the two sugar molecules, providing the hydrogen and hydroxyl groups necessary for the sugars to exist as monosaccharide. **Oligosaccharides** consist of 3 to 10 monosaccharides bonded together. The two most common oligosaccharides are raffinose (one galactose, one glucose and one fructose) and stachyose (two galactose, one glucose and one fructose). Raffinose and stachyose are readily metabolized by bacteria in the colon. **Polysaccharides**, such as glycogen and starch, consist of long chains having hundreds or thousands of monosaccharide units. The two main forms of starch are amylose (long, unbranched chains of glucose molecules) and amylopectin (branched chains of glucose molecules).

In general, fruit that is riper has higher sugar content. Before ripening, a banana is almost entirely starch. After ripening, the dessert varieties are almost entirely sugar.

Dietary fiber refers to non-starch polysaccharides in plant cell walls (and inside plant cells) that are resistant to digestive enzymes, leaving some residue in the digestive tract. There are two basic forms of dietary fiber: soluble (e.g. pectin) and insoluble (e.g. cellulose). **Soluble dietary fiber** may be metabolized in the large intestine. **Insoluble dietary fiber** passes through the entire gastrointestinal tract without being metabolized.

The term '**simple carbohydrate**' usually refers to refined, highly processed carbohydrate that has largely been broken down into dissaccharides and monosaccharides. The term '**complex carbo-hydrate**' is commonly used to refer to carbohydrate that is mainly in the polysaccharide form. It is in the natural, unrefined state and is consequently found in combination with vitamins, minerals and dietary fiber. When fiber intake increases so should water intake to prevent the stool from becoming hard and impacted. A sudden increase in fiber intake can cause flatus and bloating. Dietary fiber may bind the following minerals in the gastro-intestinal tract: zinc, calcium, magnesium and iron, thus preventing them from being absorbed. A diet rich in complex carbohydrate decreases the risk of certain kinds of cancer.

Non-nutritive sweeteners are substances with little or no caloric value that are added to food and drink in order to impart sweetness. Non-nutritive sweeteners are 200 to 700 times sweeter than sucrose. In the USA, the Food and Drug Administration (FDA) has approved of four non-nutritive sweeteners: acesulfane K, aspartame,

saccharin and sucralose. **Nutritive sweeteners**, such as honey and high fructose corn syrup, have high caloric value.

See also DIET; FLATUS; GLUCOSE; GLYCEMIC INDEX; LACTOSE.

CARBOHYDRATE-ELECTROLYTE DRINKS
See under FLUID REPLACEMENT.

CARBOHYDRATE LOADING   Glycogen supercompensation. It is an ergogenic aid that was developed in the 1960s and has been used by athletes with the aim of increasing glycogen concentration to more than twice that of normal. The original procedure involved the athlete doing a fast long-distance run seven days before an endurance race in order to deplete the glycogen stores. Over the following three days, training would be continued on an almost carbohydrate-free diet. The three days after that, including the day of the race, the athlete would 'load' with carbohydrate. This procedure takes advantage not only of the high carbohydrate intake, but also of the fact that the muscle enzyme glycogen synthetase is stimulated following the glycogen depletion. It is now believed that the depletion phase is not necessary in trained athletes. In fact, it has often caused serious side effects, including a period of depression and lethargy. A modified procedure consists of three days of a mixed diet together with training followed by three days of using a taper and a high carbohydrate intake. Glycogen storage requires water retention, thus extra water is required to prevent dehydration. After repeated attempts at carbohydrate loading, it seems that the body adapts to any change in enzymatic activity and the supercompensation effect is diminished. It is now thought that endurance-trained athletes are able to achieve maximal glycogen storage simply by resting for 48 to 72 hours and eating 8 to 10 g carbohydrate per kg body mass.

Elevated pre-exercise levels of muscle glycogen will postpone fatigue by about 20% in endurance events lasting more than 90 minutes. As exhaustion from such exercise usually coincides with critically low muscle glycogen, it seems that the supply of energy from glycogen utilization cannot be replaced by an increased oxidation of blood glucose.

There is little or no benefit of glycogen supercompensation for either moderate-intensity running or cycling lasting 60 to 90 minutes, or for a single exhaustive bout of high-intensity exercise lasting less than five minutes.

There is evidence that females may have a decreased ability to increase muscle glycogen during a period of dietary carbohydrate loading, but this may be due to lower energy intake in female athletes.

Chronology

•1969 • UK athlete Ron Hill used 'carbohydrate loading' as an ergogenic aid before his victory in the marathon of the European Championship in Athens.

Bibliography

Hargreaves, M., Hawley, J.A. and Jeukendrup, A. (2004). Pre-exercise carbohydrate and fat ingestion. Effects on metabolism and performance. *Journal of Sports Sciences* 22, 31-38.

Hawley, J.A. et al. (1997). Carbohydrate-loading and exercise performance. An update. *Sports Medicine* 24(2), 73-81.

CARBOHYDRATE PROCESSING DIS-ORDERS *See* GLYCOGEN STORAGE DISEASES.

CARBAMINO EFFECT *See under* CARBON DIOXIDE.

CARBON DIOXIDE A gas that is a waste product of internal respiration. Carbon dioxide moves out of body tissues by diffusion. About 60 to 80% of the total carbon dioxide diffuses into red blood cells, where it combines with water to form **carbonic acid** in a reaction catalyzed by the enzyme carbonic anhydrase. Carbonic acid dissociates into hydrogen ions and bicarbonate ions. The hydrogen ions are buffered by hemoglobin. It is the excess hydrogen ions that cause respiratory acidosis. The bicarbonate ions diffuse into the blood plasma in exchange for chloride ions. This ionic exchange process is called the chloride shift. In the lungs, bicarbonate ions and hydrogen ions are joined to form carbonic acid, which then dissociates into carbon dioxide and water. The carbon dioxide is expired. Although the carbonic anhydrase reaction also occurs in plasma, it is about a thousand times faster in red blood cells because, unlike plasma, they contain carbonic anhydrase. The hydrogen ions released during the carbonic anhydrase reaction bind to hemoglobin, triggering the Bohr effect. Because of the buffering effect of hemoglobin, the liberated hydrogen ions cause little change in pH under resting conditions. About 20 to 30% of carbon dioxide is transported to the lungs by compounds formed when carbon dioxide reacts with parts of hemoglobin and other proteins. Since carbon dioxide binds directly to the amino acids of globin (and not to the heme), carbon dioxide transport in red blood cells does not compete with oxyhemoglobin (or the nitric oxide) transport mechanism. The loading and unloading of carbon dioxide to and from hemoglobin are directly influenced by the partial pressure of carbon dioxide and the degree of oxygenation of hemoglobin. About 5 to 10% of the carbon dioxide travels to the lungs dissolved in blood plasma.

As carbon dioxide enters the systemic bloodstream, it causes more oxygen to dissociate from hemoglobin (**Bohr effect**). In turn, this allows more carbon dioxide to combine with hemoglobin and more bicarbonate ions to be formed (**Haldane effect**). In the pulmonary circulation, the situation is reversed. As hemoglobin becomes saturated with oxygen, the hydrogen ions released combine with bicarbonate ions, helping to unload carbon dioxide from the pulmonary blood.

During internal respiration, when partial pressure of oxygen is low and partial pressure of carbon dioxide is high, the Haldane effect promotes the loading of carbon dioxide onto the hemoglobin, while both the Bohr effect and the carbamino effect work to promote oxygen unloading. When carbon dioxide is bound to hemoglobin, the **carbamino effect** changes hemoglobin's conformation and decreases its affinity for oxygen.

Carbon dioxide output is the amount of carbon dioxide expired from the body into the atmosphere per unit time. This differs from carbon dioxide production rate under conditions in which additional carbon dioxide may be evolved from the body's stores or carbon dioxide is added to the body's stores. In the steady state, carbon dioxide output equals carbon dioxide production. If carbon dioxide is measured at (or converted to) STPD conditions, then the fraction of carbon dioxide in expired air is the fraction of dry gas volume; the fraction of carbon dioxide in inspired air is negligible.

At a sea-level atmospheric pressure of 760 mm Hg, the partial pressure of carbon dioxide is 0.3 mmHg. **End-tidal partial pressure of carbon dioxide** is the partial pressure of carbon dioxide measured at the end of an exhalation. It is usually the highest partial pressure of carbon dioxide measured during the alveolar phase of the exhalation.

Arterial end-tidal partial pressure of carbon dioxide difference is the difference between the mean arterial partial pressure of carbon dioxide and the end-tidal partial pressure of carbon dioxide. It is positive when the arterial partial pressure of carbon dioxide is higher than the end-tidal partial pressure of carbon dioxide.

When alveolar ventilation decreases, alveolar carbon dioxide increases. The increase of carbon dioxide content above normal excites the respiratory center in the brain. As a result, alveolar ventilation is increased. A similar process takes place when alveolar carbon dioxide content decreases below normal.

Bibliography

Powers, S.K. and Beadle, R.E. (1985). Control of ventilation during submaximal exercise: A brief review. *Journal of Sports Sciences* 3, 51-65.

CARBONIC ACID   *See under* CARBON DIOXIDE.

CARBON MONOXIDE   *See under* AIR POLLUTION.

CARBONYL GROUP   A functional group that consists of an oxygen atom joined by a double bond to a carbon atom. If the carbonyl group is joined only to alkyl groups or aryl groups, the compound is a ketone. If it is joined to at least one hydrogen atom, the compound is an aldehyde.

CARBOXYL   Carboxy. The acid group (-COOH)

found in most organic acids.

CARBUNCLE   *See under* SKIN

CARCINOGENIC   Cancer causing.

CARDIAC ARREST   A cardiac emergency; it is when the heart does not function at all. In the USA, sudden cardiac arrest accounts for approximately 220,000 deaths each year. A quarter of these deaths can be prevented if an automated external defibrillator is available at the time of the emergency. 75% of all cardiac arrests happen in people's homes. Sudden cardiac arrest is the leading cause of death in adults and it occurs twice as frequently in men compared to women.

CARDIAC ARRHYTHMIAS   These are caused by one or more of the following abnormalities in the rhythmicity-conduction system of the heart: abnormal rhythmicity of the pacemaker, shift of the pacemaker from the sinus node to another place in the heart, blocks at different points in the spread of the impulse throughout the heart, abnormal pathways of impulse transmission through the heart, and spontaneous generation of spurious impulses in almost any part of the heart.

Ventricular arrhythmias in the athlete generally occur in the setting of structural heart disease, which is genetically determined (e.g. hypertrophic cardiomyopathy) or acquired (e.g. coronary artery disease). **Ventricular fibrillation** is a disturbance of the electrical activity in the heart's ventricular muscle. Most cases of ventricular fibrillation during exercise in the general population are fatal, because they are not identified and treated. **Ventricular tachycardia** is a rapid arrhythmia of the ventricles that can degenerate to ventricular fibrillation, which usually suggests a myocardial scar rather than myocardial ischemia.

See ATRIAL FIBRILLATION; BRADYCARDIA; TACHYCARDIA

Bibliography

Guyton, A.C. and Hall, J.E. (2000). *Textbook of medical physiology*. 10th ed. Philadelphia, PA: W.B. Saunders Co.

Link, M.S., Homoud, M.K., Wang, P.J. and Estes, N.A. (2001). Cardiac arrhythmias in the athlete. *Cardiology in Review* 9(1), 21-30.

CARDIAC CYCLE This describes the function of the heart muscle (myocardium), which is to move blood through the circulatory system. The purposes of the cardiovascular system are transport of oxygen to the tissues and removal of waste products, transport of nutrients to tissues, and thermoregulation. The contractile system is similar to that of skeletal muscle in that there are thick and thin filaments that interdigitate and slide among each other during contraction. Unlike skeletal muscle, cardiac muscle cannot sustain an oxygen debt and never rests for more than a second. The heartbeat does not depend on stimulation from nerves. Under normal conditions, an electrical impulse is initiated by the specialized neuromuscular tissue in the posterior wall of the right atrium of the heart (**sinoatrial node; sinus node**).

The cardiac cycle can be subdivided into two stages: systole and diastole. During **systole**, blood is forced from the ventricles (the upper chambers of the heart) into the arterial system. It starts with ventricular pressure overcoming atrial pressure and the atrioventricular valves closing. A period of isometric contraction of the heart follows in which ventricular pressure increases while atrioventricular valves and aortic valves (on the left side) are closed. Blood is ejected from the ventricles when the ventricular myocardium generates ventricular pressures that exceed arterial pressures and the aortic valve opens. This causes a short time interval where contraction is occurring, but no blood is ejected (**isovolumetric contraction**). In the period of maximal ejection, ventricular pressure continues to rise. It then falls during the period of decreased ejection, when the aortic valve is open and the atrioventricular valves are closed.

During **diastole**, the cardiac muscle relaxes and the heart fills with blood from the veins. During the pre-diastolic phase, ventricular pressure falls until it is less than aortic pressure (on the left side), when the aortic valve closes. During the isometric relaxation phase, ventricular pressure continues to fall rapidly until it is less than atrial pressure, when the atrioventricular valves open. In the period of rapid filling ventricular pressure falls to zero. In the period of slower filling (**diastasis**) both atrial and ventricular pressures are low. Finally, atrial contraction causes an increase in both atrial and ventricular pressure.

Preload can be defined as all of the factors that contribute to passive ventricular wall stress (or tension) at the end of diastole, and the term **afterload** can be defined as all of the factors that contribute to total myocardial wall stress (or tension) during systolic ejection (Norton, 2003). **End-diastolic volume** is the volume of blood in each ventricle. End-diastolic volume may be an excellent index of preload, but it cannot be equated with preload. The end-systolic pressure and the relationship between ventricular end-systolic pressure and end-systolic volume can be used as quantifiable indices of afterload and/or myocardial contractility, but should not be equated with afterload. The greater the end-diastolic volume and the greater the stretch, the faster is the resultant ventricular myocardial contraction. This produces an increase in stroke volume and cardiac output. Increases in end-diastolic volume cause muscle fibers in the ventricular myocardium to lengthen. This is the **Frank-Starling effect** and the basis of the **Frank-Starling law**, which states that when the rate at which blood flows into the heart from the veins (i.e. venous return) changes, the heart automatically adjusts its output to match the inflow. **Contractility** is the velocity of myocardial contraction for a given end-diastolic volume. Contractility increases with increased sympathetic stimulation.

Action potentials spread rapidly throughout the ventricular myocardium, because of the diffuse presence of specialized low-resistance conducting tissue in cardiac muscle (**intercalated discs**). During ventricular systole, not all blood is ejected from each ventricle. **Ejection fraction** is stroke volume expressed as a percentage of the end-diastolic volume. The ejection fraction for a healthy heart at rest is approximately 0.6.

The recording and amplification of electric

potentials that have spread to the surface of the body from the heart is called **electrocardiography**. The resulting graphic tracing is called an electrocardiogram. It shows the sum of electrical activity of all cardiac muscle fibers during depolarization and repolarization. The '**P wave**' represents depolarization of the atria. The '**P-R interval**' represents electrical transmission from the atria to the ventricles. The '**QRS complex**' represents depolarization of the ventricles. The repolarization of the atria produces a small wave that is usually obscured by the QRS complex. The '**R wave**' represents the 'heart beat' and is used to determine heart rate. The '**T wave**' represents repolarization of the ventricles. The time from the start of the QRS interval to the start of the T wave represents systole. The time from the end of the T wave to the start of the QRS interval represents diastole.

Bibliography

Rothe, C. (2003). Toward consistent definitions for preload and afterload – revisited. *Advances in Physiology Education* 27, 44-45.

Norton, J.M. (2001). Toward consistent definitions for preload and afterload. *Advances in Physiology* 25, 53-61.

Norton, J.M. (2003). Toward consistent definitions for preload and afterload – revisited. *Advances in Physiology Education* 27, 89-90.

CARDIAC EMERGENCIES There are two general types of cardiac emergencies: myocardial infarction (heart attack) and cardiac arrest. Most people who die of heart attacks do so within 2 hours after the first signs appear. Many lives are lost because people deny they are having a heart attack and delay calling for help. *See* CARDIO-PULMONARY RESUSCITATION.

CARDIAC HYPERTROPHY An increase in the size of the heart. '**Athlete's heart**' is a benign condition consisting of physiological adaptations to the increased cardiac workload of exercise. Its primary features are hypertrophy of both ventricles, and bradycardia associated with normal systolic and diastolic function. High blood pressure puts a pressure load on the ventricles, which leads to a thickening of the ventricular walls. The blood leaving the left ventricle must overcome the large pressure and resistance in the aorta, hence the left ventricle contracts with more force than the muscles of the other chambers. Consequently, the left ventricle hypertrophies more. Athletes with the most substantial wall thickening are rowers, canoeists and cyclists who are competitive at elite levels for a substantial period of time. Twin studies suggest that hereditary factors may be important determinants of cardiac dimensions and/or the degree of cardiac adaptability to exercise training.

Isotonic (dynamic) exercise, such as running, places a volume load on the myocardium. Isotonic exercise increases venous return, and thus left ventricular end-diastolic diameter, allowing for a larger stroke volume and cardiac output. In response to a chronic volume demand, the left ventricular wall thickens proportionately in order to normalize wall stress. Changes occur according to **Laplace's law**: Wall stress = (pressure x radius)/(wall thickness x 2). The myocardium hypertrophies in an eccentric fashion such that the mass-to-volume ratio remains unchanged.

Isometric (static) exercise, such as weightlifting, places a pressure load on the myocardium by brief increases in systemic blood pressure during training. Wall thickness increases in response to a chronic pressure demand in accordance with Laplace's law. Without an increase in left ventricular end-diastolic diameter, the myocardium hypertrophies in a concentric fashion such that the mass-to-volume ratio increases. Haykowsky et al. (2002) propose that when left ventricle geometry is altered after resistance training, the pattern is usually concentric hypertrophy in Olympic weightlifters. However, the pattern of eccentric hypertrophy (increased left ventricular mass secondary to an increase in diastolic internal cavity dimension and wall thickness) is not uncommon in bodybuilders. Nearly 40% of all resistance-training athletes have normal left ventricle geometry, and these athletes are typically powerlifters. Resistance training athletes who use anabolic steroids have been shown to have significantly higher left ventricle mass compared with drug-free sport-matched athletes. Sport involves a combination of both isotonic and isometric exercises, and cardiac adaptations are usually a blend of eccentric and concentric hypertrophy. The resultant overall increase in cardiac mass is due to an increase in left ventricular diastolic cavity dimension, wall thickness, or both.

A close examination of animal studies and echocardiographic research has called into question the validity of exercise-induced cardiac hypertrophy. There is doubt as to whether observed differences in left ventricular wall thickness and end diastolic diameter exceed the technical resolution (approximately 2.2 mm) of echocardiography. For example, a comparison of 1000 athletes to 800 sedentary individuals found an average difference of 1.6 mm in left ventricular wall thickness. Perrault and Turcotte (1994) argue that it is likely that increased diastolic filling, rather than eccentric hypertrophy, explains the differences reported. Furthermore, the differences in left ventricular wall thickness between athletes and their sedentary counterparts are actually eliminated when a correction for body surface area is introduced. Illegal drug supplementation may also contribute to the cross-sectional differences reported. *See also* SUDDEN DEATH.

Bibliography

George, K.P., Wolfe, L.A. and Burggraf, G.W. (1990). The 'athletic heart syndrome:' A critical review. *Sports Medicine* 11(5), 300-330.

Hart, G. (2003). Exercise-induced cardiac hypertrophy: A substrate for sudden death in athletes. *Experimental Physiology* 88(5), 639-644.

Haykowsky, M.J. et al. (2002). Resistance training and cardiac hypertrophy: Unravelling the training effect. *Sports Medicine* 32(13), 837-849.

Maron, B.J. (1997). Hypertrophic cardiomyopathy. *Lancet* 350(9071), 127-133.

Pedoe, D. (1984). The way to an athlete's heart. *New Scientist*, 2nd August, 32-33.

Perrault, H. and Turcotte, R.A. (1994). Exercise-induced cardiac hypertrophy. Fact or fallacy? *Sports Medicine* 17(5), 288-308.

Urhausen, A. and Kindermann, W. (1992). Echocardiographic findings in strength- and endurance-trained athletes. *Sports Medicine* 13 (4), 270-284.

CARDIAC MUSCLE Myocardium. It is the heart muscle. *See under* CARDIAC CYCLE.

CARDIAC OUTPUT The amount of oxygenated blood that is pumped into the circulatory system from one ventricle per minute. It is usually measured from the left ventricle. Cardiac output is equal to stroke volume multiplied by heart rate. At rest, cardiac output is usually in the range of 4.5 to 5.5 L/min. At maximal exercise, it may increase to 20 to 30 L/min.

An improvement in cardiac output from training comes about through an increase in stroke volume. It seems that the trained individual achieves an increase in stroke volume due to a larger diastolic volume of the left ventricle and a slightly larger total heart size. The **Fick principle** states that the cardiac output equals the amount of oxygen absorbed from the lungs, divided by the arterial-mixed venous oxygen difference.

A linear relationship between cardiac output and oxygen uptake has been shown. The relationship between cardiac output and exercise intensity is also linear through a wide range of exercise intensities. Endurance training results in a significant rightward shift of this line due to improvements in stroke volume, thus heart rate becomes decreased at any submaximal exercise level.

Decreased heart rate at rest and during submaximal exercise is due to increased parasympathetic influence, decreased sympathetic influence, and lower intrinsic heart rate. Increased stroke volume is due to decreased heart rate (rest and submaximal exercise), increased blood volume, increased heart size and volume, increased cardiac contractility, increased ventricular compliance, and increased ventricular filling pressure. *See also under* GROWTH.

CARDIAC REGULATION There are two main types of regulation of heart function: chronotropic and inotropic. **Chronotropic regulation** affects heart rate. **Inotropic regulation** affects the velocity of myocardial contraction (contractility). Increased contractility results from the sympathetic neural and hormonal stimulation of the ventricular myocardium. The start of exercise stimulates both chronotropic and inotropic regulation. This causes an increased heart rate and improved abilities of the heart to function as a pump.

CARDIAC SPHINCTER   *See under* VOMITING.

CARDIAC SYNDROME X   Microvascular angina. A clinical condition defined by the presence of angina-like chest pain, often with signs of cardiac ischemia, a positive response to stress testing, and absence of coronary artery disease. It has been shown to occur in 20 to 30% of angina patients undergoing coronary arteriography. Patients with cardiac syndrome X are much less likely to develop a heart attack than those with narrowing of the major coronary arteries.

The prevalence of cardiac syndrome X is higher in women, especially peri- and postmenopausal women. It has therefore been hypothesized that estrogen deficiency may play a major role in the pathogenesis of cardiac syndrome X. Estrogen vasoactive properties involve endothelium-dependent effects.

The cause is not known, but one theory is that it is caused by a poorly-defined disorder of arteries in the cardiac muscle that are too small to be seen during catheterization. Another theory suggests a certain 'hypersensitivity' to cardiac pain.

There is some evidence that persons with cardiac syndrome X, as with those with metabolic syndrome X, have lipid abnormalities, and thus the two syndromes may be the same.

See METABOLIC SYNDROME X.

Bibliography

Kaski, J.C. (2002). Overview of gender aspects of cardiac syndrome X. *Cardiovascular Research* 53(3), 620-626.

CARDINAL SYMPTOMS   The primary or major symptoms of diagnostic importance.

CARDIOPULMONARY   RESUSCITATION
CPR. A set of procedures used on a person who is not breathing and shows no movement (coughing or response to breaths). It involves a combination of chest compressions and rescue breathing. If the victim is not breathing, the rescuer tilts the head back, pinches the nose, and gives 2 slow rescue breaths. Each breath should make the chest clearly rise.

Early CPR helps circulate blood that contains oxygen to the vital organs until an automatic external defibrillator is ready to use or emergency personnel arrive. Most victims of sudden cardiac arrest need defibrillation. A person in cardiac arrest is already clinically dead. If CPR is started within 4 minutes of collapse, and defibrillation provided within 10 minutes, a person has a 40% chance of survival. In approximately two-thirds of sudden cardiac arrest cases, the heart goes from a normal heartbeat to ventricular fibrillation. Ventricular fibrillation is fatal unless an electric shock (defibrillation) can be given. CPR does not stop ventricular fibrillation, but it does extend the window of time in which defibrillation can be effective.

The American Heart Association recommends the following procedures to determine the correct hand position for cardiac compression. Trace along the lower border of the rib cage with the middle and index fingers up to the xiphoid notch. The middle finger should be placed in the notch and the index finger next to it, in order to avoid placing any direct compressive force on the xiphoid process. The heel of the opposite hand should be positioned next to the index finger on the body of the sternum. Once the hand is positioned, the heel of the other hand is placed on top of it. The rescuer should compress the chest vertically with the fingers interlaced.

The rescuer compresses the patient's chest 15 times in about 10 seconds, and then gives 2 slow breaths. The rescuer does 3 more sets of 15 compressions and 2 breaths, rechecking breathing and movement. If there is no movement, the rescuer continues with sets of 15 compressions and 2 breaths until the ambulance arrives.

CPR for children (ages 1 to 8 years) is similar to performing quick CPR for adults, but there are 4 differences: (i) if the rescuer is alone with the child, one minute of CPR is given before calling 911; (ii) the heel of one hand is used for chest compressions; (iii) the sternum is pressed down 1 to 1.5 inches; and

(iv) one full breath is given, followed by 5 chest compressions. When a child's heart stops, it is usually the result of a breathing emergency. After giving 2 slow rescue breaths, chest compression should be made 5 times in about 3 seconds. Then one slow breath is given. Sets of 5 compressions and one breath are continued for about a minute, after which breathing and movement is checked for again. If there is no movement, sets of 5 compressions and one breath are continued until the ambulance arrives.

With an infant, chest compression is made with two fingers positioned in the center of the chest over the sternum, with the hand vertically aligned above the fingers. The chest is compressed 5 times in slightly less than 3 seconds. The infant's head is tilted back, with the mouth and nose covered by the rescuer's mouth, and one slow breath is given. Sets of 5 compressions and one breath are given for about a minute. If there is no movement, sets of 5 compressions and one breath are continued until the ambulance arrives.

Chronology

•1992 • In the USA, The Occupational Safety and Health Administrators mandated the use of barrier devices to protect the coach from transmission of blood-borne pathogens during CPR.

Bibliography

American Heart Association. Http://www.americanheart.org

American Red Cross First Aid/CPR/AED Program Participant's Booklet.

American Red Cross. Http://www.redcross.org

Eisenberg, M. Http://depts.washington.edu/learncpr/index.html

CARDIOVASCULAR Of the heart and circulatory system.

CARDIOVASCULAR CONTROL There are three cardiovascular centers located within the medulla oblongata of the brain stem. The **cardioaccelerator center** sends signals via sympathetic accelerator nerves, leading to increased heart rate and force of contraction. The **cardioinhibitor center**, also known as the **vagal nucleus**, sends signals via the vagus nerve that

results in decreased heart rate. The **vasomotor center** innervates the smooth muscles of the arterioles via sympathetic nerves. The arterioles that supply skeletal muscles vasodilate when stimulated, whereas the arterioles in visceral beds constrict under sympathetic influence.

The cardiovascular centers are influenced by several higher brain centers, including the cerebral cortex and hypothalamus. Emotional influences arising from the cerebral cortex can affect cardiovascular function at rest. Input from the motor cortex which is relayed via the hypothalamus, can influence cardiovascular function during exercise. This leads to increased heart rate and vasodilation in active muscle.

Body temperature affects the cardiovascular centers via the hypothalamus. Increased body temperature leads to increased heart rate, increased cardiac output, and vasodilation in the arterioles of the active muscle and skin.

CARDIOVASCULAR DISEASE The generic term for more than twenty different diseases of the heart and its vessels. This is the most common cause of death in the adult population of the Western world.

Coronary (ischemic) heart disease is a malfunction of the heart caused by occlusion of the two arteries that arise from the aorta and supply the heart muscle. It can cause angina pectoris, cardiac arrhythmias, myocardial infarction (heart attack), heart failure and sudden death.

The most common cause of coronary heart disease is **atherosclerosis**, which is the accumulation of lipid deposits, such as cholesterol and fat, on the walls of arteries. These fatty plaques can lead to a narrowing of arteries (and therefore ischemia) or can encourage the formation of a thrombus (blood clot). A blood clot in a narrowed artery is the immediate cause of a heart attack. **Embolism** is the plugging of a small blood vessel (such as an arteriole) by material that has been carried through the larger vessels by the blood stream. Atherosclerosis is a form of arteriosclerosis. **Arteriosclerosis** refers to the many conditions in which the arteries become thickened, hard and less elastic.

Coronary heart disease appears to begin with injury to endothelial cells, which may result from multiple causes, such as: tobacco smoke and other chemical irritants from tobacco; hypertension and the resultant turbulent blood flow and increased shear stress; hypercholesterolemia; glycated substances resulting from diabetes mellitus; vasoconstrictor substances; immune complexes; homocysteine; and viral or bacterial infection. Pathogenesis may progress as follows: injury to the endothelial cell wall of the coronary artery; fibroblastic proliferation of the inner lining (intima) of the artery; further obstruction of blood flow as lipid accumulates at the junction of the arterial intima and middle lining; cellular degeneration and subsequent formation of hyaline within the arterial intima; and calcium deposition at the edges of the hyalinated area. Platelets adhere to the injured endothelium (platelet aggregation), form small blood clots (mural thrombi), and release growth factors and vasoactive substances, such as thromboxane A2, which is a potent vasoconstrictor that may cause additional vascular injury. Monocytes from the blood may adhere to the endothelium, migrate into the intima, accumulate cholesterol, and be transformed into macrophages. Growth factors, such as platelet-derived growth factor, enhance monocyte binding to the endothelium and increase the number of LDL receptors, inducing greater LDL binding and increased deposition of cholesterol in the arterial wall and in the macrophages. As the plaque ages, an increasing amount of fibrous tissue accumulates. This may lead to the formation of a fibrous cap, which may rupture and cause a myocardial infarction.

Nearly 50% of 13.5 million cases of coronary heart disease in the USA can be accounted for by the atherosclerosis susceptibility gene, which appears on chromosome 19 (near the gene that regulates the receptor that removes LDL cholesterol from the blood). This gene apparently expresses a set of characteristics (abdominal obesity, low levels of HDL cholesterol and high levels of LDL cholesterol) that triple a person's risk of myocardial infarctions.

There is a correlation between elevated levels of plasma lipids and increased incidence of coronary artery disease. It is not known whether the correlation implies causation, nor if decreasing the level of lipids decreases the risk.

Women tend to lag 5 to 20 years behind men in the extent and severity of coronary atherosclerosis. This appears to be related to estrogen, since postmenopausal women have an accelerated course of coronary artery disease.

Persons without risk factors are much less likely to develop coronary artery disease than those who do have risk factors. Cigarette smoking is the most important of the known modifiable risk factors for cardiovascular disease. Tobacco smoke exerts a number of atherogenic effects: endothelial damage; increased platelet adhesion to the injured endothelium; increased release of platelet-derived growth factor; carbon monoxide-induced arterial wall hypoxia and proinflammatory state; promotion of LDL oxidation; increased blood catecholamine concentrations via sympathetic nervous system stimulation; decreased blood HDL cholesterol concentration; increased thrombogenicity; increased fibrinogen levels; increased whole body viscosity (secondary to polycythemia); and impaired endothelial-mediated vasodilation.

In 1992, the American Heart Association added physical inactivity (lack of regular exercise) to the list of major risk factors for the development of coronary heart disease. Other risk factors implicated in atherogenesis include hypercholesterolemia, hypertension, diabetes, obesity, increased platelet aggregation, increased levels of fibrinogen, and decreased levels of clotting factors.

There are various techniques used to treat coronary heart disease. **Percutaneous transluminal coronary angioplasty** involves inserting a catheter into a groin artery and threading it up to the blocked coronary artery. The balloon is then inflated several times, compressing the plaque against the arterial wall. **Coronary stents** – flexible, stainless steel tubes that are permanently implanted in a coronary artery to keep it propped open – are used in conjunction with angioplasty. **Coronary artery bypass surgery** involves a segment of a blood vessel from another part of the body (e.g. the saphenous vein in the leg) being used as a graft. **Atherectomy** involves either a rotating blade or drill being used to shave plaque off the artery wall. **Laser ablation** uses laser light emitted from the tip of a catheter in order to heat a probe that burns plaque away from the artery wall.

The American College of Sports Medicine has concluded that most patients with coronary artery disease should engage in individually designed exercise programs to achieve optimal physical and emotional health. *See also* ASPIRIN; HEART MURMUR; PERIPHERAL ARTERY DISEASE; STROKE.

Chronology

•1953 • In "Coronary Heart Disease and Physical Activity of Work," published in *The Lancet*, Jeremy N. Morris compared the amount of severity of coronary heart disease in London bus drivers and bus conductors. It was observed that the more sedentary drivers had more coronary heart disease than the more active conductors, and it was concluded that physical activity offers protection from coronary heart disease. Three years later Morris published further research, which reported that the conductors and drivers were dissimilar people from the outset: the bus drivers were fatter, with higher cholesterol levels and higher blood pressure.

•1977 • Jim Fixx published *The Complete Book of Running*, which focused on the physical and psychological benefits of running. It was translated into 14 languages and had sold nearly a million hardback copies by 1996. In 1984, Fixx, aged 52, was discovered dead from a heart attack beside the road. His father had died of a heart attack at 43. Until his mid-thirties, Fixx was a heavy smoker, overweight and had a high-stress executive job. At the age of 35, Fix started running. The permanent effects of these cardiovascular disease risk factors were confirmed by an autopsy showing that his left circumflex coronary artery was 99% occluded. Scar tissue indicated that three other heart attacks had occurred within 2 months of his death. Ironically, six months before his death, Fixx had been invited by Dr Kenneth Cooper to undergo a stress test. He declined the invitation.

•1987 • In the USA, the Centers for Disease Control and Prevention (CDCP) classified physical inactivity as a major cardiovascular risk factor. It presented a similar risk to cigarette smoking, hypertension, obesity, and dyslipidemia.

•1998 • The American Heart Association (AHA) added obesity to its list of primary risk factors for cardiovascular disease that already included cigarette smoking, hypertension, hypercholesterolemia and physical inactivity.

Bibliography

American College of Sports Medicine (2000). *ACSM's guidelines for exercise testing and prescription.* 6th ed. Philadelphia, PA: Lippincott Williams and Wilkins.

Heyden, S. and Fodor, G.J. (1988). Does regular exercise prolong life expectancy? *Sports Medicine* 6, 63-71.

Leon, A.S. (1997, ed). *Physical activity and cardiovascular health. A national consensus.* Champaign, IL: Human Kinetics.

Solomon, H.A. (1984). *The exercise myth.* Orlando, FL: Harcourt Brace Jovanovich.

CARDIOVASCULAR DRIFT The increase in heart rate and decrease in stroke volume that occurs during prolonged exercise. Cardiovascular drift is more pronounced during exercise in heat stress. Coyle and Gonzalez-Alonso (2001) propose that cardiovascular drift is due to increased heart rate, rather than a progressive increase in cutaneous blood flow as body temperature rises.

Bibliography

Coyle, E.F. and Gonzalez-Alonso, J. (2001). Cardiovascular drift during prolonged exercise: New perspectives. *Exercise and Sport Sciences Reviews* 29(2), 88-92.

CARDIOVASCULAR SYSTEM *See under* CARDIAC CYCLE.

CARNITINE A coenzyme that transports long-chain fatty acids into the mitochondria for beta oxidation. Carnitine combines with fatty acyl-coenzyme A (acyl-CoA) in the cytoplasm, allowing fatty acid to enter the mitochondrion. This step is catalyzed by carnitine palmitoyl transferase 1 and the trans-membrane transport is facilitated by acylcarnitine transferase. Within the mitochondrion, the action of carnitine palmitoyl transferase 2 regenerates free carnitine and the fatty acyl-CoA is released for entry into the beta-oxidation pathway. Carnitine also modulates the metabolism of coenzyme A and contributes to ketogenesis.

Carnitine is not an essential dietary nutrient, because it may be formed in the liver and kidney from other nutrients (mainly lysine and methionine). Severe carnitine deficiency disrupts lipid and protein metabolism, but most individuals consume sufficient carnitine in the daily diet. Rich sources of L-carnitine are meat, poultry, fish and dairy products. About 90% of total carnitine is located in muscle. During exercise, there is a redistribution of carnitine in muscle, but there is no loss of total carnitine. Carnitine supplementation neither enhances fatty acid oxidation, nor spares glycogen or postpones fatigue during exercise. There is currently no scientific basis for healthy individuals or athletes to use carnitine supplementation in order to improve performance. Many nutritional supplements contain D-carnitine, which is physiologically inactive in humans but may cause significant muscle weakness through mechanisms that deplete L-carnitine in tissues.

Carnitine deficiency is a metabolic state in which carnitine concentrations in plasma and tissues are less than the levels required for normal function of the body. It is a slowly progressive disorder, which causes cardiac disease and skeletal muscle weakness. It is inherited as an autosomal recessive trait. Muscle carnitine deficiency is characterized by depletion of carnitine levels in muscle with normal serum concentrations. Evidence suggests that this is caused by a defect in the muscle carnitine transporter. Carnitine deficiency may occur secondary to other metabolic disease (**secondary carnitine deficiency**), or in response to a mutation of the gene in the protein responsible for bringing carnitine into the cell (**primary carnitine deficiency**). Progression of the disease varies and carnitine supplementation is often effective.

Carnitine palmitoyl transferase deficiency is a disorder that causes muscle pain, stiffness and tenderness. There are two forms: hepatic (attributable to deficiency of carnitine palmitoyl transferase I) and muscle (attribute to deficiency of carnitine palmitoyl transferase II). It is inherited as an autosomal recessive trait. Symptoms are usually brought on by prolonged and intense exercise, especially in combination with fasting, but may not appear until several hours after activity ceases. Short periods of exercise do not usually provoke symptoms. Symptoms may also be provoked by illness, cold, stress or menstruation. Breakdown of muscle tissue during an attack can cause myoglobinuria. *See* AEROBIC ENERGY SYSTEMS.

Bibliography

Armsey, T.D. and Green, G.A. (1997). Nutrition supplements: Science vs. hype. *The Physician and Sportsmedicine* 25(6), 76-92.

Clarkson, P.M. (1996). Nutrition for improved sports performance. Current issues on ergogenic aids. *Sports Medicine* 21(6), 393-401.

Heinonen, O.J. (1996). Carnitine and physical exercise. *Sports Medicine* 22(2), 109-132.

Scaglia, F. (2004). Carnitine deficiency. Http://www.emedicine.com

CARNOSINE A dipeptide found in muscle, brain and other innervated animal and human tissues. It is formed by a process involving the enzyme carnosine-synthetase that bonds the amino acids alanine and histidine. Carnosine is a water soluble antioxidant, acting to prevent lipid peroxidation within the cell membrane.

Bibliography

Stuerenburg, H.J. (2000). The roles of carnosine in aging of skeletal muscle and in neuromuscular diseases. *Biochemistry* (Moscow) 65(7), 862-865.

CAROTENOIDS *See under* VITAMIN A.

CAROTID ARTERY The main artery supplying blood to the head from the heart. There is one on each side of the neck.

CAROTID BODY A structure containing sensory nerve endings that respond to the oxygen and carbon dioxide content of the blood. As a result, there are reflex changes in respiration.

CAROTID SINUS A widening of the carotid artery where it divides into internal and external branches. It contains carotid bodies.

CAROTID SINUS REFLEX Pressure on, or in, the carotid artery at the level of its bifurcation causing reflex slowing of the heart rate.

CARPAL BONES *See under* INTERCARPAL JOINTS.

CARPAL TUNNEL SYNDROME   Compression of the median nerve, most commonly as it passes through the carpal tunnel, in conjunction with the 9 flexor tendons of the wrist and fingers. The carpal tunnel is formed, anteriorly, by the volar (or transverse) carpal ligament (flexor retinaculum) and, posteriorly, by the carpal bones. Any process that increases pressure within the carpal tunnel leads to compressive force on the median nerve and subsequent symptoms of carpal tunnel syndrome. Acute carpal tunnel syndrome may involve compression by an invasive structure, such as intrusion of a fractured or dislocated bone, or compression from a ganglion cyst. A **wrist ganglion cyst** is a benign cyst formed by a concentration of synovial fluid just below the skin, usually just forward of the wrist crease on the top of the hand. 70% of wrist ganglion cysts occur between the second and fourth decades of life. Chronic carpal tunnel syndrome is most often associated with inflammation and subsequent swelling of the synovial sheaths that surround the flexor tendons. Carpal tunnel syndrome is the most common nerve entrapment, but occurs more commonly in the work setting than in sport. In tennis and baseball, it occurs as a result of repetitive wrist flexion/extension. It also occurs in athletes applying excessive pressure over the palmar aspect of the hand, such as during gripping a racquet.

CARPO-METACARPAL JOINT   Trapeziometa-carpal joint. The articulation of the metacarpal bone of the thumb with the trapezium bone of the carpals. It is a saddle joint.
   See HAND.

CAREER TERMINATION   Retirement from sport can be viewed as career transition. A study of Canadian Olympians found that most had experienced difficulty in the transition from being an international athlete to being an ordinary citizen. Factors involved in this transition included: an alternative to sports participation allowing redirection of energy; facilitation of transition through the feeling that goals had been reached; positive/negative effects of relationship with coaches; negative transition experiences associated with premature career termination due to injury; the negative effect of Canada deciding not to participate in the 1980 Olympics; financial problems leading to retirement and negative emotions; and the positive effect of social support. Werthner and Orlick (1986) found that 64% of the former Olympic athletes they studied felt they had little sense of personal control over their lives during their sport careers.

Most elite, female gymnasts are involved in intensive training (usually 20 to 30 hours per week) by the age of 8 or 9 years, and retire from gymnastics between the ages of 15 and 19. The fact that these gymnasts are children and adolescents during most of their athletic careers may affect the nature of the sport experience, and therefore retirement. Gymnasts who had dictator-like coaches, who yelled at them, disempowering and controlling them, were angry over what they had endured. The gymnasts' retirement experiences were marked by a pursuit or, in some cases, a struggle for identity. The preoccupation with appearance and weight in gymnastics left them feeling dissatisfied with their bodies and struggling with these issues. Kerr and Dacyshyn (2000) argue that participation in elite gymnastics may have the effect of postponing identity formation.

Bibliography

Kerr, G. and Dacyshyn, A. (2000). The retirement experiences of elite, female gymnasts. *Journal of Applied Sport Psychology* 12, 115-133.

Lavallee, D. and Wylleman, P. (2000, eds). *Career transitions in sport: International perspectives.* Morgantown, WV: Fitness Information Technology.

Ogilvie, B. and Taylor, J. (1993). Career termination issues among elite athletes. In Singer, R., Murphey, M. and Tennant, L.K. (eds). *Handbook of research on sport psychology.* pp761-775. New York: MacMillan.

Petipas, A. et al. (1997). *Athlete's guide to career planning.* Champaign, IL: Human Kinetics.

Werthner, P. and Orlick, T. (1986). Retirement experiences of successful Olympic athletes. *International Journal of Sport Psychology* 17, 337-363.

Wykeman, P. et al. (1999, eds). *Career transitions in competitive sports.* Biel, Switzerland: European Federation of Sport Psychology Monograph Series.

CARRIER   i) A substance that can pick up a group of atoms and transfer it to another compound. Examples include ATP, which carries activated phosphoryl groups, and $FADH_2$ that carry electrons (hydrogens). **ii)** A heterozygote for a recessive allele.

CARRYING ANGLE   *See under* ELBOW JOINT COMPLEX.

CARTESIAN COORDINATE SYSTEM A system whereby a point can be located in space by three coordinates, usually denoted by (x, y, z), which expresses the perpendicular distance of the point along the respective axis from an origin. The three axes are mutually perpendicular. The system is said to be right-handed if a rotation from x to y is clockwise and in the direction of positive z. A two-dimensional Cartesian coordinate system involves mutually perpendicular x- and y-axes. *See also* POLAR COORDINATE SYSTEM.

CARTILAGE A type of connective tissue found in various parts of the body that contains no blood vessels. It is a firm, but flexible tissue, which consists of a dense network of collagen and elastin fibers embedded in a ground substance (chondroitin sulfate). The collagen gives cartilage its strength, while the chondroitin sulfate gives cartilage resilience. Cartilage is avascular and has no nerves. Based on structure, there are three main forms of cartilage: hyaline cartilage, white fibrocartilage and yellow fibrocartilage.

Hyaline cartilage is elastic and makes up articular, costal and temporary cartilages. **Articular cartilage** is found on the joint surfaces of bone and its smoothness allows free movement of the bone. Articular cartilage is a viscoelastic material. **Costal cartilage** is found between the ribs, and between the ribs and the sternum. **Temporary cartilage** is found in early life before it is converted to bone.

White fibrocartilage is flexible, tough and elastic. It makes up interarticular, connecting, circumferential and stratiform fibrocartilages. **Interarticular fibrocartilage** forms menisci that are flattened plates found between the articular cartilages of certain joints. These assist in spreading

synovial fluid over load-bearing joint surfaces and increase the variety of movements at a joint. **Connecting fibrocartilages** are discs found between articular surfaces of joints that permit only limited movement and act as shock absorbers. **Circumferential fibrocartilages** surround some of the articular cavities and serve to deepen the articular surface, in order to protect its edges. **Stratiform fibrocartilages** form a thin coating on osseous grooves through which the tendons of some muscles glide and are also found in the tendons of some muscles where they glide over bones.

Yellow (elastic) fibrocartilage is found in the auricle of the outer ear, the eustachian tubes, the cornicula laryngitis and the epiglottis. It maintains the shape of structures while allowing elasticity.

Cartilage may be subject to creep. A constant compressive load causes extracellular fluid to exude from the matrix, and eventually an equilibrium compressive strain is reached. If the compressive load is released, the fluid is drawn into the matrix by the hydrophilic proteoglycans. The cylical loading and unloading of cartilage allows for a fluid flux (with accompanying nutrients and waste products) into and out of the cartilage. When cartilage is replete with water, it is easier to compress, but when densely packed with glycosaminoglycans, it is more compression resistant. *See also* CHONDRO-MALACIA.

CASCADE A series of enzyme activations serving to amplify a weak chemical signal.

CATALASE *See under* FREE RADICALS.

CATARACT Clouded or opaque spots on the lens of the eye that gradually increase in size and diminish vision, particularly in low-light conditions. Cataracts are the most common cause of blindness worldwide. Cataracts can be treated by **phakoemulsification**, which involves replacing the cloudy crystalline lens with a new clear plastic lens. Following cataract surgery, long distance vision is generally quite good, but reading glasses will be required.

CATASTROPHIC INJURY The National Center

for Catastrophic Sport Injury in the USA defines a catastrophic injury as either nonfatal (resulting in permanent severe functional brain or spinal cord disability) or serious (involving transient brain or spinal cord disability). Fatalities are either direct (resulting directly from performing the specific activities of a sport) or indirect (caused by systemic failure as a result of exertion while participating in a sport).

The prohibition of 'spearing' in American football, and the rules regarding water depth and the racing dive in swimming, are examples of how data on fatalities and catastrophic injuries can be used to help promote the safety of athletes. In swimming, catastrophic injuries occurred when swimmers struck their head on the pool bottom while doing a racing dive in the shallow end. As a consequence, safety rules regarding water depth were introduced in the early 1990s.

Between 1979 and 1999, 18 children died and 14 were seriously injured in the USA when movable soccer goals fell on them, according to the Consumer Product Safety Commission (CPSC). Safety measures include anchoring the goals, warning players to avoid climbing on them and using proper moving, maintenance, and storage techniques.

There were 88 baseball-related deaths to children in the age range of 5 to 15 years between the years 1973 and 1995 (CPSC). Of these, 43% were from commotio cordis; 24% were from direct-ball contact with the head; 15% were from impacts from bats; 10% were from direct contact with a ball impacting the neck, ears or throat; and in 8%, the mechanism of injury was unknown. Preventive measures to protect young players from direct ball contact include: the use of batting helmets and face protectors while at bat and on base; the use of special equipment for the catcher (helmet, mask, chest and neck protectors); the elimination of the on-deck circle; and protective screening of dugouts and benches.

From 1983 to 1997, high-school track and field resulted in 16 direct fatalities and 23 catastrophic injuries. The pole vault was associated with 13 of the direct fatalities in which the athlete bounced or landed out of the pit. Since 1987, the pole vault

landing area must include a common cover or pad extending over the whole of the pit. From 1983 to 1997, there were 10 direct fatalities or catastrophic injuries in high-school athletes as a result of being struck by a thrown discus, shot put or javelin.

From 1982 through 1997, 60 direct fatalities and catastrophic injuries and 25 indirect fatalities occurred among high school and college female athletes, including cheerleaders. Cheerleading accounted for 34 (57%) of the direct fatalities and catastrophic injuries. A major factor in these injuries was the change in cheerleading activity, which now involves gymnastic-type stunts such as front and back flips. Many state high-school associations have responded to these changes and the increase in injuries by banning stunts such as pyramid building.

Each year in the USA snowmobile accidents produce approximately 200 deaths and 14,000 injuries. Excess speed, alcohol, driver inexperience and poor judgment are the leading causes of accidents. Similar to motor vehicle accidents, multi-system trauma occurs frequently with head injury being the leading cause of death. Head injuries remain the leading cause of mortality and serious morbidity, arising largely from snowmobiles colliding, falling, or overturning during operation. Most deaths and serious injuries occurred as a result of the operators striking fixed objects, such as a tree. Children younger than 16 years were injured or killed when they fell from their snowmobiles, had the vehicle roll over them, or crashed the snowmobile into other snowmobiles, vehicles or stationary objects. Children are also injured while being towed in a variety of conveyances by snowmobiles. Other problems associated with snowmobile operation that were reported in the literature include hearing loss from prolonged exposure to excess engine noise and white finger syndrome arising from the effects of cold weather and hand/arm vibration from the handlebars of the snowmobiles.

Of a total of 36 persons who died while skating between 1992 and 1998 in the USA, 31 had collided with a motor vehicle. Several deaths have been caused by 'skitching' or 'truck surfing,' which refers to skating behind or alongside a vehicle while the skater holds onto the vehicle. This enables the skater to travel at the same velocity as the vehicle. It can be very dangerous, however, because the skater cannot slow down fast enough to prevent colliding with the vehicle or being thrown into oncoming traffic or the roadbed if the vehicle suddenly slows, stops or turns. The design of the skates should match the ability of the skater, with five-wheeled, extremely low-friction skates being reserved for competitive or long-distance skaters. Full protective gear needs to be used at all times, including a helmet, wrist guards, knee pads, and elbow pads. In some states, such as Oregon, it is mandatory by law for children and adolescents to wear helmets. The helmet should be certified by the American National Standards Institute, the American Society for Testing and Materials, the Snell Memorial Foundation or the Consumer Product Safety Commission. Skaters performing tricks need special protective gear.

Between 1990 and 1999, the Consumer Product Safety Commission received reports of 6 deaths involving trampolines. Victims range in age from 3 years to 21 years, although the 21-year-old died six years after being injured on a trampoline. Most deaths occurred when victims fell from the trampolines, and most involved the cervical spinal cord. In 1996, an estimated 83,400 trampoline-related injuries occurred in the USA. Most injuries were sustained on home trampolines. Many trampoline injuries occur when there are simultaneous multiple users. Some vendors offer cage-like net structures to surround trampolines for safety. This false sense of security often leads to participants doing activities beyond their capabilities and can lead to even greater risk. The mini tramp, while different in nature and purpose from the trampoline, shares its association with risk of injury, especially spinal cord injury, most notably from poorly executed somersaults. The American Academy of Pediatrics (1999) recommends that trampolines should never used in the home environment, in routine physical education classes, or in outdoor playgrounds. Design and behavioral recommendations are made for the limited use of trampolines in supervised training programs. A safety pad should cover all portions of the steel frame

and springs. The surface around the trampoline should have an impact-absorbing safety surface material. The condition of the trampoline should be regularly checked for tears, rust and detachments. Safety harnesses and spotting belts, when appropriately used, may offer added protection for athletes learning or practicing more challenging skills on the trampoline. Setting the trampoline in a pit so that the mat is at ground level should be considered. Ladders may provide unintended access to the trampoline by small children and should not be used. Even in supervised training programs, the use of trampolines for children younger than the age of 6 years should be prohibited. *See also* HEAD INJURIES.

Bibliography

American Academy of Pediatrics (1998). In-line skating injuries in children and adolescents. *Pediatrics* 101(4), 720-722.

American Academy of Pediatrics (1999). Trampolines at home, school, and recreational centers. *Pediatrics* 103(5), 1053-1056.

American Academy of Pediatrics (2000). Snowmobiling hazards. *Pediatrics* 106(5), 1142-1144.

American Academy of Pediatrics (2001). Injuries in youth soccer. A subject review. *Pediatrics* 105(3), 659-661.

American Academy of Pediatrics (2001). Risk of injury from baseball and softball in children. *Pediatrics* 107(4), 782-784.

American Sports Data, Inc. (1996). *American Sports Analysis: Summary Report*. Hartsdale, NY: American Sports Data, Inc.

Cantu, R.C. and Mueller, F.O. (1999). Fatalities and catastrophic injuries in high school and college sports, 1982-1997. *The Physician and Sportsmedicine* 27(8), 35-48.

National Association for Sport and Physical Education (2002). *The use of trampolines and mini tramps in physical education*. A position paper of the Middle and Secondary School Physical Education Council and the National Association for Sport and Physical Education. Reston, Virginia.

Pierz, J.J. (2003). Snowmobile injuries in North America. *Clinical Orthopaedics and Related Research* 409, 29-36.

CATCHING Receiving force from an object with the hands. Motor milestones in catching are: chasing a ball, but not responding to an aerial ball (2 to 3 years); responding to an aerial ball with delayed arm movements (2 to 3 years); needing to be told how to position the arms (3 to 4 years); turning the head away as a fear reaction (3 to 4 years); using the body to make a basket catch (3 years); and using the hands only to catch a small ball (5 years).

Fielders in cricket do not run to catch a ball at the place where the ball will fall and wait for it. Rather, they run at speeds that take them through the point where the ball will fall at the exact time it arrives. If the flight duration is lengthened, by increasing the angle of projection, or if the fielder starts closer to the correct location, then the fielder runs at an overall slower speed. Fielders do not explicitly select the direction or speed when running, but they move in a way that satisfies the constraints for the changes in two angles: (i) the angle of gaze elevation to the ball (*alpha*) and (ii) the horizontal gaze angle to the ball (*delta*). According to McLeod et al, fielders ensure that *alpha* increases at a decreasing rate and *delta* increases at a constant rate (unless the distance to be run is small). Allowing *delta* to increase throughout the catch minimizes the acceleration required by the fielder to reach the interception point at the same time as the ball. The origin of this strategy may be that a child watching objects that hit him or her will experience *alpha* increasing at a decreasing rate, whereas watching balls that pass by will produce a declining *alpha* and an accelerating *delta*. When the child tries to catch the ball, he or she will run in a way that reproduces previous experiences with objects that hit and avoids those from objects that missed (McLeod et al., 2003).

Bibliography

Dienes, Z. and McLeod, P. (1993). How to catch a cricket ball. *Perception* 22, 1427-1439.

McLeod, P. and Dienes, Z. (1993). Running to catch the ball. *Nature* 362, 23.

McLeod, P. and Dienes, Z. (1996). Do fielders know where to go to catch the ball or only to get there? *Journal of Experimental Psychology: Human Perception and Performance* 22, 531-543.

McLeod, P., Reed, N. and Dienes, Z. (2001). Towards a unified fielder theory: What we do not yet know about how fielders run to catch the ball. *Journal of Experimental Psychology: Human Perception and Performance* 27, 1347-1355.

McLeod, P., Reed, N. and Dienes, Z. (2003). How fielders arrive in time to catch the ball. *Nature* 246, 244-245.

Payne, V.G. and Isaacs, L.D. (2002). *Human motor development: A lifespan approach.* 5th ed. Boston, MA: McGraw-Hill.

CATCH-UP *See under* GROWTH.

CATECHOLAMINES A category of substances, which includes epinephrine, norepinephrine and dopamine. **Dopamine** is an intermediate in the biosynthesis of norepinephrine and epinephrine.

CATHETER A hollow, tubular device that can be inserted into a cavity, duct or vessel to permit injection or withdrawal of fluid. A catheter can be inserted into an artery and left in for a period of time to make repeated sampling of arterial blood easier, faster and painless. A catheter can also be used for continuous monitoring of blood pressure during exercise.

CATIONS *See* POSITIVE IONS.

CAT SCAN *See* COMPUTED AXIAL TOMOGRAPHY.

CAUDA EQUINA A bundle of nerve roots caudal to the level of spinal cord termination. These nerve roots are particularly susceptible to injury, since they have a poorly developed epineurium. **Cauda equina syndrome** may result from any lesion that compresses the cauda equina roots. Symptoms include severe back pain and rapidly progressing motor weakness. There are many causes of cauda equina syndrome, including trauma, disk herniation and spinal stenosis. Cauda equina syndrome is uncommon, whether by traumatic or nontraumatic causes.

Bibliography

Beeson, M.S. (2003). Cauda equina syndrome. Http://www.emedicine.com

CAUDAL Pertaining to the tail. *See* CEPHALOCAUDAL.

CAULIFLOWER EAR Hematoma of the pinna. Auricular hematoma. In contact sports, one or more episodes of trauma to the pinna of the ear may result in subperichondral hemorrhage, with pressure or infection destroying the cartilage underlying the pinna. If a hematoma develops, it should be drained under aseptic conditions as soon as possible. If left untreated, the hematoma forms a fibrosis in the overlying skin, leading to necrosis of the auricular cartilage and the cauliflower appearance. It is common in wrestlers, but is preventable by wearing proper headgear at all times when on the mat.

CAVUM SEPTI PELLUCIDI *See under* HEAD INJURIES.

CELEBRITY A person who is known for his or her well-knowness. The **hero** is distinguished by his or her achievements; the celebrity by his or her image or trademark. The hero created him or herself; the celebrity is created by the media. Sporting celebrities include Michael Jordan, Tiger Woods, David Beckham, Anna Kournikova and Tonya Harding.

Chronology

•1994 • While in Detroit preparing for the US National Figure Skating Championship, Nancy Kerrigan was struck on her knee by an amateur hitman who was hired by rival skater Tonya Harding's bodyguard, Shawn Eckhard and ex-husband Jeff Gillooly. It is not known who suggested using violence against Kerrigan. Harding pleaded guilty to hindering the investigation of the attack on Kerrigan. Penalties included three years suspended probation, a $100,000 fine, a $50,000 fund to benefit Special Olympics, $10,000 court costs and 500 hours community service work. Harding was banned for life from the US Figure Skating Association. Harding had a difficult upbringing, 13 homes in 16 years, and a very poor family. She married Gillooly in 1990 and three years later a petition for a restraining order read, "It has been an abusive relationship for the past two years, and he has assaulted me physically with his open hand."

•2000 • Tonya Harding served three days in jail after pleading guilty to disorderly conduct and an alleged attack on a former boyfriend.

•2002 • Tonya Harding participated in "Celebrity Boxing" on the Fox network, fighting against Paula Jones of "Clinton Scandal" fame. She was originally billed to fight against Amy Fisher, but the New York State Parole Board refused to release Fisher, who had fired a gunshot into the head of Joey Buttafouco's wife ten years earlier. Fisher had a relationship with Buttafouco when she was 16 years old.

Bibliography

Andrews, D.L. and Jackson, S.J. (2001, eds). *Sport stars. The cultural politics of sporting celebrity*. London: Routledge.

Foote, S. (2003). Making sport of Tonya. Class performance and social punishment. *Journal of Sport and Social Issues* 27(1), 3-17.

CELL The basic structural and functional unit of all living things. **Protoplasm** is the substance within and including the plasma membrane of a cell. **Cytoplasm** is the protoplasm excluding the nucleus. The **plasma membrane** (**cell membrane**) is the membrane immediately surrounding the cytoplasm of a cell. It is a double layer of phospholipids, which selectively allow both fatty and water substances into the cell. It contains the receptors for hormones and other regulatory compounds. In plants, and some microorganisms, the cell membrane is surrounded by a rigid **cell wall**. The **nucleus** is the control center of the cell and contains the chromosomes of the eukaryotic cell. Every nucleus has originated from a previous nucleus. The **nucleolus** is a nuclear organelle in which ribosomal RNA is made and ribosomes are partially synthesized. It is usually associated with the nucleolar organizer region. A nucleus may contain several nucleoli.

See BACTERIA; TISSUE.

CELL DEATH *See* APOPTOSIS; NECROSIS.

CELL PROLIFERATION Rapid reproduction of tissue, i.e. high rates of cell division and growth. Cancer cells are very prolific.

CELLULITE Gynoid lipodystrophy. A phenomenon associated with the fat in adipose tissue under the skin (subcutaneous fat). It is characterized by a bulged, rippled, 'orange peel' appearance of the skin. It is found most often on the hips, thighs and buttocks. The cause is unknown, but it is thought that fat cells may bulge as they fill with fat due to restrictions imposed by the connective tissue that ensheathes each fat cell and separates them into compartments. According to the American Society for Dermatologic Surgery, cellulite affects 85% to 90% of post-adolescent American women.

Cellulite tends to afflict women more than men because their fat compartments are larger, their outer layer of skin is thinner and their fat tends to be concentrated on the hips, thighs and buttocks. Men lay less fat on their thighs, have differently arranged connective tissue and thicker skin, which is less likely to be deformed by underlying fat. Unlike male hormones, female hormones such as estrogen can cause a change in the shape of fat cells. Only a small percentage of men are affected by cellulite and this is usually due to a build up of toxins in the body. Cellulite tends to increase with age due to loss of flexibility and thinning of the outer layer of skin. There may be a genetic predisposition toward cellulite. There is controversy as to whether treatment should be directed toward the fat cells or the adjacent connective tissue. Cellulite should not be confused with **cellulitis**, which is an inflammation in cellular tissue and usually refers to infection in subcutaneous tissue. *See also* LIPOSUCTION; STRETCH MARKS.

Bibliography

American Society of Dermatologic Surgery. Http://www.asds-net.org

Draelos, Z.D. and Marenus, K.D. (1997). Cellulite – etiology and purported treatment. *Dermatologic Surgery* 23(12), 1177-1181.

Hexsel, D.M. and Mazzuco, R. (2000). Subcision: A treatment for cellulite. *International Journal of Dermatology* 39(7), 539-544.

Rossi, A.B. and Vergnanini, A.L. (2000). Cellulite: A review. *Journal of the European Academy of Dermatology and Venereology* 14(4), 251-262.

Stamford, B. (1986). What is cellulite? *The Physician and Sportsmedicine* 14(11), 226.

CENTRAL CORE DISEASE   A type of myopathy with inheritance that is autosomal dominant. It appears in early infancy to childhood, and symptoms include delayed motor development. Severity and progression varies, but it may be disabling.

CENTRAL NERVOUS SYSTEM   *See under* NERVOUS SYSTEM.

CENTRAL VENOUS PRESSURE   *See under* VENOUS RETURN.

CENTER OF BUOYANCY   *See under* BUOYANCY.

CENTER OF GRAVITY   A fixed point in a body through which the resultant force of gravitational attraction acts. If the gravitational field is uniform, which it generally is on earth, the gravitational forces acting on each particle of the body are parallel. Furthermore, their resultant also passes through the center of mass. The **center of mass** (**center of inertia**; **centroid**) is defined as a point of a body or system of bodies that moves as though the system's total mass existed at that point and all external forces were applied at that point. A body's center of gravity changes as the parts of the body move. The center of gravity can also be thought of as the **balance point** of a system, since the system's mass balances out on all sides of this point. The **line of gravity** is an imaginary vertical line that passes through the center of gravity.

If a person lowers one arm from a position of both arms extended overhead, then the center of gravity is lowered by the same amount that his reach with the other arm is increased. The center of gravity need not lie within the physical limits of a body. It is thus possible for a pole-vaulter to clear the bar even though his center of gravity passes under the bar.

The act of standing motionless involves a continual process of minute adjustments of body position to keep the center of gravity over the base of support. The smaller the base (such as standing on one foot instead of two feet), the more accurate those adjustments must be for stability to be maintained. Alternating contraction and relaxation of the ankle extensors results in postural sway. The amplitude of sway is less precisely regulated in the absence of visual and/or auditory cues. With increased sway, the labyrinthine organs of the inner ear, which are sensitive to displacement and acceleration changes in head position, invoke reflex compensatory movements. When a body segment deviates from the desired postural position, one or more of five 'righting reflexes' will cause muscle contractions to counteract the deviation. Head-righting reflexes must be voluntarily suppressed during inversion skills such as headstands and handstands. The stability of athletes while they perform various maneuvers depends on the position of the center of mass in relation to the base of support. The lower a body's center of gravity, the greater is its stability. In gymnastics, short height can be a disadvantage. When pivoting at the end of a beam, the shorter gymnast will fall faster from side to side than a taller gymnast.

'Hang time' (appearance of mid-air suspension) in basketball jump shots is an illusion that results from a high-velocity takeoff with extended body posture, a combination of horizontal and vertical speeds, keeping the center of gravity higher during descent, and landing with the knees flexed. Furthermore, an outstanding player, like Michael Jordan, also has the skill to release the ball well after reaching his vertical peak. Most players can only shoot effectively while rising or at the peak of the vertical leap.

Segmental analysis is a method used to determine the location of the center of gravity for the whole body and involves estimating the mass and the location of the center of gravity for each body segment. *See also* REFLEXES.

Chronology

•1968 • Dick Fosbury broke the world record in high jump using a technique that was subsequently called the 'Fosbury flop.' He jumped 2.22 meters at the Olympic Games in Mexico City after missing his first two attempts. He began experimenting with the technique when he was 16 years old. At a time when the scissors motion was predominant, Fosbury had accidentally discovered that when the human body is arched backward, the center of mass can be made to move to just outside the back. In this position, a jumper's body can clear the bar while his center of mass travels beneath it. Thus, for the same energy expenditure, an athlete doing the Fosbury flop can clear a higher bar. At the 1980 Olympic Games, 12 of the 13 of the finalists used the Fosbury flop.

•1984 • In the javelin, Uwe Hohn of East Germany set a new world record of 104.80 meters (343.83 feet) with a throw that exceeded the safe throwing area within a stadium. Hohn used a 'fatter' javelin, with very little taper from either end to the grip, which had an increased surface area and got more support from the air. With the center of gravity shifted back toward the midpoint, the javelin would follow a much flatter and longer trajectory.

•1986 • The International Amateur Athletics Federation (IAAF) pushed the allowable center of gravity in a javelin four centimeters forward, and put specific control on the shape and taper of the javelin. This had the effect of making the javelin nose-dive earlier in its flight, thus shortening the distance thrown.

Bibliography
Zumerchik, J. (1997, ed). *Encyclopedia of sports science*. New York: Macmillan Library Reference.

CENTER OF MASS   *See under* CENTER OF GRAVITY.

CENTER OF PRESSURE   *See under* FORCE PLATE.

CENTRIFUGAL FORCE   *See under* CENTRIPETAL FORCE.

CENTRIPETAL ACCELERATION   Radial acceleration. The component of the linear acceleration directed towards the axis of rotation. It is calculated as the ratio of the square of the tangential linear velocity to the radius of rotation. *See also* TANGENTIAL ACCELERATION.

CENTRIPETAL FORCE   The force required to keep a body moving in a circular path. It is a radial force because it is directed toward the center of the circle (a tangential force acts at right angles to the radius of a given circle). Centripetal force is proportional to the square of the angular velocity of the body.

Centrifugal force is an imaginary or pseudo force, which acts outwards in a frame of reference that is rotating with respect to a stationary frame of reference. It is equal and opposite to centripetal force and was introduced to validate Newton's 3rd law of motion in a moving frame of reference.

In tennis, when a player swings a racquet through the air along an angular path, the hand gripping the racquet supplies the centripetal force that keeps the racquet exerting a centrifugal force on the hand.

When an athlete swings a heavy object such as a hammer, the amounts of centripetal and centrifugal force are proportionally increased so that the athlete must lean away from the rotating hammer to avoid being pulled off balance by the centrifugal force.

In going around curves on a track, a cyclist must lean inward and press outward on the ground (centrifugal force by the cyclist on ground) to generate centripetal ground reaction force (by the ground on the cyclist/cycle system) to be able to travel in a curved path. If the cyclist travels too fast, however, the centripetal friction force is not great enough, and he slips. This friction problem is alleviated by banked curves that permit cyclists to press into a 'wall' when they turn. The smaller the radius of curvature (the tighter the curve), the more difficult it is for a cyclist to negotiate a curve at high velocity.

When making a turn, a skier exerts a centripetal force by leaning or falling inward. A skier leans on the outside edge of one ski and the inside edge of the other, and increases the pressure on the skis by increasing the muscle force exerted by the legs. This is necessary to counterbalance the outward and downward force, a centrifugal force created by inertia and gravity. When the skier turns, the body's inertial tendency is to keep going straight down the hill. The skier approximately doubles his initial rotational velocity by moving from a squatting velocity to a standing position. Then, as he comes out of the turn, the skier approximately halves his rotational velocity by bending lower and spreading his arms.

Bibliography

Zumerchik, J. (1997, ed). *Encyclopedia of sports science*. New York: Macmillan Library Reference.

CENTROID Center of volume. The **centroidal axis** is a line through the center of mass.

CEPHALIN A phospholipid, similar to lecithin, present in the brain of mammals.

CEPHALOCAUDAL *See under* DEVELOP-MENT.

CEREBELLUM *See under* BRAIN.

CEREBRAL BLOOD FLOW *See under* VALSALVA'S MANEUVER.

CEREBRAL INJURIES *See under* HEAD INJURIES.

CEREBRAL PALSY A chronic, neurologic disorder of movement and posture, which is neither hereditary nor progressive. It is caused by a lesion of the immature brain, accompanied by associated dysfunction. The term 'immature brain' usually means up to the age of 5 years. Cerebral palsy is usually not diagnosed until a child is about 2 to 3 years of age.

About 2 to 3 children in 1,000 over the age of 3 years have cerebral palsy. In the USA, there are about 500,000 children and adults with cerebral palsy. It is more common among females and also among first born. It is the orthopedic impairment most often found in American public schools.

The disorder varies from mild (generalized clumsiness or a slight limp) to severe (dominated by reflexes, unable to ambulate except in a motorized chair, inability to speak, and almost no control of motor function). Many children with cerebral palsy use the muscle synergies of various reflexes in functional movements. An example is the use of the asymmetric tonic neck reflex for reaching and for postural stability in sitting and walking.

Three types of cerebral palsy are now recognized: spasticity, athetosis and ataxia. Most individuals have mixed types, with the diagnosis indicating which is most prominent (approximately 70% spasticity, 20% athetosis and 10% ataxia). Hypotonia is a temporary diagnosis associated with floppy baby syndrome and coma.

Spastic diplegia is a common manifestation of cerebral palsy. It is when both legs are affected and a child may have difficulty walking because tight muscles in the hips and legs cause the legs to turn inward and cross at the knees so that the legs move awkwardly and stiffly (thus causing the scissors gait). **Spastic hemiplegia** is when one side of the body is affected and often the arm is more severely affected than the leg. Spastic quadriplegia is most severe and involves all four limbs, often along with the muscles controlling the mouth and tongue. Children with spastic quadriplegia usually have mental retardation, difficulty in speaking and other problems. For some children with spasticity affecting both legs, a surgical technique called **selective dorsal rhizotomy** may permanently decrease spasticity and improve the ability to sit, stand and walk. According to United Cerebral Palsy, this procedure is usually recommended only for children with severe leg spasticity who have not responded well to other treatments.

About 90% of brain damage that causes cerebral palsy occurs before or during birth. Common prenatal causes are maternal infections (e.g. AIDS), chemical toxins (e.g. alcohol) and injuries to the mother that affect fetal development. About 10% of children with cerebral palsy acquire it after birth due to brain injuries that occur during the first 2 years of life. The most common causes of postnatal cerebral palsy are brain infections (e.g. meningitis), cranial traumas from accidents/child abuse (e.g. shaken baby syndrome), chemical toxins (airborne or ingested) and oxygen deprivation (e.g. hypoxia). Maternal age is associated with cerebral palsy, with the risk increased for mothers under age 20 years or over age 34 years. Prematurity and low birth-weight are also risk factors.

Persons with cerebral palsy should be encouraged to move as independently as possible. Decreased muscular strength, flexibility and cardiovascular endurance are common in persons with cerebral palsy.

About half of the athletes in the US Cerebral Palsy Athletic Association (USCPAA) are in wheelchairs because of reflex and postural reaction abnormalities. An additional 20 to 35% have coordination problems related to reflexes, even though the individuals are ambulatory. Spasticity, athetosis and exaggerated reflex action are associated with mechanical inefficiency. The asymmetrical tonic neck reflex can prevent effective use of implements such as bats. The symmetrical tonic neck reflex can affect the ability to perform activities requiring the chin to be tucked toward the chest, such as stopping a rolling ball. Difficulty in kicking from a standing position can be affected by the crossed extension and positive supporting reflexes. Sporting activities that include a speed component can be difficult for persons with cerebral palsy because quickly performed movements tend to activate the stretch reflex. Because of abnormal postures and movements, persons with cerebral palsy have difficulty with controlling balance and body coordination. Loud noises and stressful situations increase the amount of electrical stimulation from the brain to the muscles; this tends to increase abnormal and extraneous movements.

Over 25% of USCPAA athletes take medication to control seizures. Persons with cerebral palsy perform better in individual sports than in team activities.

The Cerebral Palsy International Sport and Recreation Association (CP-ISRA) classes are as follows: 1) Movement difficulties strongly affecting the whole body; 2) Movement difficulties affecting the whole body; 3) Wheelchair user with one upper limb affected; 4) Wheelchair user with unaffected arms; 5) Ambulant athlete with both legs affected; 6) Ambulant athlete with all four limbs affected; 7) Ambulant athlete with arm and leg one side affected; and 8) Minimal disability. See also TRAUMATIC BRAIN INJURY.

Chronology

•1968 • The first international games for persons with cerebral palsy were held in France.

•1978 • The National Association of Sports for Cerebral Palsy was founded. The name was changed in 1986 to the US Cerebral Palsy Athletic Association.

Bibliography

Cerebral Palsy International Sport and Recreation Association. Http://www.cpisra.org

March of Dimes. Http://marchofdimes.com

Sherill, C. (2004). *Adapted physical activity, recreation, and sport: Crossdisciplinary and lifespan.* 6th ed. Boston, MA: McGraw-Hill.

United Cerebral Palsy. Http://www.ucpa.org

US Cerebral Palsy Athletic Association. Http://www.uscpaa.org

Winnick, J.P. (2000, ed). *Adapted physical education and sport.* 3rd ed. Champaign, IL: Human Kinetics.

CEREBROSPINAL FLUID A solution containing small molecules of blood in low concentration, which fills the cavities in the central nervous system and the space between the two membranes that ensheath the central nervous system. It is secreted by the **choroid plexuses** and reabsorbed by veins of the surface of the brain. *See under* RESPIRATORY FREQUENCY.

CEREBROVASCULAR ACCIDENT   *See under* STROKE.

CEREBRUM   *See under* BRAIN.

CERUMEN   The waxy secretion of the ceruminous glands of the external auditory meatus of the ear.

CERVICALE   An anatomical landmark that is the most posterior point on the spinous process of the seventh cervical vertebra.

CERVICAL SPINAL STENOSIS   Narrowing of the spinal canal, which results in nerves becoming irritated or squeezed. The flow of cerebrospinal fluid may also be obstructed.   Congenital conditions, injuries to the spine, cervical disc disease and age-related degeneration can be instigators of cervical spinal stenosis.

CERVICAL SPINE INJURIES   *See* NECK INJURIES.

CHAFING   An injury that results from long-term friction; mechanical rubbing of the skin by other body parts or by clothing. '**Jogger's nipple**' is produced by persistent friction at the nipples and areolae of runners. It is more common in men than women, probably because most women wear some type of soft, protective sports bra. A circular piece of tape, cut to the size of the areola, may be the best preventive measure.

Bibliography

Basler, R.S., Hunzeker, C.M. and Garcia, M.A. (2004). Athletic skin injuries. Combating pressure and friction. *The Physician and Sportsmedicine* 32(5).

CHARACTER BUILDING   This concerns morality, which can be defined as an ethical concern for honesty, fairness, justice and generosity in human relations.

Around the middle of the nineteenth century, influential Christian men in England and New England ('muscular Christians'), promoted the idea that the physical condition of one's body had religious significance. Organizations such as the YMCA organized sports because their leaders believed that sport participation developed moral character.

Game playing in the English public schools of the nineteenth century was associated with the ideology of '**athleticism**.' This ideology was based on the belief that sport enables the development of desirable moral virtues, and that the moral training associated with game playing would have a beneficial effect on life skills in general. Olympic ideology and amateurism are strongly related to athleticism.

Empirical research evidence suggests that sport in Western, industrialized societies is at best not a significant contributor, and at worst may be detrimental, to moral development. Pro-social behavior, such as sharing and helping, are negatively associated with most sport participation. Antisocial behaviors such as aggression are positively associated with participation. Exceptions to the above may be possible if sport is intentionally organized to encompass experiences designed to promote moral development. In terms of Nicholls' (1984) developmental theory of motivation, it has been suggested that there is an emphasis on fair play when a child's motivation is 'task-oriented.' As a child develops 'ego-oriented' motivation, there may be a decreased emphasis on fair play and an increased emphasis on defeating an opponent at any cost.

There is substantial evidence that individuals who participate in interscholastic sports have higher educational aspirations than non-athletes (even when account is taken for intelligence, academic performance, socioeconomic status of the parents and parental academic encouragement). A slight positive correlation has been found between sport participation and educational attainment.

In criminology, it is generally accepted that attainment of some degree of success within the educational system acts as a deterrent to delinquency. The hypothesis that interscholastic sport participation should act as a deterrent to juvenile delinquency has been supported by research evidence. It seems that rates of deviance among athletes are similar or lower than those of non-athletes. The conviction that athletic participation imparts desirable educational, social and personal values has been the basis for including recreational sports in remedial programs for juvenile delinquents.

Chronology

•c. 700 BC • Homer's poems demonstrate the moral and ethical conduct valued by the ancient Greeks through the display of arête, an ancient Greek term that embodies the cultural ideal of excellence, goodness, manliness, valor, nobility and virtue. It refers to the drive to excel, to be victorious and to perform deeds of heroism.

•564 BC • In the 54th Olympiad, Arrhachion (Arrhichion) of Philagia displayed arête in the pankration and became an Olympic champion despite being strangled to death. In the second century AD, Pausanias wrote that, "…his opponent, whoever he was, got a grip first and held Arrhachion with his legs squeezed around Arrachion's midsection and his hands squeezing around his neck at the same time. Meanwhile, Arrhachion dislocated a toe on his opponent's foot but was strangled and expired. At the same instant, however, Arrhachion's opponent gave up because of the pain in this toe. The Eleans proclaimed Arrhachion the victor and crowned his corpse." Pankration was introduced to the Ancient Olympic Games in 648 BC. It became the most popular and demanding of all athletic events. The Greeks distinguished two styles of wrestling: 'upright wrestling' (wrestling proper; the only wrestling admitted in the pentathlon and wrestling competitions) and 'ground wrestling' (that was part of the pankration). Pankration was extremely brutal, with few rules, and included kicks to the groin. There were no weight division or time limits. The 'ring' was smaller than a 12 to 14 foot square. Philostratus described the pankration as the "worthiest contest in the Olympiads and the most important for preparation of warriors." Pankration was basic to the majority of the Greek warriors who served under Alexander the Great during his invasion of India in 326 BC. The Romans later adopted pankration, but degraded it into a blood sport with the fighters being armed with spiked gloves.

•1828 • In England, Thomas Arnold became headmaster of Rugby School where he instilled moral and religious principles. He promoted games playing at the school, where a stone can be found that "commemorates the exploit of William Webb Ellis who, with a fine disregard for the rules of football as played in his time, first took the ball in his arms and ran with it, thus originating the distinctive feature of the Rugby game A.D. 1823." Arnold actually "cared little for sports and had no faith in them as ethical inculcators" (Guttman, 1988, p73). For moral reform he relied on sermons replete with Christian doctrine. It was Arnold's admiring student, Thomas Hughes, who misconstrued his preceptors's message and dramatized it in one of the nineteenth century's classic boys' books, *Tom Brown's School Days* (1856). It was Hughes, rather than Arnold, who imagined that piety and manhood were learned on the playing fields. In *Athleticism in the Victorian and Edwardian Public School* (1981), Tony Mangan showed that by the 1890s there was hardly an English school where the 'games ethic' did not reign supreme.

•1857 • The term 'muscular Christianity' was coined by T.C. Sander in a *Saturday Review* notice of Charles Kingsley's novel *Two Years Ago*. Kingsley preached about muscular Christianity in sermons and assumed that morality was a function of muscularity as well as piety, and that the best sort of Christians was physically fit. He wrote, "Games conduce not merely to physical, but to moral health; in the playing-field boys acquire virtues which no books can give; not merely daring and endurance, but, better still, temper, self-restraint, fairness, honour, unenvious approbation of another's success."

•1864 • In Britain, the Royal Commission on Public Schools, chaired by the Earl of Clarendon, emphasized the importance of team games, rather than gymnastic exercises, such as cricket for character training.

•1881 • Princeton organized the first faculty athletic committee with Harvard following suit the next year. Of prime concern was the number of days that athletes were spending away from their classes for intercollegiate matches.

•1882 • At a convention in Springfield, a rule was adopted for intercollegiate football that "no man shall be allowed in championship games for a longer period than five years." In 1889, the presence of graduate players on the teams became such an open abuse that the newspapers took notice.

•1889 • Luther H. Gulick was appointed as supervisor of physical training for the Young Men's Christian Association (YMCA) School for Christian Workers in Springfield, Massachusetts, which opened in 1885. In 1890, it changed its name to the International YMCA Training School, and later renamed to Springfield College. Gulick was strongly influenced by muscular Christianity and promoted the use of games and sport for educational purposes.

Gulick, who was one of Sargent's students at Harvard, used the notion of an inseparable link between a sound mind and sound body from the pagan Greeks. He reconciled the Christian mission of the YMCA with Greek paganism by arguing that there had been no Christ in Ancient Greece. Higgs (1995) argues that Gulick, like so many muscular Christians after him, "transformed the body of Christ into a Hercules or Apollo, for which there is no scriptural foundation."

•1891 • Canadian James Naismith invented basketball, as an alumnus and faculty member of the YMCA at Springfield, Massachusetts, after Luther Gulick, director of the YMCA had given him the task of finding an inexpensive game that could be played indoors in the winter: "The immediate purpose of basketball was to provide exercise and amusement for eighteen young men who were bored by calisthenics and too rambunctious for indoor football. Ultimately, however, basketball was meant as an instrument to bring these young men to Christ." (Guttman, 1988, p73)

•1892 • Amos "Alonzo" Stagg played in the first public basketball game as a faculty member at Springfield College scoring the faculty team's only basket in a 5-1 loss. He took basketball from Springfield to Chicago where it became a major sport. 5-man basketball was his brainchild. Stagg was one of many Christian football coaches from the eastern colleges who brought muscular Christianity to the West and South. Basketball became one of America's most popular sports in the 1920s and 1930s, especially in metropolitan high schools and colleges.

•1892 • Senda Berenson became Director of the Gymnasium and Instructor of Physical Culture at Smith College, where she introduced Swedish gymnastics supplemented by organized athletic contests in sports such as volleyball, fencing, field hockey and basketball, all intended to build character in her female students. Trained at the Boston Normal School of Gymnastics, Berenson was hired at Smith College one month after the game had been invented in nearby Springfield, MA.

• 1893 • Senda Berenson organized the first women's college basketball game. The only man allowed in the gymnasium was the president of the College who was thought to be too old to get erotically aroused. She modified Naismith's rules with his consent. She soon adapted the rules to avoid the roughness of the men's game.

•1894 • In the dedication address for the gymnasium of the Training School at Springfield College, American psychologist G. Stanley Hall endorsed muscular Christianity. The philosophy of Stanley Hall was based upon a scientific and muscular interpretation of Christianity: "We are soldiers of Christ, strengthening our muscles not against a foreign foe, but against sin within and without us."

•1894 • Football was banned from the Kansas Methodist Conference, after a group of ministers were offended by the questionable recruiting practices of Baker University in Kansas.

•1895 • William Morgan came to the YMCA at Springfield under the influence of James Naismith (See 1891). Finding basketball too strenuous for businessmen in his evening gymnastic class, Morgan developed a game called "mintonette" (later called volleyball).

•1896 • The YMCA organized the Athletic League of North America to coordinate its expanding athletic interests and to maintain the high profile of competition. Under the direction of Luther Gulick, it stated, "the idea that Christ's kingdom should include the athletic world, that the influence of athletics upon character must be on the side of Christian courtesy."

•1898 • At Brown University, all the colleges of the present-day Ivy League with the exception of Yale met to discuss intercollegiate athletics. The Brown Conference Committee Report spoke out for the sport model found at Oxford and Cambridge: "We should not seek perfection in our games, but, rather, good sport." The Brown Conference failed to solve major athletic problems.

•1898 • F. A. Kellor wrote an essay entitled "A Psychological Basis for Physical Culture," in which she advocated that women in American colleges should place less emphasis on formal gymnastics in their physical education classes and place more emphasis on participation in various sports and games.

•1899 • Edward W. Scripture, director of the psychological laboratory at Yale University published a study in *Popular Science Monthly* stating that desirable personality traits could be fostered through participation in sport and that these traits would transfer to other areas of a person's life.

•1900 • In Britain, the Board of Education (set up in 1899) first instructed inspectors that games were officially a suitable alternative to Swedish drill or physical exercises.

•1907 • The Athletic Research Society was founded to study social and moral aspects of the rapidly expanding school and college athletic programs in America.

•1934 • In Moray (Scotland), Kurt Hahn founded Gordonstoun as a public (i.e. independent secondary) school. Hahn, a Jew who fled Nazi Germany and read classics at Oxford, based the school on the ideal was that the intellectual, cultural, physical, social and spiritual attributes of his pupils should be simultaneously developed. The aim of Hahn's physical education was to produce healthy living habits, rather than develop competitive performance, with an outdoors ethos. It inspired the "Outward Bound" movement that emphasizes working in groups of 8 to 12 participants, physical and mental challenges, community service work, and a period of wilderness solitude.

•1936 • In the long jump competition at the Olympic Games, Jesse Owens fouled on his first two jumps, but he was stunned when officials counted a practice run down the runway and into the pit as an attempt. With one jump remaining, Luz Long, a German long jumper who was Owens' biggest rival, introduced himself to Owens and suggested that Owens made a mark several inches before the takeoff board and jump from there to play it safe. Owens took the advice and qualified. Long was killed in World War II.

•1936 • The undefeated Joe Louis was knocked out in twelve rounds at the Yankee Stadium by Germany's Max Schmeling. German Minister of Propaganda Joseph Goebbels proclaimed Schmeling's victory as a victory for Hitler's regime and Germany. In a 1938 rematch, Louis defeated Schmeling in one round. Schmeling opposed the Nazis. He became a personal friend of Louis and paid for a part of Louis' funeral in 1981.

Bibliography

Arnold, P.J. (1986). Moral aspects of an education in movement. In: Stull, G.A. and Eckert, H.M. (eds). *Effects of physical activity on children*. pp14-21. Champaign, IL: Human Kinetics.

Bredemeier, B.J. (1988). The moral of the youth sport story. In Brown, E.W. and Banton, C.F. (eds). *Competitive sports for children and youth*. pp285-296. Champaign, IL: Human Kinetics.

Coakley, J. (1993). Sport and socialization. *Exercise and Sport Sciences Reviews* 21, 169-200.

Coakley, J. (2004). *Sports in society. Issues and controversies*. 8th ed. Boston, MA: McGraw-Hill.

Guttmann, A. (1988). *A whole new ball game. An interpretation of American sports*. Chapel Hill: University of North Carolina Press.

Higgs, R.J. (1995). *God in the stadium. Sport and religion in America*. Lexington: University of Kentucky Press.

Hodge, K.P. (1989). Character building in sport: Fact or fiction? *New Zealand Journal of Sports Medicine* 17(2), 23-25.

Hodge, K.P. and Tod, D.A. (1993). Ethics of childhood sport. *Sports Medicine* 15(5), 291-298.

Shields, D.L.L. and Bredemeier, B.J.L. (1995). *Character development and physical activity*. Champaign, IL: Human Kinetics.

Weiss, M.R. and Bredemeier, B.J. (1990). Moral development in sport. *Exercise and Sport Sciences Reviews* 18, 331-78.

Wiggins, D.K. (1987). A history of organized play and highly competitive sport for American children. In: Gould, D. and Weiss, M. (eds). *Advances in pediatric sport sciences*. Vol. 2: Behavioral issues. pp1-24. Champaign, IL: Human Kinetics.

CHARCOT-MARIE-TOOTH SYNDROME *See under* HEREDITARY MOTOR AND SENSORY NEUROPATHY.

CHARLES' LAW *See under* GAS.

CHELATE The ring structure formed by the reaction of two or more groups on a ligand with a metal ion.

CHEMICAL REACTIONS The breaking of chemical bonds in reactant molecules, followed by the making of new chemical bonds to form product molecules. In order for a chemical reaction to occur, the reactant molecules must acquire enough energy – the **activation energy** – to enter an activated state in which chemical bonds can be broken and formed. The activation energy does not alter the difference in energy content between the reactants and final products, since this energy is released when the products are formed. The types of chemical reactions that are most important in biochemistry are oxidation-reduction (redox), condensation and hydrolysis.

The **equilibrium constant** is the point of equilibrium for any chemical reaction, i.e. the point at which the forward and reverse reactions of molar concentrations of the reactants and products will be equal. This point is unique to each chemical reaction. At chemical equilibrium, there is no longer any net change from reactant to product; there is no further potential to do work. **Rate constant** is a constant of proportionality relating the single step of a reaction to the concentrations of the reactants. The **mass action law** states that the rate of a chemical reaction for a uniform system at constant temperature is proportional to the concentrations of the substances reacting. *See also* ENZYMES.

CHEMICAL STRUCTURE The spatial configuration of the atoms contained in a molecule.

Many molecules can exist in more than one form. Compounds with identical molecular formulae, but with differences in the nature of sequence of their chemical bonds, or with differences in the spatial arrangements of their atoms, are referred to as **isomers**.

Isomers may be either structural isomers or stereoisomers. **Structural (constitutional) isomers** have molecules with the same components, but different constitutions (sequence of atoms). An example is glucose 6-phosphate and glucose 1-phosphate, which are interconverted by the enzyme phosphoglucomutase. A **stereoisomer** is an isomer of a reference molecule that has the same atom-to-atom connections as the reference molecule, but has a shape that is nonsuperimposable with it.

An **epimer** is one of two stereoisomers that differ only in the configuration of a single atom, at one chiral center; e.g. the -OH group points 'upward' at carbon 17 in testosterone, but 'downward' in epitestosterone. A **chiral** is a compound that cannot be superimposed on its mirror image.

Optical isomers are distinguished by the characteristic rotation of the plane of polarized light falling on the molecule, either rotation to the right (dextrarotatory, D or + form) or to the left (laevorotatory, L, or – form). This occurs because of the asymmetrical structure imposed on the carbon atom when it forms bonds with different groups. All amino acids (except glycine) have four different groups attached to their alpha carbon. Because of this, the alpha carbon is asymmetric, with two different ways of arranging these groups, i.e. two different configurations. Optical isomerism reflects the shape of the molecule that determines its ability to interact with other molecules.

CHEMIOSMOTIC COUPLING   *See under* ELECTRON TRANSPORT CHAIN.

CHEMORECEPTOR   A sensory receptor that responds to substances according to their chemical structure. Chemoreceptors are located in the aortic and carotid arteries. They are sensitive to the partial pressure of oxygen, partial pressure of carbon dioxide, and concentration of hydrogen ions in arterial blood. Increased partial pressure of carbon dioxide and hydrogen ions, or decreased partial pressure of oxygen, leads to reflex vasoconstriction of arterioles. *See under* RESPIRATION.

CHEMOTAXIS   The release of chemicals by microbes and inflamed tissues that attract phagocytes.

CHEST DEVIATIONS   *See under* PECTUS DEFORMITIES.

CHEST INJURIES   A direct blow to the chest may result in injuries such as rib fractures, costochondral separations or myocardial contusion.

CHILDHOOD DISINTEGRATIVE DISORDER An extremely rare pervasive developmental disorder with the following diagnostic criteria: A) Apparently normal development for at least the first 2 years after birth as manifested by the presence of age-appropriate verbal and nonverbal communication, social relationships, play, and adaptive behavior. B) Clinically significant loss of previously acquired skills (before the age of 10 years) in at least two of the following areas: expressive or receptive language, social skills or adaptive behavior, bowel or bladder control, play and motor skills. C) Abnormalities of functioning in at least two of the following areas: qualitative impairment in social interaction (e.g. impairment in nonverbal behaviors); qualitative impairments in communication (e.g. delay or lack of spoken language); and restricted, repetitive and stereotyped patterns of behavior, interests and activities. D) The disturbance is not accounted for better by another pervasive developmental disorder or by schizophrenia.

Bibliography

American Psychiatric Association. (1994). *Diagnostic and statistical manual of mental disorders*. 4th ed. Washington, DC: American Psychiatric Association.

CHILL FACTOR   *See* WINDCHILL.

CHLORINE   An element, which as a 'macromineral' and electrolyte in the human body, is involved in regulating osmotic pressure between extracellular and intracellular compartments. Chloride is the major anion in the extracellular fluid, occurring mostly in combination with sodium. Less than 15% of the total body chloride is intracellular. The '**chloride shift**' is a process in which bicarbonate ions diffuse out of red blood cells in exchange for chloride as hemoglobin exchanges oxygen for carbon dioxide. The chloride shift is the primary homeostatic mechanism for the control of blood pH and the maintenance of osmolarity of the extracellular fluid.

CHOKING   *See under* STRESS.

CHOLESTEROL   The most abundant steroid in the body. The liver manufactures most of the cholesterol in the body, but the intestine contributes significant amounts and all cells synthesize some cholesterol. At least a gram of cholesterol is produced in the body per day, more than what is found in the average diet. Cholesterol is a precursor of five major classes of sterol hormones: progesterones, glucocorticoids, mineralocorticoids, androgens and estrogens. Cholesterol is transported around the body on lipoproteins, which have a core of triglycerides and cholesterol esters surrounded by a shell of phospholipids with embedded proteins and cholesterol. In general, as the proportion of triglyceride drops, the density of the lipoprotein increases.

Apolipoprotein is protein embedded in the outer shell of lipoproteins that helps other enzymes function, acts as lipid transfer protein, or helps binding to a receptor. There are at least 9 types of apolipoproteins. **Chylomicrons** are large blood lipoproteins that contain about 90% triglycerides, some phospholipids and a small amount of proteins. **Apolipoprotein B-48** is the primary protein of chylomicrons. Chylomicrons are synthesized in the intestinal mucosa cells from products of lipid digestion and are distributed to body tissues via the lymphatic vessels, thoracic duct and, finally, blood vessels. As they circulate through capillaries,

chylomicrons gradually give up their triglycerides. **Lipoprotein lipase** is an enzyme located in the endothelium of capillaries. It attacks chylomicrons and removes triglyceride, breaking it into free fatty acids and glycerol that can enter adipose cells in order to be reassembled into triglycerides. Chylomicrons may remain in circulation, though, with the free fatty acids bound to albumin. The liver picks up chylomicron remnants and uses them to build very low-density lipoproteins.

Very low-density lipoprotein (VLDL) is composed mainly of triglyceride and carries cholesterol from the liver into the blood stream. VLDL has a very low density, because it is comprised about 65% fat. Lipoprotein lipase splits off and hydrolyses triglycerides from VLDL cholesterol as it circulates through capillaries.

Intermediate-density lipoprotein (IDL) is comprised of about 40% triglycerides. As IDL travels through the bloodstream, it acquires cholesterol from another lipoprotein and circulating enzymes remove some phospholipids.

Low-density lipoprotein (LDL) is derived from VLDL by the action of lipoprotein lipase. It supplies most parts of the body with cholesterol. **Apolipoprotein B** is the major protein in LDL. Moderate levels of LDL in the blood are necessary for health. LDL delivers cholesterol to body cells, which use it to synthesize membranes, hormones and other vital components. The cell engulfs and ingests the LDL via endocytosis. Inside the cell, LDL is broken down into its component parts. Liver cells also have LDL receptors that bind LDL and control blood cholesterol levels. Saturated fats appear to block these receptors. This explains why saturated fats tend to increase blood cholesterol levels: a lack of LDL receptors decreases uptake of cholesterol, forcing it to remain in circulation at dangerously high levels. LDL is also picked up by scavenger receptors that have a particular affinity for oxidized LDL. When blood vessel walls are damaged (e.g. by smoking), white blood cells are mobilized and travel to the site of the injury where they bury themselves in the blood vessel wall. Certain white blood cells with scavenger receptors bind and ingest LDL. As LDL degrades, it releases its cholesterol.

Accumulation of cholesterol leads to development of plaque and thus atherosclerosis. Regarding how cholesterol sticks to the walls of arteries, it is believed that LDL becomes oxidized and then damages the lining of the artery. This damage allows the cholesterol a place to join on to and build up, ultimately narrowing the artery. Antioxidants, such as vitamin E, may help protect against the oxidation of LDL cholesterol and prevent the build up of plaque in the arteries.

Lipoprotein (a) is LDL with apolipoprotein B-100 linked to apolipoprotein (a). It is a low-density lipoprotein that at high levels seems especially harmful, preventing the normal break up of blood clots that cause heart attack or stroke. Lipoprotein (a) is taken up by macrophages and interferes with clot lysis by inhibiting the conversion of plasminogen to plasmin. It is proatherogenic and prothrombic at concentrations of approximately 20 mg/dL or greater. It is an independent risk factor for cardiovascular disease and is considerably higher in African Americans than Caucasians.

High-density lipoprotein (HDL) is made by the liver and intestines. Its trigylceride content of about 5% is similar to LDL, but it has only about 20% cholesterol (LDL has 50%). **Apolipoprotein A-1** is the major protein of HDL. **Reverse cholesterol transport** involves the take up of cholesterol by HDL from cells and from other lipoproteins (especially IDL) through the action of enzymes that physically transfer molecules from one place to another. HDL carries cholesterol away from the cells, back to the liver, thus promoting its excretion from the body. HDL is thought to help clear blood vessels by picking up cholesterol released by dying cells and from cell membranes as they are renewed. HDL also picks up cholesterol from arterial plaques, decreasing their accumulation. A high level of HDL relative to that of LDL in the circulation is thought to be beneficial with regard to protection from coronary heart disease. A person who increases the amount of fat and cholesterol in their diet (e.g. by consuming a high-protein diet) may increase their HDL, because their body is trying to get rid of the extra 'garbage' (fat and cholesterol) by increasing the number of available 'garbage

trucks' (HDL). HDL is predictive of relative heart disease risk only in populations in which everyone is eating a similar high-fat diet.

In 2001, the National Cholesterol Education Program (NCEP) of the National Heart, Lung and Blood Institute (NHLBI) in the USA released new guidelines for decreasing heart disease risk. Changes from earlier guidelines included: treating high cholesterol more aggressively in people with diabetes; a cholesterol test every 5 years for all adults over age 20; defining low HDL as being less than 40 mg/dL compared to the earlier value of 35 mg/dL; intensifying the use of nutrition, physical activity and weight control in the treatment of elevated blood cholesterol; identifying a 'metabolic syndrome' of risk factors linked to insulin resistance and dramatically increase the risk of heart attack; and more aggressive treatment for elevated triglycerides. Lowering cholesterol intake does help some people, but for most the result is variable and less effective than lowering intake of saturated fats. It is currently recommended that total fat and saturated fat intake is lowered, while keeping body weight normal. Within total fat limits, monounsaturated oils should be the fat source of choice.

Total cholesterol should be less than 200 mg/dL of blood, LDL cholesterol should be less than 100 mg/dL and HDL cholesterol should be greater than 40 mg/dL. Total trigylcerides should be less than 150 mg/dL.

After menopause, women have less favorable lipid profiles than before menopause. While regular exercise improves lipid metabolism in men, the specifics for doing so in pre- and post-menopausal women are not fully understood. Higher-volume exercise programs increase HDL cholesterol levels in both pre- and post-menopausal women.

Exercise training can decrease total blood cholesterol and LDL cholesterol, but only modestly. People who have the highest cholesterol levels before training show the greatest improvement. Exercising for longer periods is more effective than shorter periods.

There is evidence that those who consume modest amounts of alcohol have a lower risk of coronary artery disease than those who drink no alcohol. Alcohol consumption may raise the fraction of HDL cholesterol. However, alcohol may not increase HDL cholesterol levels in people who are already very active.

See also CARDIOVASCULAR DISEASE; HYPERLIPIDIMIA; NUTRITION.

Chronology

•1999 • Mark Spitz was prescribed a statin, called lipitor, which was able to lower his cholesterol level in about 30 days from 303 mg/dL to below 200 mg/dL. After 18 months on the drug, his cholesterol had decreased to 177 mg/dL.

•2001 • The National Cholesterol Education Program (NCEP) released their third report on the detection, evaluation and treatment of high blood cholesterol.

Bibliography

Berg, A. et al. (1994). Physical activity and lipoprotein lipid disorders. *Sports Medicine* 17(1), 6-21.

Dowling, E. (2001). How exercise affects lipid profiles in women. What to recommend for patients. *The Physician and Sportsmedicine* 29(9).

Franklin, B.A. (1993). Can exercise help lower cholesterol? *The Physician and Sportsmedicine* 21(10), 103-104.

Goldberg, L. and Elliot, D.L. (1987). The effect of exercise on lipid metabolism in men and women. *Sports Medicine* 4, 307-321.

Mitchell, T.L, Mitchell, M.D., and Gibbons, L.W. (1998). Controlling blood lipids. Part 1: A practical role for diet and exercise. *The Physician and Sportsmedicine* 26(10), 41-53.

Ornish, D. (2004). Was Dr. Atkins right? *Journal of the American Dietetic Association* 104(4), 537-542.

Stamford, B. (1990). What cholesterol means to you? *The Physician and Sportsmedicine* 18(1), 149-150.

CHOLINE An amine and a constituent of phospholipids found in plant and animal foods. Choline is a critical part of lecithin and sphingomyelin, both of which are constituents of the cell membrane. Choline is also needed for the synthesis of acetylcholine; the body synthesizes it from methionine. Most choline in foods is found in the form of phosphatidylcholine (lecithin). Milk, eggs, liver and peanuts are rich sources of choline. Lecithins added during food processing may increase the daily consumption of choline by about 115 mg/day. The main criterion for establishing the Adequate Intake for choline is the prevention of liver damage. The adequate intake for adults is 550 mg (males) and 425 mg/day (females).

Bibliography

Oregon State University. The Linus Pauling Institute. Micronutrient Information Center. Http://lpi.oregonstate.edu/infocenter

CHOLINERGIC *See under* AUTONOMIC NERVOUS SYSTEM.

CHONDROCYTE A cell that produces cartilage.

CHONDROLYSIS The disappearance of articular cartilage as a result of disintegration or dissolution of the cartilage matrix and cells.

CHONDROMALACIA Pathologically softened cartilage. When normal cartilage (such as on the patella) is exposed to excessive pressure or shear, isolated chondrocyte necrosis can occur, resulting in loss of matrix and softening of the articular surface. **Chondromalacia patellae** occurs in two distinct age-groups. In people over the age of 40 years, it occurs when articular cartilage breaks down as part of the age-related, wear-and-tear process that occurs with the rest of the body. In teenagers (especially girls), it occurs when the articular cartilage softens in response to excessive and uneven pressure on the cartilage, due to structural changes in the legs with rapid growth and muscle imbalance around the knee. Unless there is actual softening or breakdown of cartilage, the knee pain in the teenager is more likely to be patellofemoral pain syndrome than chondromalacia patellae.

CHOREA A type of dyskinesia characterized by repetitive, brief, jerky, large-scale, dancing-like, involuntary uncontrolled movements that start in one part of the body and move abruptly, unpredictably, and often continuously to another part.

CHOROID PLEXUSES Structures, located in the

four large fluid cavities of the brain, which secrete cerebrospinal fluid.

CHROMATIN This is the 'storage' form of DNA inside the nucleus of a cell. It is a highly condensed form of DNA. Enormous lengths of chromosomes are tightly packed, but it permits specific genes to be accessed and activated when the cell needs them to perform their assigned functions. **Chromatin diseases** represent failures of the cell to control the timing of activity of certain chromatin genes during growth and development.

CHROMATOGRAPHY A method of separating and analyzing mixtures of chemical substances.

CHROMIUM An element that, as a 'trace element' in the human body, is involved in the regulation of carbohydrate and lipid metabolism and is a cofactor with insulin in glucose metabolism. It also plays a role in the metabolism of nucleic acids and in immune function and growth.

Relatively rich sources of chromium in food include whole grain products, broccoli and processed meats. Broccoli (half a cup) contains 11 mcg of chromium. Processed turkey ham (3 oz) contains 10.4 mcg of chromium. The Food and Nutrition Board has set an Adequate Intake (AI) based on chromium content in normal diets. The AI for adults (19-50 years) is 35 mcg (males) and 25 mcg (females); for adults (51 years and older) it is 30 mcg (males) and 20 mcg/day (females).

Picolinate is a natural derivative of tryptophan and apparently facilitates the absorption of chromium into the body. Chromium picolinate is used by athletes with the belief that it will act as an anabolic agent. In animal studies, chromium supplementation has been associated with increased lean mass, decreased body fat, improved insulin metabolism, improved immunity and increased longevity. Clancy et al. (1994) found that 9 weeks of chromium supplementation (200 _g) in a double-blind design in football players was ineffective in bringing about changes in body composition or strength during a program of intensive weight-lifting training. It is possible that the small differences

reported in lean body mass between the chromium-supplemented group and the placebo group in this experiment may have been due to errors in the measurement techniques; easily done when skinfold and girth measurements are used.

Bibliography

Campbell, W.W. and Anderson, R.A. (1987). Effects of aerobic exercise and training on the trace minerals chromium, zinc and copper. *Sports Medicine* 9, 9-18.

Clancy, S.P. et al. (1994). Effects of chromium picolinate supplementation on body composition, strength, and urinary chromium loss in football players. *International Journal of Sport Nutrition* 4(2), 142-153.

Clarkson, P.M. (1991). Nutritional ergogenic aids: Chromium, exercise and muscle mass. *International Journal of Sport Nutrition* 1(3), 289-293.

Lukski, H.C. (1999). Chromium as a supplement. *Annual Review of Nutrition* 19, 279-302.

Oregon State University. The Linus Pauling Institute. Micronutrient Information Center. Http://lpi.oregonstate.edu/infocenter

Williams, M.H. (1999). *Nutrition for fitness and sport.* 5th ed. Boston, MA: McGraw-Hill.

CHROMOSOME *See under* HEREDITY.

CHRONIC Of long duration. The opposite of chronic is acute.

CHRONIC FATIGUE SYNDROME An illness characterized by persistent or relapsing, debilitating fatigue of an unknown origin, resulting in moderate to severe disability. In general, patients are not clinically immunocompromised; they do not develop opportunistic infections. The fatigue is disproportionate to the intensity of effort that is undertaken, has persisted for six months or longer, and has no obvious cause. The hallmark of chronic fatigue syndrome is an increase in symptoms following exercise, usually high intensity or prolonged exercise. For many patients, minimal exertion can exacerbate symptoms from 6 hours to as long as 5 days afterward. Patients with the syndrome are not as likely to push themselves to their true maximum, because they do not want to worsen symptoms.

Shephard (2001) concludes that chronic fatigue syndrome is a syndrome rather than a clear-cut disease, defined by a symptom-complex rather than clear physiological and biochemical manifestations. It affects both athletes and sedentary individuals. There have been reports of associations with overtraining, nutritional deficiencies, immune disturbances, autonomic and endocrine dysfunction, and viral infection. It is likely, however, that these represent precipitants or consequences rather than underlying causes of the syndrome. The study of etiology and treatment of chronic fatigue syndrome has been hampered by the low prevalence of the disease (less than 0.1% of the general population) and (until recently) a lack of clear and standardized diagnostic criteria. Current treatments for chronic fatigue syndrome are symptom-based, with psychological, pharmacological and rehabilitation treatments providing some relief, but no cure. Immunological and nutritional treatments have been tried but none has provided reproducible benefits.

In chronic fatigue syndrome, dysfunction of the autonomic nervous system is generally manifested as a suppression of parasympathetic function and the development of exertional hypotension. Given the major influence of training on cardiac performance and peripheral venous tone, the rest or decreased training commonly recommended for patients with chronic fatigue syndrome could, in itself, predispose to a shift in sympathetic/parasympathetic balance and susceptibility to orthostatic hypotension (Shephard, 2001). A low blood pressure has been noted as one feature of the parasympathetic form of overtraining. It is possible that autonomic dysfunction could trigger chronic fatigue syndrome in a proportion of cases.

Recently known as myalgic encephalomyopathy, 'yuppie flu,' 'postviral fatigue syndrome' or 'postinfection fatigue syndrome,' the concept of chronic fatigue syndrome developed as the convergence of certain other conditions including fibromyalgia syndrome, mononucleosis and myalgic encephalomyelitis. **Mononucleosis** is an acute viral infection in which the patient develops a sore throat, swollen lymph glands and fever. Epstein-Barr virus is the cause of most cases of acute mononucleosis. There is evidence that Epstein-Barr virus may be reactivated more often in patients with chronic fatigue syndrome than in healthy individuals. Epstein-Barr virus is a herpes virus that is carried by 90% of adults in Western societies, and in at least half of those who are infected it gives rise to no symptoms. Epstein-Barr virus becomes incorporated into the DNA of lymphocytes and the epithelial cells of the oropharynx. High levels of Epstein-Barr specific T-memory cells seem to be important to the control of infection. Immunosuppression by intensive exercise and/or stress could impair the activity of these specific memory cells, explaining how the virus could suddenly induce chronic fatigue syndrome. **Myalgic encephalomyelitis** (ME) is a syndrome in which tiredness, muscle pain, lack of concentration, panic attacks, memory loss and depression occur. It often occurs after viral infections of the upper respiratory tract or gut.

Most studies report chronic fatigue syndrome patients to have normal muscle strength and either normal or slightly decreased muscle endurance. Chronic fatigue syndrome patients have been found to have either no impairment or mild impairment of the aerobic energy systems. Moderate exercise can often be performed without exacerbating symptoms and sometimes it leads to an improvement in the immediate condition. Patients can perform a progressive cycle ergometer test to exhaustion. Little is known about the long-term effects of exercise on chronic fatigue syndrome. A number of researchers have suggested that chronic fatigue syndrome may involve alterations in the central nervous system, rather than in the peripheral muscles. This is supported by research evidence that patients have increased perception of fatigue in response to exercise. A case study of an elite ultra-endurance cyclist suffering from chronic fatigue syndrome suggested that decreases in performance were the result of detraining, rather than impairment of aerobic metabolism due to chronic fatigue syndrome per se. Rowbottom et al. (1998) proposed that central factors influence fatigue perception in chronic fatigue syndrome sufferers.

See FIBROMYALGIA SYNDROME.

Bibliography

McCully, K.K., Ann Sisto, S. and Natelson, B.H. (1996). Use of exercise for treatment of chronic fatigue syndrome. *Sports Medicine* 21(1), 35-48.

Rowbottom, D.G. et al. (1998). The case history of an elite ultra-endurance cyclist who developed chronic fatigue syndrome. *Medicine and Science in Sports and Exercise* 30(9), 1345-1348.

Shephard, R.J. (2001). Chronic fatigue syndrome. An update. *Sports Medicine* 31(3), 167-194.

Skinner, J.S. (2004). Chronic fatigue syndrome. Matching exercise to symptom fluctuations. *The Physician and Sportsmedicine* 32(2).

CHRONIC OBSTRUCTIVE PULMONARY DISEASE   Chronic airflow limitation. Chronic destructive lung disease. A group of diseases of the respiratory tract that produce an obstruction to airflow and ultimately compromise gas exchange at the alveoloar level. Major diseases classed as chronic obstructive pulmonary disease are bronchitis, bronchiectasis, emphysema, asthma and cystic fibrosis. Treatment for chronic obstructive pulmonary disease includes bronchodilators (such as $beta_2$ adrenergic receptor agonists) and anti-inflammatory drugs (such as corticosteroids).

Breathlessness and exercise intolerance are the most common symptoms of chronic obstructive pulmonary disease. In flow-limited patients during exercise, air trapping is inevitable and causes further dynamic lung hyperinflation, above the already increased resting volumes. Dynamic lung hyperinflation causes elastic and inspiratory threshold loading of inspiratory muscles already burdened with increased work against resistance, with the result that tidal volume increases are constrained. Dynamic lung hyperinflation compromises the ability of the inspiratory muscles to generate pressure, and the positive intrathoracic pressures likely contribute to cardiac impairment during exercise.

Therapeutic interventions that decrease operational lung volumes during exercise, by improving lung emptying or by decreasing ventilatory demand (which delays the rate of dynamic lung hyperinflation), may improve endurance of patients with chronic obstructive pulmonary disease during exercise. Functional weakening of the inspiratory muscles in response to dynamic lung hyperinflation appears to be a central component of dyspnea. After respiratory muscle training, a decrease in the intensity of respiratory effort sensation, during exercise and loaded breathing, has been observed in patients with obstructive lung disease (as well as healthy individuals).

Bibliography

Aliverti, A. and Macklem, P.T. (2001). How and why exercise is impaired in COPD. *Respiration* 68(3), 229-239.

American College of Sports Medicine (2001). *ACSM's resource manual for Guidelines for Exercise Testing & Prescription.* 4th ed. Philadelphia, PA: Lippincott Williams & Wilkins.

McConnell, A.K. and Romer, L.M. (2004). Dyspnea in health and obstructive pulmonary disease: The role of respiratory muscle function and training. *Sports Medicine* 34(2), 117-132.

O'Donnell, D.E. (2001). Ventilatory limitations in chronic obstructive pulmonary disease. *Medicine and Science in Sports and Exercise* 33(7S), S647-S655.

CHRONOTROPIC   A term that refers to the rate of rhythmic movements such as the heart beat.

CHYLOMICRON   *See under* CHOLESTEROL.

CHYME   *See under* GASTRO-INTESTINAL SYSTEM.

CIGARETTE SMOKING   This is the most preventable cause of death in the USA, where the government estimates that there are about 400,000 premature deaths each year due to cigarette smoking. Approximately 90% of lung cancers, 80% of emphysema, 75% of bronchitis and 30% of coronary heart disease are attributable to smoking. Tobacco smoke contains more than 4000 chemicals, 60 of which have been identified as carcinogenic. Smokers of low-yield cigarettes compensate for the low delivery of nicotine by inhaling the smoke more deeply and by smoking more intensely. Consequently, the peripheral lung is exposed to increased amounts of smoke carcinogens, which are suspected to lead to lung adenocarcinoma. In addition to lung cancer, cigarette smoking can cause cancer of the esophagus, larynx, lip, mouth, pharynx, tongue, kidney, pancreas, urinary bladder and uterine cervix.

Many of the gases and condensed tar particles emitted from tobacco smoking are oxidants and pro-oxidants capable of producing free radicals, thus enhancing lipid peroxidation in biological membranes. Cadmium, naturally found in tobacco, decreases the bioavailability of selenium and acts antagonistically to zinc, a cofactor for superoxide dismutase. Smoking has been shown to lower the level of vitamin C and beta-carotene in plasma. Vitamin E may be at suboptimal levels in tissues of smokers. In heavy smokers, however, increased intake of beta-carotene and vitamin E has been found to increase the incidence of lung cancer. A possible explanation is that antioxidants interfere with important processes needed to kill cancer cells. Nearly 40% of cardiovascular deaths are attributable to smoking. The main mechanisms that affect the development of heart disease are the effects of carbon monoxide. The risk of heart disease is directly related to the number of cigarettes smoked. Smoking one pack per day doubles the risk compared to nonsmoking; smoking more than one pack per day triples the risk. After 2.5 years of not smoking, the risk of lung cancer is decreased by 50%. Within 3 to 5 years of not smoking, risk of a heart attack is similar to that of a nonsmoker's, and within 5 to 10 years, risk of major health problems decreases to levels only slightly greater than those who have never smoked. Cigarette smoking also increases the risk of osteoporosis, and precipitates premature hearing loss and vision problems. Smokers are at greater risk of complications during and after surgery.

Smoking prevalence decreased from 42.4% in 1965 to 24.7% in 1997. Most smokers quit a number of times before achieving long-term abstinence. Most smokers who relapse do so within 6 months of quitting. Most people who have quit smoking report doing so without the help of a health professional.

See also CARBON MONOXIDE; MARIJUANA; NICOTINE.

Chronology

•2004 • In the UK, the Scientific Committee on Tobacco and Health updated their previous warning (in 1988) of the health risks of passive smoking with respect to lung cancer and cardiovascular disease. This committee advocated a total ban on smoking in public places.

Bibliography

American College of Sports Medicine (2001). *Resource manual for Guidelines for exercise testing and prescription.* 4th ed. Philadelphia, PA: Lippincott, Williams and Wilkins.

Preston, A.M. (1991). Cigarette smoking – nutritional implications. *Progress in Food and Nutrition Sciences* 15(4), 183-217.

CIRCADIAN RHYTHMS   *See under* BIO-LOGICAL RHYTHMS.

CIRCULATORY SYSTEM   The system of blood vessels. **Systemic circulation** is the circulation of blood from the left ventricle through all parts of the body except the lungs, and its return to the right atrium. **Pulmonary circulation** is the circulation of blood from the right ventricle to the lungs and its return to the left atrium.

About 72% of the resistance of the circulatory system at rest arises in the arterial system (mainly the arterioles) and only 28% in the venous system. During exercise, total resistance may be decreased by more than 50%.

According to **Poiseuille's law**, cardiac output is proportional to the fourth power of the vessel radius. The greater the pressure gradient, the larger is the radius. The lower the viscosity and length of the vessel, the greater is the flow. For the systemic circulation, where arteries are longer, a greater pressure difference is required to maintain a given flow. When the radius is decreased, such as during vasoconstriction, this has a large influence on decreasing flow because of the fourth power function.

CIRCUMDUCTION   A limb movement that is a combination of rotation, extension/flexion, and abduction/adduction.

CITRIC ACID CYCLE   *See* KREBS CYCLE.

CLASSICAL CONDITIONING   It is a type of learning, conditioning or behavioral intervention, which is based on the association between a conditioned stimulus and an unconditioned stimulus. A conditioned (neutral) stimulus comes to elicit a conditioned response, which before conditioning was elicited as an unconditioned response only by some other unconditioned stimulus. Classical conditioning is mainly a function of the contingency between the conditioned stimulus and the unconditioned stimulus during the learning trials. The conditioned stimulus comes to substitute for the unconditioned stimulus. Classical conditioning is generally most effective when the conditioned stimulus and the unconditioned stimulus occur close to each other temporally and spatially (the 'principle of contiguity').

Pavlov's famous experiments involved dogs salivating with food in the mouth, a response that is not due to learning. The food is the unconditioned stimulus, salivation is the unconditioned response and the conditioned stimulus is the signal that the unconditioned stimulus is about to appear (a bell). After a dog had been brought to the laboratory a number of times, it would start to salivate before the food was placed in its mouth. The sight of the food dish, which had not previously elicited salivation, became a conditioned stimulus for salivation. Salivation at the conditioned stimulus is a conditioned response. The sight of food (conditioned stimulus) substitutes for the food (unconditioned stimulus).

Since Pavlov, many other automatic, involuntary responses (such as emotions) have been classically conditioned. Classical conditioning can lead to pleasant or unpleasant responses. An example of a pleasant response is: stirring music (unconditioned stimulus) leads to positive emotion (unconditioned response), a neutral stimulus such as national flag plus stirring music (conditioned stimulus) leads to positive emotion (unconditioned response), and finally the national flag (conditioned stimulus) leads to positive emotion (conditioned response). An example of an unpleasant response is: the sight of a needle for injection (unconditioned stimulus) leads to nausea (unconditioned response), a neutral stimulus (smell of hospital) plus an unconditioned stimulus leads to an unconditioned response, and finally the smell of hospital (conditioned stimulus) leads to nausea (conditioned response).

Extinction is the weakening and eventual disappearance of a learned response. In classical conditioning, it occurs when the conditioned stimulus is no longer paired with the unconditioned stimulus. Extinction is not the same as unlearning or forgetting. The reappearance of a response, spontaneous recovery, accounts for why the complete elimination of a conditioned response usually requires more than one extinction session.

Higher-order conditioning is a procedure in which a neutral stimulus becomes a conditioned stimulus through association with an already established conditioned stimulus. Higher-order conditioning may explain why some words trigger emotional responses in us.

Stimulus discrimination is the tendency to respond differently to two or more similar stimuli. In classical conditioning, it occurs when a stimulus similar to the conditioned stimulus fails to evoke the conditioned response.

Counter-conditioning is the process of pairing a conditioned stimulus with a stimulus that elicits a response that is incompatible with an unwanted conditioned response.
See SYSTEMATIC DESENSITIZATION; PSYCHOLOGICAL SKILLS TRAINING.

CLAUDICATION   *See under* PERIPHERAL ARTERIAL DISEASE.

CLAVICLE   The upper extremity's only bony articulation with the appendicular skeleton. It prevents the shoulder from dropping across the chest and thus helps maintain the distance between the upper arm and the sternum. The length of the clavicle influences habitual posture of the shoulders. A relatively long clavicle will force the shoulder back, whereas a relatively short clavicle will require the scapulae to lie forward and to the side, and will cause the shoulders to be brought forward.

Injuries to the clavicle and its two articulations

are common in athletes. Most injuries are acute traumatic injuries to the clavicle, the acromioclavicular joint and the sternoclavicular joint. Fractures of the clavicle may occur indirectly following a fall onto an outstretched hand or the tip of the shoulder, or from direct trauma in contact sports. Osteolysis of the distal end of the clavicle occurs when the acromioclavicular joint is highly stressed, such as in gymnastics. Atraumatic osteolysis of the distal clavicle may result from hyperextension of the shoulder during a bench press (i.e. dropping the elbows below the body line during the eccentric phase of movement) that puts excessive stress on the acromioclavicular joint. A '**shoulder pointer**' is a contusion to the distal end of the clavicle.

Bibliography
Reeves, R.K., Laskowski, E.R. and Smith, J. (1998). Weight training injuries: Part 2: Diagnosing and managing chronic conditions. *The Physician and Sportsmedicine* 26(3), 54-73.

CLAW FOOT *See* PES CAVUS.

CLAW TOE A deformity involving hyperextension of the metatarsophalangeal joint and a hyperflexion of the interphalangeal joint. It may be either congenital, or a result of muscle imbalances or neurological disorders.

CLENBUTEROL A beta-2 adrenergic agonist prescribed as a bronchodilator in Europe, but not in the USA. In doses far greater than those required for bronchodilation, clenbuterol has been found to increase lean mass and retard deposition of adipose tissue in chickens and cattle. Clenbuterol may promote muscle hypertrophy by stimulating protein metabolism in the cell via increased calcium transport, increased cyclic AMP levels and an activation of protein kinase. The effect on adipose tissue is related to enhanced lipolysis. Clenbuterol is available in Europe as an over-the-counter asthma medication and has been used by athletes, though it would have minimal effects as a 'nutrient partitioning agent' (i.e. a drug that simultaneously increases lean muscle and decreases fat deposition) in the dosages commonly used by athletes. High doses of clenbuterol cause the usual side effects of an adrenergic agent, such as tachycardia, muscle tremors, nausea and fever. Myocardial infarction has also been reported. The World Anti-Doping Agency (WADA) does not permit the use of clenbuterol. *See* ASTHMA; DIETING DRUGS.

Bibliography
Dodd, S.L. et al. (1996). Effects of clenbuterol on contractile and biochemical properties of skeletal muscle. *Medicine and Science in Sports and Exercise* 28(6), 669-676.

Prather, I.D. (1995). Clenbuterol: A substitute of anabolic steroids? *Medicine and Science in Sports and Exercise* 27(8), 1118-1121.

World Anti-Doping Agency. Http://www.wada-ama.org

CLIMBER'S ELBOW *See under* BRACHIALIS MUSCLE.

CLINODACTYLY A congenital condition where the little finger is curved towards the ring finger. It can occur in isolation, or be associated with chromosomal abnormalities like Down syndrome.

CLONUS A type of convulsion characterized by rapid, alternate contraction and relaxation of a muscle.

CLOSED-CIRCUIT SPIROMETRY *See under* CALORIMETRY.

CLOSED-LOOP CONTROL *See under* MOTOR LEARNING.

CLOSED SKILL *See under* MOTOR SKILL.

CLUBFOOT *See* TALIPES.

CLUMSINESS *See* DEVELOPMENTAL COORDINATION DISORDER.

CLUMSY TEENAGER PHENOMENON A condition associated with a temporary deterioration in bodily stability (balance) that may occur at the time of peak height velocity. The irregular and uncoordinated growth patterns of different body segments that occur during this period may require temporary adjustments in the interpretation of proprioceptive signals.

COACHING   With respect to a planned, coordinated and integrated program of preparation and competition, Lyle (2002) stated that four fundamental roles for the coach are: direct intervention (purposeful activities that are focused on performance enhancement); intervention support (coaching activities that support or prepare for the direct intervention, such as planning); constraints management (attempts to manage the situational factors to the best advantage of the athlete and the coaching process); and strategic coordination (ensuring a continuous overview of the progress of the coaching process in relation to the stated objectives).

A distinction can be made between autocratic and democratic coaching. **Autocratic coaching** is characterized by: the primacy of the coach in decision making; a dominating, directive approach to interpersonal behavior; one-way transmission of knowledge in teaching; coach-determined rules, rewards, standards and application; rigidity and lack of personal empathy. **Democratic coaching** is characterized by: a participative decision-making style; an interactive communication process; human values incorporated into goals and evaluations; active involvement in teaching-learning process; and flexibility, empathy and support in personal relationships.

Smith and Smoll (1996) distinguish between a positive and negative approach to coaching. The **positive approach** attempts to strengthen the desired behaviors by motivating players to perform them and by reinforcing them when they occur. The **negative approach** attempts to eliminate unwanted behaviors through punishment and criticism. Most coaches use both approaches, but punishment should be minimized.

The legendary John Wooden, basketball coach to University of California at Los Angeles (UCLA), was observed for 30 hours during practice by Tharp and Gallimore (1976). Most of Wooden's behaviors related to instruction: 50.3% were instructions

(what to do, how to do it); 12.7% were hustles (activate or intensify previous instructed behavior); 8% were "Woodens" (scold, modeling-positive, followed by modeling-negative, ending with modeling-positive); 6.9% were praises (compliments); 6.6% were reproofs (scolds; expressions of displeasure); 2.8% were modeling-positive (demonstration of how to perform); 1.6% were modeling negative (demonstration of how not to perform); 1.2% were nonverbal reward (smiles, pats etc.); and less than 1% were nonverbal punishment (scowls, despairing gestures, temporary removal of player from scrimmage). What Gallimore and Tharp (2004) call a "Wooden," Coach Wooden himself describes as a "sandwich approach." Gallimore and Tharp (2004) argue that what Wooden calls a "sandwich" may not overlap with what Smith et al. (1977) describe as a "positive sandwich" (a positive reinforcement for effort or some part of a skill executed correctly, a future-oriented positive instruction focusing on the good thing that will happen if corrective instruction is followed, and encouragement designed to increase self-efficacy). Citing Scanlan and Scanlan (2003), Gallimore and Tharp note that a "future-oriented" statement can imply criticism couched in positive terms.

In reanalyzing their original data, along with published sources of Wooden's work and interviews with Wooden himself, Gallimore and Tharp (2004) concluded that exquisite and diligent planning lay behind the heavy information load, economy of talk and practice organization. Wooden viewed learning in terms of explanation, demonstration, imitation and repetition. Teaching according to the whole-part method, he emphasized the use of drill and repetition. Wooden's use of praise was minimal, and he used praise that was specific and informative rather than general and noninformative.

In a study of football coaches at collegiate and high school level, Anshel and Straub (1991) identified a total of 31 undesirable coaching behaviors and classified them into the following seven categories (in order of frequency): lack of effective communication between coach and athlete (e.g. coach makes statements that embarrass athletes in presence of peers); not explaining to players the rationale for strategies; expression of anger toward athletes; not defining the role or status of nonstarters; inappropriate content in pre-game and half-time talks; failure to treat players as individuals (e.g. coach disregards an athlete's pain, injury, frustration, or depression); and ineffective use of assistant coaches.

The **Coaching Behavior Assessment System** (Smith, Smoll and Hunt, 1977) distinguishes between reactive and spontaneous behaviors. **Reactive behaviors** involve responses to: desirable performance (reinforcement or non-reinforcement); mistakes (mistake-contingent encouragement, mistake-contingent technical instruction, punishment, punitive technical instruction or ignoring mistakes); and misbehavior (keeping control). **Spontaneous behaviors** involve game-related instruction (general technical instruction, general encouragement or organization) and game-irrelevant responses (general communication).

Coach Effectiveness Training, based on the Coaching Behavior Assessment System, has been adopted by many youth sport coaches. Its guidelines for coaches are: provide a positive developmental context with emphasis on giving maximum effort and making improvement; make liberal use of positive reinforcement, encouragement and sound technical instruction (e.g. sandwich a positive, action-oriented instruction between two encouragement statements); establish norms that emphasize athletes' mutual obligations to help and support one another; involve athletes in decision making and compliance reinforcement; obtain behavioral feedback; and engage in self monitoring.

The National Standards for Athletic Coaches have been established by the National Association for Sport and Physical Education (NASPE). These standards address eight domains: (i) injury care and prevention; (ii) risk management; (iii) knowledge of growth and development; (iv) training, conditioning and nutrition; (v) the social/psychological aspects of coaching; (vi) skills, tactics and strategies; (vii) teaching and administration; and (viii) professional preparation and development. *See also* EXPERTISE; INTRINSIC MOTIVATION; LEADERSHIP; OPERANT CONDITIONING; SPORTS PSYCHOLOGY; SPORTS SCIENCE.

Chronology

•300 AD • *De Ante Gymnastica*, the manual on physical training by Philostratus, is the only one of many such manuals from antiquity that appears to have survived. It was discovered near Constantinople in 1844. Philostratus, who considered gymnastics to be a science, criticized trainers who indiscriminately applied hard-and-fast rules about diet and training techniques without regard to age or individual differences. He described ideal body types for different sports and also referred to the "tetrad system" of training - a cycle of four days in which something different is done each day: Day 1 Prepare the athlete; Day 2 Intense exercise; Day 3 Relax; and Day 4 Moderation. The trainer (i.e. coach) had great power over the athlete in ancient Greece. Philostratus justifies the killing of an athlete by a coach using a sharp instrument because the athlete did not exert himself to win.

•1864 • Yale hired the first professional coach in American collegiate athletics, William Wood, to enable the Yale crew to defeat Harvard.

•1914 • Sam A. Mussabini's *The Complete Athletic Trainer* was published. Mussabini argued that Britain required training methods of professional trainers. Scipio Africanus ("Sam") Mussabini was born in London of Arab-Turkish-Italian-French ancestry and became known for his analytic approach and enthusiasm. In five Olympic Games, his protégées won 11 medals. As featured in the movie *Chariots of Fire*, Harold Abrahams won gold in 100 meters and silver in 4 x 100 meters at the 1924 Olympic Games in Paris. Mussabini was ostracized, because he was a paid coach in the amateur era. Seeing the difference between being a masseur and a technical adviser, he was adamant that he should be called a coach and not (as was the usual terminology) a trainer. Mussabini also wrote on the technicalities of billiards and launched a billiards journal in 1902.

•1919 • At the University of Illinois, George Huff developed the first degree-program in coaching. By the 1930s, coaching courses had become the primary focus of many physical education departments that offered undergraduate degrees.

•1934 • In the UK, the course in athletics held at Loughborough College, under the auspices of the Amateur Athletics Association, marked the beginning of a movement to study the techniques of many sports and to work out systematic ways of coaching them in schools and clubs.

•1961 • In Canada, the Fitness and Amateur Sport Act (Bill C-131) was enacted as a result of concern about Canada's mediocre performance in international competition and the intensive drive mounted by physical education and sport organizations. It led to the establishment of the National Advisory Council on Fitness and Amateur Sport and included training for coaches.

•1964 • Under Coach John Wooden, the University of California Los Angeles (UCLA) Men's Basketball team began a run of 10 National Collegiate Athletic Association (NCAA) Championships in 12 years. No other school in the history of the sport has won more than four.

•1969 • In Australia, a coaching accreditation course was started under the auspices of the National Fitness Council of Western Australia.

•1981 • The American Coaching Effectiveness Program (ACEP) delivered its first course. ACEP was founded at the University of Illinois, Urbana-Champaign in 1976 by Rainer Martens. By 1986, there 1,400 certified instructors who had trained more than 50,000 coaches. In 1994, the scope of the program was broadened to include parents and administrators, and it was renamed the American Sport Education Program (ASEP). It is now a division of Human Kinetics Publishers, Inc. Its motto is "Athletes first, winning second."

•1981 • The National Youth Sporting Coaches Association (NYSCA) training program was founded in West Palm Beach, Florida. In 1993, it was expanded to form the National Alliance for Youth Sports (NAYS) to include parents, administrators, and officials as well as coaches. More than one million youth coaches have participated in this program.

•1990 • The American Sport Education Program (ASEP) began a partnership with the National Federation of State High School Associations (NFHS) to develop and deliver the NFHS Coaches Education Program for high school coaches. Thirty-five states now require NFHS Coaches Education Program courses for their high school coaches, and more than 75 universities use NFHS/ASEP courses and resources.

• 1992 • The National Association for Sport and Physical Education (NASPE) appointed a special task force to consider ways to improve the quality of coaching, building on all previous initiatives over the past 30 years. The standards were officially released in 1995.

•2000 • In the Women's Korea Basketball League, Coach Jin Song Ho of the Hyundai Hyperion, lined up the team in the changing room and smacked three players, one of who suffered a ruptured eardrum. At the end of the season, his coaching license was revoked by the League. Cho Seung Youn, executive director the league, was quoted as saying: "Coaches know that hitting players is the fastest and easiest way to improve their skills. However, Jin has tarnished the reputation of the league and we can't accept his harsh actions." (Http://www.time.com/time/asia/magazine/2000/0814/korea.bbcoach.html)

Bibliography

Anshel, M.H. (2003). *Sport psychology: From theory to practice*. 4th ed. San Francisco: Benjamin Cummings.

Anshel, M.H. and Straub, W.B. (1991). Congruence between players' and coaches perceptions of coaching behavior. *Applied Research in Coaching and Athletics Annual* 1991, 49-65.

Gallimore, R. and Tharp, R. (2004). What a coach can teach a teacher, 1975-2004: Reflections and reanalysis of John Wooden's teaching practices. *The Sport Psychologist* 18, 119-137.

Johnson, N.L. (2003). *The John Wooden Pyramid of Success*. 2nd ed. Los Angeles, CA: Cool Titles.

Lyle, J. (2002). *Sports coaching concepts. A framework for coaches' behavior*. London: Routledge.

National Association for Sport & Physical Education. Http://www.aahperd.org/naspe

Scanlan, T. and Scanlan, L. (2003). Personal communications to Gallimore and Tharp. Cited in Gallimore and Tharp (2004).

Smith, R.E. (2001). Positive reinforcement, performance feedback, and performance enhancement. In Williams, J.M. (ed.) *Applied sport psychology: Personal growth to peak performance*. 4th ed. pp29-42. Boston, MA: McGraw-Hill.

Smith, R.E., Smoll, F.L. and Hunt, E.B. (1977). A system for behavioral assessment of athletic coaches. Research Quarterly 48, 401-407.

Smith, R.E., Smoll, F.L. and Hunt, E. (1977). A system for the behavioral assessment of athletic coaches. *Research Quarterly* 48, 401-407.

Smith, R.E. Smoll, F.L. and Curtis, B. (1979). Coach Effectiveness Training: A cognitive-behavioral approach to enhancing relationship skills in youth sport coaches. *Journal of Sport Psychology* 1, 59-75.

Smith, R.E. and Smoll, F.L. (1996). *Way to go, Coach: A scientifically-proven approach to coaching effectiveness*. Portola Valley, CA: Warde Publishers.

Smith, R.E. and Smoll, F.L. (1997). Coaching the coaches: Youth sports as a scientific and applied behavioral setting. *Current Directions in Psychological Science* 6, 16-21.

Smith, R. (2003); Smoll, F.L. (2003). Personal communications to Gallimore and Tharp. Cited in Gallimore and Tharp (2004).

Tharp, R.G. and Gallimore, R. (1976). What a coach can teach a teacher. *Psychology Today* 9 (Jan), 74-78. Cited in Weinberg,

R.S. and Gould, D. (1999). *Foundations of sport and exercise psychology*. 2nd ed. Champaign, IL: Human Kinetics.

Wooden, J.R. with Jamison, S. (1997). *Wooden: A lifetime of observations and reflections on and off the court*. Lincolnwood, IL: Contemporary Books.

COACH-ATHLETE RELATIONSHIPS Athletes tend to be uncomfortable with the coach who tries to be 'good friends' with the players, but mentoring is an important part of a healthy coach-athlete relationship. **Mentoring** involves a trusted and experienced person taking an interest in the personal and professional development of a younger or less experienced person. *See also under* INTRINSIC MOTIVATION.

Bibliography

Anshel, M.H. (2003). *Sport psychology: From theory to practice*. 4th ed. San Francisco: Benjamin Cummings.

COACTIVATION *See under* KINETIC CHAIN EXERCISE; MUSCLE ACTION, MULTI-JOINT.

COAGULATION FACTORS *See under* THROMBOSIS.

COCAINE An alkaloid compound derived from the *Erythroxylon coca* shrub native to the South American Andes. The purified powder form of cocaine is prepared by dissolving the alkaloid complex in hydrochloric acid to form a soluble salt known as cocaine hydrochloride. Cocaine was used as a local anesthetic before the development of synthetic local anesthetics, when its potential for abuse was realized. It is usually snorted through the nose. '**Free basing**' is conversion of cocaine into its alkaline form for smoking as **crack cocaine**. It is more powerful than cocaine in hydrochloride form.

Like amphetamine, cocaine promotes the release of dopamine or norepinephrine and increases arousal. As a stimulant, it causes a transient feeling of energy, alertness and euphoria. The physiological effects are similar to amphetamine, but the mood effects are more profound. The 'high' that occurs for up to 30 minutes after inhalation is followed by depression. It is unlikely that this drug would have any beneficial effects on athletic performance. It can be addictive and has a number of short- and long-term health risks. Cocaine is very toxic to the heart and can cause fatal cardiomyopathy.

Over the last ten years, there has been a dramatic increase in the number of pregnant women who use cocaine. The US Department of Health and Human Services has estimated that between 50,000 and 375,000 cocaine-exposed babies are born each year in the USA. Cocaine use can cause the placenta to pull away from the wall of the uterus before labor begins. This condition is called **placental abruption** and can lead to extensive bleeding, which may be fatal for both the mother and her baby. Babies of women who use cocaine regularly during pregnancy are between three and six times more likely to be born at a low birth weight (less than 5.5 pounds) than babies of women who do not use cocaine. Maternal use of crack or cocaine results in smaller than normal infants who require immediate treatment for addiction. These '**crack babies**' may exhibit combined mental retardation-cerebral palsy patterns as they grow.

See also FETAL ALCOHOL SYNDROME; TERATOGEN.

Chronology

•1869 • Cyclists were known to be using 'speedballs' of heroine and cocaine.

•1986 • Don Rogers, a standout defensive back for the Cleveland Browns in the National Football League, died from cardiac arrhythmia brought about by chronic cocaine use.

•1993 • Reggie Lewis of the Boston Celtics died after fainting while practicing jump shots. There was more than $15 million in insurance coverage of Lewis' contract that could be paid out to the Lewis family and the Celtics, but only if no link to drugs was shown. It is not known whether Lewis died from a heart damaged by cocaine, but it was strongly suspected. The official cause of death was adenovirus 2 (a common virus that causes the common cold) that led to inflammation of Lewis' heart, widespread scarring of tissue and, ultimately, a fatal cardiac arrest. Three months earlier Lewis had collapsed during a playoff game and medical opinion was divided as to whether he was suffering from ventricular tachycardia, the most dangerous form of arrhythmia, caused by focal cardiomyopathy; or a neurocardiogenic fainting disorder (vasovagal syncope).

Bibliography

Keller, D. and Todd, G.L. (1994). How cocaine kills athletes. *International Journal of Cardiology* 44(1), 19-28.

McDonough, W. (1993). Lewis died of heart abnormality myocarditis, State autopsy says. *The Boston Globe*, August 4, Sports Page 1.

COCCYX   Vestigial tailbone consisting of (usually) four fused vertebrae. Coccygeal fractures can occur when an athlete falls in a sitting position, and sustains a direct blow to the coccyx. It is most common in horse riding. Direct blows can lead to contusions and fractures. Prolonged or chronic pain may also result from irritation of the coccygeal nerve plexus (**coccygodynia**).

COCHLEAR IMPLANT   A device that replaces part or all of a person's inner ear, when the organ's malfunction is causing a severe to profound hearing loss. An otolaryngologist must drill behind and into the inner ear and mastoid bone, creating a space or cavity to house the implant. The cochlear implant is placed in this inner ear cavity and secured to the skull, and then the cavity is closed with an incision. Sounds enter the cochlear implant device through a microphone that is worn behind the ear. The sounds are then sent from the microphone via a thin cable to an external speech-processor that is often attached to a belt or worn in a shirt pocket. Implants enable auditory nerve fibers to remain functional even when the hair cells in the inner ear cochlea are damaged or decreased in number. **Hearing aids** amplify sounds, but cochlear implants increase the user's opportunity to perceive sound by stimulating nerve fibers and hair cells in the cochlea. The perceived sound and speech are then altered to electrical signals that travel, via the auditory nerve, to the brain for interpretation.

Approximately 60,000 individuals worldwide use cochlear implants. Implantation is occurring at a rate of approximately 3,000 new devices per year. The current practice is to implant only one ear.

Demapping causes the implant to be disabled and eliminates any chance of hearing in the implanted ear. It is usually caused by static electricity from sources such as clothes, plastic play equipment, computer screens, and painted or varnished surfaces. Cold temperatures may create uncomfortable sensations around the head, neck and ear regions for the individual with the implant.

Protection for the student with a cochlear implant is necessary in activities that can result in head injuries. In general, an individual with a cochlear implant should not participate in any contact activities or sports, such as football, hockey, rugby, soccer and wrestling. For baseball, basketball and swimming, the cochlear implant device should be removed and necessary headgear and precautions used.

Bibliography

Hilgenbrinck, L.C., Pyfer, J. and Castle, N. (2004). Students with cochlear implants. Teaching con-siderations for physical educators. *Journal of Physical Education, Recreation and Dance* 75(4), 28-33.

COCHLEOPUPILLARY REFLEX   A reaction of the iris, which in which there is contraction of the pupil followed by dilation in response to a loud sound.

COEFFICIENT OF RESTITUTION   It is an index of elasticity for colliding bodies: the ratio of the relative velocity of the two bodies after impact to the relative velocity before impact. The closer the coefficient of restitution is to one, the more elastic the impact. The closer the coefficient of restitution is to zero, the more plastic the impact. In tennis, a ball dropped from a height of 100 inches onto a hard surface rebounds only to a height of about 55 inches. Indeed, that is the official specification for the manufacture of a tennis ball. About 45% of the energy is lost. For an official major league baseball, the required coefficient of restitution is 0.546 +/- 0.032. The variation of 0.032 means that the distance traveled by two identically hit baseballs can vary by 4.5 meters. Due to modern baseball manufacturing and testing methods, the actual variation among regulation baseballs is much less than 0.032.

Chronology

•1997 • Following independent research, the National Collegiate Athletic Association (NCAA) in the USA instituted an interim standard for baseball bat performance that a ball cannot rebound more than 15 per cent faster off a stationary bat than off a solid wall.

Bibliography

Zumerchik, J. (1997, ed). *Encyclopedia of sports science*. New York: Macmillan Library Reference.

CO-ENZYME   Vitamin-derived cofactors. Dissociable cofactors. The non-protein part of an enzyme functions as an acceptor of electrons or functional groups. The two major coenzymes involved in most cell redox reactions are FAD and NAD^+. The coenzyme FAD can accept two hydrogen atoms to become $FADH_2$ (i.e. the reduced form of FAD). The coenzyme NAD^+ accepts a hydride ion, becoming NADH.

CO-FACTOR   A specific substance required for the activity of an enzyme, e.g. a co-enzyme. Co-enzyme A (Co-A) was the first such factor discovered. Coenzymes and metal ions (e.g. magnesium ions) are cofactors.

COGNITIVE DEVELOPMENT   Movement is a primary agent in the acquisition of increased cognitive structures, especially during infancy and early childhood. **Adaptation** requires a child to adjustment to environmental conditions and to intellectualize adjustments through the complementary processes of accommodation and assimilation. **Accommodation** is adaptation that the child must make to the environment when new or incongruent information is added to his or her repertoire of possible responses. **Assimilation** involves interpretation of new information based on present interpretation. This means taking in information from the environment and incorporating it into the individual's existing cognitive structures.

Piaget proposed the following stages of cognitive development: sensorimotor stage, preoperational stage, concrete operational stage and formal operational stage. The **sensorimotor stage** (0 to 2 years) can be described as 'thinking by bodily movement' and involves development of: ability to differentiate between self and other; recognition of objects that exist even though they are no longer in the visual field; and mental imagery that allows contemplation of past and future. The **preoperational stage** (2 to 7 years) involves development of: language; manipulation and locomotion leading to increased exploration of the environment; and imaginary play, parallel play and an increase in social participation. The **concrete operational stage** (7 to 11 years) is reached when attention can be dissociated from one or more aspects of a problem-solving situation and there is awareness of alternative solutions. It is 'concrete' because the child's mental activities are still tied to concrete objects. Play is used to understand the physical and social world. **Reversibility** refers to the capacity of the child to understand that any change of shape, order, position or number can be mentally reversed and returned to its original shape, order, position or number. The **formal operational stage** (12 years and later) reflects the highest level of cognitive ability. There is a systematic approach to problem solving. It involves the ability to think hypothetically and to make judgments by implication. Piaget believed that highly sophisticated intellectual capabilities were developed by about 15 years.

Contemporary developmental psychologists have noted flaws in Piaget's work. Piaget believed that new reasoning abilities depend on the emergence of previous ones, but cognitive abilities seem to develop in overlapping waves rather than discrete steps or stages. Preschoolers are not as egocentric as Piaget thought – most 3- and 4-year olds can take another person's speech. When 4-year olds play with 2-year olds, for example, they modify and simplify their speech so that the younger children will understand. By ages 3 to 4 years, children develop a theory of mind, a system of beliefs about how their own and other people's minds work and how people are affected by their beliefs and emotions. Cognitive development also depends on the child's education and culture. Contrary to Piaget's beliefs, contemporary evidence in psychology suggests that cognitive development depends not only on age, but also on life experiences and continued practice. *See* EXPERTISE.

Bibliography

Payne, V.G. and Isaacs, L.D. (2004). *Human motor development: A lifespan approach*. 6th ed. Boston, MA: McGraw-Hill.

COGNITIVE DISSONANCE   A state that exists whenever an individual holds incompatible cognitions. Festinger's (1957) Cognitive Dissonance theory has been used to explain psychological consequences of exercise. An individual who initially did not enjoy exercise may find a way to justify the time and effort expended to continue exercise. In doing so, the person's attitude and mood would shift in a more positive direction. The more effort and hard work that is put in by the individual, the greater the dissonance and the greater the likelihood that the person will feel better about the activity. *See also* EXERCISE ADHERENCE.

Bibliography

Festinger, L. (1957). *A theory of cognitive dissonance*. Stanford, CA: Stanford University Press.

COGNITIVE INTERVENTIONS   Developing or restructuring thoughts and images that guide behavior. One of the most popular interventions is Ellis' (1962) Rational Emotive Therapy, which is based on the premise that behavioral problems arise through distorted or irrational thinking. The aim of Rational Emotive Therapy is to identify and challenge such maladaptive thinking. Common cognitive distortions include: unwarranted generalization from the particular to the general; guessing rather than reasoning about what might happen; concentrating on the negative aspects of oneself; minimizing one's achievement; negative feelings dominating one's thoughts; and perfectionism.

Perfectionism involves the setting of excessively high standards of performance in conjunction with a tendency to make overly critical self-evaluations. A perfectionist has difficulty in discriminating between realistic and idealized standards. It has been suggested that perfectionist athletes fear failure and mistakes to such an extent that their enjoyment of sport may be diminished and their performance compromised.

Ellis (1982) identifies four basic irrational beliefs that can negatively affect an athlete's performance: (i) "I must at all times perform outstandingly well;" (ii) "Others whom I hold significant to me have to approve and love me;" (iii) "Everyone has got to treat me kindly and fairly;" and (iv) "The conditions of my life, particularly my life in sports, absolutely must be arranged so that I get what I want when I want." Ellis (1984) argues that exercise and sports avoidance are usually motivated by low frustration tolerance and/or irrational fears of failure.

Rational emotive therapy involves a variety of interventions, such as logical and empirical questioning of irrational thinking, role-playing, modeling, relaxation, operant conditioning and skills training. Other cognitive interventions include attributional retraining and social learning interventions.

Bibliography

Ellis, A. (1962). *Reason and emotion in psychotherapy*. New York: Lyle Stuart.

Ellis, A. (1982). Self-direction in sport and life. In: Orlick, T., Partington, J. and Salmela, J. (eds). *Mental training for coaches and athletes*. pp10-17. Ottawa, ON: Coaching Association of Canada.

Ellis, A. (1984). The sport of avoiding sports and exercise: A Rational Emotive Behavior therapy perspective. *The Sport Psychologist* 8, 248-261.

Frost, R.O. and Henderson, K.J. (1991). Perfectionism and reactions to athletic competition. *Journal of Sport and Exercise Psychology* 13, 323-335.

COGNITIVE PSYCHOLOGY   A broad discipline, with many branches, concerned with mental processes. Much research has been done since the 1950s using an information-processing approach based on a computer metaphor in which cognitive (mental) processes are modeled using analogies to computers. This is reflected in the types of theories used in motor learning. Neisser (1976) pointed out disadvantages of the information processing approach, in particular that it treats cognition too abstractly and that human beings have important differences to machines. Neisser argued for an ecological approach, in which the relation of humans to their environment is considered.

A distinction can be made between cognitive psychology and cognitivism. Cognitive psychology is based on mentalism, i.e. that which is internal, private and laden with meaning. **Cognitivism** is a subset of mentalism and refers to an approach in which cognitive processes are based on rule-based relationships between symbolic representations. Cognitive approaches based on the traditional computer metaphor are cognitivist.

Social-cognitive theories emphasize how behavior is learned and maintained through observation and imitation of others, positive consequences, and cognitive processes such as plans, expectations and beliefs. *See also* MOTOR LEARNING.

Bibliography

Marteniuk, R.G. (1976). *Information processing in motor skills*. New York: Holt, Rinehart and Winston.

Neisser, U. (1976). *Cognition and reality. Principles and implications of cognitive psychology*. San Francisco: W.H. Freeman.

Straub, W.F. and Williams, J.M. (1984). *Cognitive sport psychology*. Lansing, New York: Sport Science Associates.

COGNITIVE STYLE A link between cognition and personality. In sport psychology, the most popular theory of cognitive style has been the 'left/right dichotomy of cognitive functioning,' which was popularized by Ornstein (1972). The dichotomy is based on research with 'split-brain' patients whose hemispheres were disconnected by surgical removal of the corpus callosum, which joins the hemispheres.

Lateralization refers to the consolidation of cerebral functions within the left and right hemispheres. Language may be lateralized to the left hemisphere from birth. Prior to about 6 years of age, the hemispheres appear relatively plastic in their ability to develop specific functions. If the left hemisphere is damaged beyond this age, the right hemisphere is much less likely to develop normal language functions. If the left hemisphere is damaged after language has been acquired, the person may never again be capable of fluent speech, because the critical period for right hemisphere substitution has been passed. The left hemisphere specializes in verbal, logical and analytical functions and processes information in a serial manner. Conversely, the right hemisphere specializes in spatial perception and processes information in a holistic, parallel manner.

Hemisphericity is a strong bias towards either left or right hemisphere processing. It has been suggested by authors such as Blakeslee (1980) that there is an overemphasis on left hemisphere functioning in Western society, to the extent that there is a suppression of right hemisphere capabilities. From this viewpoint, it has been argued that visual and kinesthetic information inherent in sport is often processed inappropriately by the left hemisphere. It follows that if the left hemisphere can be shut down before and during certain phases of performance, the capabilities of the right hemisphere can be released. Peak performance can be explained as periods when the two hemispheres of the brain work in perfect harmony with each other, with regard to the specific task and situational demands. There is a widespread belief in sport psychology that an individual's preferred processing bias necessitates a complementary mode for the teaching of motor skills. *See also under* PEAK EXPERIENCE.

Bibliography

Blakeslee, T.R. (1980). *The right brain: A new understanding of the unconscious mind and its creative powers*. New York: Anchor Press/ Doubleday.

Boutcher, S.H. and Rotella, R.J. (1987). A psychological skills educational program for closed-skill performance enhancement. *The Sport Psychologist* 1, 127-137.

Fairweather, M.M. and Sidaway, B. (1994). Implications of hemispheric function for the effective teaching of motor skills. *Quest* 46, 281-298.

Hall, E.G. and Hardy, C.J. (1982). Using the 'right' brain in sport. In: Salmela, J.H., Partington, J.T. and Orlick, T. (eds). *New paths of sport learning and excellence*. pp104-108. Ottawa: Sport in Perspectives.

Ornstein, R.E. (1972). *The psychology of consciousness*. New York: Harcourt, Brace, Joranovich.

COHESION Cohesiveness. The tendency of team or group members to 'stick together' and remain united in pursuit of its goals and objectives. It involves loyalty, commitment and a willingness to make individual sacrifices for the benefit of the group. The subjective experience of cohesion is team spirit.

Sociometric cohesion refers to the amount of 'liking' amongst group members. **Task cohesion** refers to the group members' satisfaction with the group, in terms of its ability to allow a person to obtain desired goals. The research evidence suggests that performance has more of an effect on cohesion than cohesion has on performance.

In addition to cohesiveness, teams develop syntality and synergy. **Syntality** is to a group what personality is to an individual, and communicates what the team is to itself and to others. It includes what members have created as a team culture, ethic, image, and vision, as well as what they themselves are. **Synergy** is a special kind of energy that moves a team. It is a combination of the drives, needs, motives and vitality of the members.

Rowing is a coacting sport, requiring less interdependence for team success than other types of sports. In rowing, crew members can successfully meet their goals without extensively affiliating with others. This was shown by Lenk (1969) to be the case with a German rowing crew, which became Olympic champions despite strong internal conflicts. *See also* TEAM.

Bibliography

Anshel, M.H. (2003). *Sport psychology: From theory to practice*. 4th ed. San Francisco: Benjamin Cummings.

Brawley, L.R. (1990). Group cohesion: Status, problems, and future directions. *International Journal of Sport Psychology* 21(4), 355-379.

Carron, A.V. (1984). Cohesion in sport teams. In: Silva, J.M. and Weinberg, R.S. (eds). *Psychological foundations of sport*. pp340-352. Champaign, Illinois: Human Kinetics.

Carron, A.V. et al. (2002). Cohesion and performance in sport: A meta-analysis. *Journal of Sport and Exercise Psychology* 24(2), 168-188.

Lenk, H. (1969). Top performance despite internal conflict. An antithesis to a functional proposition. In Loy, J. and Kenyon, G. (eds). *Sport, culture and society: A reader on the sociology of sport*. Toronto, ON: MacMillan.

Lumsden, D.L. and Lumsden, G. (1999). *Communicating in groups and teams: Sharing leadership*. Belmont, CA: Wadsworth.

Syer, J. (1986). *Team spirit*. London: Kingswood Press.

COLD *See under* COLD STRESS; UPPER RESPIRATORY TRACT INFECTION.

COLD PRESSOR REFLEX Immersion of the hand in ice water for several minutes causes vasoconstriction, tachycardia and transient hypertension due to activation of the sympathetic nervous system.

COLD STRESS Stimulation of cold receptors in the skin causes constriction of peripheral blood vessels and a redirection of blood flow to the warmer core and away from the cooler periphery. Thus, core temperature rises and skin temperature falls. The hypothalamus begins to lose its thermoregulatory ability when core temperature falls below 34.5 degrees Celsius. Dehydration decreases blood flow to the skin, which can lead to cold injury. The skin and subcutaneous fat provides insulation.

The main mechanisms for avoiding excessive cooling of the body are shivering, non-shivering thermogenesis and peripheral vasoconstriction. **Shivering** is controlled by somatic nerves and involves involuntary muscular contractions. It is initiated at the spinal level, as well as by neurons in the anterior hypothalamus. During exercise in the cold, shivering may not be necessary due to the elevated metabolism associated with exercise. **Non-shivering thermogenesis** involves stimulation of metabolism by the sympathetic nervous system. Peripheral vasoconstriction occurs as a result of sympathetic stimulation of smooth muscle surrounding the arterioles in the skin. This stimulation causes the muscle to contract, constricting the arterioles and decreasing the blood flow from the core to the periphery in order to prevent unnecessary heat loss. The metabolic rate of skin cells also decreases as the skin's temperature falls, so that the skin requires less oxygen.

An increase in exercise intensity may not help maintain body temperature, because of increased heat lost by evaporation from the respiratory passages, increased air or water movement over the surface of the body and a pumping of air or water under the clothing.

Repeated exposure to cold may alter peripheral

blood flow and skin temperatures, allowing greater tolerance of cold stress. Acclimatization to cold stress takes about ten days. Following acclimatiza-tion, shivering begins at a lower skin temperature. This is because cold-acclimatized individuals maintain heat production by increasing non-shivering thermogenesis at the expense of shivering. Cold acclimatization seems to result in improved intermittent peripheral vasodilation to increase the flow of blood and heat to both the hands and feet. In this way, cold-acclimatized individuals are able to maintain a higher average hand-and-foot tempera-ture during cold stress when compared to unacclimatized individuals. Cold acclimatization enables individuals to sleep better in cold environments due to increased non-shivering thermogenesis. Shivering makes it difficult for unacclimatized individuals to sleep in cold environments.

In extreme cold, the greater surface-area-to-mass ratio in children results in a higher rate of heat loss. The lower body fat in girls, compared with women, provides lower insulation and is disadvantageous in a cold environment. In a cold environment, children are characterized by lower skin temperatures, reflecting greater vasoconstriction. Their metabolic heat is increased in the cold to a greater extent than that of adults and this appears to be sufficient to maintain their body temperature during exercise, but not during prolonged rest. There is limited evidence that training may improve thermo-regulation during cold exposure in children.

In cold weather, clothing should be impermeable to heat loss by evaporation. Insulation is increased by wearing several layers of clothing. This traps more air next to the skin than is possible with a single layer of clothing. The air trapped by the cloth fibers becomes warm. The inner layer of clothing should insulate and wick moisture to the outer layer where it can evaporate. Polypropylene 'long johns' (tight underwear) have good wicking and insulation properties. **Wicking** is a capillary action that takes sweat away from the body surface, decreasing the cooling effect of evaporation, thus improving clothing's effectiveness for conserving body heat. Dupont has designed a fabric called CoolMax®, which wicks moisture away from the skin better than

wool and polypropylene. Relative humidity is the most important factor determining the effectiveness of evaporative heat loss. Cotton is not suitable, because it soaks up moisture and keeps it by the skin. For the middle layer, wool can be used because it is a good insulator even when wet. When clothing becomes wet, insulation is decreased and heat loss (especially from evaporation) is greatly increased. The outer layer should be a windproof and water repellent, but breathable fabric such as *Gore-Tex*. Head gear enhances the conservation of heat, because up to 40% of body heat can be lost through the head. The following factors affect the insulation value of clothing: wind speed (increased speed disturbs the zone of insulation), body movements (oscillatory actions of the arms and legs disturb the zone of insulation), chimney effect (loosely hanging clothing ventilates the trapped air layers away from the body), bellows effect (vigorous body movements increase ventilation of air layers for conserving body heat), water vapor transfer (clothing resists the passage of water vapor and thus decreases body heat loss by evaporative cooling) and permeation efficiency factor (how well clothing absorbs liquid sweat by wicking).

The **clo unit** is an index of thermal resistance. It indicates the insulating capacity provided by any layer of trapped air between the skin and clothing, including the clothing's insulation value. Assuming an environment with negligible air movement and body movement to disturb the circulatory layer of air about the body, one clo unit maintains a sedentary person at 1 MET indefinitely in an environment of 21 degrees Celsius (68.8 Fahrenheit) and 50% relative humidity.

Frostnip and frostbite are freezing injuries. In **frostnip**, only the outer layer of skin is frozen. **Superficial frostbite** injures the outer layer of skin, plus some underlying tissue. **Severe frostbite** involves crystallization of fluid in the skin. The crystals pierce skin cell membranes, resulting in necrosis. There are a number of non-freezing injuries, including **chilblain (pernio)**, which is an exaggerated cold-induced vasoconstriction that results in cell ischemia and limb edema. *See also* WIND CHILL.

Bibliography

Armstrong, L.E. (2000). *Performing in extreme environments*. Champaign, IL: Human Kinetics.

Doubt, T.J. (1991). Physiology of exercise in the cold. *Sports Medicine* 11(6), 367-381.

Falk, B. (1998). Effects of thermal stress during rest and exercise in the pediatric population. *Sports Medicine* 25(4), 221-240.

Gavin, T.P. (2003). Clothing and thermoregulation during exercise. *Sports Medicine* 33(13), 941-947.

Noakes, T.D. (2000). Exercise and the cold. *Ergonomics* 43(10), 1461-1479.

Rowland, T.W. (1996). *Developmental exercise physiology*. Champaign, IL: Human Kinetics.

Shephard, R.J. (1985). Adaptation to exercise in the cold. *Sports Medicine* 2, 59-71.

Stamford, B. (1994). Hot tips for cold-weather workouts. *The Physician and Sportsmedicine* 22(1), 111-112.

COLLAGEN   A fibrous protein that serves as the major component of certain connective tissues such as ligaments and tendons. Zyderm® and Zyplast® implants are made of purified bovine (cow) collagen that is used to replenish the skin's natural collagen and to smooth facial lines and wrinkles. The implants contain a numbing agent called lidocaine that is used to help ensure patients' comfort during the injection procedure. Risks include an allergic reaction to collagen. *See also* VITAMIN C.

COLLECTIVE EFFICACY   *See under* TEAM.

COLLES' FRACTURE   *See under* ELBOW FRACTURES.

COLLINEAR FORCES   Forces having lines of action lie along the same line.

COLON   *See under* GASTROINTESTINAL SYSTEM.

COLUBOMA   A birth defect that causes a cleft in the pupil, iris, lens, retina, choroids or optic nerve. It can result in decreased acuity and field loss if the damage extends to the retina.

COMMERCIALISM   The development of commercialism in the USA can be traced back to the urbanization and liberal attitude in the nineteenth century. Among the most important factors that made possible commercialization of sports in the USA are the unique legal standing of the professional sports leagues and the heavy involvement of the media. The US government allowed the professional leagues to function as monopolies, without breaking the anti-trust laws. The strong connection between television and sport came about primarily through the growing trend towards passive sports intake.

The Olympics can be understood in terms of the inter-relationships between nationalism, commercialism and amateurism. Whannel (1992) argued that the globalization of sport should be termed "Americanization." For the 1988 Olympic Games at Seoul, the American television networks requested, and succeeded in changing, the schedule of events for prime-time television in order to ensure they made a profit from broadcasting the Olympic Games. This further accelerated the commercialization of the Olympics.

Media emphasis on the 'bottom line' of wins and losses reveals the business nature of sport. Competitive individualism appears to be the salient theme in media portrayals of sport, regardless of whether or not the text focuses on individual or team sports. From a content analysis of the sportscasters' commentary during a televised Super Bowl football game, it was concluded that the dominant values communicated were those of individualism and achievement, and that the salience of the sportscasters' specific comments provided a vehicle for value transmission. Three ways in which individual athletes are highlighted in media coverage include the focus on star players when teams are discussed, the focus on one or two star performers in individual events and the use of star athletes as commentators.

The poor performance of America at the 1984 Olympic Games was attributed by the media to character flaws of the athletes. Holding people individually responsible for the hardships they endure is a common way to explain failure in capitalist societies. Success is thought to be available to all those who work hard, and those who fail have only themselves to blame. While teamwork and competitive individualism seem to be contradictory themes, they are both an important part of capitalist society. The media portrayal of teamwork in sport is often defined in terms of obedience to authority, maintaining loyalty to the group and placing the good of the group above individual interest.

Chronology

•1926 • John Logie Baird invented the television.

•1936 • In the UK, the first televised soccer match was shown: Arsenal versus Everton.

•1939 • Columbia versus Princeton in baseball was the first sporting event ever to be televised in the USA. The single camera, placed on a large platform, close to the home plate with a range of 50 feet, focused on the batter, catcher and umpire. Only 400 sets could pick up the game.

•1948 • The Olympic Games were held in London. It was the first Games to be widely televised in the UK, but only 80,000 people had televisions in their home.

•1956 • CBS became the first network to broadcast some NFL regular-season games to selected television markets.

•1962 • The NFL entered into a single-network agreement with CBS for telecasting all regular-season games for $4.65 million annually.

•1963 • The Army versus Navy football game facilitated the development of professional football as a made-for-TV sport. In the same year, instant replay was made available when Ampex introduced the industry-standard EDITEC electronic video editor allowing frame-by-frame recording control.

•1968 • Color television pictures of the Olympic Games were produced for the first time.

•1970 • Monday Night Football started when the American Broadcasting Company (ABC) acquired the rights to televise 13 NFL regular-season Monday night games in 1970, 1971 and 1972.

•1976 • Ozzie and Dan Silna, owners of the Spirits of St. Louis from the American Basketball Association (ABA) pulled off one of the most incredible business deals ever when the ABA merged with the National Basketball Association (NBA). In 1975, it had been agreed by the ABA owners that no less than six teams should be taken in a possible merger and that the seventh team should be paid off in a proper manner. However, only four ABA teams were allowed into the NBA. At the end of the 1974-5 season, the Virginia Squires folded and John Y. Brown, the Kentucky Fried Chicken owner who also owned the Kentucky Colonels accepted a $3 million buyout (which he used later to buy the Boston

Celtics). Ozzie Silna then had representatives from the other four teams – the Denver Nuggets, Indiana Pacers, New York Nets and San Antonio Spurs sign an agreement to share one-seventh of their national television revenues in perpetuity with the Silnas. At that time NBA television revenues were very small, but with the arrival of Larry Bird, Magic Johnson and Michael Jordan the revenues grew substantially and the Silnas have collected approximately $100 million from the NBA.

•1992 • Worldwide coverage of Olympic basketball provided the NBA with publicity worth many millions of dollars. The NBA finals are now televised in about 200 countries.

Bibliography

Bailey, C.I. and Sage, G.H. (1988). Values communicated by a sports event: The case of the Super Bowl. *Journal of Sport Behavior* 11(3), 126-143.

Hargreaves, J. (1992). Olympism and nationalism: Some preliminary considerations. *International Review for the Sociology of Sport* 27(2), 119-137.

Kinkema, K.M. and Harris, J.C. (1992). Sport and the mass media. *Exercise and Sport Sciences Reviews* 20, 127-59.

Lobmeyer, H. and Weidinger, L. (1992). Commercialism as a dominant factor in the American sport scene: Sources, developments, perspectives. *International Review for the Sociology of Sport* 27(4), 309-327.

Min, G. (1987). Over-commercialization of the Olympics 1988: The role of the US television networks. *International Review for the Sociology of Sport* 22(2), 137-142.

Sage, G.H. (1990). *Power and ideology in American sport*. Champaign, IL: Human Kinetics.

Seppaenen, P. (1984). The Olympics: A sociological perspective. *International Review for the Sociology of Sport* 19(2), 145-156.

Whannel, G. (1992). *Fields of vision: Television, sport and cultural transformation*. London: Routledge.

COMMOTIO CORDIS Arrhythmia or sudden death from low-impact, blunt trauma to the chest without apparent heart injury. It is believed to involve a precordial blow that occurs during a period of electrically vulnerable ventricular repolarization. Ventricular fibrillation is the most commonly associated arrhythmia. In baseball, it occurs when a batter is struck in the chest by a pitched ball or when the catcher is struck by a foul-tipped baseball. It has also been reported in other sports including hockey and softball. Only about 10% of reported victims of *commotio cordis* are known to survive. There are 2 to 4 deaths per year. In young athletes, the narrower anteroposterior diameter of the thorax and greater compliance of the chest wall are risk factors.

Preventive measures include education of participants and coaches, chest protection for catchers and possibly batters, and softer baseballs. Because a softer baseball may allow a greater proportion of the ball to enter the eye's orbit, it is precluded from being a measure used to prevent *commotio cordis. See also under* CATASTROPHIC INJURIES.

COMMUNICATION   It is the process of using verbal and nonverbal cues to negotiate a mutually acceptable meaning between two or more people within a particular context and environment. **Assertiveness** involves a person communicating openly and honestly, expressing thoughts, feelings and beliefs in a socially appropriate way that does not violate or infringe on the rights of others. It includes being able to say no; and being able to initiate, continue and finish general conversation. In the context of sport, it can mean not being pushed around or having opponents gain the upper hand, at the same time as being respectful of opponents.

Bibliography

Lumsden, G. and Lumsden, D. (2000). *Communicating in groups and teams: Sharing leadership.* Belmont, CA: Wadsworth.

Connelly, D. and Rotella, R.J. (1991). The social psychology of assertive communication: Issues in teaching assertiveness skills to athletes. *The Sport Psychologist* 5, 73-87.

Spears, L.C. (1998, ed). *Insights on leadership: Service, stewardship, spirit, and servant leadership.* New York: John Wiley & Sons.

COMPARTMENT SYNDROME   *See* LOWER LEG, COMPARTMENT SYNDROME.

COMPENSATION   *See under* MISALIGNMENTS.

COMPETITION   A process in which the comparison of an individual's or team's performance is made with respect to some standard in the presence of at least one other person who is aware of the criterion for comparison and can evaluate the comparison process. While some authors argue that one can compete against oneself, Martens (1975) disagrees, stating that a competitive context excludes the comparison of a person's performance with his previous performance in the absence of an evaluative other. *See* ACHIEVEMENT MOTIVA-TION; SPORT.

Chronology

•1875 • William G. Sumnor taught one of the first sociology courses at Yale University. He was America's leading proponent of Social Darwinism, the social philosophy that justified the 'success ethic' and the 'gospel of wealth.' Social Darwinism is attributed to British sociologist Herbert Spencer, who used Charles Darwin's principles of survival of the fittest in his book *Education: Intellectual, Moral and Physical* (1860). (Charles Darwin's *Origin of Species* was published in 1859.) Sumnor viewed winning as the just reward of hard work from the superior individual, while losing was viewed as the overt manifestation of inferiority. Although Social Darwinism repudiated the humane and Christian principles on which democratic tradition rested, Spencer's theories had great popularity and markedly penetrated North American thought. The rise of highly organized sport coincided with the emergent popularity of Social Darwinism.

•1947 • A Joint Statement of Policy on Interscholastic Athletics by the National Federation of High School Athletic Associations and the American Association for Health, Physical Education and Recreation (AAHPER) recommended that the competitive needs of elementary-age children be met with a balanced intramural program. Two years later, AAHPER and its Society of State Directors of Health, Physical Education and Recreation joined with representatives from the Department of Elementary School Principals, the National Education Association and the National Council of State Consultants in Elementary School Principals to form the Joint Committee on Athletic Competition for Children of Elementary and Junior High School Age.

•1950 • The President's Committee on Interschool Competition in the Elementary School, representing AAHPER, found that 60% of schools surveyed had no competition for elementary-age children. Of the 40% that did have some competitive sport, none had competition below the fourth-grade level.

•1969 • Paul Weiss, Sterling Professor of Philosophy at Yale University, published *Sport: A Philosophic Inquiry.* Weiss argued that sport provides humans with their greatest opportunity to excel. Indeed, the first chapter was entitled "Concern for Excellence" about which Weiss stated, "Illustrating perfection, [excellence] gives us a measure of whatever else we do."

Bibliography

Martens, (1975). *Social psychology and physical activity*. New York: Harper Row.

Martens, R. (1977). *Sport Competition Anxiety Test*. Champaign, IL: Human Kinetics.

COMPLEMENT PROTEINS   Proteins (inactive enzymes) that come from the blood and serve to stimulate phagocytes and basophils, rupture bacteria and increase inflammation. The **complement system** is a non-specific defence mechanism that complements the action of specific antibodies. *See under* IMMUNITY.

COMPLEX   A term used to refer to an ordered aggregate of molecules, as in energy-substrate complex.

COMPLIANCE   The reciprocal of stiffness. It is the amount of elongation per unit of force. *See* BLOOD VESSEL COMPLIANCE.

COMPOSITES   *See under* MATERIALS.

COMPOUNDS   Chemicals that contain two or more elements chemically combined. A compound has a fixed composition, as specified by its chemical formula. *See also under* ELECTRON.

COMPRESSION   Compressive force. Collinear forces act in opposite directions to push a material together. During compressive loading, equal and opposite loads are applied toward the surface of the structure. Compressive stress can be thought of as many small forces directed into the surface of the structure. Compressive stress and strain result inside the structure. Maximal compressive stress occurs on a plane that is perpendicular to the applied load. Under compressive loading, the structure shortens and widens. *See under* BENDING; BONE; ELASTIC MODULI; FRACTURES; MUSCLE ACTION; MUSCLE STRAIN.

COMPULSIONS   *See under* ANXIETY DISORDERS.

COMPUTED AXIAL TOMOGRAPHY An x-ray test of a body organ, such as the brain, that uses computer reconstruction of multiple images at different planes. It is commonly referred to as a CAT scan.

CONCENTRATION   Amount of substance per unit volume (mol/m^3).

CONCENTRIC MUSCLE ACTION   *See under* MUSCLE ACTION.

CONCUSSION   *See under* HEAD INJURIES.

CONDENSATION   i) Transformation from a gas to a liquid. ii) A type of chemical reaction in which two or more molecules join together to form a larger molecule.

CONDUCTANCE   The reciprocal of resistance, thus the ease with which charged particles move through an object.

CONDUCT DISORDER   A pattern of persistent and repetitive behaviors that violate the basic rights of others and/or major age-appropriate societal norms or rules. These behaviors can be categorized as follows: aggressive conduct that causes or threatens physical harm to other people or animals; destruction of property, deceitfulness, lying, or theft; and serious violations of major rules or laws (e.g. truancy from school).

The prevalence of conduct disorder for males ranges from 6 to 16%, while those for females range from 2 to 9%. Attention-deficit hyperactivity disorder is often diagnosed in children with conduct disorder. Individuals with conduct disorder are considered to be at risk of several adult disorders, including substance-related abuse, mood disorders and anxiety disorders. Without effective interventions, many individuals with conduct disorder become juvenile delinquents.

Juvenile mania can be very similar to conduct disorder, but is distinguished by its episodic nature. Adults with conduct disorder are usually given the diagnosis of antisocial personality disorder.

Bibliography

American Psychiatric Association (1994). *Diagnostic and Statistical Manual of Mental Disorders*. 4ᵗʰ ed. Washington, DC: American Psychiatric Association.

CONDUCTION   *See under* THERMO-REGULATION.

CONFLICT   *See under* SOCIOLOGY; TEAM.

CONFORMITY   *See under* TEAM.

CONGENITAL   Of, or pertaining to something (e.g. a defect), which is present in a person at birth, but is not necessarily innate.

CONGENITAL ADRENAL HYPERPLASIA   It is a group of inherited disorders that can cause lifelong disorders and even death. It is inherited as an autosomal recessive trait.

A distinction can be made between classical and nonclassical types of congenital adrenal hyperplasia. The effects of **classical congenital adrenal hyperplasia** occur as a result of imbalance of cortisol, aldosterone and androgens. Lack of aldosterone production occurs in 3 out of 4 cases of the classical type, and results in a life-threatening difficulty in retaining salt. Girls with the classical type are born with masculine appearing external genitals due to high levels of androgens *in utero*. Although their internal organs are normal, excess androgens may affect puberty and result in irregular menstrual periods, excessive hair growth and infertility. The classical type occurs in one in every 15,000 persons.

Nonclassical congenital adrenal hyperplasia is a mild version of the classical form of the disease. The same gene is affected, but defects are much less severe. The nonclassical type occurs in at least one in every 1,000 people, but its incidence is higher in certain ethnic groups, such as Hispanics.

Bibliography

Congenital Adrenal Hyperplasia. Http://www.congenitaladrenalhyperplasia.org

The Endocrine Society. Http://www.endo-society.org

CONJUGATED PROTEIN   A protein containing a prosthetic group. A metal or organic group (but not an amino acid), which is bound to a protein and serves as its active group. Examples are lipoproteins and glycoproteins.

CONJUNCTIVA   The membrane between the inner lining of the eyelid and anterior eyeball. **Conjunctivitis** ('pink eye') is inflammation, often due to chlorine irritation in swimming pools, or bacterial infection of the conjunctiva. **Subconjunctival hemorrhage** is caused by direct trauma and results in rupture of several small capillaries, making the white sclera of the eye appear red, blotchy and inflamed.

CONNECTIVE TISSUE   A number of different tissues come under the category of connective tissue due to their common function of connecting and supporting other tissues. It is the most abundant and widespread tissue in the body.

Cells, extracellular matrix and tissue fluid are the structural elements of connective tissues. **Fibroblasts** are large, flat, spindle-shaped cells that produce the extracellular matrix. In connective tissues, the extracellular matrix is a blend of components, including protein fibers (collagen and elastin), simple and complex matrix glycoproteins, and tissue fluid (filtrate of the blood that resides in the interstitial spaces). When a fibroblast becomes mature, it is also known as a **fibrocyte**.

Embryonic connective tissue is found primarily in the embryo or fetus. **Mesenchyme** is the undifferentiated embryonic tissue that develops into the mature connective tissue. It is composed of a semi-fluid ground substance that contains reticular fibers. Embedded in this matrix are star-shaped embryonic cells. Mesenchyme arises during the early weeks of embryological development and eventually differentiates into all other connective tissues.

Mature connective tissue can be classified as loose connective tissue, dense connective tissue, cartilage, bone tissue and vascular (blood) tissue. **Loose connective tissue** comprises loosely woven protein fibers and many cells. The loose connective tissues are areolar connective tissue, adipose tissue and reticular connective tissue. **Areolar connective tissue** comprises an extracellular matrix of a semi-fluid ground substance. The most abundant cells are the fibroblasts. Areolar connective tissue also contains white blood cells, especially macrophages. Areolar connective tissue is soft and pliable. It ensheathes organs, blood vessels and nerves. It also forms the subcutaneous layer below the skin. **Adipose tissue** contains large numbers of adipocytes (fat cells), which develop from fibroblasts. Adipose tissue is found wherever areolar connective tissue is found. It is found in the subcutaneous layer below the skin (where it acts as a shock absorber and insulates against heat loss), the abdomen (primarily in men), hips and thighs (primarily in women), bone marrow, around the kidney and heart, behind the eyeballs and around joints. Adipose tissue is also a major energy reserve for the body. **Reticular connective tissue** consists of a network of interlacing reticular fibers. It is included in the supporting framework (stroma) for many soft organs, including the liver and spleen.

Dense connective tissue consists of numerous fibers that are densely packed in its matrix. It has fewer fibroblasts and other cells. It includes dense regular connective tissue, dense irregular tissue and elastic connective tissue. **Dense regular connective tissue** contains bundles of collagen fibers, arranged parallel to each other, enabling the connective tissue to resist tension in one direction. Dense regular connective tissue makes up tendons and most ligaments. **Dense irregular connective tissue** contains randomly arranged collagen fibers, enabling the connective tissue to resist tension in all directions. It is found in the dermis (deep layer) of the skin. It also forms fibrous capsules around joints and organs such as the kidneys and liver. **Elastic connective tissue** contains most elastic fibers. It forms the ligaments between vertebrae, the vocal cords, and is also found in lung tissue.

Resistance exercise training also provides growth of and/or increases the strength of connective tissues such as ligaments, tendons, tendon to bone and ligament-to-bone junctions, articular cartilage, fascia and bones. Resistance training has been shown to increase the thickness of hyaline cartilage on the articular surfaces of bone. Increasing the thickness of this cartilage may facilitate improved shock absorption between the bony surfaces of a joint. It seems that to most effectively stimulate the growth of connective tissues, high-intensity exercise should be used and anti-gravity muscles should be active. Load-bearing activities may be most effective in stimulating bone formation. There is evidence that various types of overuse injuries may be decreased by specific resistance training. Overtraining may adversely affect connective tissue growth. *See also* BLOOD; BONE; CARTILAGE; DURA MATER; FASCIA; JOINT CAPSULES; LIGAMENTS; STRETCHING; TENDONS.

Bibliography

Stone, M.H. (1992). Connective tissue and bone response to strength training. In: Komi, P.V. (ed). *Strength and power in sport.* pp279-290. Oxford: Blackwell Scientific Publications.

CONSCIOUSNESS i) The quality of being aware of objects in the environment or being aware of some of one's thoughts, perceptions or emotions. ii) The condition of a person such that he or she is alert and able to act, i.e. awake rather than asleep or unconscious. **Readiness potential** is a gradual negative shift in electrical potential. Voluntary acts are preceded by a readiness potential about 550 ms before the action occurs, and about 200 ms before subjects record a conscious intent to act. This suggests that consciousness is constructed well after the fact, and even that consciousness may be unimportant. Libet (1985) argued that the function of consciousness is to veto unconsciously initiated actions – whether or not the action actually takes place or not can still be decided consciously by a subject.

See ALTERED STATES OF CONSCIOUSNESS; AROUSAL; ATTENTION

Bibliography

Libet, B. (1985). Unconscious cerebral initiative and the role of conscious will in voluntary action. *Behavioral and Brain Sciences* 8, 528-566.

Libet, B. (1987). Are the mental experiences of will and self-control significant for the performance of a voluntary act? *Behavioral and Brain Sciences* 10, 783-786.

Libet, B. (1989). The timing of a subjective experience. *Behavioral and Brain Sciences* 12, 183-185.

CONSTIPATION   *See under* GASTRO-INTESTINAL SYSTEM.

CONTACT LENSES   A **scleral lens** is a large diameter contact lens that goes beyond the cornea to cover the sclera (white portion of the eye). Modern scleral lenses are made of plastics, such as polymethylacrylate, silicone-acrylate and fluoro-silicone acrylate, and are designed to allow oxygen to enter the cornea and to allow the lens to become wet in the eye. Relatively tight, large diameter, medium thickness, low water content lenses will provide the greatest in-eye stability, which appears to be an important pre-requisite for most sports.

When swimming, scleral lenses stick to the cornea in fresh water (hypotonic), probably due to an osmotic effect rather than a tightening of the lens. A lens that has been splashed is thus unsafe for removal for at least 20 minutes after leaving the pool. The main risks with wearing contact lenses are from **Acanthamoeba keratitis**, a protozoan that can get underneath a contact lens and cause inflammation of the cornea. In salt water (hypertonic), soft lenses float as freely as they would in the tearing eye. It is recommended that people who wear contact lenses either remove their lenses for swimming or wear non-prescription swimming goggles.

Gas permeable lenses do not dry out, because they do not contain water, thus are useful for athletes, such as ice-hockey goalkeepers, who need to keep their eyes open without blinking. Their permeability allows oxygen to reach the eye better than soft lenses. They are good for correcting astigmatism, because they hold their shape on the eye.

In shooting or archery, small movements of the contact lens and drying out of the front surface of the eye can be visually disturbing.

Bibliography

All About Vision. Http://www.allaboutvision.com

D & J Brower Opticians. Http://www.brower.co.uk

CONTEXTUAL INTERFERENCE   *See under* PRACTICE.

CONTRACEPTIVE PILL   *See* ORAL CONTRA-CEPTIVES.

CONTRACTURE   Shortening of tissue that may produce distortion or deformity, and abnormal limitation of movement of a joint. **Physiologic contracture** results from mechanical, chemical or other agents acting directly on the contractile mechanism of skeletal muscle, without involving an action potential, such as when a working muscle becomes fatigued. **Myostatic contracture** is a fibrotic condition of the supporting connective tissues of a muscle or joint, resulting from immobilization of the muscle in the short position while the nerve-muscle unit remains intact. Myostatic contracture occurs after a limb has been immobilized in a cast, after a tendon has been severed or detached, or after antagonistic muscles have been paralyzed. Among persons who spend most of their time in wheelchairs or able-bodied people who sit for prolonged periods of time, hip, knee, and ankle flexors tend to become excessively shortened.

CONTRAST   Subjective assessment of the difference in appearance of two parts of a field of view seen simultaneously or successively.

CONTRAST SENSITIVITY   Measurements of contrast sensitivity give an indication of visual sensitivity to detail and how well the eyes see during different weather and lighting conditions. Contrast sensitivity allows a person to see fine details from a distance, e.g. the subtle contours on a golf course.

Some people have difficulty in discriminating between red and green, or between blue and yellow. A reddish-brown football on a green field could be a problem for a player who has color deficiency. This color deficiency is found in about 8% to 10% of males and less than 1% of females. Tests for color deficiency include cards on which are printed random dot patterns in a particular pattern, with an object printed in a different color, and the person has to distinguish the object.

CONTRECOUP INJURY   *See under* HEAD INJURIES.

CONTUSION   An acute injury resulting from a direct, but blunt trauma to a soft tissue (e.g. skin). It usually results in pain, edema and mild-to-severe extravastation of blood into surrounding tissues. Contusions occur more frequently over bony prominences. Chronic blows to the anterior arm or near the distal attachment of the deltoid muscle, where the humerus is least padded by muscle tissue, may lead to development of ectopic bone in either the belly of a muscle (myositis ossificans) or as a bony outgrowth (exostosis) of the underlying bone.

See under HEAD INJURIES; HIP POINTER; HUMERUS; MUSCLE CONTUSION.

CONVECTION   *See under* THERMO-REGULATION.

CONVERGENCE   In vision, movement of the eyes turning inwards or towards each other.

CONVULSION   *See under* EPILEPSY.

COOL DOWN   *See* ACTIVE RECOVERY.

COORDINATION   The patterning of body and limb movements relative to the patterning of environmental objects and events. In terms of motor behavior, it involves various muscles working together in order to constrain the body's limitless movement possibilities (degrees of freedom) into one efficient, functional unit. Between the ages of 2 and 6 years, the child improves gross motor coordination.

Bibliography
Payne, V.G. and Isaacs, L.D. (2004). *Human motor development. A lifespan approach*. 6th ed. Boston, MA: McGraw-Hill.

COPPER   An element that as a 'trace element' in the human body is involved in electron transport and iron metabolism. Copper contributes to cellular antioxidant protection as a co-factor for the antioxidant enzyme, copper-zinc superoxide dismutase. This enzyme, located in the cytosol of cells, is responsible for eliminating superoxide radicals.

Copper is found in a wide variety of foods, but is most plentiful in organ meats, shellfish, nuts and seeds. Liver (1 oz, beef, cooked) contains 1,265 mcg of copper. Cashew nuts (1 oz) contain 629 mcg of copper. The recommended daily allowance (RDA) for copper is based on the prevention of deficiency. In adults, the RDA for copper is 900 mcg/day. To protect against possible liver damage, the tolerable upper intake level (UL) was set at 10 mg per day.

Bibliography
Campbell, W.W. and Anderson, R.A. (1987). Effects of aerobic exercise and training on the trace minerals chromium, zinc and copper. *Sports Medicine* 9, 9-18.

Oregon State University. The Linus Pauling Institute. Micronutrient Information Center. Http://lpi.oregonstate.edu/infocenter

CORE STRENGTH   *See under* INTRA-ABDOMINAL PRESSURE.

CORI CYCLE   The cyclic group of biochemical reactions whereby glycogen is broken down and resynthesized. Muscle glycogen is broken down into lactic acid, which is transported to the liver in the blood. Lactic acid is converted to glycogen and then to glucose. The glucose is transported in the blood to muscle where it is converted into glycogen.

See GLUCONEOGENESIS.

CORIOLIS ACCELERATION   The acceleration that is acting when a body moves with respect to a rotating reference frame.

CORN   A thickening of skin in response to pressure of the skin against a bony prominence. A **hard corn** (*heloma durum; clavus durus*) results from pressure of the toe against the top of a tight-fitting shoe, and is most common along the lateral aspect of the fifth toe at the condyle of the dorsal aspect of the proximal interphalangeal joint. A **soft corn** (*heloma molle; clavus mollis*) results from pressure of the bony prominence of one toe against the bony prominence of an adjacent toe, and is most common at the point of contact between the lateral base of the proximal phalanx of the fourth toe and the medial condyle of the proximal phalanx of the fifth toe.

A **plantar keratosis** is a painful corn caused by pressure on a specific point, especially a minor skeletal defect of the foot. It can be treated with daily filing and by wearing a doughnut-shaped pad.

CORNEA   The transparent anterior portion of the fibrous coat of the globe of the eye. The cornea is the first and most important refracting surface of the eye. *See under* EYE INJURIES.

CORONAL PLANE   *See* FRONTAL PLANE.

CORONARY ARTERY   One of the two arteries that arise from the aorta and supply blood to the muscle of the heart wall. *See* ANGINA PECTORIS.

CORONARY BLOOD FLOW   The main macrovascular vessels comprising the coronary circulation are the left main coronary artery that divides into the left anterior descending and circumflex branches, and the right main coronary artery. These vessels, lying on the epicardial surface of the heart, serve primarily as low resistance, distribution vessels. Branching off these vessels are smaller vessels that enter into the myocardium and become the microvascular resistance vessels, which regulate coronary blood flow and its distribution. These microvascular vessels give rise to a dense capillary network so that each cardiac muscle fiber has several capillaries running parallel to it. The high capillary-to-fiber density ensures short diffusion distances to maximize oxygen transport into the cells and removal of metabolic waste products such as carbon dioxide from the cells.

In disease-free coronary vessels, an increase in cardiac activity and oxygen consumption is accompanied by an increase in coronary blood flow (active hyperemia), which is nearly proportionate to the increase in oxygen consumption. Adenosine and nitric oxide are important regulators of coronary blood flow.

Bibliography

American College of Sports Medicine (2001). *ACSM's resource manual for Guidelines for Exercise Testing & Prescription*. 4th ed. Philadelphia, PA: Lippincott Williams & Wilkins.

CORONARY HEART DISEASE   *See under* CARDIOVASCULAR DISEASE.

CORTEX   *See under* ADRENAL GLANDS; BRAIN.

CORTICAL   *See under* BRAIN.

CORTICOSTEROIDS   Glucocorticosteroids. Any of the hormones produced by the adrenal cortex and their synthetic equivalents. Aldosterone, desoxycorticosterone and corticosterone are classed as mineralocorticoids. Cortisol, cortisone and corticosterone are classed as glucocorticoids. Corticosterone affects carbohydrate, potassium and sodium metabolism. **Cortisol** is the major glucocorticoid (cortisone is released in lesser amounts). Cortisol assists in maintaining blood glucose levels by stimulating the release of amino acids from muscle, by stimulating gluconeogenesis in the liver, and by helping mobilize free fatty acids from adipose tissue. Cortisol also affects connective tissue development and the amount of water in the body. Systemic corticosteroids (glucocorticoids) are synthetic derivatives of the natural steroid, cortisol. Examples are prednisone, prednisolone and hydrocortisone.

Corticotropin (adrenocorticotropic hormone) is a polypeptide released from the corticotrope cells of the anterior pituitary gland. **Tetracosactrin** (e.g. Synacthen) is the synthesized form with full biological activity. Clinically, tetracosactrin is used for the differential diagnosis of adrenocortical failure. A decline in blood glucose level stimulates the hypothalamus to secrete corticotropin-releasing factor, which then stimulates the anterior pituitary gland to release corticotropin, which, in turn, causes the adrenal cortex to release cortisol into the circulation. There is increased secretion of cortisol as exercise intensity increases. Trained individuals usually have higher levels. The secretion of corticotropin is controlled by hypothalamic releasing factor and cortisol. It stimulates the production and release of adrenal hormones, including cortisol and aldosterone. It seems to be secreted more during exercise, due to the increased secretion of cortisol during exercise. Trained individuals usually have higher levels of corticotropin.

Cortisone is largely inactive in humans until it is converted to 17-hydrocortisone (cortisol). As the acetate ester, cortisone is used as an anti-inflammatory and immunosuppresant and for replacement therapy in adrenocortical insufficiency.

Therapeutic use of corticosteroids may be particularly beneficial in the treatment of local inflammation and pain associated with sports injuries. Corticosteroids are lipid soluble and block the body's natural response to inflammation by inhibiting the synthesis of chemical mediators such as prostaglandins, leukotrienes and histamine. Exogenous corticosteroids, such as cortisol and hydrocortisone, have generally been shown to adversely affect the healing of acute strains and contusions. Injection of corticosteroid inside tendons has a deleterious effect on the tendon tissue and is strictly contraindicated. With proper indications, there are only few and trivial complications that may occur with corticosteroid injections. Based on data from one NFL team for all hamstring injuries requiring treatment between 1985 and 1998, it was found that 58 players (13%) sustained severe, discrete injuries with a palpable defect within the substance of the muscle and were treated with intramuscular injection of corticosteroid and anesthetic. There were no complications related to the injection of corticosteroid. Only 9 players (16%) missed any games as a result of their injury.

Corticosteroids are prohibited in all sports by the World Anti-Doping Agency (WADA) when administered orally, rectally, or by intravenous or intramuscular administration. All other routes of administration require a medical notification in accordance with section 8 of the International Standard for Therapeutic Use Exemptions. For the World Anti-Doping Agency Prohibited List 2005, dermatological preparations of glucocorticoids were no longer prohibited (no Therapeutic Use Exemptions required). *See also* ASPIRIN; NON-STEROIDAL ANTI-INFLAMMATORY DRUGS; OVERTRAINING; STEROIDS.

Bibliography

Almekinders, L.C. (1999). Anti-inflammatory treatment of muscular injuries in sport. An update of recent studies. *Sports Medicine* 28(6), 383-388.

Fredberg, U. (1997). Local corticosteroid injection in sport: Review of literature and guidelines for treatment. *Scandanavian Journal of Medicine and Science in Sport* 7(3), 131-139.

Levine, W.N. et al. (2000). Intramuscular corticosteroid injections for hamstring injuries. A 13-year experience in the National Football League. *American Journal of Sports Medicine* 28(3), 297-300.

World Anti-Doping Agency. Http://www.wada-ama.org

COSINE In a right-angled triangle, it is the ratio of the side adjacent to the angle in question to the side that is the hypotenuse.

COSTOCHONDRAL INJURY Injury to cartilage of the ribs. It may occur during collision with another object or as a result of a severe twisting motion of the thorax. This leads to sprain or separation of the costal cartilage where it attaches to the rib or sternum.

COSTO-VERTEBRAL JOINTS Two sets of gliding joints where the ribs articulate with the vertebral column. The first set involves articulation of the heads of the ribs with the bodies of the vertebrae in the thoracic region. The second set involves the articulation of the tubercles of the ribs with the transverse processes of the vertebrae. A slight gliding of the articular surfaces on each other is the only movement at these joints. This results in elevation of the front and middle parts of the ribs.

COUGH A non-respiratory gas movement that occurs from taking a deep breath, closing the glottis and forcing air superiorly from the lungs against the glottis. The glottis opens suddenly and a blast of air rushes upward. It may dislodge foreign particles or mucus from the lower respiratory tract, propelling such matter superiorly. A **sneeze** is similar to a cough, but expelled air is directed through the nasal cavities as well as through the oral cavity. Sneezing clears the upper respiratory tract.

COUGH REFLEX The sequence of events initiated by the sensitivity of the lining of the airways and mediated by the medulla in the brain as a consequence of impulses transmitted by the vagus nerve, resulting in coughing. The **laryngeal reflex** is a type of cough reflex in which irritation of the fauces and larynx causes cough. The **fauces** is the space between the cavity of the mouth and the pharynx, bounded by the soft palate and the base of the tongue.

COUP INJURY *See under* HEAD INJURIES.

COUPLE Two equal and oppositely directed, parallel (but not collinear) forces acting upon a body. In terms of translation, the net effect of these forces is zero and they cause rotation only. For example, the oblique abdominal muscles serve as a force couple to rotate the trunk. The moment of a couple is torque. The moment arm is the equal to the product of the size of the forces and the perpendicular distance between their lines of action.

COUPLED REACTION Two chemical reactions having a common intermediate that acts as a vehicle by which energy can be transferred from one set of reactants to the other (e.g. the production of creatine from creatine phosphate coupled with the production of ATP from ADP). An exergonic reaction drives an endergonic reaction. *See* THERMODYNAMICS.

COVALENT COMPOUNDS *See under* ELECTRON.

COXA VALGA *See under* FEMORAL NECK.

COXA VARA *See under* FEMORAL NECK.

CRACK *See under* COCAINE.

CRAMP A type of immediate muscle soreness. It is a sustained contraction of skeletal muscle that is involuntary, intense and painful. The exact cause is not known.

Night (nocturnal) cramp is any cramp that occurs when an individual is at rest, but it may be due to contractions (perhaps during REM sleep) of the *gastrocnemius* muscle while in the plantar-flexed position.

Heat cramp is associated with dehydration and electrolyte imbalance. It is more common at the beginning of the summer, when people are not yet acclimatized to the heat and lose more electrolytes in their sweat. Adequate hydration and intake of electrolytes from the diet should prevent heat cramp. It may be associated with an underlying condition such as diabetes.

Exercise-associated muscle cramping can be defined as a painful, spasmodic, involuntary contraction of skeletal muscle, which occurs during or immediately after exercise. Important risk factors include muscle fatigue and poor stretching habits. Poor stretching habits could lead to an exaggerated stretch reflex, thereby increasing muscle spindle activity. Schwellnus et al. (1997) hypothesized that exercise-associated muscle cramping is caused by sustained abnormal spinal reflex activity that appears to be secondary to muscle fatigue. Local muscle fatigue is therefore responsible for increased activity of muscle spindles and decreased activity of Golgi tendon organs. Multi-articular muscles can more easily be placed in shortened positions during exercise and would therefore decrease the Golgi tendon organ afferent activity. Sustained abnormal reflex activity would explain increased baseline EMG activity between acute bouts of cramp. Passive stretching invokes afferent activity from the Golgi tendon organ, thereby relieving the cramp and decreasing EMG activity.

Bibliography

Joekes, A.M. (1981). Cramp: A review. *Journal of the Royal Society of Medicine* 75, 546-549.

Levin, S. (1993). Investigating the cause of muscle cramps. *The Physician and Sportsmedicine* 21(7), 111-113.

Schwellnus, M.P., Derman, E.W. and Noakes, T.D. (1997). Aetiology of skeletal muscle 'cramps' during exercise: A novel hypothesis. *Journal of Sports Sciences* 15(3), 277-285.

Stamford, B. (1993). Muscle cramps. Untying the knots. *The Physician and Sportsmedicine* 21(7), 115-116.

CRANIAL FRACTURES   *See under* HEAD INJURIES.

CRANIAL NERVES *See under* BRAIN.

CRANIOSTENOSIS *See under* BRAIN.

CRAWLING   *See under* MOTOR DEVELOP-MENT.

CRAWLING REFLEX   A postural reflex that is believed to be essential for development of sufficient muscle tone for future voluntary creeping. The reflex is elicited by stroking the soles of the feet alternately while the infant lies prone on the floor, causing the legs and arms to move in a crawling-like action. The crawling reflex operates from birth to around 4 months.

C-REACTIVE PROTEIN   A protein that is released by the body in response to acute injury, infection or other inflammatory stimuli. The level of C-reactive protein reflects the amount of inflammation related to atherogenesis, but it is not clear whether it plays a direct role in the process.

CREATINE A substance that is mainly (95%) found in skeletal muscle, with the remainder being mostly found in the heart, brain and testes. About 40% of the creatine found in skeletal muscle is in its free form, the remainder is in its phosphorylated form (i.e. creatine phosphate). The estimated average of creatine obtained from a mixed diet – but especially from meat and fish – is about 1 g per day. Dietary creatine intake accounts for about half of the body's daily need for creatine, with the remainder obtained through endogenous creatine synthesis in the liver, pancreas and kidneys from the following amino-acids: arginine, glycine and methionine. Creatine is excreted in the urine as creatinine. Daily turnover of creatine to creatinine is about 1.6% per day; this amounts to about 2 g per day for a 70 kg male. Creatine is transported into the muscle from the bloodstream.

In the early 1990s, creatine became a popular dietary supplement used by athletes. Creatine supplementation in humans is possible by oral administration of creatine monohydrate, a white powder that is soluble in warm water. Exogenous creatine supplements are often consumed by athletes in amounts of up to 20 g/day for a few days, followed by 1 to 10 g/day for weeks, months or even years.

On a normal diet, muscle total creatine is about 120 to 125 mmol/kg dm (dry mass). Creatine supplementation has been reported to increase creatine stores to as much as 160 mmol/kg dm.

There appear to be wide individual differences in response to creatine supplementation. For some individuals, muscle creatine concentrations increase only slightly. It has been found that creatine levels in skeletal muscle can be increased, and performance of high-intensity intermittent exercise enhanced, following a period of creatine supplementation (20 g/day; 5 g taken 4 times/day for 5 days). One study found that skeletal muscle creatine phosphate could be increased by more than 20%. There is no conclusive evidence that differences in skeletal muscle creatine levels exist between trained and untrained individuals. Vegetarians, with low muscle creatine levels, may gain more benefit from creatine supplementation than people on a normal mixed diet. In controlled laboratory studies, oral creatine supplementation has been shown to be ergogenic in repeated stationary cycling sprints, weight lifting, repetitive sets of muscle contractions (such as knee extensions) and kayak ergometry. The strongest support for the ergogenic potential of creatine supplementation is in repeated maximal bursts of activity, specifically 6- to 30-second bouts of stationary cycling with 20 seconds to 5 minutes rest between bouts. Of approximately 300 studies that have evaluated the ergogenic value of creatine supplementation, about 70% of these studies report statistically significant results while remaining studies generally report non-significant gains in performance. No study reports a statistically ergolytic effect. There is no evidence of an effect of gender or training status on effect size following creatine supplementation. Improvements in performance during high-intensity, intermittent exercise following creatine supplementation may be partly explained by a greater availability of creatine phosphate in the working muscle before each exercise period. This could be a result of a higher pre-exercise concentration, a smaller decrease in muscle pH and a higher rate of resynthesis during recovery periods. Neither maximal oxygen uptake nor endurance exercise performance appears to be enhanced.

The weight gain following creatine ingestion is most likely due to water retention. It has been suggested, however, that creatine may stimulate protein synthesis. It is possible that there is a link between hyperhydration of muscle to increase the water content and acceleration of protein synthesis. Human studies have largely failed to detect any specific effect of creatine ingestion on skeletal muscle protein turnover.

Gastrointestinal disturbances and muscle cramps have been reported occasionally in healthy individuals following use of creatine monohydrate, but the reports are anecdotal. Poortmans and Francaux (2000) found no adverse effects on renal function of creatine supplementation in the short-term (5 days), medium-term (9 days) or long term (up to 5 years). The effects of ingesting megadoses of creatine are not known. Creatine is a small water-soluble molecule easily cleared by the kidney, and the additional nitrogen load resulting from supplementation is small. From limited scientific research, there is no evidence that chronic use of creatine causes adverse changes in renal function. More than 90% of the ingested creatine is removed from the plasma by the kidney and excreted in the urine.

Creatine monohydrate supplementation may increase strength in some types of muscular dystrophy, but Tarnopolsky et al. (2004) did not find that it increased strength of patients with muscular dystrophy type 1.

A major point that relates to the quality of creatine products is the amount of creatine ingested in relation to the amount of contaminants present. During the production of creatine from primary starting materials (e.g. sarcosine), variable amounts of contaminants (dicyandiamide, dihydrotriazines, creatinine, ions) are generated, thus their tolerable concentrations must be defined by specific toxicological research. *See also under* GROWTH.

Chronology

•1832 • French scientist Michel E. Chevreul discovered a new organic constituent in meat that he named creatine.

•1847 • German chemist Justus von Liebig confirmed that creatine was a regular constituent of meat and that the meat of wild foxes killed in the chase contained 10 times the amount of creatine as that of foxes in captivity. He thus concluded that physical work results in the accumulation of creatine.

Bibliography

Balsom, P.D., Soderlund, K. and Ekblom, B. (1994). Creatine in humans with special reference to creatine supplementation. *Sports Medicine* 18(4), 268-280.

Benzi, G. (2000). Is there a rationale for the use of creatine either as nutritional supplementation or drug administration in humans participating in a sport? *Pharmacological Research* 41(3), 255-264.

Benzi, G. and Ceci, A. (2001). Creatine as nutritional supplementation and medicinal product. *Journal of Sports Medicine and Physical Fitness* 41(1), 1-10.

Branch, J.D. (2003). Effect of creatine supplementation on body composition and performance: A meta-analysis. *International Journal of Sport Nutrition and Exercise Metabolism* 13(2), 198-226.

Demant, T.W. and Rhodes, E.C. (1999). Effects of creatine supplementation on exercise performance. *Sports Medicine* 28(1), 49-60.

Farquhar, W.B. and Zambraski, E.J. (2002). Effects of creatine use on the athlete's kidney. *Current Sports Medicine Reports* 1, 103-106.

Kreider, R.B. (2003). Effects of creatine supplementation on performance and training adaptations. *Molecular and Cell Biochemistry* 244, 89-94.

Maughan, R.J. (1995). Creatine supplementation and exercise performance. *International Journal of Sport Nutrition* 5, 94-101.

Maughan, R.J., King, D.S. and Lea, T. (2004). Dietary supplements. *Journal of Sports Sciences* 22, 95-113.

Mesa, J.L. et al. (2002). Oral creatine supplementation and skeletal muscle metabolism in physical exercise. *Sports Medicine* 32(14), 903-944.

Poortmans, J.R. and Francaux, M. (2000). Adverse effects of creatine supplementation. Fact or fiction? *Sports Medicine* 30(3), 155-170.

Spriet, L.L. and Gibala, M.J. (2004). Nutritional strategies to influence adaptations to training. *Journal of Sports Sciences* 22, 127-141.

Tarnopolsky, M. et al. (2004). Creatine monohydrate supplementation does not increase muscle strength, lean body mass, or muscle phosphocreatine in patients with myotonic dystrophy type 1. *Muscle and Nerve* 29(1), 51-58.

Williams, M.H, Kreider, R.B. and Branch, D.J. (1999). *Creatine: The power supplement*. Champaign, IL: Human Kinetics.

CREATINE PHOSPHATE   Phosphocreatine. A substance found in muscle cells and involved in one of the anaerobic energy systems, i.e. the **alactacid system** (also known as the **creatine phosphate system** or **phosphocreatine system**). The alactacid system is the immediate energy system and uses ATP and creatine phosphate that is stored in cells. There is about 3 to 4 times more creatine phosphate than ATP in skeletal muscle. Creatine phosphate cannot be used as an immediate source of energy, but it can rapidly replenish ATP. In order to supply sufficient ATP to support explosive sprint performance, ATP must be generated from creatine phosphate in a reaction catalyzed by the enzyme **creatine kinase**. With high-intensity exercise, the creatine phosphate stores in a skeletal muscle could be totally depleted within 10 seconds. The rate of creatine phosphate degradation has been shown to be higher in Type II muscle fibers than in Type I fibers. There is evidence that creatine phosphate is used even during steady-state metabolic conditions. Energy for the resynthesis of creatine phosphate comes from oxidation of hydrogen atoms, which are available from glycolysis and the Krebs cycle. Replenishment of creatine phosphate has been linked to the fast component excess post-exercise oxygen consumption and to power recovery in repeated bouts. About 50% of creatine phosphate (i.e. its half life) is replenished in 30 seconds with full replenishment taking about 2 minutes. It appears that high-intensity exercise, involving larger muscle mass, displays a stronger relationship between maximal oxygen uptake and creatine phosphate resynthesis than does intense exercise utilizing small muscle mass. The alactacid system resynthesizes more quickly during complete rest. Following exercise that results in the depletion creatine phosphate stores and an increase in lactate and hydrogen ion accumulation (from the lactic acid

system), it will require longer to return to the pre-exercise state.

The **creatine phosphate shuttle** is the transfer of inorganic phosphate from ATP in the mitochondria to creatine and ADP in the cytosol. The source of the phosphate is the terminal phosphate of ATP formed from glycolysis and mitochondrial respiration. The presence of creatine kinase, a mitochondrial-bound enzyme, is important for the creatine phosphate shuttle to provide a rapid means of phosphate transfer from the mitochondria to the cytosol. The transfer of phosphate molecules is thought to occur in concert with the activities of the adenylate kinase and respective ATPase enzymes. If muscle contraction is too intense for mitochondrial respiration to restore the cytosolic creatine phosphate concentration, a decrease in creatine phosphate and an increased stimulation of mitochondrial respiration will occur. Severe decreases in creatine phosphate lead to further increases in production of ADP, slight decreases in production of ATP, production of AMP and a decreased cytosolic phosphorylation potential. Creatine phosphate buffers the intracellular hydrogen ions associated with lactate production and muscle fatigue during exercise.

CREATININE   A metabolite that is produced in muscle cells from the breakdown of creatine phosphate. While creatine can be resynthesized to creatine phosphate, the production of creatinine from creatine is irreversible. *See also under* BODY COMPOSITION; CREATINE.

CREEP   The phenomenon that occurs in a viscoelastic material when it is loaded, under constant stress, for a prolonged period of time. The greater the load, the faster the material will deform toward failure. If the load is removed, the material gradually regains its original size and shape. Repetitive loading will lead to cumulative creep.
    See CARTILAGE; STRESS RELAXATION.

CREPITUS   Crepitation. (i) A dry, crackling sound or sensation heard along with the breath sounds in various lung diseases. (ii) A 'crackling' sound that is usually caused by a tendon's tendency to stick to the surrounding structure while it slides back and forth. This sticking is due primarily to the chemical products of inflammation that accumulate on the irritated tendons. (iii) A clicking sound often heard in movements of joints, e.g. the temporomandibular joint as a result of joint irregularities. (iv) The discharge of flatus from the bowels.

CRITICAL PERIOD   Sensitive period. In the context of human development, it is the time of particular sensitivity to environmental stimuli. An **epigenic period** is a prenatal period during which there is particular sensitivity to environmental harm. It appears that there are critical periods for all aspects of human behavior. Inadequate nutrition, prolonged stress, inconsistent nurturing or a lack of appropriate learning experiences may have a more negative impact on development if they occur early in life rather than at a later age. Appropriate intervention during a specific period tends to facilitate more positive forms of development at later stages than if the intervention occurs at another time.

Readiness refers to the maximum sensitivity or readiness for the development of a particular pattern or skill. There are no signs, however, that indicate that a child is ready. Some individuals are ready to learn new skills when others are not. Hence, the tendency to exhibit individual differences is closely related to the concept of readiness.   *See* TERATOGEN.

Chronology
•1999 • The Youth Sport Coalition of the National Association for Sport and Physical Education (NASPE) produced a document entitled "Choosing the Right Sport or Physical Activity for your Child," which encouraged parents and guardians to consider the following in order to evaluation school- or community-based programs: i) administration and organization of the program; ii) safety considerations; iii) child's readiness to participate; iv) parent/guardian commitment to child's participation; and v) evaluation of the program.

CROSSED ADDUCTOR REFLEX   Adduction of one leg when an attempt is made to elicit the knee jerk reflex on the opposite side.

CROSSED-EXTENSOR REFLEX   *See under* WITHDRAWAL REFLEX.

CROSS TRAINING   A form of training that is either 'dissimilar mode' (participation in an alternative training, which is not task- or sport-specific) or 'similar mode' (combining an alternative training mode with task- or sport-specific training). Highly trained athletes gain more from similar-mode cross training, while individuals with low aerobic capacity gain more from dissimilar-mode cross training. Research evidence suggests that within each fitness level, a higher aerobic capacity is associated with a smaller relative improvement from cross training. Similar-mode cross training may be useful to athletes who are injured or who are looking for an alternative activity during the off-season.

Bibliography
Loy, S.F., Hoffman, J.J. and Holland, G.J. (1995). Benefits and practical use of cross training in sports. *Sports Medicine* 19(1), 1-8.

Moran, G.T. and McGlynn, G.H. (1997). *Cross training for sports*. Champaign, IL: Human Kinetics.

CRURAL INDEX   The ratio of lower leg length to thigh length. A high crural index allows application of force against the ground for a greater period of time than a lower crural index. Jumping athletes (such as in basketball) and sprint swimmers tend to have above-average crural indices. Long-distance runners, gymnasts and weightlifters tend to have below-average crural indices.   *See* PROPORTIONALITY.

CUBITAL TUNNEL SYNDROME   Irritation or compression of the ulnar nerve within the cubital tunnel at the elbow. It is the second most common compressive neuropathy of the upper extremity after carpal tunnel syndrome, and is common in competitive cyclists. The ulnar nerve runs along the medial edge of the elbow, just behind the epicondyle, to the common flexor origin. Cubital tunnel syndrome may be caused by direct trauma to the ulnar nerve in the cubital tunnel, repetitive elbow flexion, hypermobility of the ulnar nerve, excessive valgus of the elbow, or impingement of the ulnar nerve by osteophytes or loose bodies. The cubital tunnel narrows as the elbow is flexed, and intraneural pressure is increased about six fold.

See also PERIPHERAL NERVE INJURIES.

CULTURE   Shared beliefs, values and expectations about appropriate ways to behave in a social group or society. **Ethnocentrism** is the tendency to regard the group or culture one identifies with as superior to any other. It involves an inability to view life from the standpoint of a different group or culture.

Cultural studies is concerned with why and how subordinate groups accept and oppose the dominant ideologies that do not apparently benefit them. Power is central to this problem, and can be analyzed as a process of legitimizing the dominant groups' position. According to Hargreaves and McDonald (2000), one of the best exemplars of cultural studies writing on sport is James (1963) that raises questions about the role of cricket in the struggle for West Indian independence against colonial rule. *See* SOCIOLOGY OF SPORT; SUBCULTURE.

Bibliography
Crosset, T. and Beal, B. (1997). The use of 'subculture' and 'subworld' in ethnographic works on sport: A discussion of definitional distinctions. *Sociology of Sport Journal* 14(1), 73-85.

Hargreaves, J. and McDonald, I. (2000). Cultural studies and the sociology of sport. In Coakley, J. (ed). *Handbook of sports studies*. pp48-60. London: Sage.

James, C.L.R. (1963/1987). *Beyond a boundary*. London: Serpent's Tail.

Washington, R.E. and Karen, D. (2001). Sport and society. *Annual Review of Sociology* 27, 187-212.

CUNEIFORM   See TRIQUETRAL BONE.

CUSHING'S SYNDROME   Hypercortisolism. A rare endocrine disorder characterized by a variety of symptoms and physical abnormalities that occur when the body's tissues are exposed to excessive levels of cortisol for long periods of time. Most cases of Cushing's disease are not inherited. Pituitary adenomas cause most cases of Cushing's syndrome. They are benign tumors of the pituitary gland that secrete increased amounts of adrenocorticotropic hormone (ACTH). **Ectopic adrenocortico-tropic hormone syndrome** occurs when some benign or malignant tumors, which arise outside the pituitary gland, produce adrenocorticotropic hormone. Lung tumors cause over 50% of these cases. Many people suffer the symptoms of Cushing's syndrome, because they take glucocorticoid hormones (such as prednisone for asthma, rheumatoid arthritis, lupus and other inflammatory diseases) or for immunosuppression after organ transplantation.

It most commonly affects adults aged 20 to 50 years. An estimated 10 to 15 of every million people are affected each year in the USA.

Bibliography
Cushing's Support and Research Foundation, Inc. Http://www.csrf.net

CUTANEOUS RECEPTORS   Receptors in the skin. Various classes of cutaneous receptors are located in or near the junction of the dermis and the epidermis. Cutaneous receptors can be categorized as mechanoreceptors, thermal receptors or nociceptors. Pressure is not detected by cutaneous receptors, but by receptors deep in the dermis. The sensations of itch and tickle are poorly understood.

CYANOSIS   A dark bluish or purplish coloration of the skin and mucous membrane due to deficient oxygenation of the blood, evident when reduced hemoglobin in the blood exceeds 5 g per 100 ml.

CYCLIC AMP   c AMP. A form of adenosine monophosphate (AMP) formed at the surface of the cell from ATP, by the enzyme adenylate cyclase. Cyclic AMP mediates the action of beta-adrenergic hormones. See under HORMONES.

Bibliography
Palmer, W.K. (1988). Introduction to the symposium: Cyclic AMP

regulation of fuel metabolism during exercise. *Medicine and Science in Sports and Exercise* 20(6), 523-524.

CYCLIC GMP Cyclic guanosine monophosphate. It is a chemical substance that acts within cells to produce hormonal changes. It functions to allow hormones to affect only selected target cells to produce the desired changes in those cells.

CYCLIST'S PALSY *See* GUYTON'S TUNNEL SYNDROME.

CYROTHERAPY It is the therapeutic use of cold. Application of ice through a wet towel for repeated periods of 10 minutes may be most effective. The target temperature is a decrease of 10 to 15 degrees Celsius. Using repeated, rather than continuous, ice application helps sustain decreased muscle temperature without compromising the skin and allows the superficial skin temperature to return to normal, while deeper muscle temperature remains low. Cold application for less than 15 minutes causes immediate skin cooling, cooling of subcutaneous tissue after a slight delay, and a longer delay in cooling muscle tissue. Vasoconstriction at the cellular level decreases tissue metabolism that decreases secondary hypoxia. Nerve conduction decreases as the temperature of peripheral nerves decreases.

The **Hunting reaction** is the initial vasoconstriction following the application of cyrotherapy, after which vasodilation occurs. It functions to prevent tissue damage. Initially the skin tries to preserve heat by local vasoconstriction. This lasts about 10 minutes and limits any possible blood loss after trauma. When the skin gets very cold, it tries to normalize the temperature by vasodilation.

Reflex activity and motor function are impaired following ice treatment, thus patients may be more susceptible to injury for up to 30 minutes following treatment.

Bibliography

MacAuley, D.C. (2001). Ice therapy: How good is the evidence? *International Journal of Sports Medicine* 22(5), 379-384.

CYST A sac or sac-like structure that contains liquid or semi-solid matter. It is often caused by blockage of a passage. *See* BAKER'S CYST; GANGLION.

CYSTEINE A nonessential, glucogenic (glycogenic) three-carbon amino acid, which is an important amino acid in the protein of hair, the keratin of the skin, and in many enzymes and other proteins.

CYSTIC FIBROSIS A genetic disease that affects the secretion of mucus by membranes of body organs. Plugs of thick and sticky mucus cling to airway walls, leading to complications such as bronchitis and pneumonia. The symptoms resemble those of asthma, bronchitis and emphysema, and include shortness of breath and early fatigue during exercise. Viscous mucus also plugs up the pancreatic ducts, preventing digestive enzymes from reaching the small intestine and causing malnutrition.

Cystic fibrosis is inherited as an autosomal recessive trait and is the most common life-threatening genetic disorder in the Caucasian population. It is about four times less common among African Americans and nonexistent in Asian Americans.

Cystic fibrosis is managed by combined pulmonary, gastrointestinal and psychological therapy. Growth hormone treatment may have beneficial effects on both growth and exercise tolerance without serious complications in prepubertal children with cystic fibrosis.

Limitations in exercise performance appear related to the extent of lung disease and compromised nutritional status. Cystic fibrosis causes increased salt loss in sweat and can increase the risk for hyponatremia. No sports are contraindicated except scuba diving.

Bibliography

Boas, S.R. (1997). Exercise recommendations for individuals with cystic fibrosis. *Sports Medicine* 24(1), 17-37.

Cystic Fibrosis Foundation. Http://www.cff.org

Hütler, M. and Beneke, R. (2004). Growth hormone and exercise tolerance in patients with cystic fibrosis. *Sports Medicine* 34(2), 81-90.

CYSTINE   A nonessential amino acid formed from cysteine in a condensation reaction. As a separate chemical compound, it has no major function but it is important to the structure of many proteins and enzymes (e.g. insulin requires peptide chains held together by cystine residues in order to be biologically active).

CYTOCHROMES   Heme proteins that act as electron carriers in the electron transfer chain. Cytochromes pick up electrons from reduced coenzyme Q and deliver them to oxygen. All cytochromes contain a heme prosthetic group. The iron in the heme group alternates between the reduced, **ferrous** (+2) state and the oxidized, **ferric** (+3) state. This shift in valence enables cytochromes to pick up and deliver one electron, whereas NADH, FADH$_2$ and coenzyme Q handle two electrons. *See under* ELECTRON TRANSFER CHAIN.

CYTOKINES   Proteins or peptides that stimulate the proliferation of the various immune cells and are important regulators of inflammation and the immune response. Examples are interferons and interleukins. **Interferons** act as a non-specific defense mechanism and prevent the spread of viruses within the body by interfering with virus replication. **Interleukins** (e.g. interleukin-1) each act on a specific group of immune cells to divide and differentiate. Cytokines are produced by CD4 cells, natural killer cells and macrophages.

Cytokines are thought to be important in exercise immune response because certain ones (e.g. interleukin-1) are proinflammatory factors, which probably play a role in coordinating the responses to muscle damage that results from strenuous exercise. Other cytokines (e.g. interleukin-4) are anti-inflammatory. The release of anti-inflammatory cytokines follows the proinflammatory response to vigorous physical activity. *See under* IMMUNITY.

Bibliography

Moldoveanu, A.I., Shephard, R.J. and Shek, P.N. (2001). The cytokine response to physical activity and training. *Sports Medicine* 31(2), 115-144.

CYTOPLASM   *See under* CELL.

CYTOSINE   A nitrogenous, pyrimidine base found in DNA and RNA.

CYTOSOL   Fluid inside the cell membrane, excluding organelles. It is the site of glycolysis and fatty acid synthesis.

CYTOSOLIC PHOSPHORYLATION POTENTIAL   *See under* ATP.

CYTOTOXIC REACTIONS   A way in whole cells are killed, primarily by punching holes in their outer membranes. **Lysis** is a form of cytotoxic reaction in which a cell is killed by destruction of the cell membrane.

D

DACTYLION An anatomical landmark that is the tip of the middle (third) finger, or the most distal point of the middle finger when the arm is hanging and the fingers are stretched downward. The corresponding tips of the other fingers are designated the 2nd, 4th and 5th dactylions (the thumb being the first digit).

D'ALEMBERT'S PRINCIPLE   *See under* INERTIAL FORCE.

DALTON'S LAW *See under* GAS.

DAMPING See under RESILIENCE.

DANDY-WALKER CYST   Congenital hydro-cephalus caused by a blockage in the brain. It is characterized by an abnormally enlarged space at the back of the brain (cystic 4th ventricle) that interferes with the normal flow of cerebrospinal fluid through the openings between the ventricle and other parts of the brain.

Bibliography

National Organization for Rare Disorders. Http://www.rarediseases.org

DASHBOARD INJURY *See under* HIP JOINT, DISLOCATIONS; KNEE LIGAMENTS.

DEAD SPACE The theoretical volume of gas that is taken into the lung, but does not take part in gas exchange (assuming that the gases in the alveolar volume equilibrate with those of the pulmonary capillary blood as it leaves the lung). It consists of: i) anatomical dead space and ii) the volume of alveoli that are ventilated, but unperfused, in addition to a certain proportion of those alveoli that are underperfused. The **anatomical dead space** is the volume of air filling the nose, mouth, trachea and other non-diffusable parts of the respiratory tract. This volume of air does not undergo gas exchange, because it does not reach the alveoli. The dead space air is fully saturated with water vapor, similar in composition to inspired air. The alveolar gas has a relatively high concentration of carbon dioxide and low concentration of oxygen.

Dead space-to-tidal volume ratio is the proportion of the tidal volume that is made up of the dead space. It is an index of the relative inefficiency of pulmonary gas exchange. It is normally 40% at rest and progressively declines (to about 20%) during exercise. It decreases with age.

Physiologic dead space is the part of alveolar volume that has poor alveolar ventilation-to-perfusion ratio (the ratio of alveolar ventilation to pulmonary blood flow), thus does not equilibrate with gas in the pulmonary capillary blood. It is negligible in the healthy lung.

DEAF How a person 'labels' themselves in terms of their hearing loss is personal and may reflect identification with the deaf community or merely how their hearing loss affects their ability to communicate. Generally, however, the term deaf refers to those who are unable to hear well enough to rely on their hearing and use it as a means of processing information. The federal government in the USA distinguishes between deafness and hearing impairment. **Deafness** is a hearing impairment that is so severe that the child is impaired in processing linguistic information through hearing, with or without amplification, and this adversely affects a child's educational performance. **Hearing impairment** is defined as impairment in hearing, whether permanent or fluctuating, which adversely affects a child's educational performance, but that is not included under the definition of deafness. In the USA, 7 to 15% of the population has significant hearing losses. Only about 10% of deaf children have deaf parents.

Total deafness means vibrations can only be felt. **Sound waves** are vibrations, with three attributes: intensity, frequency and timbre (tone). **Intensity** refers to the perception of loudness and softness. It is measured in decibels (dB). Speech can be heard from a distance of 10 to 20 feet when the loudness is 35 to 65 dB, depending on the pitch. **Frequency** refers to the perception of high and low pitch. It is measured in hertz. Most humans can perceive frequencies from about 20 Hz to 20,000 Hz. **Timbre** refers to all the qualities besides intensity and frequency that enable us to distinguish between sounds, voices, and musical instruments.

A distinction can be made between conductive and sensorineural hearing loss. **Conductive hearing loss** is caused by anything that interferes with the transmission of sound from the outer to the inner ear. Some of the possible causes are middle ear infections (*otitis media*), collection of fluid in the middle ear, blockage of the outer ear by wax, and damage to the eardrum by infection or injury. Conductive loss results in hard of hearing, not deafness. **Sensorineural hearing loss** is due to damage to the pathway for sound impulses from the hearing cells of the inner ear to the auditory nerve and the brain. Some of the possible causes are: age-related hearing loss, injury to hair cells caused by loud noise, and infection (e.g. viral infections, meningitis). Most persons who are born deaf have sensorineural loss, and many of these are hereditary hearing losses. Meningitis carries a 1 in 5 risk of hearing loss. **Presbycusis** is the degeneration of hearing with age, and is primarily due to sensorineural rather than conductive losses. Many persons have mixed (combined) conductive and sensorineural losses.

In the USA, American Sign Language is the recognized language of deaf people who communicate manually. Federal law states that assessment, for purposes of placement, must be in the student's native language. For many deaf students, this is American Sign Language (ASL), the fourth most commonly used language in the USA. **Transliteration** is the process of transmitting information from English to ASL and vice versa. Speech reading (lip reading) is a difficult skill, because many sounds look identical, and is particularly difficult in group conversations or discussions in which the speaker is frequently changing.

55 dB is the minimum criterion for eligibility to participate in activities of the American Athletic Association for the Deaf (AAAD), and 70 dB is the accepted criterion level for distinguishing between hard of hearing and deafness. The rules, strategies and skills of deaf sport are not adapted except for communication modes. Modifications are made only in starting and stopping signals and in the ways officials communicate with the players.

Chronology

•1817 • The American School for the Deaf was established in Hartford, Connecticut.

•1864 • Gallaudet University was founded by an Act of Congress. It is the only university in which all programs and services are specifically designed to accommodate deaf and hard of hearing students.

•1924 • Comité Internationale des Sports de Sourds (CISS) was founded when two deaf Europeans, Eugène Rubens-Alcais of France and Antoine Dresse of Belgium, saw the need for an international sport governing body to stage quadrennial games for the deaf in Olympic format. The World Games for the Deaf was held in Paris. This was the first major athletic initiative for a special population.

•1945 • The American Athletic Association for the Deaf (AAAD) was established to provide, sanction and promote competitive sport opportunities for Americans with hearing impairments. In 1998, the name was changed to the USA Deaf Sports Federation (USADSF).

•1995 • The Deaf sport group withdrew from the Paralympic movement. One issue was that the Comité Internationale des Sports de Sourds (CISS) had asked the International Paralympic Committee (IPC) whether or not the IPC would make available the latest technology, such as visual devices to parallel auditory devices, to overcome communication restrictions.

Bibliography

American Athletic Association for the Deaf. Http://www.aaad.org

National Association of the Deaf. Http://www.nad.org

Sherill, C. (1998). *Adapted physical activity, recreation and sport. Cross disciplinary and lifespan*. 5th ed. Boston, MA: McGraw-Hill.

Winnick, J.P. (2000, ed). *Adapted physical education and sport*. 3rd ed. Champaign, IL: Human Kinetics.

DEAF-BLIND   It is a broad term that describes

people who have varying degrees and types of both vision and hearing loss together. Examples are: hard of hearing and visually impaired; deaf and tunnel vision; hard of hearing and blind; and totally deaf and blind. They fall into four groups: those who are born deaf and blind, which can happen if the mother suffered Rubella during pregnancy; those who were born deaf and then lost their sight; those who were born blind and then lost their hearing; and those who become deaf-blind as a result of illness, trauma, or old age. Deaf-blind ('dual sensory impaired') people have a combined sight and hearing loss, which leads to difficulties in communicating, mobility and accessing information. The federal government in the USA defines deaf-blind as concomitant hearing and visual impairments the combination of which causes such severe communication and other developmental and educational problems that they cannot be accommodated in special education programs solely for children with deafness or children with blindness. Deaf-blind people use a variety of different communication methods, including tactile American Sign Language and Braille.

Usher's syndrome is a form of retinitis pigmentosa, with associated deafness. It is the cause of approximately 10% of all hereditary deafness, with deafness existing at birth or developing soon afterward. It is inherited as an autosomal recessive trait. Eye symptoms usually appear by the age of 10 years, and start with night blindness. Visual acuity diminishes as the child grows older, and may result in complete blindness by midlife. There are two types of Usher's syndrome: type 1 and type 2. With **Type 1**, early damage to the cochlea of the ear results in deafness, which starts from birth. The retinitis also starts early with a progression from night blindness to tunnel vision within the first 10 years of life. With **Type 2**, the loss of hearing is less severe and the retinitis pigmentosa becomes more evident duding the late teens and twenties.

Persons who are deaf-blind typically engage in sports under the auspices of the US Association for Blind Athletes.

Bibliography
American Association of the Deaf-Blind. Http://www.aadb.org
Deaf Blind UK. Http://www.deafblind.org.uk
Sherill, C. (2004). *Adapted physical activity, recreation and sport. Cross disciplinary and lifespan.* 6th ed. Boston, MA: McGraw-Hill.

DEAMINATION   Removal of an amino (-NH$_2$) group from a molecule.
See AMINO ACID DEGRADATION.

DEBRANCHER ENZYME DEFICIENCY Cori's disease. Glycogenosis type 3. It is a carbohydrate processing disorder, which mainly affects the liver, causing swelling of the liver, slowing of growth, low blood glucose levels and, sometimes, seizures. In children, these symptoms often improve around puberty. Muscle weakness may develop later in life, and is most pronounced in the muscles of the forearms, hands, lower legs, and feet. Weakness is often accompanied by muscle atrophy. Cardiac problems may occur. It is inherited as an autosomal recessive trait.

DECARBOXYLATION   The removal of a carboxyl group from an amino acid. Thiamin pyrophosphate, a coenzyme, plays a key role in decarboxylation and helps drive the reaction that forms acetyl CoA from pyruvate during metabolism.

Decarboxylation of histidine produces histamine. Decarboxylation of tryptophan occurs in serotonin synthesis. In the adrenal medulla, decarboxylation of tyrosine occurs in the synthesis of norepinephrine and epinephrine. Decarboxylation of glutamate produces GABA (gamma-aminobutyrate).

DECOMPRESSION A decrease in gas pressure, e.g. in the body during ascent from deep water or ascent to high altitude. *See* HYPERBARIC PHYSIOLOGY.

DEEP VEIN THROMBOSIS   *See under* THROMBOSIS.

DEFIBRILLATION This involves attaching two large electrodes to the patient's chest and delivering an electrical shock from a defribillator machine. An

automatic external defibrillator is a small, portable device that automatically analyzes a heart rhythm and, if necessary, prompts a trained responder to deliver a life-saving shock to restore a heart's normal rhythm. The standard placement for defibrillation electrodes is one immediately to the right of the upper part of the sternum below the clavicle and the other to the left and 1 or 2 inches below the left nipple with the electrode center in the mid-axillary line. *See also* SUDDEN DEATH.

DEFLECTION Elastic movement of a structure. In a tennis racket, for example, tight strings generate less power than looser strings. If the strings have a lower tension, they will deflect more (i.e. store more energy) and the ball will deform less (i.e. dissipate less energy). In other words, the looser strings, the longer the ball will reside on the strings (the greater dwell time). Top players have tight strings because they hit the ball so hard that they can afford to string their rackets tightly to gain other advantages, such as accuracy.

Bibliography

Brody, H. (1987). *Tennis science for tennis players*. Philadelphia: University of Pennsylvania Press.

DEFORMATION A state of mechanical strain in a body.

DEGENERATION A change in tissue physiology such that it becomes less functionally active.

DEGRADATION The breakdown of a chemical compound into simpler components, e.g. the breakdown of a protein into amino acids.

DEGREES OF FREEDOM In mechanics, the number of ways in which the spatial configuration of a system may change. With respect to biomechanics of human movement, a degree of freedom can be thought of as an axis of rotation. A joint with three degrees of freedom permits rotation about three different axes. *See under* MOTOR LEARNING.

DEHYDRATION Loss of water from the body.

Insensible water loss is the continuous evaporation of water from the respiratory tract and water that passes through the skin by transepidermal diffusion and is also lost by evaporation. It is termed insensible because we are usually unaware of it. It typically accounts for about 25 to 50% of daily water loss. High altitude, low humidity and high temperatures increase these losses. An 'average' adult who expends 2,400 kcal daily loses about 2.4 liters of water per day. Fever, coughing, rapid breathing and water nasal secretions all significantly increase water loss.

Hypohydration that is induced by prior exercise has much less impact on plasma volume than hypohydration induced through diuretics or sauna exposure.

During prolonged exercise, especially in the heat, it is vital that fluid replacement takes place to maintain a good state of hydration. Even small losses of water can adversely affect work capacity and athletic performance. Negative effects on aerobic exercise performance have been demonstrated with 2% dehydration.

There is general consensus in the scientific literature that dehydration should not exceed 2% of body weight loss during most athletic events. Dehydration by 2% of body weight generally occurs during exercise lasting more than 90 minutes, and does appear to significantly impair endurance performance in environments of 20 to 21 degrees Celsius. In hot environments (31 to 32 degrees Celsius), sweating rate is higher and 60 minutes of intense exercise typically elicits dehydration of approximately 2% of body weight. Dehydrated people are less tolerant of hyperthermia and they usually collapse or fatigue at core temperatures in the range of 38.5 to 39.5 degrees Celsius.

Carbohydrate metabolism in muscle may be decreased following dehydration. Heart rate rises disproportionately during exercise, impairing the ability of the body to dissipate heat. Blood lactate levels have been found to systematically rise at a lower oxygen uptake following dehydration when compared with the same exercise protocol in a normal state of hydration. The cause of this change is not known.

Water lost from sweating is derived from all fluid compartments of the body including the blood (hypovolemia), thus causing an increase in the concentration of electrolytes in the body fluids (hypertonicity). As dehydration progresses, there is a decrease in the efficiency of the circulatory and thermoregulatory systems. A decrease in central blood volume causes a decrease in both ventricular filling pressure and stroke volume, while heart rate is increased. For every 1% of body weight loss due to dehydration, heart rate increases by 5 to 8 bpm.

At altitude, water loss is hastened by loss of water from evaporation as cool, dry air is warmed and moistened in the respiratory passages. A cross-country air flight in the USA with low cabin humidity can cause fluid losses of about 1 to 1.5 litres.

Even when fluid is consumed during exercise, dehydration may occur, because the rate at which fluid is lost as sweat can be double the rate at which ingested fluid can be absorbed. It is common for athletes to dehydrate by 2 to 6% of their body weight during exercise in the heat, even when beverages are available. Dehydration due to inadequate fluid replacement increases the frequency of gastrointestinal symptoms.

Markers of hydration status include: body mass changes; urinary indices (volume, color, protein content, specific gravity and osmolality); blood borne indices (hemoglobin concentration, hematocrit, plasma osmolality and sodium concentration, plasma testosterone, epinephrine, norepinephrine, cortisol and atrial natriuretic peptide); bioelectrical impedance analysis; and pulse rate and systolic blood pressure response to postural change. There is currently no universal hydration-status marker, particularly for the relatively moderate levels of hypohydration that frequently occur in an exercise situation. The urinary measures of color, specific gravity and osmolality are more sensitive at indicating moderate levels of hypohydration than are blood measurements of hematocrit and serum osmolality and sodium concentration. Urine color is directly proportional to the level of dehydration. The day-to-day reliability of urine color measurements is enhanced if meals,

fluid consumption during exercise, the time of urine collection and training are consistent. Urine color tracks body water or fluid fluctuations better than urine volume except when dehydrated athletes rapidly rehydrate with a large quantity of pure water or dilute fluid, resulting in one or two urine samples with a low urine color, specific gravity or osmolality, before the body water deficit has been replaced completely. An eight-color scale can be used to rate urine color. It ranges from very pale yellow (number 1) to brownish green (number 8). Normal urine specimens in healthy adults have a specific gravity in the range of 1.013 to 1.029. During dehydration or hypohydration, urine specific gravity exceeds 1.030. When excess water exists, specific gravity is typically in the range of 1.001 to 1.012.

Cumulative dehydration may develop insidiously over several days and is typically observed during the first few days of a season during practice sessions or in tournament competition. Cumulative dehydration can be detected by monitoring prepractice and postpractice weights. Blood tests appear to be the most accurate monitoring method for hydration testing of athletes, but are impractical because of cost and invasiveness.

See FLUID REPLACEMENT; GASTROINTES-TINAL SYSTEM.

Bibliography

Armstrong, L.E. (2000). *Performing in extreme environments.* Champaign, IL: Human Kinetics.

Armstrong, L.E. et al. (1998). Urinary indices during dehydration, exercise and rehydration. *International Journal of Sport Nutrition* 8, 345-355.

Barr, S.I. (1999). Effects of dehydration on exercise performance. *Canadian Journal of Applied Physiology* 24(2), 164-172.

Oppliger, R.A. and Bartok, C. (2003). Hydration testing of athletes. *Sports Medicine* 32(15), 959-971.

Shirreffs, S.M. (2000). Markers of hydration status. *Journal of Sports Medicine and Physical Fitness* 40(1), 80-84.

DEHYDROEPIANDROSTERONE *See under* ANDROGEN SUPPLEMENTS.

DEHYDROGENASE A class of enzyme that removes hydrogen atoms from a substrate and transfers them to an acceptor other than oxygen.

DEHYDROGENATION An oxidation reaction in which electrons are lost as part of hydrogen atoms or hydride ions.

DEMENTIA A broad diagnostic term for multiple cognitive deficits that involve significant change from a previous level of functioning and that can be attributed to a medical condition and/or substance. The most common dementias in older adults are those caused by Alzheimer's disease and multi-infarct dementia. In **multi-infarct dementia** (**vascular dementia**), a series of small strokes or changes in the brain's blood supply may result in the death of brain tissue. Mild cognitive impairment is different from both Alzheimer's disease and normal age-related memory change.

DEMENTIA PUGILISTICA *See under* HEAD INJURIES.

DENATURATION (i) Loss of the normal three-dimensional shape of a macromolecule without breaking covalent bonds, usually accompanied by loss of its biological activity. (ii) Conversion of DNA from the double-stranded into the single-stranded form. (iii) Unfolding of a polypeptide chain.

DE NOVO LIPOGENESIS *See under* FATTY ACID SYNTHESIS.

DENSITOMETRY Method for the assessment of total body density. *See under* BODY COMPOSITION.

DENSITY Mass per unit volume. Objects with a density greater than 1 will sink in water, but those with a density of less than 1 will float in water. The Standard International unit is kilogram per cubic meter (kg/m^3). The US Customary unit is pound per cubic foot (lb/ft^3).

DENTAL INJURIES *See under* TEETH.

DEOXYRIBONUCLEASE An enzyme that breaks sugar-phosphate bonds in DNA.

DEOXYRIBOSE The five-carbon sugar present in DNA.

DEPRESSANTS A group of drugs that produce general inhibition of central nervous system functions leading to such effects as euphoria and sedation. Alcohol, benzodiazepines and barbiturates are members of the class of depressant drugs called sedative-hypnotics. **Hypnotics** are central nervous system (CNS) depressants used to induce drowsiness and encourage sleep. **Sedatives** are CNS depressants used to relieve anxiety, fear and apprehension.

Benzodiazepines are used as sleeping pills. The specific binding sites in the brain for benzodiazepines are part of a receptor for gamma aminobutyrate (GABA). Many of the actions of benzodiazepines probably result from an enhancement of GABA's inhibitory actions. The drugs relax muscles because they inhibit some areas of the brain that control muscle tone. The tranquillizing and sleep inducing effects of benzodiazepines may be partly due to the secondary dampening of the release of other neurotransmitters such as norepinephrine and serotonin in excitatory pathways, influencing arousal and emotion. Diazepam (Valium®) is used more than any other benzodiazepine and has addictive qualities. Benzodiazepines are generally recommended now only for short-term use (up to a fortnight) because of harmful effects, including dependence and withdrawal symptoms that occurs with chronic use. Chronic use of benzodiazepines can cause depression.

Barbiturates prolong rather than intensify GABA effects and, in high concentration, can be GABA mimetic. Barbiturates also directly depress excitatory neurons. Barbiturates are clinically used to treat anxiety, convulsions and insomnia. It is unlikely that barbiturates would have beneficial effects on athletic performance. Chronic abuse is harmful to health.

Bibliography

Ashton, H. (1989). Anything for a quiet life? *New Scientist*, 6 May, 52-55.

DEPRESSION   i) A movement which consists of downward, non-angular gliding of one surface over another.

ii) The most common psychiatric disorder. It is characterized by feelings of misery that are excessive in relation to the circumstances. People with negative thinking patterns and low self-esteem are more likely to develop clinical depression. **Major depressive disorder** is having at least one major depressive episode, and five or more symptoms for at least a two-week period. With respect to the diagnostic criteria of the American Psychiatric Association, at least one of the symptoms is either: (i) depressed mood most of the day, nearly every day, as indicated by either subjective report (e.g. feels sad or empty) or observation made by others (e.g. appears tearful); or ii) markedly diminished interest or pleasure in all, or almost all, activities most of the day, nearly every day (as indicated by either subjective account or observation made by others). Other symptoms are: significant weight loss when not dieting or weight gain (e.g. a change of more than 5% of body weight in a month), or decrease or increase in appetite nearly every day, or (in children) failure to make expected weight gains; insomnia or hypersomnia nearly every day; psychomotor agitation or retardation nearly every day (observable by others, not merely subjective feelings or restlessness or being slowed down); fatigue or loss of energy nearly every day; feelings of worthlessness or excessive or inappropriate guilt (which may be delusionsal) nearly every day (not merely self reproach or guilt about being sick); diminished ability to think or concentrate, or indecisiveness, nearly every day (either by subjective account or as observed by others); recurrent thoughts of death (not just fear of dying), recurrent suicidal ideation without a specific plan, or a suicide attempt or a specific plan for committing suicide. Symptoms that are clearly due to a general medical conditions, or mood-incongruent delusions or hallucinations are excluded. The symptoms do not meet criteria for a mixed episode. The symptoms cause clinically significant distress or impairment in social, occupational, or other important areas of functioning. The symptoms are not due to the direct physiological effects of a substance (e.g. a drug of abuse, a medication) or a general medical condition (e.g. hyperthyroidism). The symptoms are not better accounted for by Bereavement, i.e. after the loss of a loved one, the symptoms persist for longer than 2 months or are characterized by marked functional impairment, morbid preoccupation with worthlessness, suicidal ideation, psychotic symptoms, or psychomotor retardation.

The diagnostic criteria for a **mixed episode** are: (A) The criteria are met for a manic episode and for a major depressive episode (except for duration) nearly every day during at least a 1-week period. (B) The mood disturbance is sufficiently severe to cause marked impairment in occupational functioning or in usual social activities or relationships with others, or to necessitate hospitalization to prevent harm to self or others, or there are psychotic features. (C) The symptoms are not due to the direct physiological effects of a substance (e.g. a drug of abuse) or a general medical condition (e.g. hyperthyroidism).

Women are nearly twice as likely than men to experience clinical depression. This may be due to hormonal changes experienced during menstruation, pregnancy, childbirth and menopause. The role of CNS serotonin activity in the pathophysiology of major depressive disorder is suggested by the efficacy of selective serotonin reuptake inhibitors in the treatment of major depressive disorder.

Postpartum blues are the mood swings, which results from the high hormonal fluctuations that occur during and immediately after childbirth. **Postpartum depression** is a major form of depression and is less common than postpartum blues.

Dysthymia is a mood disorder that has longer lasting, but milder symptoms than clinical depression. It lasts at least two years. About 3% of the American population suffers from dysthymia at some time. Women are nearly twice as likely than men to experience dysthymia.

Depression is associated with a higher risk of accidents and lapses of memory or attention. Some of the drugs used to treat depression may increase this risk. For example, there is evidence that many road accidents may be due to **tricyclic anti-depressants**, a class of drugs that inhibits the neuronal uptake of norepinephrine and serotonin to a greater or lesser extent. Tricyclic antidepressants, such as amitriptyline (Elavil), boost norepinephrine and serotonin levels by preventing the normal reabsorption, or reuptake, of these substances by the cells that have released them. Although these drugs are most effective in the treatment of major depression, there are numerous side effects relating to multiple-receptor systems. Adverse effects include sedation, confusion, dry mouth, orthostasis, constipation, urinary retention, sexual dysfunction and weight gain. Each drug in the class causes various degrees of anti-histamic, anti-muscarinic, alpha-adrenergic antagonistic and anti-cholinergic effects. The side effects of tricyclic anti-depressants, especially cardiac conduction abnormalities, preclude their use by athletes with depression.

Selective serotonin reuptake inhibitors, such as fluoxetine (Prozac), are the first-line drugs used to treat most patients with depression in the USA. These drugs have nearly exclusive effect on neural uptake of serotonin and minimal or no effect on the receptor systems affected by tricyclic anti-depressants. There is a relative lack of serious side effects (e.g. they are not as sedating as tricyclic antidepressants and therefore cause fewer accidents), but side effects include gastrointestinal upset, sexual dysfunction and changes in energy level (fatigue/restlessness). These drugs can produce ergogenic effects including prolonged running time to exhaustion, decreased central fatigue, and enhanced motivation and self-esteem.

Monoamine oxidase inhibitors such as phenelzine (Nardil) elevate the level of norepinephrine and serotonin in the brain by blocking or inhibiting an enzyme that deactivates these neurotransmitters. Patients on monoamine oxidase inhibitors must follow a low tyramine diet, due to the risk of hypertensive crisis. Monoamine oxidase inhibitors interact with foods containing tyramine, a chemical found in cheese and beer. Other adverse effects include insomnia, anxiety, orthostasis, weight gain and sexual dysfunction.

More than 80% of people who seek treatment for depression show improvement. Electroconvulsive therapy is a highly effective treatment for depression and may have a more rapid onset of action than drug treatments.

See also BIPOLAR DISORDER; MENTAL HEALTH; MOOD DISORDERS.

Bibliography

American Psychiatric Association. (1994). *Diagnostic and statistical manual of mental disorders*. 4th ed. Washington, DC: American Psychiatric Association.

Aronson, S.C. (2004). Depression. Http://www.emedicine.com

DEPTH PERCEPTION   The ability to judge the distance of an object from oneself. **Monocular depth cues** include size, texture gradient, shading, convergence, overlap, proportionality and linear perspective. **Binocular depth cues** include retinal disparity – an object of visual regard being viewed from a slightly different angle by each eye.

Infants are capable of perceiving depth cues during the first year of life. Using the visual cliff, psychologists have discovered that infants have depth perception by the age of 6 months and possibly even earlier.

DE QUERVAIN'S SYNDROME   Paratenonitis of the *abductor pollicis longus* and *extensor pollicis brevis*. It occurs in sports that require repetitive radial and ulnar deviations of the wrist, such as golf, racquet sports and javelin throwing. The extensor tendons are stabilized by a series of six separate compartments that function as tunnels and permit gliding of the tendons by keeping them fixed to the dorsum of the wrist. The sheaths of these tendons are not always in optimal alignment with the direction of pull of the tendon, due to the many degrees of freedom of wrist and hand movement. As a consequence, increased friction may occur.

DERMATOMYOSITIS One of a group of acquired muscle diseases called inflammatory myopathies. It is an autoimmune disorder with a subacute onset and appears in childhood to late adulthood. Symptoms include skin rash, weakness of neck and limb muscles, muscle pain and swelling. The disease progression and severity varies among individuals. Treatment usually consists of prednisone.

Bibliography

Myositis Association. Http://www.myositis.org

DERMATOPHYTES A fungus that causes superficial infections of the skin, hair and/or nails.

DERMATOSIS A broad term that refers to any disease of the skin, especially one that is not accompanied by inflammation.

DERMIS The deeper layers of the skin, containing hair follicles, sweat glands, sebaceous glands, nerve endings and blood vessels.

DESATURATION The act or result of making something less completely saturated. With respect to hemoglobin, it refers to a decrease in oxygen saturation.

DETRAINING Partial or complete loss of training-induced adaptations, in response to an insufficient training stimulus. A distinction can be made between short-term detraining (less than 4 weeks of insufficient training stimulus) and long-term detraining (more than 4 weeks).

Short-term detraining in highly-trained endurance athletes is characterized by a rapid decline in maximal oxygen uptake and blood volume. A loss in blood volume partially accounts for the decrease in stroke volume. Exercise heart rate increases insufficiently to counterbalance the decreased stroke volume, thus maximal cardiac output is decreased. Ventilatory efficiency and endurance performance are also impaired. These changes are more moderate in recently trained individuals. Short-term inactivity implies an increased reliance on carbohydrate metabolism during exercise, as shown by a higher exercise respiratory exchange ratio and lowered lipase activity, GLUT-4 content, glycogen level and lactate threshold. At the muscle level, capillary density and oxidative enzyme activities are decreased. Training-induced changes in the cross-sectional area of muscle fibers are reversed, but decline in strength performance is limited. Hormonal changes include decreased insulin sensitivity, lower levels of growth hormone in strength athletes and a reversal of short-term training-induced adaptations in fluid-electrolyte regulating hormones.

If a person detrains for 12 days, approximately 50% of the improvements (above the detrained level) in mitochondrial enzyme activity will be lost. If after 12 days of detraining the person is able to resume full training, it will require approximately 36 days to achieve about 93% of the previous trained levels of mitochondrial activity. It is therefore hypothesized that every 12 days of detraining requires three times the number of days retraining.

Long-term detraining is characterized by a significant decline in the maximal oxygen uptake of athletes, but remains above control values during long-term detraining, whereas recently acquired gains in maximal oxygen uptake are completely lost. This is partly due to decreased blood volume, cardiac dimensions and ventilatory efficiency, resulting in lower stroke volume and cardiac output, despite increased heart rates. Resting muscle glycogen levels return to baseline, carbohydrate utilization increases; and the lactate threshold is lowered, although it remains above untrained values in highly trained individuals. In endurance athletes, the proportion of slow-twitch muscle fibers is decreased. In strength athletes, force production declines slowly and usually remains above control values for very long periods.

In contrast to the effects of detraining, adaptations to aerobic training may be retained for at least several months through **reduced training** (when training is maintained at a decreased level), as long as training intensity is maintained and frequency decreased only moderately. Training volume can be significantly decreased. Cross training may also be effective in maintaining training-induced adaptations.

Bibliography

Houmard, J.A. (1991). Impact of reduced training on performance in endurance athletes. *Sports Medicine* 12(6), 380-393.

Mujika, I. And Padilla, S. (2000). Detraining: Loss of training-induced physiological and performance adaptations. Part I. Short term insufficient training stimulus. *Sports Medicine* 30(2), 79-87.

Mujika, I. and Padilla, S. (2000). Detraining: Loss of training-induced physiological and performance adaptations. Part II: Long term insufficient training stimulus. *Sports Medicine* 30(3), 145-154.

Mujika, I. and Padilla, S. (2001). Cardiorespiratory and metabolic characteristics of detraining in humans. *Medicine and Science in Sports and Exercise* 33(3), 413-421.

Neufer, P.D. (1989). The effect of detraining and reduced training on the physiological adaptations to aerobic exercise training. *Sports Medicine* 8(5), 302-321.

DETRUSOR HYPERREFLEXIA   *See under* AGING; URINARY INCONTINENCE.

DEVELOPMENT   *See under* GROWTH; MOTOR DEVELOPMENT.

DEVELOPMENTAL COORDINATION DISORDER   Dyspraxia. Apraxia. Clumsy child syndrome. It involves marked impairment in the development of motor coordination. It involves a breakdown between cortical and subcortical functions. Performance in daily activities that require motor coordination is substantially below that expected given the person's chronological age and measured intelligence. This may be manifested by marked delays in achieving motor milestones (e.g. walking, crawling, sitting), dropping things, 'clumsiness,' poor performance in sports or poor handwriting. This diagnosis is made only if: i) the condition significantly interferes with academic achievement or activities of daily living; and ii) the condition is not caused by a general medical disorder (e.g. cerebral palsy) or pervasive developmental disorder. If mental retardation is present, the motor difficulties are in excess of those usually associated with it. Developmental coordination disorder is a problem for many persons with learning disabilities.

Children and adolescents with developmental coordination disorder may have problems with gross motor skills, fine motor skills, or both. Some have difficulty planning movements, and executing them, others have difficulty planning movements, but not executing them, and others have difficulty executing movements but not planning them. The more complex an activity, the more likely that performance will be clumsy because of information processing and motor planning demands. It is a typical characteristic of children with learning disabilities. For the majority of those with dyspraxia, there is no known cause.

In the USA, approximately 6% of children aged 5 to 11 years have developmental coordination disorder. It may be a lifetime problem, rather than a developmental disorder.

See also CLUMSY TEENAGER PHENOMENON.

Bibliography

American Psychiatric Association. (1994). *Diagnostic and statistical manual of mental disorders*. 4th ed. Washington, DC: American Psychiatric Association.

Australian Dyspraxia Support Group and Resource Center. Http://www.dyspraxia.com.au

Cermak, S.A. and Larkin, D. (2002, eds). *Developmental coordination disorder*. Albany, NY: Delmar.

Dyspraxia Foundation. Http://www.dyspraxiafoundation.org.uk

Geuze, R.H. et al. (2001). Clinical and research diagnostic criteria for developmental coordination disorder: A review and discussion. *Human Movement Science* 20(1/2), 7-47.

Henderson, S.E. and Barnett, A.L. (1998). The classification of specific motor coordination disorders in children: Some problems to be solved. *Human Movement Science* 17, 449-469.

Le Febvre, C. and Reid, G. (1999). Prediction in ball catching by children with and without a developmental coordination disorder. *Adapted Physical Activity Quarterly* 15(4), 299-315.

Sigmundsson, H. et al. (1998). We can cure your child's clumsiness! A review of intervention methods. *Scandanavian Journal of Rehabilitation Medicine* 30, 101-106.

DEVELOPMENTAL DELAYS   According to federal legislation in the USA, developmental delays can occur in five areas: cognitive, physical, language and speech, psychosocial or emotional, and self-help skills. At risk of developmental delays are infants and toddlers who have been exposed to adverse prenatal, perinatal or postnatal factors that are likely to cause clearly identifiable delays before the age of 3 years.

See TERATOGEN.

DEVIANCE   A lack of conformity to the expectations of other people.

DEXA   *See*   DUAL-ENERGY   X-RAY ABSORPTIOMETRY.

DEXTRINS   *See* MALTODEXTRINS.

DEXTROSE   *See* GLUCOSE.

DHEA   *See* DEHYDROEPIANDROSTERONE.

DIABETES MELLITUS   A condition in which blood glucose increases to an abnormally high level (hyperglycemia) because insufficient glucose reaches the cells. Large quantities of both glucose and water are excreted in the urine (glycosuria) because the excess glucose is passed into the kidney tubules, where the glucose in the plasma filtrate causes an increase in osmotic pressure that also decreases the reabsorption of water. The excretion of excessive urine (polyuria) leads to excessive thirst (polydypsia). Most patients with diabetes develop some neuropathy after 2 to 3 years, and this is associated with poor glucose control.

The **oral glucose-tolerance test** evaluates blood glucose level, 2 hours after drinking a concentrated glucose-containing solution. Delayed removal of ingested glucose indicates diabetes. The **fasting plasma glucose** (FPG) test measures plasma glucose following an 8-hour fast. The American Diabetes Association currently recommends the FPG test. A normal result is less than 110 mg/dL, the impaired range is 110 to 125 mg/dL and diabetes is suspected if it is greater than 125 mg/dL.

Three categories of diabetes mellitus can be identified: Type-1, Type-2 and that associated with other conditions such as pancreatic disease or excess production of growth hormone. Since 1997, it has been recommended that use of the terms insulin dependent diabetes mellitus (IDDM) and non-insulin dependent diabetes mellitus (NIDDM) be discontinued because they are based on treatment, which can vary considerably, and do not indicate the underlying problem.

Type-1 diabetes (insulin-dependent or juvenile-onset diabetes) accounts for 10% of the diabetic population and develops early in life. It arises as a consequence of immunologically mediated, pancreatic islet, beta cell destruction in genetically susceptible individuals. 40 to 50% of inherited diabetes risk is accounted for by at least two genes in the human leukocyte antigen region, which is a section of a chromosome that contains several genes that are involved in immune function. One gene that is important is DR. People can inherit one form of DR from their mother and another form of DR from their father. Two forms of DR, designated DR3 and DR4, are present in 95% of type-1 diabetics, and 30% have inherited both DR3 and DR4. Only 50% of the general population have DR3 or DR4, and 1 to 3% have both. Diabetics who have inherited DR3, but not DR4, develop diabetes at an older age, and tend to have antibodies against pancreatic beta cells but not against insulin. Diabetics who have inherited DR4, but not DR3, tend to develop diabetes earlier in life and have an immune reaction against insulin. Diabetics who inherit both DR3 and DR4 develop diabetes at the youngest age and have the highest levels of antibodies against insulin.

Type-1 diabetes is characterized by severe deficiency or absence of insulin production. The Type-1 diabetic is in a similar state to that of a starved person. Insulin therapy is necessary for survival.

Without insulin, the body cannot metabolize glucose and the primary source of energy is then derived from fat. The end products of fat metabolism are ketone bodies. These ketone bodies alter the acid-base relationship, resulting in a decrease in the body's pH (ketoacidosis). In an attempt to diminish the acidosis and bring the pH of the body back to normal (7.35 to 7.45), the respiratory system tries to increase its elimination of carbon dioxide by deep sighing (**Kussmaul breathing**). Ketoacidosis and dehydration depress the nervous system, and as a consequence the person becomes confused and may lapse into diabetic coma. In diabetic coma, acetones are expired from the lungs giving the breath a fruity odor.

The predominant problem regarding exercise in Type-1 diabetes mellitus is hypoglycemia, especially for patients undergoing intensive insulin therapy. People with Type-1 diabetes are most vulnerable to severe hypoglycemia. A few Type-1 diabetics may not be able to develop the early warning symptoms. This is known as **'hypoglycemia unawareness.'** Although it seems that exercise does not improve long-term glycemic control in Type-1 diabetics, all such patients should be encouraged to participate in exercise for the same reasons as the general population. Since exercise lowers the blood glucose, any increase in the level of exercise must be compensated for by increasing food intake or by lowering the amount of hypoglycemic agent given. If compensatory changes are not made, the blood glucose will drop below normal levels (hypoglycemia) and the athlete will go into hypoglycemic shock (insulin shock).

When diabetic patients who use insulin participate in physical activity, they must make frequent insulin adjustments to maintain glycemic control, especially during higher-intensity or longer-duration exercise. A small amount of insulin is always required during exercise to counterbalance glucose-raising hormones such as catecholamines, glucagons, growth hormone and cortisol. With experience and blood glucose testing, the insulin regimen that makes an exercising diabetic individual's response closest to that of a nondiabetic individual's is **Continuous Subcutaneous Insulin Infusion (CSII) therapy** (also known as **insulin pump therapy**). The American College of Sports Medicine (ACSM) and the American Diabetes Association (ADA) have established general clinical practice recommendations for exercise and diabetes that apply to patients who use insulin pumps. The main change from previous recommendations is that patients who have pre-exercise glucose levels less than 100 mg/dL may not require a carbohydrate snack. Pump users can simply decrease or suspend basal insulin during an activity. The insulin decreases and the carbohydrate intake necessary for aerobic activity will depend on its intensity and duration. A change in either insulin (basal or bolus doses) or carbohydrate intake can often compensate for shorter, less intense activities.

Exercise is advised if blood glucose levels are less than 250 mg/dL and no ketones are detected. If blood glucose is more than 250 mg/dL, exercise is still advised if ketones are not present, but a small insulin bolus may be needed. If ketones are found and the pre-exercise blood glucose exceeds 250 mg/dL, exercise is not advised. Exercise may be possible if blood glucose is more than 300 mg/dL and ketones are not present, but extra caution is advised and an insulin bolus may be necessary.

Type-2 diabetes (adult-onset diabetes) was previously defined as non-insulin dependent, but some patients do require insulin injections. It accounts for 90% of diabetic cases and tends to occur in older people. There are two groups. Firstly, those with a primary deficit in the beta-cell, in the form of impaired capacity for insulin secretion. Sufferers tend to be lean. Secondly, those in whom the primary deficit is insulin sensitivity in muscle or liver tissue. Sufferers tend to be obese. Ketosis is rarely associated with Type-2 diabetes.

Bodyweight reduction improves the impaired metabolic control associated with Type-2 diabetes and obesity by improving both hepatic and peripheral insulin sensitivity. Oral Sulfonylureas, hypoglycemic drugs such as acetohexamide that stimulate the synthesis and release of insulin from the beta cells of the pancreas, are used to treat patients with Type-2 diabetes and can effectively lower fasting plasma glucose and decrease basal hepatic glucose production. Furthermore, when diet and sulfonylurea treatment is not sufficient, intermittent or chronic insulin treatment can be used to overcome insulin resistance and improve beta-cell responsiveness to glucose.

Unlike Type-1 diabetes, glucose regulation during exercise is not usually a problem in Type-2 diabetes. Exercise is expected to improve insulin sensitivity, thus is an important part of therapy in Type-2 diabetes. Different categories of patients with Type-2 diabetes respond differently to exercise training. The majority of younger patients without complicating diseases, and patients characterized by low insulin secretion, demonstrate impaired metabolic control. Low-intensity exercise is therefore recommended, as it is most effective for weight control and is often the only form that older patients can perform.

Long-term exercise training is beneficial for Type-2 diabetics, but not because of a continued improvement in exercise-induced insulin sensitivity. Insulin sensitivity is retained only in individuals who exercise and decrease body fat content. In fact, loss of body fat in an overweight Type-2 diabetic can decrease insulin release and increase insulin sensitivity, regardless of exercise training. Nevertheless, for individuals who exercise daily, the continued increase in exercise-stimulated insulin sensitivity is retained from one exercise session to the next, producing a meaningful improvement in the control of blood glucose. For individuals with Type-2 diabetes who are not using supplemental insulin, such strict recommendations are not necessary to maintain correct blood glucose levels during exercise. Blood glucose monitoring should be done before and after exercise. Supplemental carbohydrates are generally not needed in these patients. However, blood glucose monitoring will reveal which individuals may need additional carbohydrates to prevent hypoglycemia during and following exercise. The most immediate and serious potential risk is that exercise can result in hypoglycemia (blood glucose level of 65 mg/dL [3.6 mM] or lower). Higher than normal levels of circulating insulin, resulting from the mobilization of injected insulin during exercise, can attenuate or prevent the normal mobilization of glucose and other substrates and increase the muscle uptake of glucose. In fact, the risk of hypoglycemia during or following exercise is substantial, especially in insulin users who take a pre-set insulin dosage, unless appropriate modifications in food or insulin are made. A preventive strategy is to exercise when circulating insulin levels are lower (at least 3 to 4 hours after the last injection of short-acting insulin, and not during a dose peak). This makes insulin levels during exercise more similar to those in a non-diabetic individual. Morning exercise, especially if done before any insulin injection, usually exerts less hypoglycemic effect than the same exercise done later in the day. This results from the effects of higher circulating cortisol and other glucose-raising hormone levels early in the day (i.e. insulin

resistance is generally greater in the morning), along with lower circulating levels of insulin. Conversely, evening exercise conveys the greatest risk for nocturnal hypoglycemia, unless the patient makes preventive changes in food intake or insulin doses.

Individuals who maintain a physically active lifestyle are much less likely to develop impaired glucose tolerance and Type-2 diabetes. The protective effect of physical activity may be strongest for individuals at the highest risk of developing Type-2 diabetes. Older individuals who vigorously train on a regular basis exhibit a greater glucose tolerance and a lower insulin response to a glucose challenge than sedentary individuals of similar age and weight.

For patients with cardiovascular disease and Type-2 diabetes, possible mechanisms to explain improved exercise capacity include decreases in ventricular and vascular structural hypertrophy and compliance coupled with increased functional reserve.

Risks of exercise for diabetics include aggravating diabetic complications such as the following (precautions are shown in parentheses): retinopathy (avoid strenuous, high-intensity exercise that involves breath-holding such as isometrics and avoid activities that lower the head such as yoga or that risk jarring the head), hypertension (avoid heavy weightlifting or breath-holding), peripheral neuropathy (avoid exercise that may cause trauma to the feet, e.g. prolonged hiking) and nephropathy (avoid exercise such as heavy weightlifting that increases blood pressure). Proper footwear is essential for diabetic patients and should be emphasized for individuals with peripheral neuropathy.

Diabetes mellitus is distinguished from **diabetes insipidus**, which is a metabolic disorder caused by inadequate release of vasopressin. It is also distinguished from gestational diabetes (see under PREGNANCY). *See also* METABOLIC SYNDROME.

Chronology

•600 AD • Chaog Yuan-Fang, a prominent Chinese physician of the Sui Dynasty promoted physical activity as a valuable adjunct to the control of diabetes.

Bibliography

Albright, A. et al. (2000). American College of Sports Medicine position stand. Exercise and type 2 diabetes. *Medicine and Science in Sports and Exercise* 32, 1345-1360.

American College of Sports Medicine (2000). ACSM position stand on exercise and Type 2 diabetes. *Medicine and Science in Sports and Exercise* 32, 1345-1360.

American College of Sports Medicine and American Diabetes Association (1997). Diabetes mellitus and exercise: Joint position statement. *Medicine and Science in Sports and Exercise* 29(12), i-vi.

American Diabetes Association (2002). Position statement: Diabetes mellitus and exercise. *Diabetes Care* 25(1), S64-S68.

American Diabetes Association. Http://www.diabetes.org

Campaigne, B.N. et al. (1994). *Exercise in the clinical management of diabetes*. Champaign, IL: Human Kinetics.

Colberg, S.R. (2001). *The diabetic athlete*. Champaign, IL: Human Kinetics.

Colberg, S.R. and Swain, D.P. (2000). Exercise and diabetes control. *The Physician and Sportsmedicine*, 28(4), 63-81.

Colberg, S.R. and Walsh, J. (2002). Pumping insulin during exercise. What healthcare providers and diabetic patients need to know. *The Physician and Sportsmedicine* 30(4), 33-38.

Dorchy, H. and Poortmans, J. (1989). Sport and the diabetic child. *Sports Medicine* 7, 248-262.

Eriksson, J.G. (1999). Exercise and the treatment of Type 2 diabetes mellitus. An update. *Sports Medicine* 27(6), 381-391.

Gordon, N.F. (1993). *Diabetes: Your complete exercise guide*. The Cooper Clinic and Research Institute Fitness Series. Champaign, IL: Human Kinetics.

Ivy, J.L. (1997). Role of exercise training in the prevention and treatment of insulin resistance and non-insulin dependent diabetes mellitus. *Sports Medicine* 24(5), 321-336.

McGavock, J.M. et al. (2004). The role of exercise in the treatment of cardiovascular disease associated with Type 2 diabetes mellitus. *Sports Medicine* 34(1), 27-48.

Wallberg-Henriksson, H. (1992). Exercise and diabetes mellitus. *Exercise and Sport Sciences Reviews* 20, 339-368.

Wallberg-Henriksson, H., Rincon, J. and Zierath, J.R. (1998). Exercise in the management of non-insulin dependent diabetes mellitus. *Sports Medicine* 25(1), 25-35.

Wasserman, D.H. and Abumrad, N.N. (1989). Physiological bases for the treatment of the physically active individual with diabetes. *Sports Medicine* 7, 376-392.

Young, J.C. (1995). Exercise prescription for individuals with metabolic disorders. Practical considerations. *Sports Medicine*

19(1), 43-54.

Zierath, J.R. and Wallberg-Henriksson, H.(1992). Exercise training in obese diabetic patients. Special considerations. *Sports Medicine* 14(3), 171-187.

DIAPHRAGM See under BREATHING MUSCLES; INTRA-ABDOMINAL PRESSURE.

DIAPHYSIS *See under* EPIPHYSEAL GROWTH PLATE.

DIARRHEA *See under* FRUCTOSE; GASTRO-INTESTINAL SYSTEM.

DIASTOLE *See under* CARDIAC CYCLE.

DIET The quality, quantity and time-course of food consumption. Taste and texture are the two most important factors that influence food choices. A healthful, 'balanced diet' is achieved by eating a wide variety of foods in moderation. In the USA, the National Academies' Institute of Medicine Food and Nutrition Board recommends that carbohydrates contribute 45% to 65% of an adult's daily calories (with at least 130 grams to avoid ketosis); 20% to 35% fat (minimizing saturated fat, cholesterol and trans fat); and 10% to 35% protein. The American Heart Association recommends that carbohydrate intake should be at least 55% of total calories, with protein intake approximately 15%, and total fat not exceeding 30%.

The **Food Guide Pyramid** devised by the United States Department of Agriculture (USDA) is a graphic representation of the number of servings from the five major food groups needed daily to have a healthful diet. It is not a rigid prescription, but rather a general guide. The major food groups are (minimum servings in parentheses): fats, oil and sweets ("sparingly"); milk, yogurt and cheese (2 to 3 servings); meat, poultry and fish (2 to 3 servings); vegetables (3 to 5 servings); fruit (2 to 4 servings); and bread, cereal, rice and pasta (6 to 11 servings).

Examples of serving sizes (shown in parentheses) in each food group are: milk, yogurt and cheese (1 cup of milk or yogurt; 1.5 oz natural cheese; or 2 oz of processed cheese); meat, poultry and fish (2 to 3 oz of cooked meat, poultry or fish; ½ cup of cooked dry beans or 2 tablespoons of peanut butter count as 1 oz of lean meat); vegetables (1 cup of raw leafy vegetables; ½ cup of other vegetables – cooked or chopped raw; or ¾ cup of vegetable juice); fruit (1 medium apple, banana, orange etc; ½ cup of chopped, cooked or canned fruit; or ¾ cup of fruit juice); bread, cereal, rice and pasta (1 slice of bread; 1 oz of ready-to-eat cereal; or ½ cup of cooked cereal, rice or pasta).

An **exchange list for meal planning** is a list of foods, which in specified portions provides equivalent amounts of carbohydrate, fat, protein and energy. Any food in an exchange list can be substituted for any other without markedly affecting nutrient intake, e.g. 1 fruit exchange is 0.5 cup of orange juice or 12 grapes or 1 medium apple.

Athletes undergoing an intense, daily training program need an appropriately high-energy intake, predominantly in the form of carbohydrate, in order to replenish muscle glycogen stores on a continual basis. A high-energy diet, chosen from a variety of different foods, should ensure sufficient intake of micronutrients (vitamins and minerals). In the optimal diet for most athletes, carbohydrate is likely to contribute about 60-70% of total energy intake, protein about 12%, while fat consumption should not exceed 30% (Devlin and Williams, 1991). However, guidelines for macronutrients should not be provided in terms of percentage contributions to total dietary energy intake. Such recommendations are neither user-friendly nor strongly related to the muscle's absolute needs for fuel. Examination of dietary survey data from endurance athletes (1970-2001) provides clear evidence that carbohydrate intake expressed as a percentage of dietary energy and intake expressed as grams relative to body mass are not interchangeable concepts. The confounding issue is restricted energy intake in some individuals or groups.

It has recently been debated whether carbohydrate diets of over 60% energy intake are necessary for athletes. The generally accepted belief is that a high carbohydrate diet fills glycogen stores to enable athletes to work at higher training loads. Carbohydrates are the only substrates that can be used to produce anaerobic energy. Tour de France cyclists riding at least 6 hours each day have been reported to consume carbohydrate intakes of 12 to 13 g/kg body weight. It has been found, however, that carbohydrate intake is generally in the range of 40 to 60%. There is little scientific evidence to support the notion that carbohydrate diets in excess of 50% total energy intake enhance training in athletes with high-energy intake. Hawley et al. (1995) pointed out that if the average athlete consumes 5000 kcal per day with only 45% carbohydrate, then this athlete consumes more than 550 g of carbohydrate per day. This amount appears to be sufficient to restore muscle glycogen within a 24-hour period. Hawley et al (1995) further stated that moderate levels of carbohydrate during heavy training do not appear to diminish training capacity. Athletes, such as female distance runners and gymnasts, who increase their carbohydrate intake to 60 to 70% of total energy, but who are restricting their total energy intake, may decrease fat or protein intake to levels that compromise health and performance.

On the day of competition, athletes should leave at least a 3 to 4 hour interval between a full meal and competition to minimize gastrointestinal discomfort. This is because the digestion of food and absorption of nutrients competes with skeletal muscles for blood supply. A meal or liquid ingested 4 hours before exercise should provide 5 g carbohydrate per kg body weight. A meal or liquid ingested 1 hour before exercise should provide carbohydrate of quantity 1 to 2 g/kg bodyweight.

The ingestion of carbohydrate in the hour before exercise results in a large increase in plasma glucose and insulin concentrations. With the onset of exercise, however, there is a rapid fall in blood glucose concentration as a consequence of the combined stimulatory effects of hyperinsulinemia and contractile activity on muscle glucose uptake and inhibition of the exercise-induced rise in liver glucose output, despite ongoing absorption of the ingested carbohydrate. The occurrence of 'rebound hypoglycemia' in susceptible individuals does not appear to be related to insulin sensitivity or to the exercise intensity. The etiology of 'rebound hypoglycemia' is not known.

An enhanced uptake and oxidation of blood glucose by skeletal muscle may account for the increased carbohydrate oxidation often observed after pre-exercise carbohydrate ingestion. The increase in plasma concentrations of free fatty acids with exercise is attenuated following pre-exercise carbohydrate ingestion, as a consequence of insulin-mediated inhibition of lipolysis.

During prolonged, strenuous exercise (greater than 90 minutes), the rate of carbohydrate oxidation can be as high as 3 to 4 g/min. Thus, muscle glycogen and/or blood glucose may decrease markedly, thus coinciding with fatigue. Carbohydrate ingested during exercise appears to be readily available as a fuel for the working muscles, at least when the exercise intensity does not exceed 70 to 75% of maximal oxygen uptake. Carbohydrate is generally ingested in a liquid form during endurance events in order to simultaneously supply glucose and ensure adequate fluid replacement. The goal for optimal carbohydrate feeding during prolonged exercise is obtained by ingestion of 40 to 75 g of glucose diluted in 400 to 750 mL of water per hour of exercise. The fatigue-delaying effect of ingested carbohydrate is due to maintenance of blood glucose levels and a high rate of carbohydrate oxidation. It is not due to a slowing of muscle glycogen utilization.

In the 1980s, it was established that ingested carbohydrate and blood glucose can be oxidized at a rate of approximately 1 g/min and that this exogenous carbohydrate becomes the predominant source of carbohydrate energy late in a bout of prolonged continuous exercise. Ingesting 30 to 60 g of carbohydrate per hour does not appear to present a general physiological risk to people who do not experience gastrointestinal discomfort. The concentration of carbohydrate should not exceed 7 to 8%.

Carbohydrate ingestion during exercise would not be expected to improve performance when fatigue is due to the accumulation of hydrogen ions in skeletal muscle, as occurs during a single bout of intense exercise. Carbohydrate ingestion is not generally recommended during events that are completed in 30 to 45 minutes or less, performed either continuously or intermittently. Carbohydrate ingestion does not appear to lessen fatigue due to hyperthermia or dehydration-induced hyper-thermia, even when exercise is prolonged.

Research using stable-isotope methods has shown that not all carbohydrates are oxidized at similar rates and hence they may not be equally effective. Glucose, sucrose, maltose, maltodextrins and amylopectin are oxidized at high rates. Fructose, galactose and amylose are oxidized at rates that are 25 to 50% lower. Combinations of multiple transportable carbohydrates may increase the total carbohydrate absorption and total exogenous carbohydrate oxidation. Increasing the carbohydrate intake up to 1.0 to 1.5 g/min will increase the oxidation up to about 1.0 to 1.1 g/min. However, a further increase of the intake will not further increase the oxidation rates. Training status does not affect exogenous carbohydrate oxidation.

Increased carbohydrate intake may be useful after muscle damage caused by eccentric exercise, which typically impairs the rate of post-exercise glycogen resynthesis. Burke et al. (2004) recommend that during immediate recovery after exercise (0 to 4 hours), 1.0 to 1.2 g/kg/hour should be consumed at frequent intervals. Recommendations for daily recovery are: 5 to 7 g/kg/day (moderate duration/low-intensity training), 7 to 12 g/kg/day (moderate to heavy endurance training) or 10 to 12+ g/kg/day (extreme exercise program - 4 to 6+ hours per day)

Excess carbohydrate tends to be oxidized, leading to indirect fat accumulation via decreases in fat oxidation. Chronically high carbohydrate ingestion (without an active lifestyle) leads to muscle becoming insulin sensitive, carbohydrates being converted to fatty acids in adipose tissue and the liver increasing production of very low-density lipoproteins.

See also BODY WEIGHT REDUCTION; DIETING; GLYCEMIC INDEX; NUTRITION; VEGETARIAN DIET.

Chronology

•1995 • For the first time, one of the Dietary Guidelines for Americans was "to balance the food you eat with physical activity…"

Bibliography

Achten, J. and Jeukendrup, A.E. (2003). Effects of pre-exercise ingestion of carbohydrate on glycemic and insulinemic responses during subsequent exercise at differing intensities. *European Journal of Applied Physiology* 88, 466-471.

Berning, J. and Nelson Steen, S. (1998, eds). *Nutrition for sport and exercise.* 2nd ed. Boston, MA: McGraw-Hill.

Brotherhood, J.R. (1984). Nutrition and sports performance. *Sports Medicine* 1, 350-389.

Burke, L.M. and Deakin, V. (2000). *Clinical sports nutrition.* Roseville, NSW: McGraw-Hill Australia.

Burke, L.M. et al. (2001). Guidelines for daily carbohydrate intake: Do athletes achieve them? *Sports Medicine* 31, 267-299.

Burke, L.M., Kiens, B. and Ivy, J.L. (2004). Carbohydrates and fat for training and recovery. *Journal of Sports Sciences* 22, 15-30.

Clark, N. (2003). *Nancy Clark's sports nutrition guidebook.* 3rd ed. Champaign, IL: Human Kinetics.

Costill, D.L. and Hargreaves, M. (1992). Carbohydrate nutrition and fatigue. *Sports Medicine* 13(2), 86-92.

Coyle, E. (2004). Fluid and fuel intake during exercise. *Journal of Sports Sciences* 22, 39-55.

Devlin, J.T. and Williams, C. (eds) (1991). Final consensus statement: Foods, nutrition and sports performance. *Journal of Sports Sciences* 9S, iii.

Economos, C.D., Bortz, S.S. and Nelson, M.E. (1993). Nutritional practices of elite athletes. Practical recommendations. *Sports Medicine* 16(6), 381-399.

Graham, T.E. and Adamo, K.B. (1999). Dietary carbohydrate and its effects on metabolism and substrate stores in sedentary and active individuals. *Canadian Journal of Applied Physiology* 24(5), 393-415.

Guezennec, C.Y. (1995). Oxidation rates, complex carbohydrates and exercise. Practical recommendations. *Sports Medicine* 19(6), 365-372.

Hargreaves, M., Hawley, J.A. and Jeukendrup, A. (2004). Pre-exercise carbohydrate and fat ingestion. Effects on metabolism and performance. *Journal of Sports Sciences* 22, 31-38.

Hawley, J.A. et al (1995). Nutritional practices of athletes: Are they suboptimal? *Journal of Sports Sciences* 13, S75-S87.

Jentjens, R.L.P.G. and Jeukendrup, A.E. (2002). Prevalence of hypoglycemia following pre-exercise carbohydrate ingestion is not accompanied by higher insulin sensitivity. *International Journal of Sport Nutrition and Exercise Metabolism* 12, 444-459.

Jeukendrup, A.E. and Jentjens, R. (2000). Oxidation of carbohydrate feedings during prolonged exercise. Current thoughts, guidelines and directions for future research. *Sports Medicine* 29(6), 407-424.

Manore, M. and Thompson, J. (2000). *Sport nutrition for health and performance.* Champaign, IL: Human Kinetics.

Maughan, R.J. and Burke, L.M. (2002). *Sports nutrition. Handbook of sports medicine and science. An IOC Medical Committee publication.* Oxford: Blackwell Science.

McArdle, W.D., Katch, F.I. and Katch, V.I. (1999). *Sports and exercise nutrition.* Philadelphia, PA: Lippincott, Williams & Wilkins.

Saris, W.H.M. et al. (1989). Study on food intake and energy expenditure during extreme sustained exercise: The Tour de France. *International Journal of Sports Medicine* 10(S1), S26-S31.

Shirreffs, S.M., Armstrong, L.E. and Cheuvront, S.M. (2004). Fluid and electrolyte needs for preparation and recovery from training and competition. *Journal of Sports Sciences* 22, 57-63.

Stamford, B. (1989). Meals and the timing of exercise. *The Physician and Sportsmedicine* 17(11), 151.

Thomas, B. (1997). *Manual of dietetic practice.* 2nd ed. Oxford: Blackwell Science.

Titchenal, C.A. (1988). Exercise and food intake. What is the relationship? *Sports Medicine* 6, 135-145.

Tsintzas, K. and Williams, C. (1998). Human muscle glycogen metabolism during exercise. Effect of carbohydrate supplementation. *Sports Medicine* 25(1), 7-23.

Williams, M.H. (1999). *Nutrition for health, fitness and sport.* 5th ed. Boston, MA: McGraw-Hill.

Wolinsky, I. (1998). *Nutrition in exercise and sport.* 3rd ed. Boca Raton, FL: CRC Press.

DIETARY REFERENCE INTAKE A generic term in the USA used to refer to estimated average requirement, recommended dietary allowance, adequate intake and tolerable upper intake level.

Estimated average requirement (EAR) is the intake that meets the estimated nutrient needs of 50% of the individuals in a specific life-stage and gender group. This dietary reference value is used as the basis for developing the recommended dietary allowances and is used by policy makers in the evaluation of the adequacy of nutrient intakes of the group and for planning how much the group should consume.

Recommended dietary allowance (RDA) is the intake that meets the nutrient needs of almost all (97 to 98%) individuals in a specific life-stage group. This reference value should be used in guiding individuals to achieve nutrient intake aimed at decreasing the risk of chronic disease. It is based on estimating an average requirement plus an increase to account for the variation within a particular group.

Adequate intake (AI) is the average observed or experimentally derived intake by a defined population or subgroup that appears to sustain a defined nutritional state, such as normal circulating nutrient values, growth or other functional indicators of health. Adequate intakes have been set when sufficient scientific evidence is not available to establish an estimated average requirement. Individuals should use the adequate intake as a goal for intake where no recommended dietary allowances exist. Adequate intake is not equivalent to recommended dietary allowance.

Tolerable upper intake level (UL) is the maximum intake by an individual that is unlikely to pose risks of adverse health effects in almost all (97 to 98%) individuals in a specified life-stage group. This figure is not intended to be a recommended level of intake, and there is no established benefit for individuals to consume nutrients at levels above the recommended dietary allowance or adequate intake. For most nutrients, supplements must be consumed to reach a tolerable upper intake level.

In the UK, until 1991, **recommended daily amount** (RDA) was the level of intake of an essential nutrient considered adequate to meet the known nutritional needs of practically all healthy persons. In 1991, it was replaced by the following dietary reference values (DRVs): lower reference nutrient intake, estimated average requirement, reference nutrient intake and safe intakes. **Estimated average requirement** (EAR) is an estimate of the average requirement for energy or a nutrient; approximately 50% of a group of people will require less and 50% will require more. It assumes normal distribution of variability. **Lower reference nutrient intake** (LRNI) is 2 standard deviations below the estimated average requirement. Habitual intakes below the LRNI by an individual will almost certainly by inadequate. **Reference nutrient intake** (RNI) is 2 standard deviations above the estimated average requirement and is the

amount of a nutrient that is sufficient for almost all (97.5%) of individuals. Some nutrients are known to be important, but there is insufficient data on human requirements to set any dietary reference values. A **safe intake** is judged to be a level or range above which there is no risk of deficiency and below a level where there is a risk of undesirable effects.

Chronology

•1941 • Recommended Dietary Allowances, the nutrient intakes that meet the needs of 97 to 98% of individuals, were first published to ensure that American military troops were being fed adequately.

DIETARY SUPPLEMENT *See under* NUTRITION; NUTRITIONAL ERGOGENIC AID.

DIETING Any attempts in the name of weight loss, 'healthy eating,' or body sculpting to deny the body of the nutrients and calories it requires to function effectively. 95% of all dieters regain their lost weight and more within one to five years. Dieting actually slows down the metabolism, because the body is forced into starvation mode and slows down many of its function in order to conserve energy. It is estimated that 40 to 50% of American girls and women are trying to lose weight at any point in time.

In order to lose and maintain a desirable body weight, it is necessary to combine a restricted energy intake with increased energy expenditure through exercise. Weight-reduction programs that involve substantial weight loss in the short term will not work over the long term and may represent a significant health risk. The immediate loss in weight is due to the decrease in the carbohydrate stores in which 2.7 grams of water are bound to each gram of carbohydrate stored as glycogen. Lack of weight loss during the first three weeks of dieting by an obese person is probably due to water retention. The water that is formed as a by-product of the metabolism of the body's fat stores is not excreted immediately via the kidneys because of the obese person's increased level of anti-diuretic hormones.

Wing and Hill (2001) define successful long-term weight loss maintenance as intentionally losing at least 10% of initial body weight and keeping it off for at least one year. In the National Weight Control Registry, successful long-term weight loss maintainers (average weight loss of 30 kg for an average of 5.5 years) share common behavioral strategies, including eating a diet low in fat, frequent self-monitoring of body weight and food intake, and high levels of regular physical activity.

The American College of Sports Medicine (2001) recommends that the combination of decreases in energy intake and increases in energy expenditure, through structured exercise and other forms of physical activity, be a component of weight loss intervention programs. An energy deficit of 500 to 1000 kcal per day achieved through decreases in total energy intake is recommended. Moreover, it appears that decreasing dietary fat intake to less than 30% of total energy intake may facilitate weight loss by decreasing total energy intake. Significant health benefits can be recognized with participation in a minimum of 150 minutes of moderate intensity exercise per week; overweight and obese adults should progressively increase to this initial exercise goal. However, there may be advantages to progressively increasing exercise to 200 to 300 minutes of exercise per week, as recent scientific evidence indicates that this level of exercise facilitates the long-term maintenance of weight loss. With respect to 'fat burning,' it is the total amount of calories expended during exercise that supports increased mobilization of fat in response to a caloric deficit. To lose body fat weight, the fuel is not as important as the amount of energy expended. A caloric deficit of 500 kcal per day (3,500 kcal per week) is associated with a 1 lb (0.45 kg) per week weight loss only over large population groups, but there is considerable variability among individuals.

Very-low-calorie diets (400 to 800 kcal) appear to be safe when properly administered and supervised. Loss of fat-free body mass seems to be limited to 20 to 30% of total body weight loss unless the energy intake falls below 400 kcal/day. A minimal loss of fat-free mass from the obese state is not only unavoidable, but is actually desirable if the loss is in the form of less essential fat-free mass. The addition of exercise to very-low-calorie diets does not consistently show the ability to preserve more

fat-free mass compared to the diet alone. The exercise tolerance of the severely obese is very poor. Obese individuals show a much smaller increase in free fatty acid levels during exercise than lean individuals. This impaired free fatty acid mobilization may be due to a state of relative insulin resistance, reflected by higher insulin levels in obese than thin individuals during exercise. The mobilization of free fatty acids associated with acclimatization to cold suggests the possibility of using winter sport as a way of treating obesity.

Repeated cycles of weight loss that are followed by weight gain is known as 'yo-yo' dieting. It may lead to a greater difficulty in achieving weight loss with subsequent dieting. It may also facilitate regaining of the lost weight and constitute an independent heart disease risk factor.

In 2004, there were estimates that as many as 30 million people in the USA had tried the Atkins diet. The initial stage of the Atkins diet involves cutting out virtually all carbohydrates – dieters are allowed to eat no more than 20 g a day, which must come in the form of salad greens and other vegetables. No fruit, bread, pasta, grains or starchy vegetables are allowed during this period. Atkins believed that individuals burn more calories when the body uses fats and proteins as fuel, and originally advised that foods such as butter, meat, cheese and eggs could be eaten "liberally." Now, however, Atkins Nutritionals suggests that intake of saturated fats should be limited to 20% of calories. The American Heart Association announced that individuals who follow these diets are at risk of potential cardiac, renal, bone and liver abnormalities. A study by Fleming (2002) found that, after one year, there was a 52% decrease in LDL cholesterol on a diet with 10% fat, compared with a 6% increase in LDL cholesterol on the Atkins diet. A low-fat, whole foods diet has been shown to reverse heart disease using actual measures of coronary atherosclerosis and myocardial perfusion, but an Atkins diet worsens myocardial perfusion (Fleming and Boyd, 2000).

Another popular diet, the '**Zone (40/30/30) diet**' is based on 40% of the total calories being obtained from carbohydrates, 30% from fat, and 30% from protein. It is thus centered primarily on protein intake and purports to change the body's insulin-to-glucagon ratio via macronutrient alterations. Changes in the existing hormonal milieu are said to result in the production of more vasoactive eicosanoids, thus allowing greater oxygen delivery to exercising muscle. There is no evidence that insulin increases the amount of 'bad' eicosanoids or that glucagons make 'good' eicosanoids. The scientific literature does not support the view that a low carbohydrate diet can support or enhance athletic performance. The notion that a 40/30/30 diet can alter the pancreatic hormone response in favor of glucagon is also unfounded. Although the post-prandial insulin response is decreased when comparing a 40% with a 60% carbohydrate diet, it is still a sufficient stimulus to offset the lipolytic effects of glucagon. There is no empirical evidence that eicosanoids make any significant contribution to active muscle vasodilation in humans.

Drawing attention to the worship of a perpetually youthful and slender body in America and its "growing intolerance of even the mildest forms of body diversity," Campos (2004) argues that a "rational public health policy" would not focus on body weight, because there is a lack of convincing evidence that significant long-term weight loss is beneficial to health.

See also under OBESITY; PROTEIN.

Chronology

•1972 • Robert C. Atkins, a physician, published *Dr. Atkins' Diet Revolution*, which sold 900,000 copies in the first seventh months of publication.

•1992 • *Dr. Atkins' New Diet Revolution* was published. It has sold over 10 million copies. The American Heart Association, the American Medical Association, the American Dietetic Association, and the American Council on Preventive medicine continue to attack Atkins' theory.

•1993 • In the USA, the Federal Trade Commission announced it was launching an investigation into the advertising messages of leading weight loss programs. Unsubstantiated weight loss claims and false testimonials were found. As a result of this investigation, new guidelines were introduced, requiring weight loss programs to base their claims on typical or average weight loss of program participants.

•2003 • Robert C. Atkins, 72 years of age, died after complications following head trauma caused by slipping and falling on ice while walking to work in New York. In 2002, he was hospitalised after he went into cardiac arrest, which he stated was "in no way related to diet."

Bibliography

Atkins, R.C. (2003). *Atkins for life*. New York: St. Martin's Press.

Campos, P. (2004). *The obesity myth: Why America's obsession with weight is hazardous to your health*. New York: Gotham Books.

Cheuvront, S.N. (1999). The Zone Diet and athletic performance. *Sports Medicine* 27(4), 213-228.

Donnelly, J.E., Jakicic, J. and Gunderson, S. (1991). Diet and body composition. Effect of very low calorie diets and exercise. *Sports Medicine* 12(4), 237-249.

Fleming, R.M. (2002). The effect of high-, moderate-, and low-fat diets on weight loss and cardiovascular disease risk factors. *Preventive Cardiology* 5, 110-118.

Fleming, R. and Boyd, L.B. (2000). The effect of high-protein diets on coronary blood flow. *Angiology* 51, 817-826.

Gaesser, G.A. (1999). Thinness and weight loss: Beneficial or detrimental to longevity? *Medicine and Science in Sports and Exercise* 31(8), 1118-1128.

Hagan, R.D. (1988). Benefits of aerobic conditioning and diet for overweight adults. *Sports Medicine* 5, 144-155.

Jakicic, J.M. et al. (2001). American College of Sports Medicine position stand. Appropriate intervention strategies for weight loss and prevention of weight regain for adults. *Medicine and Science in Sports and Exercise* 33(12), 2145-2156.

King, A.C. and Tribble, D.L. (1990). The role of exercise in weight regulation in nonathletes. *Sports Medicine* 11(5), 331-349.

Marks, B.L. and Rippe, J.M. (1996). The importance of fat-free mass maintenance in weight loss programmes. *Sports Medicine* 22(5), 273-281.

National Eating Disorders Association. Http://www.NationalEatingDisorders.org

Ornish, D. (2004). Was Dr. Atkins right? *Journal of the American Dietetic Association* 104(4), 537-542.

Pacy, P.J., Webster, J. and Garrow, J.S. (1986). Exercise and obesity. *Sports Medicine* 3, 89-113.

Sears, B. (1995). *The Zone Diet: A dietary road map*. New York: Regan Books.

Wing, R.R. and Hill, J.O. (2001). Successful weight loss maintenance. *Annual Review of Nutrition* 21, 323-341.

DIFFERENTIATION *See under* MOTOR DEVELOPMENT.

DIFFUSION A form of passive transport. **Simple diffusion** involves free and continuous net movement of molecules in aqueous solution across a plasma membrane. Simple diffusion across the plasma membrane occurs for: water molecules; dissolved gases (oxygen, carbon dioxide and nitrogen); small, uncharged polar molecules, such as urea and alcohol; and various lipid-soluble molecules. Flux occurs from a region of higher pressure to one of lower pressure.

Facilitated (carrier-mediated) diffusion involves passive, highly selective binding of lipid-insoluble molecules (and other large molecules) to a lipid-soluble carrier molecule. It is faster than simple diffusion because a carrier in the cell membrane is used. The **carrier molecule**, a protein called a **transporter (permease)**, crosses the plasma membrane and facilitates the transfer of membrane-insoluble chemicals like hydrogen, sodium, calcium and potassium ions, as well as glucose and amino acids, down their concentration gradients, across the cell's plasma membrane. The **transmembrane carrier molecule** serves only to accelerate the rate at which equilibrium is attained; no energy is expended in this process. See also FILTRATION.

DIGESTION It is the breakdown of complex foodstuffs into simple compounds, by enzymes in the gastrointestinal system, which can be absorbed by the body for use in metabolism. The **coefficient of digestibility** is an index that shows the proportion of ingested food that is actually digested and absorbed to serve the metabolic needs of the body. General coefficients of digestibility are 97% for carbohydrate, 95% for lipid and 92% for protein. There is intra-nutrient variability, e.g. protein is 78% from vegetable sources and 97% from animal sources. Dietary fiber decreases the coefficient of digestibility. *See also* ENERGY YIELD OF NUTRIENTS.

DIGITAL ANGLE In the foot, it is the angle formed between the longitudinal bisection of the digits and the longitudinal bisection of the metatarsus. The angle is normally an adductus angle. The digital angle is usually equal and opposite in direction to the forefoot angle. Any irregularity or alteration to the forefoot angle will proportionately alter the digital angle in the opposite direction.

DIGITAL RAY A digit of the hand or foot and the corresponding portion of the metacarpus or metatarsus, considered as a continuous structural unit.

2,3 DIPHOSPHOGLYCERATE 2,3 DPG. A substance found in red blood cells. It is formed as a by-product in the breakdown of glycogen and glucose. It has the effect of greatly decreasing the affinity of hemoglobin for oxygen and this effect is related to the partial pressure of oxygen in the lungs. The increase in 2,3-DPG at medium and high altitude allows hemoglobin to release oxygen more readily in the tissues. With regard to 2,3-DPG, some authors have argued that 'bis' is a more exact nomenclature than 'di.' See also VITAMIN C.

Bibliography

Brown, S.P. and Keith, W.B. (1993). The effects of acute exercise on levels of erthyrocyte 2,3-bisphosphoglycerate: A brief review. *Journal of Sports Sciences* 11, 479-484.

DIPLOPIA A condition in which a single object is seen as two rather than as one.

DIRECTIONAL AWARENESS Laterality and directionality. The understanding and application of concepts such as up and down, front and back, and left and right. **Laterality** involves awareness of the body's dimensions with respect to their location and direction. **Directionality** refers to the external projection of laterality. It gives dimension to objects in space.

DISABILITY According to a revision in 2001 of the International Classification of Functioning, Disability and Health (ICF), published by the World Health Organization, disability is an umbrella term for any or all of: an impairment of body structure or function; a limitation in activities; or a restriction in participation.

Out of the total US population of 250 million, 43

million (17%) have disabilities. The US Department of Education, Office of Special Education Programs, documents services to about 5 million individuals from birth through age 21 years. This is only about 2% of this age group, although most sources indicate that 10 to 12% of individuals who are 21 years of age or younger have disabilities and could benefit from special education services, including physical education. The three most common physical disabilities among school-age persons are: cerebral palsy, spina bifida and muscular dystrophy.

The following disabilities are recognized under the Individuals with Disabilities Act (IDEA): autism, deafness, deaf-blindness, emotional disturbance, hearing impairment, learning disability, mental retardation, multiple disabilities, orthopedic impairment, other health impairment, speech or language impairment, traumatic brain injury, and visual impairment.

Adapted physical activity refers to an individualized program of developmental activities, exercises, games and sport designed to meet the unique physical education needs of individuals. Adapted physical activity may be conducted in a variety of settings, ranging from integrated settings in which individuals with disabilities interact with non-disabled participants to segregated environments in which sporting activity includes only persons with disabilities.

The six categories of disability used at the Paralympics are: amputees, cerebral palsy, intellectual disability, les autres, vision impaired and wheelchair. Within these six disability categories, athletes are then classified according to their differing level of functional impairment. Not all disability categories can compete in all 18 sports. Judo and goalball are played only by vision-impaired athletes. Soccer is played only by athletes with cerebral palsy. Swimming and athletics are open to all six disability categories. Amputees include athletes who have at least one major joint in a limb missing. Depending on the sport, some amputees compete as wheelchair athletes.

The Handicapped Scuba Association International, founded in 1981, classifies divers according to physical performance standards, rather than type of disability. Level A consists of divers who can care for themselves and others; level B are divers who need partial support; and level C are divers who need full support.

Chronology

•1780 • Clement J. Tissot, later to become surgeon-in-chief of the French armies, published his book, *Gymnastique Médicinale et Chirurgicale* (Medical and Surgical Gymnastics) in which he recommended "prescribed craft and recreational activities as therapeutic exercises for the treatment of disabled muscles and joints following disease or injury."

•1803 • Andres O. Lindfors' dissertation at the University of Lund (Sweden), *Arte Gymnastica* (On the subject of gymnastics), was the first of its kind presented as partial fulfillment of the doctorate degree in any university. Lindfors made a distinction between artificial and natural exercises. Artificial exercises were placed in three categories: i) military gymnastics, ii) pedagogical gymnastics, and iii) medical gymnastics for the prevention of physical defects. The second category included the Greek pentathlon of running, jumping, javelin and discus throwing, and wrestling and Plato's orkäsis, which consisted of games, acrobatics and dancing. Medical gymnastics was the first widely used term to refer to what is now called adapted physical education. The word 'gymnastics' was replaced with "exercises" in the early 1900s.

•1814 • Per H. Ling opened his Central Institute of Gymnastics in Stockholm and subsequently dominated Swedish physical education. Ling soon started to develop medical gymnastics for the relief and cure of physical disabilities. He believed that the medical value of gymnastics had been under emphasized and that gymnastics for the weak was as important as gymnastics for the strong. He had been interested in the therapeutic value of exercise at least since taking up horse riding in his youth for a 'chest complaint.' A post-mortem examination showed that he had suffered from tuberculosis.

•1899 • Public schooling for persons with disabilities had begun, with the earliest documentation citing 100 large cities, such as New York, with special education classes.

•1905 • The Therapeutic Section of the American Physical Education Association (APEA) began with Baroness Rose Posse as chair. This date is often used to mark the beginning of the adapted physical activity profession.

•1906 • In *Physical Education*, Dudley A. Sargent listed four aims of physical training: (i) hygiene (the consideration of the normal proportions of the individual, the anatomy and the physiological functions of various organs, and a study of the ordinary agents of health such as exercise, diet, sleep, air, bathing and clothing); ii) education (the cultivation of special powers of mind and body used in the acquisition of some skilful trade or physical accomplishment, such as golf, swimming or skating); iii) recreation (the renovation of vital energies to enable the individual to return to his daily work with vigor and accomplish his tasks with ease); and iv) remedy (the restoration of disturbed functions and the correction of physical defects and deformities.)

•1909 • In *Exercise in Education and Medicine*, R.Tait McKenzie, who was a student of Dudley A. Sargent, described deafness, blindness and mental retardation along with activities appropriate for each population. He was the first physical educator to write about serving individuals in residential facilities.

•1928 • The first textbooks to use the term corrective physical education were published: George Stafford's *Preventive and Corrective Physical Education* and Charles Lowman et al's *Corrective Physical Education for Groups*. Stafford was a physical therapist and corrections specialist; and Lowman was an orthopedic physician.

•1930 • The historic White House Conference on Child Health and Protection took place. The Committee on the Physically and Mentally Handicapped wrote the Bill of Rights for Handicapped Children.

•1937 • The British medical profession turned to physical educators for assistance in the field of rehabilitation, and it was so successful that the United States Army created a program to train corrective therapists. Trainees were army personnel with a background in physical education, coaching or athletics. The program included courses in anatomy, kinesiology, medical terminology, physiology and psychology. The major function of the graduates was to provide rehabilitation programs that would return soldiers to duty. Howard Rusk, the director of Rehabilitation Medicine at New York University, was credited with developing the rehabilitation concept based on an interdisciplinary approach including "corrective therapy." By 1946, the United States Veterans Administration officially established a medical rehabilitation program with corrective therapy as an integral part.

•1939 • *Sports for the Handicapped* by George T. Stafford of the University of Illinois was published. This was the first indicator of a trend away from corrective exercise toward sports as appropriate for programming individuals with disabilities.

•1944 • In Britain, the Disabled Persons Employment Act was passed. It led to the realization of the importance of sport for the disabled and in the same year Sir Ludwig Guttman introduced sporting activities as an essential part of medical treatment.

•1952 • The American Association for Health, Physical Education

and Recreation (AAHPER) formed a subcommittee to define the subdiscipline of adapted physical education and to give direction and guidance to professionals. Adapted physical education was defined as a diversified program of developmental activities, games, sports, and rhythms suited to the interests, capacities, and limitations of students with disabilities who may not safely or successfully engage in unrestricted participation in the rigorous activities of the general physical education program. Adapted Physical Education became the official term used by the American Alliance for Health, Physical Education and Recreation (AAHPER), but had strong opposition from many Therapeutics Section members.

•1954 • Arthur Daniels' *Adapted Physical Education* was published. It was the first textbook to use this term.

•1958 • Legislation, PL 85-926, was passed in the USA, authorizing grants for training personnel in mental retardation. This legislation marked the beginning of the federal government's commitment to the rights of persons with disabilities.

•1965 • In the USA, the Elementary and Secondary Education Act (P.L. 89-10) was passed. It provided a comprehensive plan for readdressing the inequality of educational opportunity for economically underprivileged children. It became the statutory basis upon which early special education legislation was drafted. The Elementary and Secondary Education Act Amendments (P.L. 89-313) authorized grants to state institutions and state-operated schools devoted to the education of children with disabilities.

•1966 • In the USA, the Elementary and Secondary Education Amendments (P.L. 89-750) amended Title VI of P.L. 89-10 and established the first federal grant program for the education of youth with disabilities at local school level, rather than at state-operated schools or institutions. It established the Bureau of Education of the Handicapped (BEH), which became the Office of Special Education Programs (OSEP) in 1980 and is the agency that funds university training programs in physical education and recreation for persons with disabilities.

•1969 • The first doctoral programs in adapted physical education were established at several universities with help of federal funding – the Mental Retardation Facilities and Community Mental Health Centers Construction Act (P.L. 90-170). By 1971, 24 universities offered graduate specializations designated as physical education for the handicapped or adapted, special, or developmental physical education. Of these 24, 19 were receiving federal money under P.L. 90-170.

•1970 • The National Sports Center for the Disabled (NSCD) was founded when the director of the Winter Park Resort's ski school agreed to teach skiing to a group of children with amputations from the Children's Hospital in Denver, Colorado. The NSCD is widely considered to be the largest and most successful outdoor therapeutic recreation agency in the world.

•1973 • Section 504 of the Rehabilitation Act (P.L. 93-112) was enacted, mandating nondiscrimination on the basis of disability in programs and facilities receiving federal funds. It was not implemented, however, until 1977. Often called "Civil Rights Law for the Disabled," Section 504 states: *"No otherwise qualified individual with handicaps in the United States... shall, solely by reason of his or her handicap, be excluded from the participation in, be denied the benefits of, or be subjected to discrimination under any program or activity receiving Federal financial assistance..."*It was amended by P.L. 98-221 in 1983, and by P.L. 99-506 in 1986.

•1973 • The International Federation of Adapted Physical Activity (IFAPA) was founded. IFAPA coordinates national, regional, and international functions (both governmental and nongovernmental) that pertain to sport, dance, aquatics, exercise, fitness, and wellness for individuals of all ages with disabilities or special needs. It is officially linked with several other international governing bodies, including the International Paralympic Committee (IPC) and the International Council of Sport Science and Physical Education (ICSSPE).

•1974 • The National Consortium on Physical Education and Recreation for Individuals with Disabilities (NCPERID) was formed to provide national professional leadership in relation to the development of the US Special Education Program for school age "handicapped children and youth in physical education and recreation."

•1975 • The Education for All Handicapped Children Act (P.L. 94-142) was enacted. It mandated that: i) a free, appropriate public education for all children with disabilities between the ages of three and twenty-one years; ii) an individualized education program (IEP) be developed for each student with a disability; iii) education take place in the least restrictive environment, adapting or modifying the physical education curriculum and/or instruction to address the individualized abilities of each child; iv) physical education be identified as a direct instructional service required for students with disabilities; and v) students with disabilities be included, where appropriate, in intramural and interscholastic opportunities.

•1978 • The Amateur Sports Act was passed by Congress. This act placed a major responsibility on the United States Olympic Committee (USOC) for establishing, coordinating and directing policy on amateur sports in the United States. It prohibited gender discrimination in open amateur sport in the USA. One of the purposes of this law was "to encourage and provide assistance to amateur athletic programs and competition for handicapped individuals, including, where feasible, the expansion of opportunities for meaningful participation by handicapped individuals in programs of athletic competition for able-bodied individuals." This legislation led to the establishment of the Committee on Sports for the Disabled (COSD), a standing committee of the United States Olympic Committee (USOC) representing a number of sport organizations including the American Athletic Association for the Deaf (AAAD).

•1984 • *Adapted Physical Activity Quarterly* was first published. It was the first professional journal to be devoted specifically to adapted physical education.

•1985 • Adapted physical activity became the umbrella term of choice with the merger of the Therapeutics Council and Adapted Physical Education Section of the American Alliance for Health, Physical Education, Recreation and Dance (AAHPERD) and with the growth of the International Federation of Adapted Physical Activity.

•1988 • The Paralympic Games was held in South Korea. This was the first time that all athletes with physical disabilities competed at the same venue and also in the same facilities as the Olympic Games.

•1989 • The International Paralympic Committee (IPC) was founded. The five disability-specific international sports federations of the International Paralympic Committee (IPC) are: Cerebral Palsy International Sport and Recreation (CP-ISRA), International Blind Sports Association (IBSA), International Sports Federation for Persons with Disability (INAS-FID), International Stoke Mandeville Wheelchair Sports Federation (ISMWSF), and the International Sports Organization for the Disabled (ISOD).

•1990 • The Americans with Disabilities Act (P.L. 101-336) was passed. Based on concepts of the Rehabilitation Act of 1973, this legislation extended civil rights protection for individuals with disabilities to all areas of American life. Related to adapted physical education and sport, this legislation has required that community recreational facilities including health and fitness facilities, should be accessible and, where appropriate, that reasonable accommodation should be made for persons with disabilities.

•1990 • The Education for all Handicapped Act (EHA) Amendments (P.L. 101-476) changed the name of EHA to the Individuals with Disabilities Education Act (IDEA). It expanded upon the previous EHA and amendments, including P.L. 91-230 (1970), P.L. 94-142 (1975), P.L. 98-199 (1983) and P.L. 99-457 (1986). It reauthorized and expanded the discretionary programs, mandated transition services and assistive technology services to be included in a child's or youth's individualized education program (IEP), and added autism and traumatic brain injury to the list of categories of children and youth eligible for special education and related services.

•1990 • The Developmental Disabilities Assistance and Bill of Rights Act (P.L. 101-496) authorized grants to support planning, coordination, and delivery of specialized services to persons with developmental disabilities. It provides funding for the operation of state protection and advocacy systems for persons with developmental disabilities. The original law was enacted in 1963 by P.L. 88-164.

•1992 • The International Paralympic Committee (IPC) became the governing body for the Paralympic movement. The Paralympic Games was staged for wheelchair users, amputees, blind, cerebral palsy and *les autres* in Barcelona and, for the first time, for people with intellectual disability in Madrid.

•1995 • The National Consortium for Physical Education and Recreation for Individuals with Disabilities (NCPERID) published the results of their Adapted Physical Education National Standards (APENS) Project. The purpose of the project was to ensure that physical education instruction for students with disabilities is provided by qualified physical education instructors. To achieve this end, the project developed national standards for the profession and a national certification examination to measure knowledge of these standards.

•1997 • The Individuals with Disabilities Education Act (IDEA) Amendment (P.L. 105-17) brought many changes to the law initially passed in 1975 as P.L. 94-142. In addition to free and appropriate public education, the amendments specifically cover: i) participation of children with disabilities in state and district-wide assessment programs; ii) the way evaluations are conducted; iii) parent participation in eligibility and placement decisions; iv) development and review of the individualized education plan (IEP); v) transition planning; vi) voluntary mediation; and vii) discipline of children with disabilities.

•1998 • In the USA, one of the provisions of the Workforce Investment Act (P.L. 105-220) was to develop research and demonstration projects to indicate how adapted physical education programs can develop health and related skills that improve work performance.

Bibliography

American College of Sports Medicine (1997). *ACSM's exercise management for persons with chronic diseases and disabilities*. Champaign, IL: Human Kinetics.

Compton, D.M., Eisenman, P.A. and Henderson, H.L. (1989). Exercise and fitness for persons with disabilities. *Sports Medicine* 7, 150-162.

DePauw, K.P. and Gavron, S.J. (1995). *Disability and sport*. Champaign, IL: Human Kinetics.

Doll-Tepper, G. and DePauw, K. (1996, eds). Adapted physical activity. *Sports Science Review* 5(1).

Handicapped Scuba Association International. Http://www.hsascuba.com

Horvat, M. et al. (2003). *Developmental/adapted physical education: Making ability count*. 4th ed. San Francisco, CA: Benjamin Cummings

International Paralympic Committee. Http://www.paralympic.org

Office of Special Education Programs. Http://www.ed.gov

Shephard, R.J. (1990). *Fitness in special populations*. Champaign, IL: Human Kinetics.

Sherill, C. (2004). *Adapted physical activity, recreation, and sport: Cross disciplinary and lifespan*. 6th ed. Boston, MA: McGraw-Hill.

Sherill, C. and DePauw, K.P. (1997). Adapted physical activity and education. In: Massengale, J.D. and Swanson, R.A. (eds.). *The history of exercise and sport science*. pp39-108. Champaign, IL: Human Kinetics.

Van der Ploeg, H.P. (2004). Physical activity for people with a disability: A conceptual model. *Sports Medicine* 34(10), 639-649.

Winnick, J.P. (2000, ed). *Adapted physical education and sport*. 3rd ed. Champaign, IL: Human Kinetics.

World Health Organization. International Classification of Functioning, Disability and Health. Http://www3.who.int/icf/icftemplate.cfm

DISINHIBITION In neurophysiology, it is inhibition of the inhibitor. For example, the Renshaw cell disinhibits the Ia inhibitory interneuron and calcium ions disinhibit the inhibitory effect of the regulatory proteins (troponin and tropomyosin).

DISLOCATION Rupture of a joint capsule and its ligaments. **Total dislocation** (luxation) of a joint indicates that the opposing articular surfaces have become separated and are no longer in contact with each other. Total dislocations most frequently affect the patella, shoulder, elbow and finger joints. **Partial dislocation** (subluxation) of a joint indicates that the articular surfaces remain in partial contact with each other, but are no longer correctly aligned. Partial dislocations usually affect the ankle, knee and acromioclavicular joint.

DISPLACEMENT   i) The distance from the initial to the final position of a body moved from one position to another due to the action of a force. It is a vector in that it possesses magnitude and direction. The change in position may be translational, whereby every point of the body is displaced along parallel lines; it may be rotational, with the points of the body describing concentric circles around an axis; or it may be a combination of the two. ii) The volume of fluid displaced by a body completely or partially submerged in that fluid.

DISRUPTIVE BEHAVIOR DISORDERS   A term used for a disorder where an affected individual continually interferes with the activities of others, causing them irritation or distress. The interference may be impulsive or proactive. Conduct disorder, oppositional defiant disorder and attention-deficit hyperactivity disorders are listed in this category.

DISTAL   Far from the midpoint of the body. In describing limbs, distal refers to relative locations away from the trunk or midpoint of the body. *See also* PROXIMAL.

DISTENTION   A term that is used to refer to the state of being stretched; it is movement of two surfaces away from each other. In joints, distraction refers to a form of dislocation where the two joint surfaces are separated but retain their ligamentous integrity.

DIURESIS   Excretion of an abnormally large amount of urine.

DIURETICS   Substances that increase urine and solute production by the kidney. They decrease blood plasma volume by promoting elimination of water in the urine and thus decrease blood pressure. In addition to their clinical use for treating hypertensive patients, diuretic drugs are used by athletes attempting to decrease body weight. They are also used to flush out other illegal drugs to avoid positive drug tests. Consequently, diuretic drugs are on the World Anti-Doping Agency (WADA) List of Banned Substances in- and out- of competition in all sports as masking agents. In a number of sports that use weight classification, and sports in which weight loss can enhance performance, no Therapeutic Use Exemptions are granted for use of diuretics. Examples of prohibited diuretics are acetazolamide (Diamox) and frusemide (Lasix, Urex). For athletes, diuretics have a number of adverse effects on performance including hypokalemia and dehydration, in addition to impaired strength, power and endurance.

Bibliography

Caldwell, J.E. (1987). Diuretic therapy and exercise performance. *Sports Medicine* 4, 290-304.

World Anti-Doping Agency. Http://www.wada-ama.org

Chronology

•1985 • Diuretics and beta-blockers were added to the International Olympic Committee (IOC)'s list of prohibited classes of substances.

•1987 • At the Pan American Games in Indianapolis, drug testers first discovered probenicid in the tests of many athletes. Probenicid is a diuretic drug used clinically to treat gout, but used by athletes to mask steroids. The following year, it was added to the IOC's list of banned substances.

•1999 • Ben Johnson was reinstated to sport eligibility in Canada. Independent adjudicator Graeme Mew concluded that the lifetime ban imposed on Johnson by Athletics Canada was excessive in the circumstances, but his appeal to the International Amateur Athletics Federation (IAAF) was rejected. Later in the year, Ben Johnson failed a doping test for the third time, testing positive for hydrochlorothiazide, a diuretic used to mask performance-enhancing substances.

DIURNAL   Active or occurring during daylight hours.

DIVERGENCE   In vision, movement of the eyes turning away from each other.

DIVING   *See under* HYPERBARIC PHYSIOLOGY.

DNA   Deoxyribonucleic acid. It is a macromolecule, usually composed of two polynucleotide chains in a double helix, which is the carrier of the genetic information in all cells and many viruses. In reference to DNA, **homologous** means having the same or nearly the same nucleotide sequence. A **DNA marker** is any feature of genomic DNA that differs among individuals and that can be used to distinguish homologous DNA molecules among the individuals in a population or in a pedigree. **DNA replication** is the copying of a DNA molecule. **Duplex DNA** is a double-stranded molecule of DNA. **Recombinant DNA** contains genes from various sources (often different organisms), which have been combined by genetic engineering. **Genetic engineering** is the linking of two DNA molecules by *in vitro* manipulation for the purpose of generating a novel organism with desired characteristics. A **clone** is a collection of organisms derived from a single parent and, except for new mutations, genetically identical to that parent. *See* CHROMATIN; HEREDITY.

DOLL EYE REFLEX   A primitive reflex that is present at birth and persists until one or two months of age, it is elicited when the head flexes and the eyes look up with the response that the head extends and the eyes look down. When the head is rotated laterally, the eyes deviate synergistically in the opposite direction. It is used to test the functional integrity of the oculomotor nerves and brain stem.

DOPAMINE   *See under* CATECHOLAMINES.

DOPING   *See under* DRUG.

DOUBLE BLIND   In a double-blind experimental design, neither the experimenter nor the subjects know whether the substance of interest (e.g. a drug) or a placebo (inert substance) is administered.

DOUBLE PRODUCT   Rate-pressure product. It is an index of relative cardiac work. It is the product of peak systolic blood pressure (as measured at the brachial artery) and heart rate. It is highly related to directly measured myocardial oxygen uptake and coronary blood flow in healthy subjects over a wide range of exercise intensities.

DOUGLAS BAG   *See under* OXYGEN UPTAKE, MEASUREMENT OF.

DOWAGER'S HUMP   *See under* FORWARD HEAD.

DOWN SYNDROME   Mongolism. An autosomal chromosomal condition that results in short stature, distinct facial features, and physical and cognitive differences that separates it from other manifestations of mental retardation.

There are three types of Down syndrome: trisomy 21, translocation and mosaicism. **Trisomy 21** explains 95% of Down syndrome. It is caused by nondisjunction, failure of chromosome pair 21 to separate properly before or during fertilization. The result is three chromosomes instead of two, like all the others, and cells that have 47 chromosomes instead of the normal 46.

The overall incidence of Down syndrome is about 1 in 800 live births, but this varies with maternal age. In the USA, approximately 5,000 such children are born each year. The risk more than doubles if the mother is more than 35 years of age. The **alpha-fetoprotein test** is a blood test performed at about 15 to 20 weeks into pregnancy.

In general, the degree of impairment in Down syndrome is related to the individual's mental age, rather than chronological age. Intellectual function varies widely. It involves mental retardation with a maximum average mental age of 8 years. Language and conceptualization are generally poor. About 50 to 60% of individuals with Down syndrome have significant hearing problems that may be congenital or acquired. Mild to moderate conductive losses in the high-frequency range are most common. Acquired hearing losses are associated with the high prevalence of middle ear and respiratory infections.

Prominent anatomical features may include: almond-shaped slanting eyes, often strabismic (crossed) and myopic (nearsighted); flattened facial features, including bridge of nose; flattened back of skull, short neck, with excess skin at the nape of neck; small oral cavity that contributes to mouth breathing; and tongue protrusion.

The rate of growth is slower in Down syndrome, leading to shorter stature (seldom more than 5 feet as adults) with short limbs and short, broad hands and feet. The abdomen of the adolescent and the adult generally protrudes like that of a small child. Almost 90% have umbilical hernias in early childhood, but the condition often corrects itself. Newborn infants exhibit an extreme degree of hypotonia. If large-muscle exercise is stressed, this muscular hypotonia will decrease with age. The hypotonia and lax ligaments cause joint looseness and hyperflexibility.

Breathing during strenuous exercise, swimming, and exposure to high-altitude conditions may be affected by structural abnormalities of the lungs, nasal passages, airways and chest wall. The lungs of many individuals with Down syndrome are hypoplastic (underdeveloped) with a smaller than normal number of alveoli. An abnormally short nasal passage, narrowed hypopharynx and bronchial tubes, and/or funnel or pigeon chest postural conditions results in chronic upper airway obstruction and diminished oxygen in all parts of the body. These anatomic features, coupled with hypotonia of chest and trunk muscles, make breathing particularly difficult during respiratory infections, which often develop into pneumonia. Asthma is more stressful in Down syndrome individuals, and there is increased risk of upper respiratory tract infections.

There is delay in the emergence and inhibition of primitive and postural reflexes, and also delay in reaching motor milestones. Balance is one of the abilities in which persons with Down syndrome are most deficient, lagging persons with the same level of retardation by 1 to 3 years. Deficits in balance and coordination can be explained not only by physical constraints, but also by central nervous system dysfunction. Asymmetry of strength is also common, with limbs on the left side stronger than limbs on the right. A higher percentage of individuals with Down syndrome than of non-Down syndrome peers are left handed. Walking is generally delayed by at least 2 years, with the mean age for walking of children being around 4 years.

Persons with Down syndrome perform more poorly on aerobic, strength, and motor tests than others with mental retardation, because of chromosomal differences that affect all of the body systems. Early identification and intervention programs appear to be successful in increasing motor functioning of infants and young children with Down syndrome.

Special Olympics events provide strong empirical evidence that some persons with Down syndrome can be successful in sports like gymnastics and swimming. The joint or ligamentous laxity can be an advantage in gymnastics and activities requiring flexibility, if the skeletal muscles are strong enough to provide stability and prevent dislocation. Persons with Down syndrome tend to like routine, and this has advantages in sport training. Music and other forms of rhythmic accompaniment seem to facilitate the acquisition of motor skills. Aerobic dance is useful for fitness training.

Down syndrome is associated with obesity, high blood cholesterol and low resting metabolic rate due in part to sedentary lifestyle and poor eating habits. About 40 to 60% of infants have significant congenital heart disease. The most common lesion is **atrioventricular canal defect**, an opening in the ventricular and atrial walls that normally separate the mitral and tricuspid valves. This opening causes a huge left-to-right shunt at the atrial and/or ventricular level that results in severe respiratory distress until corrected by surgery. Adults with Down syndrome have a 14 to 57% prevalence rate of mitral valve prolapse and an 11 to 14% prevalence rate of aortic regurgitation, both of which are attributed to the ligamentous laxity associated with Down syndrome. These heart conditions are generally asymptomatic and do not contraindicate participation in vigorous sports.

The age-related decline of self-care and cognitive abilities with Down syndrome is linked with early-onset Alzheimer-type neuropathology, which is present from about 40 years of age.

See also under ATLANTO-AXIAL JOINT.

Bibliography

Block, M.E. (1991). Motor development in children with Down
    syndrome: A review of the literature. *Adapted Physical Activity*

Quarterly 8(3), 179-209.

Jobling, A. (1999). Attainment of motor proficiency in school-aged children with Down syndrome. *Adapted Physical Activity Quarterly* 16(4), 344-361.

Maraj, B.K.V. et al. (2003). Verbal and visual instruction in motor skill acquisition for persons with and without Down Syndrome. *Adapted Physical Activity Quarterly* 20, 57-69.

National Down Syndrome Society. Http://www.ndss.org

Weeks, D.J., Chua, R. and Elliott, D. (2000, eds). *Perceptual-motor behavior in Down syndrome*. Champaign, IL: Human Kinetics.

2,3 DPG *See* 2,3 DIPHOSPHOGLYCERATE.

DRAG For a body in a flowing fluid, drag is the resistance caused by friction in the direction opposite to the motion of the center of gravity of that body. Drag force increases in proportion to the square of velocity. The power that is required to overcome retarding forces and drive an athlete through the air increases in proportion to the cube of the athlete's velocity.

As schematized lines of fluid flow, **streamlines** conceptually represent consecutive layers of particles in a fluid. The streamline closest to the object is the boundary layer, a thin layer (about 50 to 100 mm) of fluid that is in motion relative to that body. It is subject to viscous stresses that decrease its velocity relative to the body, and thus decrease lift and increase drag. **Boundary layer separation** is the point where the boundary layer separates from the surface of a body. The momentum of the fluid after it has overcome the viscous forces may not be great enough to allow the flow to proceed into regions of higher pressure. Consequently, eddies are formed with the breakdown of the laminar fluid flow. The fluid is then said to be turbulent. Typically, the streamline touching the object has the lowest velocity, because it is slowed down by the effect of friction between the layer of particles and the object. This effect is known as **surface drag** (**viscous drag**; **skin friction**). It increases in proportion to increases in the relative velocity of fluid, flow, the surface area of the body over which the flow occurs, the roughness of the body surface and the viscosity of the fluid. Body hair removal prior to major competition is an accepted practice in swimming.

There is evidence that it may decrease the surface drag produced as the water slides over the surface of the skin, thus decreasing the physiological demands of swimming at a given velocity.

When an object has an asymmetrical shape, such as an airfoil, or when an object such as a ball is spinning, the streamline traveling the greater distance around the object travels at a greater velocity, and the pressure on that side is less than on the other side. This effect is due to **Bernoulli's principle**, which states that fluid pressure is inversely related to fluid velocity. When the pressure on the topside of the airfoil is less because the velocity of the streamline is greater, a force pushes the airfoil upward. This effect is known as **lift** and represents the fluid resistance force that acts perpendicularly to the direction of fluid flow, generally producing vertical motion. A **foil** can thus be defined as a shape capable of generating lift in the presence of fluid flow. In swimming, however, lift generated by the hands and legs contributes to forward motion. The amount of lift that is created in swimming depends on the velocity of the hand relative to the water, the density of the water, the area of the hand, and (most importantly) the hand's angle of attack. Cupping the hand creates lift, but not as much as changing the tilt of the hand relative to the airflow. As with an airfoil, a 20 to 60 degree angle of attack creates a greater propulsive force than a flat-palm motion (0 degrees). Freestyle propulsion is primarily attributable, however, to drag forces based on Newton's Third Law of Motion; the presumed S-shaped stroke developed in Counsilman's (1971) two-dimensional biomechanical model fails to consider body rotation. Coleman (1999) notes that, "in the absence of contrary evidence from researchers, many swimming coaches had embraced the idea of lift propulsion, and incorrect changes may therefore have been made to a number of swimmers' techniques. It is interesting to note that swimming records still improved over this time, suggesting that successful coaches ignored lift forces, successful swimmers ignored their coaches, that incremental improvements from such changes in technique are relatively small, or that other aspects (such as physiological changes) outweighed the apparently inappropriate technique alterations." Recent research has shown that elite swimmers pitch their hands at about 60 degrees to the water. Propulsive drag forces, produced by the hand, stop before the hand reaches the hip. Propulsive lift forces are negligible throughout the stroke. The latest coaching theory for competitive freestyle is based on 'early catch with an early exit' and a 'straight-through pull arm stroke.'

Form drag (**profile drag**; **pressure drag**; **shape drag**) is due to turbulent flow and results from pressure differences between the front and rear sides of a body moving through a fluid. Use of streamlining through improved stroke mechanics enables highly skilled swimmers to move the separation point of the boundary layer closer to the trailing edge of the water. This is similar to what occurs when an oar slices through the water with the blade parallel rather than perpendicular to the flow of water. Stroke power in swimming has also been found to increase when the fingers are slightly spread apart rather than kept together. This is because drag between the fingers creates a larger cross-sectional area, so that the hand works more like the webbed appendage of a marine animal such as a seal. The crouched postures of downhill skiers, cyclists and speed skaters are examples of techniques used to decrease the athlete's frontal area. To minimize drag, it would make sense for a slalom skier to keep his arms at his side as he rounds each gate, but he cannot do this because his arms must help in slowing his body's rotational velocity. If two runners are positioned abreast, the drag on each is greater than the sum of their individual drag, because the combined frontal area results in a larger shared drag. In middle distance running, there is a strategy called 'drafting' in which a following runner is shielded from the effects of opposing relative airflow by a front runner. It may decrease the energy required to overcome drag by as much as 40%; this could amount to more than a second per 400 m lap at a typical middle-distance running pace. In running, streamlined apparel worn by a following runner would compound the advantage of drafting.

The International Amateur Athletics Federation (IAAF) does not recognize records attained with assisting winds greater than 2 m/s. The velocity of the wind is measured with a device placed parallel to the straight of the track that only measures the wind component in this direction. The IAAF may disallow a world record even if the wind causes an unfavorable effect at a wind direction of 130 degrees. What is allowed, however, is largely favorable wind of 5 m/s from a direction of 250 degrees. This could lead to a record with an advantage as much as almost 1 s in the 200 m sprint.

Laminar flow occurs when the streamlines move around an object and remain uniform. Turbulent flow occurs when the streamlines move around an object and become non-uniform. At a critical Reynold's number, the fluid flow changes from laminar to turbulent. The **Reynold's number** is dependent on both the viscosity and density of the fluid. It can be used in calculations involving the flight of balls, particularly when they swing. At a certain value of Reynold's number, there will be a velocity at which the flow will become turbulent. The wake found behind the body narrows dramatically and there is a decrease in drag. The **wake** is the region behind a body that is moving in a fluid. It is characterized by **turbulence** (**turbulent flow**) that involves motion of fluids in which local velocities and pressures fluctuate randomly with **eddy currents** (rotatory-like motion of a fluid that opposes the main current). In upright humans, the velocity required to generate wake narrowing is approximately 18m/s – significantly above maximum running speed, but significantly below speeds achieved in skiing, cycling and bobsledding. Golf ball dimples decrease the width of the wake and form drag by delaying the point along the object at which the streamlines become turbulent.

Wave drag occurs at the interface of two fluids such as air and water. Waves build up in front of, and form hollows behind, a body moving through a fluid. In swimming, wave drag is increased with up-and-down movement. Wave drag increases according to the cube of the velocity, whereas surface and form drag increases according to the square of the velocity. Making swimming strokes underwater minimizes wave drag in swimming events, where the rules of the sport permit. Olympic swimming pools are now all at least 7.5 feet deep and this significantly decreases wave rebound off the bottom. The walls of the pool have contoured gutters to eliminate turbulence from waves rebounding off the wall. Lane dividers have finned disks that further decrease wave turbulence. *See also* SWIMMER'S SHOULDER.

Chronology

•720 BC • According to Dionysius of Halicarnassus, Greek athletes competed in the nude during the "fifteenth Olympiad" at which time the Spartan runner, Acanthus, appeared at the Olympics without the loincloth. 200 years after Dionysius, Pausanias attributed the origin of the practice of competing in the nude to the Megarian sprinter, Orsippus, who won the one-stade foot race at the Olympics in 720 BC. Pausanias suggested that Orsippus deliberately broke with the prevailing practice, because he realized that a naked man could run faster. In the fifth century BC, coaches were also required to appear in the nude in the stadium (possibly because at one of the games a woman disguised herself as a male coach in order to see her son compete). Koroibos won the stade race in 776 BC, but it is not clear whether or not he wore shorts.

•1875 • In his second attempt to cross the English Channel, Captain Matthew Webb was successful and became the first person to do so. His waterlogged woolen swimwear weighed about 10 lb. (Modern swimming trunks weigh just a few ounces, even when soaked.) Webb was in the water, without touching a boat, for nearly 22 hours. During the swim, he complained of being stung by a jellyfish and asked for a little brandy. He had previously been supplied with some cod liver oil and hot coffee. In 1883, he was drowned while attempting to swim the Niagra rapids.

•1912 • Swimming and tennis were the only two Olympic events for women. The American women were not allowed to take part, because of the scanty nature of the swimwear and the American tennis players boycotted their event in sympathy for the swimmers. Sarah "Fanny" Durack, an Australian, wearing a long woolen swimsuit with a skirt, won the 100 meters freestyle.

•1956 • Masaru Furukawa of Japan set an Olympic record for the breaststroke by swimming underwater for 75% of the time. A year later underwater swimming was outlawed because it gave a distinct advantage and spectators wanted to see swimmers on the surface of the water.

•1958 • James "Doc" Counsilman of the USA started as Head Swimming Coach at Indiana University, where he produced 59 Olympians, including Mark Spitz. He pioneered the use of underwater photography and demonstrated the role of lift and hand-speed acceleration in swimming. He also introduced interval training, invented the pace clock, and introduced a weight-training protocol for swimmers. In 1979, at the age of 58, Counsilman became the oldest person to swim the English Channel.

•1984 • Robert Schleihauf's hydrodynamic analysis method was applied to members of the US Olympic swim team. Schleihauf promoted the idea that propulsion was probably a combination of lift and drag and that the resultant of the two was actually the source of propulsion.

•1988 • In the US Olympic Swimming trials, in what NBC swimming commentator, John Naber, called the "Berkoff Blast off," David Berkoff used 35 dolphin kicks underwater for 40 meters of the 100 meters backstroke on his way to setting a new world record of 54.95 secs. In the final, he was even faster (54.91 secs). At the preliminaries of the Olympic Games, he clocked 54.51 secs, but was beaten in the final by a Japanese swimmer, Daichi Suzuki, who emulated his innovation. La Fédération Internationale de Natation (FINA) made a rule change stating that a swimmer must surface within 10 meters from the start of the race (previously it was 15 meters). In 1991, FINA increased the distance to 15 m and swimmers were no longer required to touch the wall with his or her hand before executing the turn maneuver. After the shoulder rotates beyond the vertical toward the breast, a continuous simultaneous double-arm pull may be used to initiate the turn. There shall be no kick, arm pull, or flotation that is independent of the turn.

•1989 • Greg LeMond's success in the Tour de France was attributed to a clip-on extension on the handlebars of his bicycle that supported his elbows. By leaning forward onto this padded U-shaped extension, LeMond improved his aerodynamic shape without compromising his riding position.

•1993 • Graeme Obree of Britain set a world record of 4 min 20.894 sec in the 4,000 m single pursuit cycling at the World Track Championships in Norway. His home-made bicycle allowed him to adopt a unique riding position: chest on the handlebars, elbows stuck out, and backside off the saddle. The French sports daily *L'Equipe* described Obree as the pedaling genius who was reinventing cycling. Obree's process of innovation had started in 1986 when he noticed that riders on the road adopted a crouched position to cut wind resistance on descents. This led him to turn the drop handlebars round and rest his arms on the bar. In 1994, the United Cycling Union banned Obree-style bikes from road events because they were 'dangerous.'

•1993 • In the Women's Tour de France, Jeannie Longo of France, the world's leading female cyclist was penalized for drafting behind a motor cycle.

•1995 • Graham Obree of Britain won the 4,000 m single pursuit cycling in the World Championship in Bogota (Columbia). He used a normal bicycle with a very long stem and a Profile Aerobar (extended to its limits). His arms were stretched out, in a "Superman" position with his hands about 30 cm before the front hub. In 1996, the Union Cycliste Internationale (UCI) banned the Superman position, stating that the handlebar is not allowed to extend the front hub for more than 15 cm. Subsequently, there was a succession of rule changes In 2004, the UCI rules stated that "the handlebar extensions should extend no further than 75 cm ahead of a vertical line passing through the bottom bracket, but can be more, to a maximum of 80 cm under certain conditions for some riders. The extensions must also be no higher than the seat. These measurements do not apply to any levers, only to the points of the handlebars which may be gripped."

•1996 • The 50m breast stroke world record was broken by a German swimmer, Mark Warnecke, wearing a new costume manufactured by Speedo. About 90% of drag resistance in water is caused by the shape of a swimmer and only 10% by the friction between the skin or costume and the water. The fabric called 'Aquablade' has printed stripes that are alternatively smooth and rough and cause lanes of slow- and fast-moving water to flow over the body. Two-speed slipstreams produce vertical vortices that form a boundary layer that prevents wider turbulence. Aquablade has 8% lower surface resistance than the S2000 swimsuit that was introduced to the 1992 Olympics and 23% lower resistance than Nylon Lycra swimwear. Scientists showed that covering the skin with 'Aquablade' was even better than swimming naked. At the 1996 Olympic Games, 77% of all medals were won by Speedo wearers.

Bibliography

Coleman, S. (1999). Biomechanics and its application to coaching practice. In Cross, N. and Lyle, J. (1999). *The coaching process*. pp130-151. Oxford: Butterworth-Heinemann.

Costill, D.L., Maglischo, W.E. and Richardson, A.B. (1992). *Handbook of sports medicine and science. Swimming*. Oxford: Blackwell Scientific Publishers.

Hay, J.G., Liu, Q. and Andrews, J.G. (1993). The influence of body roll on hand path in freestyle swimming: A computer simulation study. *Journal of Applied Biomechanics* 9, 227-237.

Johnson, J.N., Gauvin, J. and Fredericson, M. (2003). Swimming biomechanics and injury prevention. New stroke techniques and medical considerations. *The Physician and Sportsmedicine* 31(1), 35-40.

Liu, Q., Hay, J.G. and Andrews, J.G. (1993). The influence of body roll on hand path in freestyle swimming: An experimental study. *Journal of Applied Biomechanics* 9, 238-253.

Nike, Inc (1989). High performance sports apparel. *The Physician and Sportsmedicine* 17(5), 143-144.

Rushall, B.S. et al. (1994). A reevaluation of forces in swimming. *Journal of Swimming Research* 10(Fall), 6-30.

Schleihauf, R.E. (1974). A biomechanical analysis of freestyle. *Swimming Technique* 11, 89-96.

van Ingen Schenau, G.J., de Koning, J.J., and de Groot, G. (1994). Optimisation of sprinting performance in running, cycling, and speed skating. *Sports Medicine* 17(4), 259-275.

DROP OUT   *See under* BURNOUT.

DRUG   A chemical substance that can alter the biochemistry of the body. An **agonist** is a drug that interacts with receptors to produce a response in a tissue or an organ. An **antagonist** (blocker) is a drug that occupies receptors without producing a response, but prevents the action of an endogenous substance or an agonist drug.

Athletes take drugs for one or more of the following reasons: therapy, recreation, performance enhancement ('pharmacological ergogenic aid') and in order to mask the presence of other drugs in the urine. **Recreational (street) drugs** are substances that people seek out and use for personal pleasure, and constitute a diverse group of drugs (e.g. cocaine, marijuana). Athletes are as likely as non-athletes to abuse recreational drugs. They are certainly more inclined to abuse drugs that are considered to be ergogenic aids. Drug taking (**doping**) is the use of drugs by athletes as ergogenic aids.

The World Anti-Doping Agency (WADA) is the official organization for doping control in sport. **Doping control** is the process including test distribution, sample collection and handling, laboratory analysis, results management, hearings and appeals. Categories of **prohibited substances** are stimulants, narcotics, cannabinoids, anabolic agents, peptide hormones, beta-2 agonists, agents with anti-estrogenic activity and masking agents. **Masking agents** are products that have the potential to impair the excretion of prohibited substances, to conceal their presence in urine or other samples used in doping control, or to change hematological parameters. Masking agents include, but are not limited to, diuretics, epitestosterone, probenecid and plasma expanders (e.g. dextran, hydroxyethyl starch).

An **analogue** is defined as a substance derived from the modification or alteration of the chemical structure of another substance while retaining a similar pharmacological effect. WADA's 2004 List of Prohibited Methods and Substances no longer required an analogue to have both a similar chemical structure and similar pharmacological effects. Designer steroids such as tetrahydrogestrinone (THG) are administered to athletes despite the lack of any scientific studies on their pharmacological effects. A **mimetic** is defined as a substance with pharmacological effect similar to that of another substance, regardless of the fact that it has a different chemical structure.

Specified substances are those that are particularly susceptible to unintentional anti-doping rule violations, because of their general availability in medicinal products or which are less likely to be successfully abused as doping agents. A doping violation involving a specified substance may result in a decreased sanction provided that the athlete can establish that the use of such a specified substance was not intended to enhance sport performance.

The International Standard for Therapeutic Use Exemptions of the World Anti-Doping Code permits athletes and their physicians to apply for **Therapeutic Use Exemptions**, i.e. permission to use, for therapeutic purposes, substances or methods contained in the List of Prohibited Substances or Methods whose use is otherwise prohibited.

The World Anti-Doping Agency (WADA) Prohibited List 2005 was organized into four sections: (I) Substances and methods prohibited at all times (in- and out-of-competition); (II) Substances and methods prohibited in-competition; (III) Substances prohibited in particular sports; (IV) Specified substances. Categories in Section I are: Anabolic agents; Hormones and related substances; Beta-2 agonists; Agents with anti-estrogenic activity; Diuretics and other masking agents; Enhancement of oxygen transfer; Chemical and physical manipulation; and Gene doping. **Enhancement of oxygen transfer** includes blood doping and the use of products that enhance the uptake, transport or deliver of oxygen (e.g. erythropoietins). **Chemical and physical manipulation** is the use of substances and methods, including masking agents, which alter, attempt to alter or may reasonably be expected to alter the integrity of specimens collected in doping controls. These include, but are not limited to, catheterization, urine substitution and/or tampering, inhibition of renal excretion and alterations of testosterone and epitestosterone concentrations. **Gene doping** is defined as the non-therapeutic use of genes, genetic elements and/or cells that have the capacity to enhance athletic performance.

Categories in Section II are all the categories under Section I, plus: Stimulants; Narcotics; Cannabinoids; and Glucocorticosteroids. Categories in Section III are: Alcohol; and Beta-blockers. For the World Anti-Doping Agency Prohibited List 2005, intravenous infusions were prohibited as a doping method. However, this was not aimed at preventing their use for legitimate acute medical purposes.

Most studies of drug effectiveness have not used athletes. The effectiveness of many drugs may be decreased in highly trained athletes, because there is a lower margin for improvement. A general problem with drug research is the large inter-individual variability in responses to a drug.

Drug addiction is a state in which either discontinuing or continuous use of a drug creates an overwhelming need, desire and craving for more of the substance to be taken.

Drug Tolerance refers to an acquired change in responsiveness of an individual as a result of exposure to a drug, such that an increased dose is necessary to produce the same degree of response, or that less effect is produced by the same dose of the drug.

See SUBSTANCE ABUSE.

Chronology

•1886 • Arthur Lindon, a British cyclist, died of an overdose of what is only known as "trimethyl" during a race between Bordeaux and Paris. It is the first recorded fatality from a performance-enhancing drug.

•1960 • Danish cyclist Kurt Jensen died during the 100 km road race at the Olympic Games. It was regarded at the time that, leading up to his death, Jensen was taking (supposedly on doctor's orders) a mixture of drugs that included Ronicol, a stimulant. Jensen was the first Olympian to die from drugs and the first athletes to die in Olympic competition since 1912.

•1962 • The International Olympic Committee (IOC) passed a resolution against doping, having set up in the previous year a Medical Commission as a result of Kurt Jensen's death in the 1960 Olympic Games.

•1963 • The Council of Europe established a definition of doping that was slightly modified and adopted by the International Olympic Committee (IOC). It defined doping as "the administration of or use by a competing athlete of any substance foreign to the body or any physiologic substance taken in abnormal quantity or taken by an abnormal route of entry into the body with the sole intention of increasing in an artificial and unfair manner his/her performance in competition. When necessity demands medical treatment with any substance which because of its nature, dosage or application is able to boost the athlete's performance in competition in an artificial and unfair manner, this too is regarded as doping."

•1965 • Arnold Beckett first applied gas chromatographic techniques to monitor drug abuse at Tour of Britain cycle races.

•1966 • Jacques Anquetil led a strike during the Tour de France in protest after doctors raided team hotels and asked for urine samples. Anquetil was the first man to win the Tour de France five times (1957, 1961-1964) and a defender of drug use, wrote in Le Journal du Dimanche: "Yes, I dope myself... you would be a fool to imagine that a professional cyclist who races 235 days a year in all temperatures and conditions can hold up without a stimulant."

•1967 • Tommy Simpson, the British cyclist, died from amphetamine-related complications, during the Tour de France.

•1967 • The Medical Commission of the International Olympic Committee (IOC) was established. Its mission was to put in place a medical control service for the 1968 Olympic Games. It published the first list of doping classes.

•1968 • Drug testing was carried out for the first time at the Winter and Summer Olympic Games. At the Summer Olympics, two pistol shooters were disqualified for taking alcohol.

•1973 • Professor Raymond Brooks of Britain, who developed the initial tests for anabolic steroids, told the International Amateur Athletics Federation (IAAF) that random dope testing outside competition should be introduced.

•1974 • East German athletes (about 10,000) were involved in a secret doping program authorized by the central committee of the Communist Party so as to promote Communism through success in sport, according to evidence uncovered in 1998 by the German historian Giselher Spitzer and published in the German weekly Der Spiegel. About 600 athletes were still registered in the doping program in 1989 when the Berlin Wall fell. Four East German sports coaches and two doctors, all of whom worked for a swimming club in Berlin, were charged with causing grievous bodily harm to 19 minors by giving them anabolic steroids.

•1978 • In the UK, the Drug Control and Teaching Centre was established at Chelsea College, University of London with funding support from the Sports Council.

•1980 • There were officially no positive dope tests at the Olympic Games in Moscow.

•1983 • At the Pan American Games in Venezuela, gas chromatography and mass spectrometry were used to test for anabolic steroids. The chromatograph takes a sample that has been vaporized and separates it into its component substances. The spectrometer then weighs the fragments to identify the specific molecule they came from. Although 19 athletes were tested positive for drugs, many athletes refused to be tested and left without competing.

•1988 • For the Olympic Games, the Soviet Union had a $2.5 million testing facility on a ship Michail Shalokhov that was floating 60 km from Seoul. Zmena, an official publication of the Communist Party of the Soviet Union, made this admission the following year.

•1996 • The International Olympic Committee (IOC) started using a new high-resolution mass spectrometer in its laboratories, saying it would provide "significant progress and more retrospectivity in the detection of anabolic steroid use." It has about 10 times the resolution of a conventional gas chromatography and mass spectrometry. The greater sensitivity means that the high-resolution unit can often detect steroid metabolites in a urine sample more than a month after the athlete has stopped taking the drugs, as opposed to perhaps two or three weeks later with conventional gas chromatography and mass spectrometry. Months after the Atlanta Games, it came to light that four test results indicating the use of the anabolic steroid methandienone were never acted upon. The results were obtained using high-resolution mass spectrometry. There was only one other positive test at the Atlanta Games and that was for stanozolol, an anabolic steroid.

•1998 • Speaking on a BBC television program, one of Britain's most experienced athletics coaches Wilf Paish attacked the existing drug-testing set up: "We should see drug-taking as an acceptable way of enhancing performance in sport. The rules simply do not work and should be scrapped." The only drugs that Paish believes should remain banned are anabolic steroids. An article by John Bryant in *The Times* (26 February) cited the above quote and argued that barriers against substances that enhance performance should remain firmly in place for health reasons. Nick Burrows, a reader of *The Times*, wrote a letter in response to Bryant's article drawing attention to three arguments for stopping drug use in sport (and problems with such arguments): i) it is inequitable (there will always be athletes with competitive advantages over other due to availability of facilities, equipment etc.); ii) it is hazardous to health (so are many training or competition practices) and iii) it is unnatural (so are other ergogenic aids such as Lycra™ clothing).

•1999 • The formation of the World Anti-Doping Agency (WADA) was announced at the World Conference on Doping. WADA was established as an independent, nongovernmental organization as a result of provisions of the Lausanne Declaration on Doping in Sport, in order to foster a doping free culture in sport. It combines the resources of sport and government to enhance, supplement and coordinate existing efforts to educate athletes about the harms of doping, reinforce the ideal of fair play, and sanction those who cheat themselves and their sport. It received its first two years of funding (US$25 million) from the Olympic Movement. Doping was defined as, "as the use of an artifice, whether substance or method, potentially dangerous to athlete's health and/or capable of enhancing their performances, or the presence in the athlete's body of a substance, or the ascertainment of the use of a method on the list annexed to the Olympic movement anti-doping code."

•2000 • On a single day within a fortnight of the Olympic Games, China dropped 27 competitors from the Games when many of them failed blood tests. The group included six female members of 'Ma's army,' coached by Ma Junren, who was one of 13 officials also omitted from the original 311-strong China delegation for the Sydney Games. China could not risk the disgrace of positive tests at the Games just as it was beginning the last year of lobbying to bring the 2008 Games to Beijing.

•2000 • At the Olympic Games in Sydney, there were 2,482 drugs tests of which 6 were positive. There were 2 out of 1,923 in 1996; 5 out of 1,848 in 1992; 10 out of 1,598 in 1988; 2 out of 1,507 in 1984; 0 out of 645 in 1980; and 11 out of 786 in 1976.

•2001 • Ma Junren was named China's deputy head coach for the world championships after three of his 'army' were selected to squad for the World Championships. Among them were Lan Lixin,

the 1998 world junior 1,500m champion and Dong Yanmei, the former 5,000 m world record holder, both dropped from the Olympics in 2000 after a blood test by the Chinese authorities indicated they might have taken erythropoietin (EPO).

Bibliography

Clarkson, P.M. and Thompson, H.S. (1997). Drugs and sport. Research findings and limitations. *Sports Medicine* 24(6), 366-384.

Cowan, D.A. (1998). Drug abuse. In: Harries, M., Williams, C., Stanish, W.D. and Micheli, L.J. (eds). *Oxford textbook of sports medicine*. pp339-365. Oxford: Oxford Medical Publishers.

Dawson, R.T. (2001). Hormones and sport. Drugs in sport – the role of the physician. *Journal of Endocrinology* 170, 55-61.

Hanson, G., Venturelli, P.J. and Fleckenstein, A.E. (2004). *Drugs and society*. 8th ed. Sudbury, MA: Jones and Bartlett Publishers.

Kulig, K., Brener, N.D. and McManus, T. (2003). Sexual activity and substance use among adolescents by category of physical activity plus team sports participation. *Archives of Pediatric and Adolescent Medicine* 157(9), 905-912.

Mottram, D.R. (1999). Banned drugs in sport. Does the International Olympic Committee (IOC) list need updating? *Sports Medicine* 27(1), 1-10.

Mottram, D.R. (2003). *Drugs in sport*. 3rd ed. London: Routledge.

Strauss, R.H. (1987). *Drugs and performance in sports*. Philadelphia: W.B. Saunders Co.

Todd, J. and Todd, T. (2001). Significant events in the history of drug testing and the Olympic movement 1960-1999. In: Wilson, W. and Derse, E. (eds). *Doping in elite sport. The politics of drugs in the Olympic movement*. pp65-128. Champaign, IL: Human Kinetics.

Voy, R. (1991). *Drugs, sport and politics*. Champaign, IL: Human Kinetics.

Wadler, G.I. and Hainlee, B. (1989). *Drugs and the athlete*. Philadelphia: F.A. Davis.

Wagner, J.C. (1991). Enhancement of athletic performance with drugs. An overview. *Sports Medicine* 12(4), 250-265.

World Anti-Doping Agency. Http://www.wada-ama.org

DUAL-ENERGY X-RAY ABSORPTIOMETRY
See under OSTEOPOROSIS.

DUCTILE MATERIAL   *See under* PLASTIC DEFORMATION.

DUODENUM   The shortest and widest part of the small intestine.

DURA MATER Connective tissue that covers the brain and spinal cord. It contains blood vessels.

DWARFISM It is a short-stature condition that is caused by a genetic condition or some kind of pathology. In general, dwarfs are at least 3 standard deviations below the mean height of the general population and shorter than 98% of their peers. The height standard for membership of adults in the Little People of America organization is 4 feet 10 inches or less, but the Dwarf Athletic Association of America uses a criterion height of 5 feet or less. Approximately 100,000 people in the USA have some type of dwarfism.

Dwarfs may be categorized as either proportionate or disproportionate. **Proportionate dwarfs** are persons whose body parts are proportionate, but abnormally short. The main cause of this is **pituitary gland dysfunction (growth hormone deficiency)**. **Disproportionate dwarfs** typically have average-sized torsos, but unusually short arms and legs. The major cause of disproportionate dwarfism is **skeletal dysplasia (chondrodystrophy)**, which is the failure of cartilage to develop into bone. This is either inherited or caused by spontaneous gene mutations.

Achondroplasia, the most common form of dwarfism, is an autosomal dominant condition that is due to a change in the genetic information for fibroblast growth factor receptor 3. It is characterized by disproportionate body structure with an average-size trunk, short limbs, short fingers and toes, and often a relatively large head. The average height for both men and women is 4 feet. Major motor milestones are frequently delayed. The limbs have **rhizomelic shortening**, i.e. there is disproportion in the length of the most proximal segment of the limbs (upper arms and thighs). The legs are straight in infancy, but when a child starts walking, they can develop a valgus (knock-kneed) posture. As the child continues to walk, the legs assume a varus (bowed-legged) appearance. With bowed legs, abnormally short femoral heads and restricted elbow extension, a waddling gait results. Surgery is occasionally used to correct the leg malalignments. Incidence of achondroplasia is between 1 in 10,000 and 1 in 40,000 births. Infants and children often have motor delays, but cognitive delays are not present. Aerobic fitness may be limited by small chest size and narrow nasal passages. In general, however, persons with achondroplasia are of normal intelligence and can be excellent athletes.

Pseudoachondroplasia, a short-limbed dwarfism, is inherited as an autosomal dominant trait. Clinically, it bears little resemblence to achondroplasia. **Hypochondroplasia** is the term for the tallest dwarfs. These individuals are often recruited into sport. **Diastrophic dysplasia** is the most disabling of the common forms of dwarfism, and is caused by failure of nourishment during prenatal bone growth and failure of nerve centers that innervate and/or failure of blood supply that carries nutrients. It typically involves spinal deformity (usually scoliosis), clubfoot, hand deformities, and frequent hip and knee dislocations. These conditions are resistant to corrective surgery. **Spondyloepiphyseal dysplasia** involves abnormal development of the growth plates within the vertebrae, causing a disproportionately short trunk with various spinal and limb irregularities. Nonachondroplasia dwarfism is associated with atlantoaxial instability.

Chronology

•1985 • The Dwarf Athletic Association of American (DAAA) was founded. DAAA especially promotes basketball, volleyball, powerlifting, track, field, swimming, bowling and boccia. Boccia is an accuracy sport in which players take turns throwing small balls toward a target ball. Internationally, dwarfs compete with *les autres*. The classification system used is considered to be unfair by many dwarfs. An international organization has been founded so that, in addition to Paralympic sport, dwarfs can compete against one another.

Bibliography

Achondroplsaia UK. Http://www.achondroplasia.co.uk

American Academy of Pediatrics (1995). Health supervision for children with achondroplasia. *Pediatrics* 95(3), 443-451.

Dwarf Athletic Association of America. Http://www.daaa.org

Low, L.J., Knudsen, M.J. and Sherrill, C. (1996). Dwarfism: New interest area for adapted physical activity. *Adapted Physical Activity Quarterly* 13, 1-15.

Sherill, C. (2004). *Adapted physical activity, recreation, and sport: Crossdisciplinary and lifespan.* 6th ed. Boston, MA: McGraw-Hill.

DYSEQUILIBRIUM   Any disturbance of balance.

DYSKINESIA   Difficulty with movement. *See* HUNTINGTON'S CHOREA.

DYSLIPIDEMIA   Disorders in lipoprotein metabolism, such as hypercholesterolemia.

DYSMETRIA   Inability to control the accuracy of body movements.

DYSMORPHIC   Not in normal form.

DYSPLASIA   Abnormal tissue development.

DYSPNEA   *See under* BREATHING.

DYSPRAXIA   *See* DEVELOPMENTAL COORDI-NATION DISORDER.

DYSTHMIA   *See under* DEPRESSION.

DYSTONIA   A neurological movement disorder characterized by involuntary muscle contractions, which force certain parts of the body into abnormal, sometimes painful, movements or postures. In the USA, dystonia is the third most common movement disorder after Parkinson's disease and tremor. It appears that dystonia is caused by overactivity in several areas of the brain – the basal ganglia, thalamus and cerebral cortex. Dystonia may be considered as the production of one pattern of muscle activity when a different pattern was intended. It usually only occurs during voluntary movement or with voluntary maintenance of a posture of the limbs or body. A dystonic movement of one limb may be triggered by attempted movement of a different limb. Tremor is not a primary symptom of dystonia.

Dystonia can affect any part of the body. **Focal dystonia** affects only one body part. **Segmental dystonia** affects at least two or more areas of the body that are adjacent. **Multifocal dystonia** appears in two or more areas of the body that are not adjacent. **Generalized dystonia** involves several body areas on both sides of the body. **Hemidystonia** affects either the left or the right side of the body.

Primary dystonia is defined by the existence of dystonia without any underlying disorder, and includes hereditary and sporadic forms of dystonia. In 1997, the DYT1 gene was identified. In people with early-onset dystonia, the DYT1 gene has a mutation that causes the deletion of three nucleotides called GAG in the genetic code. **Secondary dystonia** arises from, and can be attributed to, numerous causes, such as birth injury, trauma, stroke or drugs. A large number of drugs are capable of causing dystonia. In most cases, the dystonia is transient but in some patients exposed to neuroleptics, such as Haldol, the dystonia may be persistent. This disorder is known as **tardive dystonia**.

Treatment for dystonia is designed to lessen the symptoms of spasms, pain, and disturbed postures and functions. Most therapies are symptomatic, attempting to cover up or release the dystonic spasms. Sensory tricks can relieve a dystonic spasm, e.g. the 'geste' in spasmodic torticollis where a finger is lightly placed on the face will neutralize the spasm. Torticollis is dystonia involving the muscles of the neck.

Musician's cramp is a primary, focal, task specific dystonia that affects a highly specialized, professional skilled motor act. It involves unintended, simultaneous activity of agonists and antagonists, inducing abnormal movements and/or postures (dystonia), mainly of the hands and fingers. The case of a professional tennis player with bilateral segmental dystonia has been reported. The symptoms were expressed in involuntary movements when he intended to hit the ball and in a progredient tremor, initially in one hand, later in both, making him unable to write.

See also TORTICOLLIS; YIPS.

Bibliography

Dystonia Medical Research Foundation. Http://www.dystonia-foundation.org

Elbert, T. et al. (1998). Alteration of digital representation in somatosensory cortex in focal hand dystonia. *NeuroReport* 9(16), 3571-3575.

Mayer, F. et al. (1999). Bilateral segmental dystonia in a professional tennis player. *Medicine and Science in Sports and Exercise* 31(8), 1085-1087.

E

EAR For hearing to take place, a sound wave passes into the external ear and through an inch-long canal to strike an oval-shaped membrane called the **tymphanic membrane (ear drum)**. A sound wave causes the eardrum to vibrate with the same frequency and amplitude as the sound wave itself.

The **middle ear** is the small space between the eardrum and the bony capsule of the inner ear. It includes the **ossicles** (**malleus, incus** and **stapes**), the small bones shaped like a hammer, anvil and stirrup, respectively. These bones transmit sound waves to the inner ear. The middle ear also contains the **eustachian tube**, which connects the back of the nose to the middle ear and is a selective valve that allows air to enter behind the sealed ear drum. The eustachian tube replaces the air the body absorbs from the middle ear. The eustachian tube also equalizes pressure changes in the outside air and causes the 'popping' that occurs when a person experiences a change in altitude, such as in an airplane. The eustachian tube is much affected by colds, sinus infections and allergies.

The **inner ear** is the inner most chamber of the ear. It is filled with fluid and contains the cochlea and the vestibular apparatus. The **cochlea** is a snail-shaped structure within the inner ear. The **organ of Corti**, a chamber inside the cochlea, is responsible for hearing. It contains hair cells that serve as the receptors for hearing. The **vestibular apparatus** is the organ of balance. Each vestibular apparatus contains 3 semi-circular canals designated as the horizontal, anterior and posterior canals. The **semicircular canals** are responsible for detecting rotational motion of the head. The canals are hoop-shaped structures that are arranged roughly at right angles with each other so that they represent all three planes of movement. The same arrangement of semicircular canals is mirrored on both sides of the head. It is important for the canals on both sides to agree as to what the head is doing. If there is disagreement, then the person will experience vertigo.

Otology is the branch of medical science concerned with the ear and related structures. Damage to the internal ear mechanism may occur in any sport, especially diving and scuba diving, but also sports such as soccer (e.g. when a player is hit on the ear by a ball). In some sports, such as shooting, hearing-protection devices are worn. **Non-explosive blast injury of the ear** refers to the otological trauma caused by a blow to the ear that seals the external auditory meatus. It results in a sudden increase of air pressure within the air canal that strikes the tympanic membrane. In a study of 91 patients with non-explosive blast injury of the ear, it was found that 60 cases were caused by a slap or a punch, 13 cases were from sports accidents (mostly in ball games), and 18 cases were from aquatic activities such as swimming. The common symptoms were hearing loss, earache, tinnitus, vertigo and otorrhea (discharge from the ear).

See also CAULIFLOWER EAR; COCHLEAR IMPLANT; DEAF; OTITIS MEDIA; PROPRIO-CEPTIVE FEEDBACK; SWIMMER'S EAR.

Bibliography

Berger, G., Finkelstein, Y. and Harell, M. (1994). Non-explosive blast injury of the ear. *Journal of Laryngology and Otology* 108(5), 395-398.

EATING DISORDERS A group of conditions characterized by abnormal dietary patterns and distorted body image. Estimates of the prevalence of symptoms of eating disorders and the existence of eating disorders among athletic populations vary from less than 1% to as high as 39%.

The term '**disordered eating**' refers to a spectrum of abnormal behavior, which at its extreme includes anorexia nervosa and bulimia nervosa. Disordered eating occurs when a person's attitudes about food, weight, and body size leads to very rigid eating and exercise habits that jeopardize one's health, happiness and safety. Disordered eating can become an obsession and may even turn into an eating disorder.

Anorexia athletica is a subclinical eating disorder in that there are significant symptoms of eating disorders, but they do not meet clinical diagnostic criteria such as those of the American Psychiatric Association. It is characterized by intense fear of gaining weight or becoming fat even though an individual is already lean (at least 5% less than expected normal weight for age and height for the general female population). Many cases of anorexia nervosa and bulimia nervosa begin as subclinical variants of these disorders. Symptoms of anorexia athletica include: exercising beyond the requirements for good health; being fanatical about weight and diet; stealing time from work, school and relationships to exercise; focusing on challenge and forgetting that physical activity can be fun; defining self-worth in terms of performance; rarely or never being satisfied with athletic achievements; always pushing on to the next challenge; and justifying excessive behavior by defining self as an athlete or insisting that their behavior is healthy. Gymnasts, distance runners, body builders, rowers, wrestlers, jockeys, dancers and swimmers are particularly vulnerable to eating disorders, because their sports necessitate weight restriction.

The greater the extent to which an athlete's body deviates from the ideal for a particular sport, then the greater the risk the athlete will develop an eating disorder. Athletes with eating disorders tend to start sport-specific training earlier than athletes who have not met the criteria for eating disorders. Starting sport-specific training at prepubertal age may prevent athletes from choosing the sport most suitable for their adult body type.

In Western culture, there are unrealistically low standards of bodyweight for girls and women that is perpetuated by the portrayal of the ideal woman in the mass media. Female self-esteem is highly related to body image. Dieting during adolescence is virtually a norm and potentially dangerous methods of body-weight reduction are often used. The proportion of female athletes engaging in at least one method of unhealthy weight control ranged from 15.4% to 61.9% across different studies and athletic activities.

Eating disorders in males are clinically similar to, if not indistinguishable from, eating disorders in females. Homosexuals are over-represented, commonly twice as high or greater, in many samples of eating disordered men. Homosexual men may be at an increased risk for developing an eating disorder because of cultural pressures within the homosexual community to be thin. Conflict over gender identity or sexual orientation may precipitate the development of an eating disorder in many males.

A meta-analysis by Sullivan (1995) from 42 studies of patient mortality found 178 deaths in 3,006 patients. 54% died from complications of eating disorders, 27% committed suicide and 19% died of other or unknown causes. Mortality increases with the duration of symptoms.

Throughout the process of detection, referral, and recovery, the focus should be on the person feeling healthy and functioning effectively, not on their weight, shape or morality. Treatment of eating disorders can be effective. For example, Reas et al. (2000) found in patients with bulimia nervosa that if treated within the first 5 years, the recovery rate is 80%; if not treated until after 15 years of symptoms, the recovery rate falls to 20%.

See also ANOREXIA NERVOSA; BIGOREXIA; BULIMIA NERVOSA; EXERCISE DEPENDENCE; FEMALE ATHLETE TRIAD; PICA; RUMINATION DISORDER; SEROTONIN.

Bibliography

Abrahams, S. and Llewellyn-Jones, D. (1997). *Eating disorders. The facts.* 4th ed. Oxford: Oxford University Press.

Beals, K.A. and Manore, M.M. (1994). The prevalence and consequence of eating disorders in female athletes. *International Journal of Sport Nutrition* 4, 175-195.

Beals, K.A. (2004). *Disordered eating among athletes. A comprehensive guide for health professionals.* Champaign, IL: Human Kinetics.

Brownell, K.D., Rodin, J. and Wilmore, J.H. (1992). *Eating, bodyweight and performance in athletics. Disorders of modern society.* Philadelphia: Lea and Febiger.

Byrne, S. and McLean, N. (2002). Elite athletes: Effects of the pressure to be thin. *Journal of Science and Medicine in Sport* 5(2), 80-94.

Crisp, A.H. (1983). Some aspect of the psychopathology of anorexia nervosa. In P.L. Darby et al. (eds). *Anorexia nervosa:*

Recent developments in research. pp15-28. New York: 15-28.

Herzog, D.B. et al. (1990). Sexuality in males with eating disorders. In A. Anderson (ed). *Males with eating disorders.* New York: Brunner/Mazel.

Leon, G.R. (1991). Eating disorders in female athletes. *Sports Medicine* 12(4), 219-227.

National Eating Disorders Association. Http://www.NationalEatingDisorders.org

Noden, M. (1994). Dying to win. *Sports Illustrated*, 8 August, 52-60.

Pipher, M. (1995). *Hunger pains.* New York: Ballantine Books.

Reas, D.L. et al. (2000). Duration of illness predicts outcome for bulimia nervosa: A long-term follow-up study. *International Journal of Eating Disorders* 27(4), 428-434.

Schneider, J.A. and Agras, W.S. (1987). Bulimia in males: A matched comparison with females. *International Journal of Eating Disorders* 6, 235-242.

Sullivan, P.F. (1995). Mortality in anorexia nervosa. *American Journal of Psychiatry* 152(7), 1073-1074.

Sundgot-Borgen, J. (1994). Eating disorders in female athletes. *Sports Medicine* 17(3), 176-188.

Thompson, R.A. and Sherman, R.T. (1993). *Helping athletes with eating disorders.* Champaign, IL: Human Kinetics.

Wilmore, J.H. (1991). Eating and weight disorders in the female athlete. *International Journal of Sport Nutrition* 1(2), 104-17.

ECCENTRIC FORCE   Any force (or resultant of a force system) that is non-zero and does not act through the center of mass of an object. It is the most common way of generating motion.

ECCENTRIC MUSCLE ACTION   *See under* MUSCLE ACTION.

ECCRINE GLAND   *See under* THERMO-REGULATION.

ECG   *See* ELECTROCARDIOGRAPHY.

ECHOCARDIOGRAPHY   Recording of the position and motion of the heart wall or internal structures of the heart and neighboring tissue by the echo obtained from beams of ultrasonic waves directed through the chest wall. Echocardiography is particularly sensitive for detecting hypertrophic cardiomyopathy. *See under* CARDIAC HYPER-TROPHY; SUDDEN DEATH.

ECSTASY   *See under* AMPHETAMINE.

ECTOMORPHY   *See under* SOMATOTYPE.

EDEMA   Local or generalized swelling due to accumulation of fluid in the interstitial spaces as a result of fluid leaking into tissues from vascular or lymphatic spaces. *See* ANGIOEDEMA; HEAD INJURIES.

EFFECTOR   (i) A molecule that brings about a regulatory change in a cell, as by induction. (ii) A peripheral tissue that receives nerve impulses and makes a response such as contraction (muscle) or secretion (gland).

EFFERENT NEURON   Any neuron that conducts impulses away from the central nervous system to an effector organ (muscle or gland). *See under* NERVOUS SYSTEM.

EFFICIENCY   The proportion of energy input that appears as useful work. In biological systems, energy exchange for work done is not a completely efficient process. The energy that is not used for work is not lost, but appears as heat. **Gross efficiency** is calculated as work output divided by energy expenditure. **Net efficiency** is calculated as work output divided by energy expenditure above that at rest.

In the context of sport, **mechanical efficiency** is the ratio of the mechanical work to the total energy expended to produce that work. Under favorable circumstances, it is 20 to 25%, but there are wide individual differences. When drag is high, however, it may be less than 20%. Mechanical efficiency depends on both **muscle efficiency** (the efficiency with which muscles convert chemical energy into mechanical energy) and **neuro-muscular skill** (the degree to which the individual has learned to recruit only those motor units required to produce maximal power output in a skilful way). Muscle efficiency has two components: the efficiency with which chemical energy is converted to ATP (the process of ATP synthesis is about 40% efficient, whereas 60% of the energy is lost as heat) and the efficiency with which energy released from ATP hydrolysis (breakdown) is converted to muscle fiber shortening. The efficiency of ATP hydrolysis is dependent on the velocities of muscle contraction. For example, slow-twitch muscle fibers are significantly more efficient than fast-twitch muscle fibers at converting ATP into mechanical work when cycling at 80 rpm. There is little that an individual can do to improve muscle efficiency because the chemical efficiency of converting fuels to ATP and the proportion of slow-twitch fibers involved in various movements are largely determined by heredity.

A distinction can be made between efficiency and economy. The most **efficient** performance occurs when the greatest amount of work is done for a given change in energy. The most **economical** performance occurs when the smallest change in energy is used to perform a given amount of work. In human movement, economy of movement is particularly associated with the body utilizing reactive and external forces rather than recruiting active muscles.

In archery, efficiency is measured as the ratio of kinetic energy of the arrow as it leaves the strings, to the energy imparted to the bow to bring it to full draw. Some of the stored bow energy is lost as kinetic energy of the limbs, the bowstring and oscillations of the moving arrow. Bowstring waves are minimized by using synthetic bowstrings made of resilient, low-stretch, high-strength fibers such as Kevlar. The heavier the arrow, the more energy the bow transfers to it. A more efficient transfer of energy does not necessarily result in greater arrow velocity.

In cycling, **gears** are machines that enable cyclists to continue pedaling at a constant rate regardless of terrain changes. For the chain sprocket, a larger diameter means that a greater torque is necessary to accelerate the pedal. For the rear sprockets, a larger size means that less torque is necessary to accelerate the pedal. With a big chain sprocket and a small rear sprocket (i.e. when the cycle is in a high gear), a cyclist travels farther for each pedal revolution. Lower gears (i.e. smaller chain sprocket, larger rear sprocket) require less effort to turn the pedal, but the cyclist must pedal more to maintain the same speed. The most efficient pedaling cadence is usually 90 to 100 rpm.

Cleated shoes, used in conjunction with toe clips, also increase pedaling efficiency by allowing for improved flexor muscle utilization during the backstroke and by distributing the workload and peak demand on the *quadriceps femoris* muscles.

Swimming requires four-times the energy for the same distance covered by running. This is because of the need to maintain buoyancy and to overcome drag forces. Women have an energy cost about 30% lower than men in swimming. The optimal water temperature for most competitive swimming averages 28 to 30 degrees Celsius.

Self-selected walking speed has been shown to be about the most metabolically inexpensive speed. *See also* MACHINE; RUNNING ECONOMY.

Bibliography

Lamb, D.R. (1995). Basic principles for improving sport performance. *Gatorade Sports Science Exchange* 8(2).

Zumerchik, J. (1997, ed). *Encyclopedia of sports science.* New York: Macmillan Library Reference.

EFFORT THROMBOSIS *See under* THROMBOSIS.

EFFUSION A pouring out of any fluid into a body cavity or tissue.

EHLERS-DANLOS SYNDROME An inherited condition, of which there are six major types, characterized by hyperextensibility of joints, with predisposition for dislocation at the shoulder girdle, shoulder, elbow, hip and knee joints. It is a collagen defect similar to osteogenesis imperfecta, but does not cause bones to break. Other features are loose and/or hyperextensible skin, slow wound healing with inadequate scar tissue and fragility of blood vessel walls. Special emphasis is given to blister prevention and hand protection.

Ehlers-Danlos syndrome (classic type) manifests with an under-recognized tendency to develop dilation of the ascending aorta. The classic type probably affects fewer than 1 in 20,000 to 1 in 40,000 people. There are at least five gene mutations that cause the classic type, four of which are concerned with the assembly of collagen molecules. Alterations in the COL1A1 gene are most common, accounting for 30 to 50% of cases. The classic type if usually inherited as an autosomal dominant trait, but rarely it is inherited it as an autosomal recessive trait.

Many people with classic Ehlers-Danlos syndrome have mitral valve prolapse that is occasionally associated with mitral regurgitation, dysrhythmia or both. Persons with classic type Ehlers-Danlos syndrome should have a screening echocardiogram before they participate in competitive athletics.

Vascular and viscous fragility is the main concern in the vascular form of Ehlers-Danlos syndrome. This condition is due to functional or relative deficiency of type-3 collagen and is inherited most often as an autosomal dominant trait. Rupture of the bowel, uterus and bladder can occur either spontaneously or with minimal blunt trauma. Most affected individuals also have skin fragility, easy bruising and poor wound healing. The most feared complication, however, is arterial rupture. The vessels at most risk include the descending aorta and all its major branches. People with vascular type Ehlers-Danlos syndrome should avoid strenuous exertion, including pregnancy (during which risk of arterial or uterine rupture is quite high) as well as activities that carry a risk of collision.

Bibliography

Ehlers-Danlos National Foundation. Http://www.ednf.org

Pyeritz, R.E. (2001). Disorders of vascular fragility. Implications for active patients. *The Physician and Sportsmedicine.* 29(6), 53-59.

EICOSANOIDS   Prostanoids. This is a class of compounds that includes prostaglandins, thromboxanes and leukotrienes. Eicosanoids are synthesized from unsaturated long-chain fatty acids (such as arachodonic acid and alpha-linolenic acid) from membrane phospholipids or circulating free fatty acids. The liver elongates these fatty acids by 2 carbons at a time until the carbon chains have 20 or 22 carbons. Elongation alternates with desaturation. Eicosanoids are called **paracrines** ('**local hormones'**) because they are short lived and alter the activities of the cells in their immediate vicinity and the cells from which they are derived. It is believed that eicosanoids play a role in platelet aggregation, vasoconstriction, immunologic and allergic reactions, and inflammatory conditions. Eicosanoids can have opposing physiologic effects depending on whether they are derived from omega-3, omega-6 or omega-9 fatty acids.

ELASTIC BANDS   Thera-Band® elastic bands and tubing have become popular as part of an exercise program for both post-injury rehabilitation and fitness. Elastic resistive exercise requires maximal muscle activation throughout the range of motion, because patients are not able to use momentum to complete the exercise. It provides multi-planar, low-impact resistance, and plyometric exercises may be performed. Elastic bands and tubing also require neuromuscular coordination and stabilization to maintain proper posture and motion patterns. Force is dependent on elongation regardless of initial length.

Bibliography

Page, P. Developing resistive exercise programs using Thera-Band® elastic bands and tubing. Http://www.thera-bandacademy.com

Page, P. and Ellenbecker, T.S. (2003, eds). *The scientific and clinical application of elastic resistance.* Champaign, IL: Human Kinetics.

ELASTICITY   The property of a material that enables it to return to its original length after being stretched. Elastic materials are good at storing and releasing energy. The **elastic limit** is defined as the maximum stress a solid can sustain without undergoing permanent deformation. *See* DEFLECTION; STRETCHING.

ELASTIC MODULUS   The modulus of elasticity for linear stress and strain is **Young's modulus**. Because it is the ratio of stress to strain, and strain is dimensionless, modulus of elasticity has the units of stress.

Stress is load (force) per unit area acting on a given plane within a material. Stress refers to how much force the atoms at any given point in a solid are being pulled apart. The Standard International unit is Newton per meter per meter (N/m^2) or Pascals (Pa). The US Customary unit is pound force per square inch (psi). Tensile stress and compressive stress are also known as **normal stresses**, i.e. they act perpendicular to a given plane. Shear stress acts parallel to a given plane.

Strain is the deformation resulting from a stress. It is measured as the ratio of the change to the total value of a dimension (such as length in which the change occurred). Strain refers to how far the atoms are being pulled apart; i.e. by what proportion the bonds between the atoms are being stretched. When strain is directly proportional to stress, for all or part of the stress-strain curve, the material is said to obey **Hooke's Law**. The **Hookean region** is the linear region of a stress-strain curve in the elastic range. The **proportional limit** is the upper limit of the Hookean region. **Elastic limit (yield point)** is the upper limit of the elastic range. The **elastic range** is the strain range within which a material remains perfectly elastic. As strain is a ratio of two lengths, it has no unit of measurement. **Shear strain** is a measure of the change in angle between two lines drawn on a surface and it is measured in radians. **Strain rate** is the speed at which a strain-producing load is applied. Because most tissue is viscoelastic, the properties will be rate dependent. **Strain energy** is the energy that a material can absorb as a result of the change of shape resulting from applied stress. Graphically, the area under a load-deformation curve represents the strain energy stored in the material during the application of stress. The Standard International units are newton meters (N.m). The US Customary Units are foot pound force (ft.lbf). A **tangent modulus of elasticity** may be used where a non-linear elastic response exists for any portion of the curve that approximates linearity. It also has the units Newton per meter per meter (N/m^2) or Pascals (Pa). The **shearing modulus of elasticity** (or **modulus of rigidity**), G, is the ratio of shear stress to shear strain, and has the units N/m^2 or Pa.

Young's modulus is a measure of the stiffness of the material within the elastic region of the linear stress-strain curve. The larger the Young's modulus, the greater is the stiffness of that material. The **stiffness (stress per unit strain)** of a material is the property indicating the amount of deformation that occurs in proportion to the load applied. A stiff material has a high Young's modulus and changes its shape only slightly under elastic loads (e.g. diamond). A flexible material has a low Young's modulus and changes its shape considerably (e.g. rubbers).

Strain isotropy exists when the Young's modulus of a material is the same in tension, compression and shear. **Strain anisotropy** exists when the Young's modulus of a material is different in tension, compression and shear. Most materials with a physical grain, such as wood, bone, tendon, ligament and cartilage, exhibit strain anisotrophy. Bone (for example) is stiffer in compression than in tension and stiffer in tension than in shear. **Specific stiffness (specific modulus)** is given by Young's modulus divided by density. Compliance is the reciprocal of stiffness, i.e. strain per unit stress.

Ultimate stress (material strength) is the stress exerted on a material immediately prior to failure. Strength is thus the ability to withstand stress and strain without breaking. A stiff material requires high loads to elastically deform it, whereas a strong material requires high loads to permanently deform (or break) it. The **yield strength** of a material is the stress at which there is no longer linear proportionality between stress and strain. It is the point at which the material is first permanently deformed. **Specific strength**, or strength-to-weight ratio, of a material is obtained by dividing its yield strength by its density.

Although it takes nearly five times as much force to break concrete as wood, it takes only three times as much energy. The reason is wood's greater elasticity. Wood has a higher elastic modulus; 16 times greater than that of concrete. It takes relatively more energy to break wood, because energy is wasted in the bending of wood before it breaks (much of it is transmitted throughout the wood and back through the person as vibrational energy).

Karate experts have demonstrated that human bone is better able to withstand compression than wood or concrete. The ability to distribute the impact makes the rupture modulus of the hand bone more than 40-times greater than that of concrete. A karate expert tries to maximize his hand speed in order to maximize the potential transfer of kinetic energy, because the kinetic energy of a moving object is proportional to the square of its speed.

See also BULK MODULUS; MATERIALS; PLASTIC DEFORMATION.

Bibliography

Zumerchik, J. (1997, ed). *Encyclopedia of sports science*. New York: Macmillan Library Reference.

ELBOW JOINT COMPLEX A joint comprising three synovial joints enclosed in a common capsule: the humero-ulnar joint, humero-radial joint and superior radio-ulnar joint.

The **humero-ulnar joint (elbow joint)** is a hinge joint between the trochlear fossa of the humerus and the trochlear notch of the ulna. The humero-ulnar joint permits flexion and extension. Muscles that produce flexion: *Brachialis, biceps brachii, brachioradialis* and *pronator teres*. Muscles that produce extension: *Triceps brachii* and *anconeous*. The **humero-radial joint (radio-humeral joint; radio-capitellar joint)** is a gliding joint between the capitellum of the humerus and the radius.

The elbow joint complex has good stability because of the interlocking configuration of the articulating surfaces. The **coronoid process** provides an important barrier against posterior displacement as the elbow joint flexes. The joint capsule surrounds all three joints and provides significant restraint to varus and valgus forces when the elbow is extended. The **ulnar (medial) collateral ligament** is the strongest ligament supporting the elbow complex and provides a restraint to valgus forces. The **radial (lateral) collateral ligament** provides restraint to varus forces, but is not as strong as the ulnar collateral ligament. The *anconeus* muscle, which has its origin on the lateral aspect of the elbow, provides additional stability against varus stress. An **interosseus membrane** connects the radial and ulnar shafts through the forearm.

The **superior (proximal) radio-ulnar joint** is a pivot joint that is formed by the convex medial rim of the head of the radius and the concave radial notch of the proximal ulna. The annular ligament completely surrounds the radial head, thus holding the radial head against the ulna. The **inferior radio-ulnar joint** is not part of the elbow joint complex, but is located at the wrist. It is a pivot joint that is formed by the head of the ulna being received into the sigmoid cavity at the medial side of the distal radius. The articular surfaces are connected together by three ligaments. The inferior radial-ulnar joint is stabilized intrinsically by the triangular fibrocartilage complex, and extrinsically by the interosseus membrane and the *extensor carpi ulnaris, flexor carpi ulnaris* and *pronator quadratus* muscles. In athletes, injuries to the triangular fibrocartilage complex may be caused by acute trauma or as a result of repetitive microtrauma. The radio-ulnar joints permit the movements of supination and pronation. In pronation, the radius rolls over a relatively fixed ulna, i.e. turning the palm of the hand downwards. The axis of the radio-ulnar joint is an oblique line that connects the superior and inferior radio-ulnar joints. Muscles that produce pronation: *pronator quadratus* and *pronator teres*. The reverse occurs in supination when the radius returns to its anatomical position, i.e. turning the palm of the hand upwards. Muscles that produce supination: *supinator* and *biceps brachii*. In addition to the superior and inferior radio-ulnar joints, there is the **middle radio-ulnar joint** that is a syndesmosis.

The **carrying angle** is formed by the interception of the long axes of the humerus and the ulna with the elbow fully extended and the forearm supinated. In the anatomical position, the forearm is abducted in relation to the humerus. It is an alignment that is caused by the angle of articulation of the humerus and ulna at the elbow joint. It is usually 10 to 15 degrees in males and 20 to 25 degrees in females.

ELBOW JOINT COMPLEX, DISLOCATION

The elbow is the most commonly dislocated joint in

children. The majority of elbow dislocations are posterior; the elbow's bony configuration provides strong resistance to anterior dislocation. **Posterior dislocations** occur as a result of a posterolateral force being applied to the elbow from a fall on the outstretched hand with the elbow in extension or hyperextension. The axial force effectively levers the ulna out of the trochlea, causing capsular and ligament rupture, hence dislocation. **Anterior dislocations** generally result from a direct blow to the posterior elbow. **Posterolateral rotatory instability** is caused by a laxity or injury (such as a fall on an outstretched hand) to the lateral collateral ligament complex, especially the lateral ulnar collateral ligament, which then allows a transient rotatory subluxation of the humero-ulnar joint (and secondary dislocation of the radio-humeral joint).

ELBOW JOINT COMPLEX, FRACTURES

Radial head fractures most often result from either longitudinal loading of the radius as a result of a fall, or as a result of elbow dislocation. Occasionally, the radial head is fractured as the result of a severe valgus force that tears the ulnar (medial) collateral ligament, and places compressive and shearing stress on the radial head. Fracture of the distal third of the radius and dislocation of the distal radio-ulnar joint is called a **Galeazzi fracture**. It occurs most often from a fall on an outstretched arm or a direct blow to the dorsolateral side of the wrist. Other common fractures to the distal radius in the general population include Colles,' Smith's and Barton's fractures. **Colles' fracture** is a low energy, extra-articular fracture of the distal radius, which occurs in elderly adults. It is usually caused by a fall on the dorsal-flexed hand of an outstretched arm. The dorsal surface undergoes compression, while the volar surface undergoes tension. **Smith's fracture** is an extra-articular, palmar-displaced distal radius fracture. Volar angulation of the fracture is a **'garden spade' deformity (reversed Colles' fracture)**. It results from a fall on the palm of an outstretched hand, causing pronation of the upper extremity while the hand is fixed to the ground. A **volar Barton's fracture** is a fracture of the volar margin of the carpal surface of the radius that is associated with subluxation of the radio-carpal joint. A **dorsal Barton's fracture** is a distal radius fracture with dislocation of the radio-carpal joint. A **Monteggia fracture** involves both the radial head and the ulna. It is most commonly a fracture of the proximal third of the ulna and anterior dislocation (or fracture) of the radial head. Common mechanisms of injury include a direct blow, hyperpronation or hyperextension. **Olecranon fractures** occur either from a direct blow to the elbow, or indirectly through a vigorous contraction of the *triceps brachii* muscle after a fall onto a flexed elbow during the flexed upper extremity. **Supracondylar fractures**, on the distal humerus, usually result from a fall on the outstretched hand or a direct blow to the posterior aspect of the elbow. They are more common in children with open physes. **Intercondylar fractures** also occur on the distal humerus, but require a higher energy mechanism. **Coronoid process fractures** typically occur in conjunction with elbow dislocations.

See also under STRESS FRACTURES.

ELBOW JOINT INJURIES   *See* ANTERIOR INTEROSSEUS SYNDROME; BICEPS TENDON INJURY; LATERAL EPICONDYLITIS; LITTLE LEAGUER'S ELBOW; MEDIAL EPICONDYLITIS; MEDIAN NERVE; OLECRANON BURSITIS; OSTEOCHONDRITIS DISSECANS; OSTEO-CHONDROSIS; PANNER'S DISEASE; PRONATOR SYNDROME; RADIAL TUNNEL SYNDROME; ULNAR COLLATERAL LIGA-MENT; ULNAR NERVE; VALGUS EXTENSION OVERLOAD SYNDROME; WRIST DROP.

ELBOW JOINT, THROWING INJURIES During the wind-up of the throw, the shoulder is hyperextended, externally rotated, and abducted; and the anterior structures of the shoulder are placed under tensile stress. The elbow is flexed to an angle of about 45 degrees and the flexor/extensor muscles around the elbow are contracted. In the acceleration phase of throwing, the humerus is whipped forward ahead of the flexed elbow resulting in medial valgus tension and lateral compression. The harder the ball is thrown, the further the forearm lags behind the upper arm, and the greater the valgus stresses.

Medially, excessive tension may damage the anterior band of the ulnar collateral ligament that is the primary restraint to valgus stress in the acceleration phase of throwing. **Acute rupture of the ulnar collateral ligament** occurs in throwers, especially as a result of chronic sprain. This leads to valgus instability. Poor technique, characterized by dropping the elbow in the acceleration phase, increases valgus stresses. Injury to the ulnar collateral ligament causes medial instability that may result in traction on the ulnar nerve.

Laterally, excessive compressive loads may damage the radio-humeral joint. As the forward momentum in the throwing action is transferred from the humerus to the forearm and wrist, the elbow rapidly extends. This may cause posterior olecranon impingement. The large valgus force generated during the late cocking and acceleration phases of throwing creates significant tensile forces in the flexor-pronator muscle group. This muscle group has its origin on the medial condyle, and serves as a secondary stabilizer to the ulnar collateral ligament. When fatigued, the flexor-pronator muscles may suffer micro- or macro-trauma. Healing with scar tissue may produce muscle contractures that prevent full elbow extension. Anterior interosseus nerve syndrome may occur along with flexor-pronator overuse injuries.

Little Leaguer's elbow is a term that refers to injuries affecting the skeletally immature elbow from repetitive stresses as a result of pitching and other overhead exercise. Injury to the epiphysis of the medial epicondyle of the humerus is the most common problem of the Little League baseball pitcher. A medial traction apophysitis, which occurs as a result of valgus stress, leads to hypertrophy of the medial epicondyle, microtearing of the flexor-pronator group and fragmentation (and even separation) of the medial epicondylar apophysis. Most cases are caused by training errors such as excessive throwing and poor pitching technique. It occurs primarily in young baseball pitchers between the ages of 9 and 12 years, but may also occur in

other throwing athletes and gymnasts. The medial epicondyle ossifies near the age of 6 years, but does not fuse until the age of 17 years. Associated pathology includes Panner's disease, osteochondritis of the capitulum, osteochondral lesions of the radial head and medial epicondylar fracture. Injury to the lateral compartment rarely occurs in the younger athlete. Safety guidelines for youth pitching recommend throwing more than 300 but less than 600 pitches per season. All throwers should avoid the side-arm throwing style. Pitchers should not play in multiple leagues, should not play hard-throwing positions when not pitching, and should not pitch when having elbow or shoulder pain.

See also LITTLE LEAGUER'S SHOULDER; VALGUS EXTENSION OVERLOAD SYNDROME.

Chronology

•1960 • B.G. Brogdon and N.E. Crow observed that in young pitchers, repetitive valgus microtrauma produced medial apophysitis. In the *American Journal of Roentgenography*, they labeled the condition 'Little Leaguer's elbow.'

•1974 • Orthopedic surgeon, Frank Jobe, extracted a tendon from Tommy John's right arm and used it to replace the torn ulnar collateral ligament on his left, pitching arm. 12 to 13% of patients do not have an accessory tendon in either arm, and a tendon is taken from the leg or toe. Transplanted tendons have three times the amount of collagen than the original ligament. The operation has a 70 to 80% success rate in terms of players returning to the game. John went on to win 170 more games, with his best season being in 1979 with the New York Yankees.

Bibliography

American Academy of Pediatrics (2001). Risk of injury from baseball and softball in children. *Pediatrics* 107(4), 782-784.

ELECTRIC CURRENT   The rate of flow of charged particles.

ELECTROCARDIOGRAPHY   ECG. It is the recording and amplification of electric potentials that have spread to the surface of the body from the heart. The resulting graphic tracing is called an **electrocardiogram**. *See under* CARDIAC CYCLE.

ELECTROENCEPHALOGRAPHY   EEG. This

involves the recording of electric potentials that have spread to the surface of the head from the brain. The potentials are amplified to give a graphic tracing (**electroencephalogram**), which shows the electrical activity of the brain over time. Two of the waves that can be identified are alpha and beta. **Alpha waves** are large amplitude, low frequency (12 to 18 cycles per second) waves associated with relaxed wakefulness. **Beta waves** are small amplitude, high frequency (13 to 30 cycles per second), desynchronized waves and are associated with cognitive activity.

In a study of small-bore rifle shooters, it was found that experts exhibited a significantly longer quiet eye period preceding shot execution than did nonexperts. During the preparatory period just prior to the shot, experts demonstrated a significant increase in left-hemisphere alpha and beta power accompanied by a decrease in right-hemisphere alpha and beta power. Nonexperts exhibited similar asymmetry, but to a lesser extent than did experts. Janelle et al. (2000) argued that these findings reflect more optimal organization of the neural structures needed to achieve high-level performance.

Bibliography

Janelle, C.M. et al. (2000). Expertise differences in cortical activation and gaze behavior during rifle shooting. *Journal of Sport and Exercise Psychology* 22(2), 167-182.

ELECTROLYTE *See under* MINERALS.

ELECTROMYOGRAPHY EMG. The recording of the electrical activity of muscle, either by inserting needle electrodes into the muscle or placing electrodes on the surface of the skin over the muscle. An **electromyogram** is the graphic tracing drawn by an electromyograph. It provides a representation of the summated electrical activation pattern of the muscle near the electrode. In isometric movements, the EMG signal is proportional to the amount of force generated by the muscle. The relationship between force and EMG in concentric, eccentric and isokinetic muscle actions is poorly understood, because it is complicated by the length-tension relationship and the force-velocity relationship. *See also* ACCOUSTOMYOGRAPHY.

Bibliography

Basmajian, J.V. and DeLuca, C.J. (1985). *Muscles alive:Their function revealed by electromyography*. 5th ed. Baltimore, MD: Williams & Wilkins.

Clarys, J.P. and Cabri, J. (1993). Electromyography and the study of sports movements. *Journal of Sports Sciences* 11, 379-448.

Hof, A.L. (1984). EMG and muscle force: An introduction. *Human Movement Science* 3, 119-153.

Smith, L.K., Weiss, E.L. and Lehmkuhl, L.D. (1996). *Brunnstrom's clinical kinesiology*. 5th ed. Philadelphia: FA Davis Co.

ELECTRON A small particle having a unit negative charge. The distance of an electron from the nucleus of an atom is determined by the amount of potential energy the electron possesses. The electrons are arranged in energy order (from low to high) in sub-shells starting with the sub-shell in which the electrons are most tightly bound and which is closest to the nucleus.

Ionic compounds are compounds that form between metals and non-metals when positively and negatively charged ions attract. The metals lose one or more electrons to non-metals, thus the metal becomes a positively charged ion (cation) and the non-metal becomes a negatively charged ion (anion). When dissolved in water, ionic compounds lose their solid crystal structure and the individual ions are dispersed. When calcium chloride (for example) is dissolved in water, a solution of calcium ions and chloride ions are formed in which the chloride ions are twice as abundant as calcium ions.

Covalent compounds are non-electrolyte and do not consist of ions and therefore do not conduct electricity. Covalent compounds are formed when neighboring atoms share electrons. A **single covalent bond** results when a pair of electrons is shared. A **double covalent bond** results when two pairs of electrons are shared. A **polar covalent bond** is a bond in which a pair of electrons is shared in common between two atoms, but the pair is held more closely by one of the atoms. The O-H bond of a hydroxyl group, for example, is polar, because the shared electrons are pulled towards the oxygen atom. The C-C bond is non-polar, because the atoms at the end of the bond are the same. There is no preferential pull of electrons to either end.

Substances with mainly non-polar bonds, such as lipids, will tend to be hydrophobic or insoluble in water. Most compounds in living organisms contain carbon with four covalent bonds, i.e. four single bonds, two single and one double bond, or two double bonds. Nitrogen has three single bonds or one double and one single bond. Oxygen has two single bonds or a double bond. Hydrogen has only a single bond. Water has two hydrogen atoms that each share an electron with an oxygen atom. Carbon dioxide has a carbon atom that shares two electrons with each of the two oxygen atoms. *See also* ELEMENT.

Bibliography

Curtis, H. and Barnes, N.S. (1989). *Biology.* 5th ed. New York: Worth Publishes, Inc.

ELECTRON TRANSPORT CHAIN   Electron transfer chain. Respiratory chain. An organized series of carrier molecules located in the inner mitochondrial membrane that shuttles electrons from NADH and $FADH_2$ to oxygen. Electron acceptors in the electron transport chain donate their electrons to other electron acceptors, which pass them on to other electron acceptors, and so on. Each time electrons move from one component to the next, they lose some energy that is ultimately used in making ATP. The electrons move along in a series of redox reactions, because each successive carrier has a greater affinity (force of attraction) for them than the preceding one in the sequence. Oxygen has the greatest affinity of all for electrons and acts as the final acceptor. Most of the components of the electron transport chain carry free electrons rather than actual hydrogen atoms.

NADH arrives at flavoprotein 1 and transfers electrons and protons from the hydrogen across the inner mitochondrial membrane. Protons are released and deposited in the intermembrane space. If $FADH_2$ is the hydrogen carrier, the transfer of electrons and protons occurs at flavoprotein 2 instead of flavoprotein 1. The high-energy electrons from $FADH_2$ enter the electron transport chain at a later point than electrons from NADH, they travel through fewer reactions and thus generate fewer ATP. $FADH_2$ donates its electrons to Coenzyme Q. The electrons shuttle down cytochromes, alternately causing the cytochromes to gain and lose electrons. In this process, they also move across the width of the inner membrane, shuttling protons from the mitochondrial matrix to the inner membrane space. Oxygen accepts the electrons. The outer shell of oxygen has room for 8 electrons, but contains only 6 electrons. Thus it can accept 2 electrons at the end of the electron transport chain. When oxygen accepts these 2 electrons, it then has a double negative charge. 2 protons are thus attracted and water is formed.

Chemiosmotic coupling is the process that couples the electron transport chain to ATP synthesis. It uses energy released in the electron transport chain to transport protons across the inner mitochondrial membrane against their concentration gradient. The energy stored in this concentration gradient is used for ATP synthesis.

The inner mitochondrial membrane contains four distinct complexes containing components of the electron transport chain. Complexes I, III and IV are able to function as both electron carriers and to transport protons from the mitochondrial matrix into the intermembrane space. This movement of protons creates a concentration gradient across the inner mitochondrial membrane such that the concentration outside is higher than inside the matrix. The concentration gradient represents a store of potential energy. The [potential] energy of the concentration gradient is the **chemiosmotic potential** or **proton motive force** and is the sum of the concentration difference of protons across the membrane and the difference in electrical charge across the membrane.

The potential energy of the concentration gradient is increased by a difference in electrical potential across the membrane. The protons are moved via proton pumps into the intermembrane space. The concentration of protons in the mitochondrial matrix is much lower than in the intermembrane space. This generates a voltage across the membrane that is negative on the matrix side and positive between the mitochondrial membranes. Both these conditions strongly attract the protons back into the matrix. The only areas of the membrane that are freely permeable to protons, however, are enzyme complexes called **ATP synthases**. The movement of protons creates an electric current, the energy of which is harnessed by ATP synthase in order to catalyze ATP synthesis. The several subunits of ATP synthase appear to work together like gears: as the core of the enzyme complex rotates, ADP and phosphorus are pulled into the mitochondrial matrix and ATP is pushed out. The concentration gradient also supplies energy to pump metabolites (e.g. ADP) and calcium ions across the relatively impermeable inner mitochondrial membrane. The outer mitochondrial membrane is quite freely permeable to these substances.

The best current estimates for the number of ATP formed from NADH and $FADH_2$ in ATP in the electron transfer chain are 2.5 and 1.5, respectively (rather than the old estimates of 3 and 2).

See AEROBIC ENERGY SYSTEMS; FATTY ACID DEGRADATION; GLYCOLYSIS.

Bibliography

Houston, M.E (2001). *Biochemistry primer for exercise science.* 2nd ed. Champaign, IL: Human Kinetics.

Insel, P., Turner, R.E. and Ross, D. (2002). *Nutrition.* Sudbury, MA: Jones and Bartlett.

Robergs, R.A. and Roberts, S.O. (2000). *Fundamental principles of exercise physiology.* Boston, MA: McGraw-Hill.

Stryer, L, Berg, J. and Tymoczko, J. (2002). *Biochemistry.* 5th ed. New York: W.H. Freeman.

ELEMENT A substance consisting only of atoms of the same type and of the same atomic number (number of protons). Elements can be classified into metallic and non-metallic, with some exceptions. **Non-metals** have high ionization energies and electronegativities; are generally poor conductors of heat and electricity; are generally brittle; and have the ability to gain electrons easily. Metals have low ionization and electronegativities (due to the fact that the electrons in the valence shell can be removed easily); are generally good conductors of heat and electricity; and can be deformed without breaking, having the property of being able to be hammered into shapes (malleability) and to be drawn into wire (ductility). A **metalloid** is an element with some of the properties of metals and some of the properties of non-metals, e.g. arsenic, boron and silicon. The electronegativities and ionization energies of the metalloids are between those of the metals and nonmetals, so the metalloids exhibit characteristics of metals and nonmetals.

In many elements, two or more atoms join to form molecules; e.g. oxygen gas is formed from two oxygen atoms. All gases consist of molecules. Of the 92 naturally occurring elements, six make up some 99% of living tissue: carbon, hydrogen, nitrogen, oxygen, phosphorus and sulfur.

Atoms are made of even smaller particles: protons, neutrons and electrons. The mass of an atom depends on the number of protons and neutrons it contains. The electrons in an atom contribute very little to its mass. The number of protons and electrons together is called the **mass number**. Whole atoms are uncharged, because the number of electrons in an atom is the same as the number of protons. The number of protons is the **atomic number (proton number)**. The lightest of atoms is an atom of hydrogen. It consists of one proton and one electron. The masses of other atoms are compared with that of a hydrogen atom.

Relative atomic mass is the mass of one atom of an element, divided by the mass of one atom of hydrogen. The nucleus of an atom, with the exception of hydrogen, contains neutrons as well as protons. A **neutron** is a subatomic particle with no electrical charge. A **proton** is the positively charged unit that forms part of the nucleus of an atom around which electrons orbit. The nucleus is minute in volume compared with the volume of the atom. The electrons occupy the space outside the nucleus. The electrons orbit the nucleus.

See also CHEMICAL REACTIONS; FREE RADICALS; MOLE.

EMBDEN–MYERHOF PATHWAY *See under* GLYCOLYSIS.

EMBOLUS A blood clot that forms in a blood vessel in one part of the body and then is carried to another part of the body. See under HYPERBARIC PHYSIOLOGY; THROMBOSIS.

EMBRYO The developing human from conception through the first two months of pregnancy. See also STEM CELLS.

EMG *See* ELECTROMYOGRAPHY.

EMOTION A complex function of a number of interacting factors: the degree of arousal change from some baseline level; the cognitive appraisal of the situation producing the change in arousal; appraisal of the arousal change, which may in turn affect the cognitive appraisal of the situation; and the specific physiological pattern of the arousal. The interaction of cognitive appraisal, the subjective (conscious) experience of emotion and arousal is not clearly understood. Emotions have two major dimensions: the qualitative dimension of pleasant-unpleasant and the quantitative dimension of intensity. The difference between being annoyed and being angry, for example, is mainly one of intensity. The difference between fear and excitement, for example, is mainly one of pleasantness. Presentation (or lack of presentation) of emotions can be either self-regulative, e.g. suppressing showing obvious signs of anger even though anger is being expressed) or social regulative, e.g. showing emotions in an attempt to motivate teammates, intimidate opponents, or deceive opponents (Hackford, 1993).

Vallerand (1987) emphasizes the role of intuitive appraisal (minimal cognition) rather than reflective appraisal (deliberate cognitive processing), and argues that the former often precedes the latter in the enactment of an emotion. Attributions are a form of reflective appraisal.

See also MOOD.

Bibliography

Hackford, D. (1993). Functional attributions to emotions in sport. In J.R. Nitsch and R. Seiler (eds.). *Movement in sport: Psychological foundations and effects. Proceedings of the VIIIth European Congress of Sport Psychology. Vol. 1.* pp143-149. Sankt Augustin, Germany: Academia Verlag.

Hanin, Y.L. (2000, ed). *Emotions in sport.* Champaign, IL: Human Kinetics.

Vallerand, R.J. (1983). On emotion in sport. Theoretical and social psychological perspectives. *Journal of Sport Psychology* 5, 197-215.

Vallerand, R.J. (1987). Antecedents of self-related affects in sport: Preliminary evidence on the intuitive-reflective appraisal model. *Journal of Sport Psychology* 9, 161-182.

EMOTIONAL DISTURBANCE A condition exhibiting one or more of the following characteristics over a long period of time and to a marked degree, which adversely affects educational performance: an inability to learn that cannot be explained by intellectual, sensory, or health factors; an inability to build or maintain satisfactory interpersonal relationships with peers and teachers; inappropriate types of behavior or feelings under normal circumstances; a general pervasive mood of unhappiness or depression; or a tendency to develop physical symptoms or fears associated with personal or school problems.

In the USA, P.L. 105-17, the IDEA Amendments of 1997, changed "Serious Emotional Disturbance" to "Emotional Disturbance," because of the negative connotation of the term "Serious." Until 1981, "Serious Emotional Disturbance" included autism. Persons with autism were then included in the official definition of "Other Health Impaired." In 1990, Autism was recognized as an independent diagnostic category. *See also* MENTAL HEALTH.

EMPHYSEMA Disease of the lungs in which there is permanent dilation of alveoli and destruction of airway walls. One theory about the tissue destruction suggests that it results from the action of **proteases**, enzymes secreted by macrophages and other white blood cells during chronic inflammation. Proteases destroy tissue by breaking down proteins, including those in elastic connective tissue. Consequently, the lungs lose elasticity and compliance increases.

A **bulla** is an enlarged airspace due to emphysema, usually greater than 1 cm in diameter, located immediately adjacent to the visceral pleura.

Bullae may be found in combination with any of the four anatomic subtypes of emphysema. The term 'bleb' is frequently used inappropriately to designate a small bulla. In the strict sense, blebs are interstitial air cysts that result from dissection of air into interstitial connective tissue.

Smokers demonstrate significantly increased pulmonary proteolytic activities, possibly related to accumulation of inflammatory cells (neutrophils, macrophages) containing a high concentration of protease enzymes. Persons with a genetic deficiency of alpha-1-antitrypsin, a potent antiprotease, are prone to develop severe emphysema at an early age even if they never smoke.

Patients with emphysema can expel a larger volume during a slow exhalation than during a maximal forced exhalation, because intrathoracic pressure is less positive and airway compression is minimized during a slow exhalation. Patients can minimize air trapping and dyspnea by pursed-lip breathing, in which the lips are puckered (drawn together) during exhalation. This creates external resistance to flow and maintains a more positive intra-airway pressure during exhalation retarding small airway compression.

Bibliography

American College of Sports Medicine (2001). *ACSM's resource manual for Guidelines for Exercise Testing & Prescription*. 4th ed. Philadelphia, PA: Lippincott Williams & Wilkins.

EMULSIFIER An agent that blends fatty and watery liquids by promoting the break up of fat into small particles and stabilizing their suspension in aqueous solution.

ENCEPHALOPATHY Any disorder of the brain.

ENCOPRESIS A condition in which a person repeatedly soils inappropriate places such as clothing with feces. It may be voluntary or involuntary. There are two types: encopresis with constipation (overflow incontinence) and encopresis without constipation. The former is usually involuntary. In the latter there may be a co-existing mental disorder.

END-DIASTOLIC VOLUME *See under* CARDIAC CYCLE.

ENDERGONIC *See under* THERMODYNAMICS.

ENDOCARDITIS Infection of a structure on the inside of the heart such as the mitral valve.

ENDOCHONDRAL OSSIFICATION Bone formation in which a cartilage model is replaced by bone.

ENDOCRINE SYSTEM *See under* HORMONES.

ENDOCYTOSIS *See under* ACTIVE TRANSPORT.

ENDOGENOUS Derived or originating internally.

ENDOMETRITIS An infection of the endometrium or deciduas, with extension into the myometrium and parametrial tissues. It is the most common cause of fever during the postpartum period.

ENDOMETRIUM The mucus membrane that lines the uterus. It thickens under hormonal control and (if pregnancy does not occur) is shed in menstruation. If pregnancy does occur, it is shed along with the placenta at parturition.

In **endometriosis**, tissue like the endometrium is found outside the uterus, in other areas of the body. In these locations outside the uterus, the endometrial tissue develops into tumors that can cause pain, infertility and other problems. The most common locations of endometrial tumors are in the abdomen and involve the ovaries, fallopian tubes, the ligaments supporting the uterus, the area between the vagina and the rectum, the outer surface of the uterus, and the lining of the pelvic cavity. Endometrial tumors are generally not malignant. Complications, depending on the location of the tumors include: rupture of tumors, which can spread endometriosis to new areas; the formation of adhesions; intestinal bleeding or obstruction, if the growths are in or near the intestines; interference with bladder function, if the growths are on or in the bladder; and other problems. The most common symptoms of endometriosis are pain before and during periods (usually worse than 'normal' menstrual cramps), during or after sexual activity, infertility, and heavy or irregular bleeding. Other symptoms may include: fatigue; painful bowel movements with periods; low-back pain with periods; diarrhea and constipation; and other intestinal distress with some periods. Some women with endometriosis have no symptoms.

Endometriosis affects 1 out of 7 women of reproductive age, and is estimated to be responsible for up to 40% of fertility problems. Infertility affects about 30 to 40% of women with endometriosis and is a common consequence with progression of the disease. In general, menopause ends the activity of mild or moderate endometriosis.

The cause of endometriosis is not known. One theory is that during menstruation some of the menstrual tissue backs up through the fallopian tubes, implants in the abdomen, and grows. Another theory suggests that remnants of tissue from when the woman was an embryo may later develop into endometriosis or that some adult tissues retain the ability they had in the embryo stage to transform into reproductive tissue under certain circumstances.

Conservative surgery involves removal or destruction of tumors, but recurrences are common. Radical surgery, involving hysterectomy and removal of all tumors and the ovaries becomes necessary in chronic cases. In the USA, surgery through laproscopy is rapidly replacing major abdominal surgery. It is recurrent and usually requires a long-term treatment plan.

Bibliography
Endometriosis Association. Http://www.endometriosisassn.org

ENDOMORPHY See under SOMATOTYPE.

ENDONEURIUM See under PERIPHERAL NERVES.

ENDOPLASMIC RETICULUM An extensive system in the cytosol that consists of interconnected tubes and parallel membranes. There are two types: rough and smooth. **Rough endoplasmic reticulum** contains ribosomes. The **smooth endoplasmic reticulum** is so named because it contains no ribosomes, is the site for synthesis of lipids (including triglycerides and steroids), and is also the site for storage of calcium ions. Closely associated with, but physically separate from, the endoplasmic reticulum, is the **Golgi apparatus** consisting of membrane-bound flattened sacs called **cisternae** that process molecules synthesized in the endoplasmic reticulum and prepares them for transport.

ENDORPHINS Opioid peptides that arise from beta lipotrophin. **Beta lipotrophin** is primarily synthesised in the anterior pituitary gland from the precursor, pro-opiomelanocortin. It can be released into the circulation from the pituitary gland or it can project into areas of the brain through nerve fibers. The term '**opioid**' usually refers to endogenous substances, with 'opiate' referring to exogenous substances. The term '**endorphin**' comes from 'endogenous morphins.' Opioids can be divided into three types (in order of potency, from least to greatest): enkephalin, endorphin and dynorphin. High levels of enkephalin are found in the hypothalamus, limbic system, basal ganglia and spinal cord. High levels of endorphin are found in the hypothalamus, spinal cord and the peripheral nervous system. High levels of dynorphin are found in the hypothalamus and posterior pituitary gland. Only endorphin is able to cross the blood-brain barrier.

Opioids function as neurohormones and neurotransmitters. By acting on specific opioid receptor sites in the brain, they are thought to block pain and produce feelings of exhilaration ('**runner's high**'). The secretion of endorphins has also been implicated in the decrease of anxiety, anger and confusion. It also seems that opioids can affect a number of other body functions, such as thermoregulation, metabolism, respiration and learning. Opioids also play a role in the regulation of various hormones involved in control of the menstrual cycle such as luteinizing hormone. Opioids inhibit release of luteinizing hormone from the pituitary gland. It is thought that opioids modulate the secretion of corticotropin-releasing factor, which mediates the release of adrenocorticotropic hormone by the pituitary gland.

Exercise appears to stimulate endogenous opioids more significantly than any other single stimulus. Exercise must be of intensity greater than 75% of maximal oxygen uptake in order for endorphins to be released in the peripheral nervous system. There seems to be wide intra- and inter-individual differences in this response. Endorphin levels probably remain elevated for 15 to 60 minutes following exercise.

Bibliography

American College of Sports Medicine (1985). Endorphins in exercise. *Medicine and Science in Sports and Exercise* 17(1), 73-105.

Goldfarb, A.H. and Jamurtas, A.Z. (1997). Beta-endorphin response to exercise: An update. *Sports Medicine* 24, 8-16.

Harber, V.J. and Sutton, J.R. (1984). Endorphins and exercise. *Sports Medicine* 1, 154-171.

Schwarz, L. and Kindermann, W. (1992). Changes in beta-endorphin levels in response to aerobic and anaerobic exercise. *Sports Medicine* 13(1), 25-36.

Sforzo, G.A. (1988). Opioids and exercise. *Sports Medicine* 7, 109-124.

ENDOSTEAL   Relating to endostosis.

ENDOSTOSIS   A process of bone formation in which ossification takes place within the substance of the cartilage.

ENDOTHELIN-1   A hormone that is released by endothelial cells in response to various chemical signals and mechanical stimuli and causes vasoconstriction.

ENDOTHELIUM   The membrane lining various vessels and cavities of the body. Vascular smooth muscles contract and relax in response to chemical substances released by the endothelium.

See also ENDOTHELIN-1; NITRIC OXIDE; PROSTACYCLIN; PROSTAGLANDINS.

ENDOTHERMIC   *See under* THERMO-DYNAMICS.

END-TIDAL PARTIAL PRESSURE OF OXYGEN   The partial pressure of oxygen measured at the end of an exhalation. It is usually the lowest partial pressure of oxygen measured during the alveolar phase of the exhalation.

ENDURANCE   Stamina. It is the capacity to sustain a given velocity or power output for the longest amount of time. **Aerobic endurance** is the ability to sustain exercise that is predominantly aerobic, and is often referred to as **cardiorespiratory/cardiovascular endurance**, which collectively is the degree to which the heart, vascular system and respiratory system can provide the oxygen necessary for exercise to be continued. The limits of human cardiorespiratory endurance are determined by both physiological/biochemical factors (oxygen transport and the metabolic capacity of the relevant muscle tissue) and psychological factors (e.g. motivation and perceived exertion).

Local muscular endurance is the degree to which specific muscle groups can continue contracting against a given load in a given period of time or for a given number of repetitions. Simple field tests such as push-ups are used to test muscular endurance.   Factors affecting local muscular endurance include the type and speed of muscular contraction, the cadence of repetitions, and the magnitude of the resistance. The limiting factor is not cardiorespiratory/cardiovascular endurance, but the physiological limitations within the muscle groups being exercised and the neuromuscular control. Three methods used to improve local muscle endurance ('strength-endurance') are traditional heavy weight training, high repetition training and variable-load training. With regard to heavy weight training, there is a strong direct relationship between muscular strength and endurance, so that a stronger muscle will have a greater endurance capacity when it is compared to a weaker one. For high-repetition training, between 30 and 50 repetitions are performed using 30 to 50% of the one-repetition maximum (1-RM), for 3 or 4 sets. Alternatively, this training involves performing as many repetitions as possible in a specified time period. Repeated exposure to high lactate levels enhances the athlete's tolerance to the fatiguing effects of lactic acid. Both heavy weight training and high-repetition methods result in similar improvements in local muscle endurance. Variable-load training involves a combination of the other two methods. A relatively large load (about 70% of 1-RM) and a relatively high number of repetitions (about 30) are used. According to Bloomfield et al (1994), variable load training appears to be the best form of training for the development of local muscle endurance.

See also RESISTANCE TRAINING; TRAINING FOR DISTANCE RUNNING.

Bibliography

Bloomfield, J., Ackland, T.R., and Elliott, B.C. (1994). *Applied anatomy and biomechanics in sport*. Melbourne: Blackwell Scientific Publications.

ENERGY The capacity to do work. It is the physical quality that imbues an object with the ability to exert a force. The units for energy are the same as for work. The six forms of energy are chemical, mechanical, heat (thermal), light (radiant), electric and nuclear. Energy can be converted or transformed into another form. For example, chemical energy from food can be converted into mechanical energy for generation of force by muscle with the breakdown of adenosine triphosphate (ATP). Energy exists in either potential or kinetic form. **Potential energy** is energy due to the position of one body with respect to another body or to the relative parts of the same body. In the context of sport and exercise science, the most common types of potential energy are gravitational energy and elastic strain energy. **Gravitational energy** is due to the location of an object or system in a gravitational field above some baseline, such as the height of an object above ground level. The greater distance a mass is raised above the ground, the greater will be its potential energy. **Elastic (strain) energy** is due to the stretch of an object or tissue beyond its resting length. Biological tissue has a tendency to return to its pre-stretch length. **Kinetic energy** is energy due to motion. It is proportional to the square of the velocity. **Energetics** is the branch of science that deals with energy exchanges in living things.

See also THERMODYNAMICS.

ENERGY BALANCE The difference between energy (caloric) intake and energy (caloric) expenditure. Macronutrients are metabolized differently and stored separately, so that the conversion of one macronutrient into another for storage does not represent important metabolic pathways. An athlete needs to manage fat, protein and carbohydrate balances separately to achieve sport-specific body size, body composition and energy store objectives.

In athletes, body weight is not a reliable indicator of either energy or macronutrient balance. Because protein and glycogen stores are associated with much more body water than are fat stores, for example, a weight gain due to small increases in protein or glycogen energy stores can counterbalance the weight loss due to larger decreases in fat energy stores during negative energy balance.

It is not feasible for athletes to measure their energy intake and expenditure accurately on a day-to-day basis as a method for managing their training. Separately managing fat, protein and carbohydrate balances will be even less practical than managing energy balance if athletes attempt to estimate fat, protein and carbohydrate intakes and expenditures in place of energy intake and expenditure. Research is required to validate specific, accurate and practical biomarkers for answering questions about macronutrient balances. Skinfold fat is a candidate biomarker for fat mass. The most convenient indicator of sustained carbohydrate deficiency may be urinary ketone bodies. 'Keto-sticks' can be purchased inexpensively in most pharmacies in order for athletes to monitor ketone bodies in their urine. Studies comparing data from the dietary records of female athletes to estimations or measurements of their energy expenditure have repeatedly found apparently very large negative balances in athletes with stable body weights. However, a meta-analysis of studies comparing dietary assessments to measurement of energy expenditure by double-labeled water found that women do not under-report more than men.

Bibliography

Loucks, A.B. (2004). Energy balance and body composition in sports and exercise. *Journal of Sports Sciences* 22, 1-14.

Trabulsi, J. and Schoeller, D.A. (2001). Evaluation of dietary assessment against doubly labeled water, a biomarker of habitual energy intake. *American Journal of Physiology: Endocrinology and Metabolism* 281, E891-E899.

ENERGY EXPENDITURE Energy output. **Total daily energy expenditure** generally refers to the sum of the following components: resting energy expenditure, diet-induced thermogenesis (thermic effect of feeding) and the energy cost of physical activities (thermic effect of activity). Total daily energy expenditure of an individual engaged in normal daily activity ranges from 1,800 to 3,000 kcal. Some athletes, such as Tour de France cyclists, exceed 10,000 kcal. Body weight appears to be regulated around a given set point, in a similar way that body temperature is regulated. The sympathetic nervous system may play a major role in this regulation. The body adapts to changes in energy intake by adjusting any or all of the three components. With very low calorie diets, for example, all three decrease. Resting energy expenditure typically constitutes 60 to 75% of daily energy expenditure, diet-induced thermogenesis constitutes approximately 10% and energy cost of physical activities - the most variable component - can constitute 15 to 30%. **Gross energy expenditure** is the total value of energy expenditure, including resting energy expenditure. **Net energy expenditure** is the energy cost of the activity, excluding the resting value.

A distinction can be made between basal and resting metabolic rate. **Basal metabolic rate** is the minimum rate of energy expenditure immediately after awakening from sleep. It is determined with the subject free of fever and anxiety, having abstained from food and heavy physical activity for at least 12 to 18 hours and resting in a relaxed supine position for at least 30 minutes in a quiet thermoneutral environment. **Resting metabolic rate** is determined in either the sitting or prone position at any time of day some 4 hours after a light meal and light physical activity (both unspecified). All other conditions are as indicated for basal metabolic rate.

The **Harris-Benedict equations** use body weight, height and age for males and females to estimate resting energy expenditure, but they tend to overestimate this figure, especially for obese people. More recent equations based on larger groups of subjects estimate resting energy rate from age, sex and body weight. Height is excluded, because it was not found to influence results appreciably. On average, resting metabolic rate is about 1 kcal/kg body weight/min for men and 0.9 kcal/kg bodyweight/min for women. The difference reflects different body composition.

The more fat-free mass a person has, the greater is total daily energy expenditure. Resting energy expenditure is also related to body surface area. The greater the body surface area, the greater is the loss of heat from the body, thus resting metabolic rate will increase to maintain body temperature. Other factors affecting resting energy expenditure include: age (gradually decreases with increasing age); body temperature (increases with increasing tempera-ture); stress (increases with increased activity of the sympathetic nervous system); and hormones (increases through action of the thyroid hormones and epinephrine).

Resting metabolic rate is modulated by the amount of calories consumed in the diet relative to energy expenditure. Excessive consumption of energy appears to increase resting metabolic rate, but fasting and very low calorie dieting cause resting metabolic rate to decrease. Since the resting metabolic rate is the primary component of daily energy expenditure, its decrease with caloric restriction makes it difficult for obese individuals to lose weight and to maintain weight that is lost.

Exercise may influence resting metabolic rate in four ways: i) the direct energy cost of exercise; ii) a prolonged increase in post-exercise metabolic rate from an acute exercise challenge; iii) a chronic increase in resting metabolic rate associated with exercise training; and iv) a possible increase in energy expenditure during non-exercising time.

It is not clear whether exercise has a carryover effect on resting metabolic rate. The following evidence suggests that energy intake and daily exercise can modulate resting metabolic rate: i) bed rest in sedentary individuals leads to a decrease in resting metabolic rate; ii) the resting metabolic rate of highly trained runners is lowered by about 7 to 10% when they cease daily exercise training; and iii) resting metabolic rate is depressed in previously sedentary obese individuals on a very low calorie diet, but it quickly returns to the pre-dieting level when exercise of sufficient frequency, intensity and duration is undertaken while dieting. On the other hand, there is evidence that exercising at 90% of maximal oxygen uptake until exhaustion significantly increases oxygen uptake for only fifteen minutes after the exercise.

The thermic effect of feeding can be subdivided into obligatory and facultative. **Obligatory thermic effect of feeding** results from the energy-requiring processes of digestion, absorption and assimilation of nutrients. **Facultative thermic effect of feeding** is related to the activation of the sympathetic nervous system and its stimulating effect on metabolism. The thermic effect of feeding reaches a peak one hour after a meal. The thermic effect of protein is much higher than that of carbohydrate, and that of dietary fat is minimal. The digestion of protein increases the metabolic rate dramatically, because of the amount of energy the liver expends processing the large amino acids. The thermic effect of feeding is minimal in obese people (the cause of this is unknown). It is not clear whether the thermic effect of feeding is significantly altered by exercise or training.

It has been hypothesized that combining diet and exercise will accelerate fat loss, preserve fat-free weight and prevent or decelerate the decline in resting metabolic rate more effectively than with diet restriction alone. The optimal combination of diet and exercise is not known, but it does seem that the combination of a large quantity of aerobic exercise with a very low calorie diet resulting in substantial loss of bodyweight may actually accelerate the decline in resting metabolic rate. *See also* CALORIE; DIET; EFFICIENCY; ENERGY YIELD OF NUTRIENTS; METABOLIC EQUIVALENT; OBESITY.

Bibliography

Clark, N. (1994). Are you a slow burner? Set your metabolism in motion. *The Physician and Sportsmedicine* 22(1), 33-36.

Mole, P.A. (1990). Impact of energy intake and exercise on resting metabolic rate. *Sports Medicine* 10(2), 72-87.

Montoye, H.J. (1996). *Measuring physical activity and energy expenditure*. Champaign, IL: Human Kinetics.

Poehlman, E.T. (1989). A review: Exercise and its influence on resting energy metabolism in man. *Medicine and Science in Sports and Exercise* 21(5), 515-525.

Poehlman, E.T., Melby, C.L. and Goran, M.I. (1991). The impact of exercise and diet restriction on daily energy expenditure. *Sports Medicine* 11(2), 78-101.

Stamford, B. (1994). Burning calories - naturally. *The Physician and Sportsmedicine* 22(4), 115-116.

Van Zant, R.S. (1992). Influence of diet and exercise on energy expenditure - A review. *International Journal of Sport Nutrition* 2(1), 1-19.

ENERGY LEVEL The total mechanical energy of a body or system. This total represents the sum of the translational and rotational kinetic energy and the potential energy.

ENERGY SUBSTRATE UTILIZATION At rest, muscle energy requirements are provided largely by fatty acid oxidation, with 10% of oxygen consumption due to glucose oxidation. Plasma free fatty acids are the major circulating lipid fuel. Other potential sources of fatty acids include circulating very low-density lipoprotein (VLDL), triglycerides and intramuscular triglycerides. At rest, the brain consumes about 60% of the energy consumed by the whole body.

During short-term exercise of maximal intensity, carbohydrates (glycogen and blood glucose) may account for at least 80% of the energy, and muscle uptake of fatty acids may even be inhibited. Blood glucose is increased by glycogenolysis in the liver. Studies involving one-legged cycling have shown that exhausting exercise depletes glycogen content in active muscle, but not in inactive muscle.

During submaximal exercise (40 to 60% of maximal oxygen uptake) the contributions from fat and carbohydrate (glycogen and blood glucose) are approximately equal. In the trained state, there is a greater reliance on free fatty acid oxidation during submaximal exercise, with a sparing of carbohydrate. Exercise training results in an increased capacity to release free fatty acids from adipocytes. More total fat is metabolized during moderate-intensity (c. 50% maximal oxygen uptake) than low or high intensity exercise.

As exercise intensity increases beyond 40 to 60% of maximal oxygen uptake, there is an increase in carbohydrate utilization. Initially, local muscle glycogenolysis provides the major substrate. But as the duration of exercise increases, and muscle glycogen depletes, blood glucose becomes increasingly important. There is an increase in glucose utilization by each active muscle fiber and/or an increase in the number of active muscle fibers.

During prolonged exercise, liver glycogen may be depleted. Blood glucose then becomes dependent on gluconeogenesis. The rate of gluconeogenesis is increased not only when exercise is prolonged, but also when it is preceded by a restricted carbohydrate intake or when it is performed with the arms.

Intramuscular triglyceride can provide energy for intense exercise at less than one third of the rate attributed to muscle glycogen. The turnover of plasma free fatty acids is sufficiently rapid to account for most of the fat metabolized during low intensity exercise (25 to 40% maximal oxygen uptake). However, an exercise intensity of 65% maximal oxygen uptake results in a slight decrease in the amount of plasma free fatty acid uptake by muscle tissue.

During prolonged exercise, intramuscular triglycerides become the predominant source of energy obtained from fat. Oxidation of intramuscular triglycerides is associated with a decrease in muscle glycogen utilization and with improved endurance performance. Like glycogen, intramuscular triglyceride formation may be

relatively rapid and its storage predominates under conditions that promote minimal glycogen formation. This suggests that the role of intramuscular triglycerides is to maintain a readily available substrate to ensure that physical activity of a moderate nature can be performed when glycogen availability is not optimal. Training increases intramuscular triglyceride content, possibly due to enhanced insulin sensitivity, which regulates movement of free fatty acids into cells.

Bibliography

Coggan, A.R. (1991). Plasma glucose metabolism during exercise in humans. *Sports Medicine* 11(2), 102-124.

Coggan, A.R. and Coyle, E.F. (1991). Carbohydrate ingestion during prolonged exercise: Effects on metabolism and performance. *Exercise and Sport Sciences Reviews* 19, 1-40.

Coyle, E. (1995). Fat metabolism during exercise. *Gatorade Sports Science Exchange* 8(6).

Jensen, M.D. (2003). Fate of fatty acids at rest and during exercise: Regulatory mechanisms. *Acta Physiologica Scandanavia* 178(4), 385-390.

Johnson, N.A., Stannard, S.R. and Thompson, M.W. (2004). Muscle triglyceride and glycogen in endurance exercise: Implications for performance. *Sports Medicine* 34(3), 151-164.

ENERGY SYSTEMS The metabolic pathways that are used to resynthesize ATP. Newsholme et al. (1992) estimated the relative contribution of each energy system in a variety of running events as follows: 100 m (50% creatine phosphate, 50% anaerobic glycolysis); 200 m (25% creatine phosphate, 65% anaerobic glycolysis, 10% aerobic glycolysis); 400 m (12.5% creatine phosphate, 62.5% anaerobic glycolysis, 25% aerobic glycolysis); 800 m (6% creatine phosphate, 50% anaerobic glycolysis, 44% aerobic glycolysis); 1500 m (25% anaerobic glycolysis, 75% aerobic glycolysis); 5000 m (12.5% anaerobic glycolysis, 87.5% aerobic glycolysis); 10,000 m (3% anaerobic glycolysis, 97% aerobic glycolysis); marathon (75% aerobic glycolysis, 5% blood glucose, 20% triglyceride); 80K (35% aerobic glycolysis, 5% blood glucose, 60% triglyceride); and 24 hr run (10% aerobic glycolysis, 5% blood glucose, 60% triglyceride). In the 1500 m, 5000 m and 10,000 m the creatine phosphate system is used for a few seconds at the start and for the sprint finish.

Two misconceptions about the energy systems are that they respond to the demands of intense exercise in an almost sequential manner and that the aerobic system responds slowly to these energy demands, thereby playing little role in determining performance over short durations (Gastin, 2001). Recent research suggests that energy is derived from each of the energy-producing pathways during almost all exercise activities. The duration of maximal exercise at which equal contributions are derived from the anaerobic and aerobic energy systems appears to occur between 1 to 2 minutes and mostly around 75 seconds, a time that is considerably earlier than has traditionally been suggested. The balance between aerobic and anaerobic energy systems depends on exercise intensity in relation to the person's maximal oxygen uptake.

See AEROBIC ENERGY SYSTEMS; ANAEROBIC ENERGY SYSTEMS.

Bibliography

Gastin, P.B. (2001). Energy system interaction and relative contribution during maximal exercise. *Sports Medicine* 31(10), 725-741.

Newsholme, E.A. et al. (1992). Physical and mental fatigue: Metabolic mechanisms and importance of plasma amino acids. *British Medical Bulletin* 48, 477.

Newsholme, E., Leech, A. and Duester, G. (1994). *Keep on running. The science of training and performance.* Chichester, W. Sussex: John Wiley.

ENERGY TRANSFER *See under* RIGID BODY.

ENERGY YIELD OF NUTRIENTS The **caloric value of food** is the amount of potential energy stored in the molecule's covalent bonds. The proportion of hydrocarbon in the molecular structure contributes to the caloric value of foods, as does the proportionate content of water. Foods containing a high proportion of water (and also fiber) possess a lower caloric density than that of food with a low water content and with a proportionately higher content of fats or oils.

The energy content of food can be determined using a **bomb calorimeter**, a device that typically consists of a heavy insulated metal shell, a capsule for the food sample to be combusted, a water bath pressurized with at least 20 atmospheres of oxygen, a thermometer to measure the water temperature and an electric fuse to ignite the food sample. The number of calories used to combust (literally explode) the food is determined by the increase in water temperature. If a given quantity of carbohydrate, fat or protein is combusted, then given amounts of oxygen consumption, carbon dioxide production and heat release can be measured. The **heat of combustion** for one gram of carbohydrate, lipid or protein is 4.2 kcal, 9.45 kcal or 5.65 kcal, respectively. These are average values; the exact value for each type of carbohydrate, fat or protein depends on its particular chemical structure. The products of carbohydrate and fat catabolism in the body are similar to those for combustion. For nitrogen catabolism, however, the products of metabolism are different from those of combustion. Catabolism of protein in the body yields carbon dioxide, water, urea, nitrogen waste in feces, and additional carbon compounds in urine and feces such as creatinine. In the body, nitrogen atoms combine with hydrogen to form urea, which is excreted by the kidneys in the urine. The excreted nitrogen and carbon compounds accompanying protein metabolism represent a loss (of about 19%) in potential heat release, and thus need to be subtracted from caloric equivalents for protein derived from bomb calorimetry. Thus the energy yield from protein is decreased to 4.6 kcal per gram.

Typically 97% of carbohydrate, 92% of protein and 95% of lipids are digested and absorbed. After digestive efficiencies have been taken into account, the net caloric yield values (**Atwater general factors**) for one gram of carbohydrate, lipid or protein are 4 kcal, 9 kcal or 4 kcal respectively. If the composition and weight of food are known, the caloric content of any portion of food or an entire meal can be determined using the Atwater general factors, which represent the energy available from ingested food nutrients. In practice, however, food composition tables and databases can be used instead of calculating the percentage composition of each energy-giving nutrient.

Studies using the bomb calorimeter have shown that about 4.82 kcal is liberated when a blend of carbohydrate, lipid and protein is burned in one liter of oxygen. This caloric value for oxygen varies only slightly even with large variations in the metabolic mixture. A rounded value of 5 kcal per liter of oxygen consumed can be used as an approximate conversion factor for estimating the body's energy expenditure under steady-state conditions. *See also* ALCOHOL.

Bibliography

McArdle, W.D., Katch, F.I. and Katch, V.I. (1996). *Exercise physiology: Energy, nutrition and human performance*. Philadelphia, PA: Lippincott, Williams & Wilkins.

Roe, M.A., Finglas, P.M. and Church, S.M. (2002). McCance and Widowson's *The composition of foods*. 6th ed. London, UK: Royal Society of Chemistry and the Food Standards Agency.

Robergs, R.A. and Roberts, S.O. (2000). *Fundamental principles of exercise physiology*. Boston, MA: McGraw-Hill.

ENJOYMENT   *See under* FLOW.

ENTERIC CANAL   *See* ALIMENTARY CANAL.

ENTERIC NERVOUS SYSTEM   *See under* GASTROINTESTINAL SYSTEM.

ENTEROGASTRIC REFLEX   Inhibition of gastric motility when irritants enter the duodenum.

ENTHALPY   *See under* THERMODYNAMICS.

ENTHESOPATHY   *See under* TENDON.

ENTROPY   *See under* THERMODYNAMICS.

ENURESIS   The term used when an individual repeatedly urinates in bed or on clothing. It may occur day and/or night.

ENZYME   A protein that acts as a catalyst. A **catalyst** increases the reactivity of a specific substance without itself being used up in the reaction. The substance that is catalyzed is called a **substrate**. The chemical reactions that take place in human metabolism are completely dependent on enzymes. Enzymes speed up reactions by lowering the energy barrier to the reaction (**energy of activation**), so that they take place at the lower temperature of an organism (37 degrees Celsius for humans). An enzyme allows the reaction to reach equilibrium faster than if the enzyme were absent, but the position of the equilibrium remains the same. In a **reversible reaction**, given sufficient time, equilibrium is established with the ratio of product concentration to substrate concentration at a constant described by the **equilibrium constant**. In a reversible reaction, the product is also a substrate for the reverse reaction. Enzymes are highly specific, catalyzing a single reaction or type of reaction. Enzymes can be inhibited by a variety of substances. Biochemists describe the relationship between temperature and reaction rate by the quotient Q_{10}, the relative increase in enzyme activity with a 10-degree increase in temperature. The Q_{10} value for most enzyme-catalyzed reactions is within the range of 1.5 to 2.5, indicating that an increase in temperature of 10 degrees Celsius approximately doubles the rate of an enzyme-catalyzed reaction.

Regulatory (rate-limiting) enzymes are enzymes that are critical in controlling the rate and direction of energy production along a metabolic pathway. They are generally found early in a metabolic pathway. If the rate-limiting enzyme were located at the end of a pathway, products might accumulate.

Certain enzyme molecules possess a binding site called the regulatory site, which is specific for molecules known as **modulators** that increase or decrease enzyme activity. A **modulator** induces a change in an enzyme's conformation, altering the shape of the active site, thus causing a change in the enzyme's activity by altering its catalytic rate, its affinity for substrate or both. Enzymes that are regulated by modulators are called **allosteric enzymes**. **Allosterism** refers to the fact that modulators change the spatial orientation, or shapes, of parts of the enzymes. Modulators may either increase enzymatic activity (**stimulators**), e.g. ADP + phosphorus; or decrease enzymatic activity (**inhibitors**) e.g. ATP. The build up of ATP serves to inhibit rate-limiting enzymes, which, in turn, slow down the reactions involved in the pathway. Two important allosteric enzymes in skeletal muscle are phosphorylase and phosphofructokinase, which are involved in glycolysis.

Most enzymes have a pH optimum, i.e. a particular pH or narrow pH range where enzyme activity is maximal. Enzyme activity is also influenced by the need for cofactors and coenzymes, substrate concentrations, enzyme concentrations, the type of isozyme and, if allosteric, activator concentrations. **Isozymes** are enzymes from the same source with identical catalytic properties, but with slightly different chemical, physical or kinetic properties.

Oxidoreductases are enzymes that catalyze redox reactions (e.g. lactate dehydrogenase). **Transferases** are enzymes catalyzing the transference of a chemical group from one compound to another (e.g. glycogen phosphorylase). **Hydrolases** are enzymes that catalyze the cleavage of certain bonds producing water as a by-product (e.g. acetylcholinesterase). **Lyases** are enzymes that catalyze the cleavage of certain bonds leaving double bonds or rings, or catalyze the addition of groups to double bonds (e.g. citrase oxaloacetate-lyase). **Isomerases** are enzymes that catalyze geometric or structural changes within one molecule (e.g. glucose 6-phosphate isomerase). **Ligases** are enzymes that catalyse the joining of two molecules coupled with the hydrolysis of a pyrophosphate bond of a triphosphate (e.g. pyruvate carboxylase).

Enzyme adaptations occur as a result of sprint training, with enzymes of all three energy systems showing signs of adaptation to training and some evidence of return to a baseline level with detraining. Myokinase and creatine phosphokinase have shown increases as a result of short-sprint training in some studies. Elite sprinters appear better able to breakdown creatine phosphate than the sub-elite sprinters. No changes in these enzyme levels have been reported as a result of detraining.

Similarly, glycolytic enzyme activity (notably lactate dehydrogenase, phosphofructokinase and glycogen phosphorylase) has been shown to increase after training consisting of either long (greater than 10-second) or short (less than 10-second) sprints. Evidence suggests that these enzymes return to pre-training levels some time between 7 weeks and 6 months of detraining.

Mitochondrial enzyme activity also increases after sprint training, particularly when long sprints or short recovery between short sprints are used as the training stimulus.

See under MUSCLE SORENESS.

Bibliography

Houston, M.E (2001). *Biochemistry primer for exercise science*. 2nd ed. Champaign, IL: Human Kinetics.

Noakes, T.D. (1987). Effect of exercise on serum enzyme activities in humans. *Sports Medicine* 4, 245-267.

Ross, A. and Leveritt, M. (2001). Long-term metabolic and skeletal muscle adaptations to short-sprint training: Implications for sprint training and tapering. *Sports Medicine* 31(5), 1063-1082.

EOSINOPHIL   A type of leucocyte that comes from bone marrow and is a weak phagocyte, in addition to being a detoxifier.

EOSINOPHILIA-MYALGIA SYNDROME   *See under* AMINO ACIDS.

EPHEDRINE   It is the most well known of the sympathomimetic amines, which is a category of stimulant drugs. **Ephedra** is a plant with varieties growing in Asia, Australia, Europe and North America. It is called *Ma Huang* in China. Ephedra contains two alkaloids, ephedrine and pseudo-ephedrine (an isomer of ephedrine). Ephedra has been found in about 200 dietary supplements sold over the counter.

Up until 2003, although products with ephedra made up less than 1% of dietary supplement sales, it accounted for 64% of the serious side effects that have been reported to the Centers for Disease Control and Prevention in association with dietary supplements. 155 deaths and 16,000 adverse effects were reported.

Ephedrine has been used in over-the-counter drugs for common colds and sinus infections. It is used as a decongestant in nasal drops and sprays in order to unblock stuffy noses and to help breathing. It decreases mucous secretion in the nasal passages, usually by vasoconstriction of the nasal mucosa. It is an effective bronchodilator due to its stimulation of beta-2 receptors in the lungs. In the treatment of asthma, however, drugs that are more selective beta-2 agonists than ephedrine are generally preferred.

Ephedrine exerts its effect indirectly on the sympathetic nervous system by displacing norepinephrine and certain other neurotransmitters from storage sites. The release of norepinephrine stimulates the release of adenosine and the synthesis of prostaglandins by the activated tissue. Adenosine and prostaglandins both inhibit the effect of norepinephrine. Caffeine opposes the effect of adenosine, thus increasing the release of norepinephrine. Aspirin inhibits the synthesis of prostaglandins, thus enhancing the effect of norepinephrine.

In clinical trials, ephedrine or ephedra promote modest short-term weight loss (approximately 0.9 kg/month more than placebo). There is no data regarding long-term weight loss. Ephedrine enhances thermogenesis. A synergy has been observed using a combination of ephedrine, caffeine and aspirin, i.e. the effect of all three together is greater than the sum of the activities of each separate compound. The 'ephedrine-caffeine-aspirin stack' is used as a weight loss agent. It may promote weight loss by increasing thermogenesis and resting energy expenditure via stimulation of beta-2 receptors in muscle. Use of ephedra or ephedrine and caffeine is associated with increased risk of psychiatric, autonomic or gastrointestinal symptoms, and heart palpitations.

Doses of 200 mg have been effective in increasing arousal, but doses above 400 mg may increase anxiety and essential tremor. Unlike epinephrine, ephedrine is active orally and it has ten times the duration of epinephrine. It is less likely to cause tachycardia, but causes greater central nervous system stimulation than epinephrine. Ephedrine decreases perception of fatigue, but it may increase the risk of developing a heat injury during exercise in warm weather. Other effects may include dizziness, headache, gastrointestinal distress, arrhythmia, heart palpitations, heart attack, stroke, seizures, psychosis and death.

Chronology

•1988 • At the Olympic Games, UK athlete Linford Christie was tested positive for pseudoephedrine, an isomer of ephedrine, which was present in a 'ginseng tea' he consumed. He was not disqualified, but rather gained silver medal after Ben Johnson was disqualified from the gold medal and Carl Lewis was awarded the gold medal. In 2003, Sports Illustrated obtained revelatory information concerning the United States Olympic Committee (USOC) from Wade Exum, who was director of the USOC anti-doping service in 1991-2000. As a result, Carl Lewis admitted, in an interview with the newspaper Orange County Register, *that before the 1988 Olympic Games he* had been caught using the following banned substances, all stimulants: pseudo-ephedrine, ephedrine and phenylpropanilamine, but received no ban from competition. Lewis claimed that the prohibited substances that he used "gave him no advantages at the competition." USOC decided that the athlete doped unintentionally: they said he had no notion that a cold medicine that he used contained some prohibited components.

•1998 • A 23-year-old UK bodybuilder, Joanne Amies-Winter, who was judged the world's second strongest woman, died from heart failure and fluid-filled lungs caused by a cocaine overdose. A post-mortem also found small quantities of the anti-depressant Prozac and larger quantities of the stimulant ephedrine and the narcotic analgesic Nubain. Her husband said that she was always worried about her appearance and took ephedrine as a dietary aid to stop her putting on body fat.

•2000 • 16-year old Romanian gymnast, Andrea Raducan, was stripped of her gold medal for the individual all-round title at the Olympics after testing positive for pseudoephedrine that was in a cold remedy she took.

•2003 • After a work out for the Baltimore Orioles at Spring training in February, in which ambient conditions were 81 degrees Fahrenheit and 74% humidity, 23 year-old pitcher Steve Bechler died in hospital of multiple organ failure from heat stroke. His core temperature rose to 108 degrees Fahrenheit. Toxicology reports did not confirm that Bechler had taken an ephedra supplement before practice. Bechler had the following risk factors for heat stroke: a priory history of heat illness episodes while in high school; a family history of sudden death following exercise (his half-brother died of an aneurysm at the age of 20 years after overheating from playing baseball); a history of hypertension and liver problems; he had not eaten solid food for a day or two, in an apparent attempt to lose weight; he was apparently not adequately acclimatized to training in the heat and humidity of South Florida; it appeared that he was wearing two or three layers of clothing during workouts, in an attempt to lose weight; he was overweight and did not have a sufficiently high level of fitness to make it through conditioning drills; and he was allowed to exercise until he collapsed with a core temperature reportedly of 106 degrees Fahrenheit before being removed from the field (Kreider, 2003). Some of Bechler's teammates claimed that he usually took three supplement capsules (1.5 servings) in the morning. According to that product' label, that would have provided 30 mg of herbal ephedra. This is one third of the dose shown in long-term clinical trials to be safe. There is no scientific or medical evidence to indicate that ephedra/caffeine supplementation significantly increases thermal stress (increases core temperature 2 to 3 degrees above normal) during exercise, that it promotes dehydration, or increases the incidence of heat illness. From the above evidence, Kreider et al. (2003) argued that Bechler's death was likely caused by poor supervision and screening of athletes rather than inappropriate use of a dietary supplement.

•2003 • In December, the Food and Drug Administration (FDA) in the USA told customers to stop using ephedra immediately.

•2004 • From April, ephedra was no longer available over-the-counter. It is the first time the US government has banned a dietary supplement.

Bibliography

Dullo, A.G. (1993). Ephedrine, xanthines and prostaglandin-inhibitors: Actions and interactions in the stimulation of thermogenesis. *International Journal of Obesity* 17(1), S35-S40.

Haller, C.A. and Benowitz, N.L. (2000). Adverse cardiovascular and central nervous system events associated with dietary supplements containing ephedra alkaloids. *New England Journal of Medicine* 343(25), 1833-1838.

Kreider, R.B. et al. (2003). What really killed Steve Bechler? Http://www.bodybuilding.com/fun/ephbay.htm

Magkos, F. and Kavouras, S.A. (2004). Caffeine and ephedrine: Physiological, metabolic and performance-enhancing effects. *Sports Medicine* 34(13), 871-889.

Shekelle, P.G. et al. (2003). Efficacy and safety of ephedra and ephedrine for weight loss and athletic performance: A meta-analysis. *Journal of the American Medical Association* 289(12), 1537-1545.

Wagner, J.C. (1991). Enhancement of athletic performance with drugs. An overview. *Sports Medicine* 12(4), 250-65.

EPICONDYLITIS   *See* LATERAL EPICONDY-LITIS; MEDIAL EPICONDYLITIS.

EPIDEMIOLOGY   The study of the distribution and determinants of health-related states or events in specified populations and the application of this study to the control of health problems, such as sports injuries. In descriptive epidemiology, the researcher attempts to quantify the occurrence of injury. **Prevalence** is the number of cases with a specific condition (such as injury or disease) in a specific population at a given time. **Incidence** is the number of new cases that occur in a population at risk over a specified period of time. **Relative risk** is the ratio of the occurrence rate of events (morbidity or mortality) of one population compared with the same rate in another population.

A **cohort** is a well-defined group of people who have had a common experience or exposure. **Prospective cohort design** consists of subjects assembled at baseline and measured on variables that are hypothesized to be related to an injury or disease (i.e. risk factors). The cohort is then followed prospectively for a period of time during which the occurrence of injury and (ideally) exposure is monitored and recorded. **Retrospective cohort design** is similar to prospective cohort design, but the cohorts have already been exposed to the risk of injury prior to the study, and injuries have already been incurred by some of them sometime in the past. Thus data are collected retrospectively.

A **primary risk factor** is one that exerts an independent effect on a disease (or injury). A **secondary risk factor** is one that increases risk when another primary risk factor is present. Until it has been subjected to rigorous empirical investigation and statistical tests, a risk factor cannot be regarded as a predictor variable. A cause and effect relationship does not have to be present in order for a particular factor to be labeled as a risk to health. However, some form of statistical relationship (such as correlation) between the risk factor and the presence of the disease (or injury) in a given population group should be evident. A correlational (rather than causal) relationship may be due to some, as yet undetermined, variable (confounder) that the risk factor and the disease (or injury) have in common. For example, shin guards will attenuate the force of impact to the tibia. Because wearing shin guards is positively related to injury incidence in soccer, level of play may be a confounder.

See CARDIOVASCULAR DISEASE; INJURY RISK FACTORS.

Bibliography

Bir, C.A. et al (1995). An analysis and comparison of soccer shin guards. *Clinical Journal of Sports Medicine* 5(2), 95-99.

Brown, S.P. (2001). *Introduction to exercise science*. Philadelphia: Lippincott Williams and Wilkins.

Caine, D. et al. (1994). *Epidemiology of sports injuries*. Champaign, IL: Human Kinetics.

Dishman, R.K., Heath, G.W. and Washburn, R. (2004). *Physical activity epidemiology*. Champaign, IL: Human Kinetics.

Inklaar, H. (1994). Soccer injuries II: Aetiology and prevention. *Sports Medicine* 18(2), 81-93.

EPIDERMIS   The outer layer of skin that provides a watertight protective covering for the body.

EPIDURAL HEMATOMA   *See under* HEAD INJURIES.

EPIGASTRALE   An anatomical landmark that is the point located on the anterior surface of the trunk at the intersection of the midsagittal plane and transverse plane through the most inferior point on the tenth ribs.

EPIGASTRIC   Relating to the upper middle area of the abdomen. The **epigastrium** is the part of the abdominal wall above the umbilicus (belly button).

EPIGASTRIC REFLEX   Contraction of the abdominal muscles caused by stimulating the skin of the epigastrum or over the fifth and sixth intercostals spaces near the axilla.

EPIGENIC PERIOD   *See under* CRITICAL PERIOD.

EPIGLOTTIS   A flap of cartilage that covers the superior opening of the larynx. While swallowing, the epiglottis bends down, helping to prevent food and drink flowing down the larynx and trachea. *See* GLOTTIS.

EPILEPSY   The terms epilepsy, **seizure disorders** and **convulsive disorders** are used interchangeably to denote a chronic condition of the central nervous system (CNS) that is characterized by recurrent seizures.

Common causes of **childhood-onset epilepsy** are birth and neonatal injuries (58%), followed by CNS infections (15%) and head trauma (12%). Common causes of **adult-onset epilepsy** are vascular lesions such as infarction hemorrhage (60%), metastatic tumors (10%), and CNS infections (9%).

A **seizure** is a sudden, involuntary alteration in perception or behavior caused by an abnormal synchronized discharge of cortical neurons in the CNS. Muscle activity in a seizure may be **clonic** (jerky or intermittent), **tonic** (continuous, stiff or rigid) or **tonic-clonic** (both tonic and clonic). Seizures are either **partial** (involving onset from a discrete area of the brain that may or may not generalize to the rest of the brain) or **primary generalized** (involving simultaneous onset from both hemispheres).

A **convulsion** is a type of seizure consisting of a series of involuntary contractions of the voluntary muscles. Such seizures are symptomatic of some neurologic disorder, but they are not in themselves a disease entity. Convulsions can be produced by: many chemical disorders; metabolic and hormonal imbalances; brain cell injury from head trauma, tumors, degenerative neural disease and stroke; anoxia and hemorrhage; acute cerebral edema; and infection and high fever (febrile convulsion). Epilepsy is one of the most common of all disorders associated with convulsions.

There are currently more than twenty documented types of seizures, and no two people who have the disorder are affected in precisely the same manner. 35 to 40% of epilepsy is a combination of absence and tonic-clonic seizures.

Absence seizures (previously called *petit mal*)

are characterized by symptoms so subtle that an inexperienced observer seldom notices the seizure. There is an impairment of consciousness, never more than 30 seconds, in which the person seems dazed. The eyes may roll upward and there may be rapid blinking and some chewing movements. If the person is talking at the time, there is a momentary silence and then continuation, with no loss of unity in thought. These seizures are rare before age of 3 years and often disappear after puberty. There is unawareness of what's going on during the seizure, but full awareness is restored once the seizure has stopped. It may result in learning difficulties if not recognized and treated.

Tonic-clonic seizures (previously called *grand mal*) are the most dramatic and easily recognized. They have 3 or 4 phases. About 50% of persons have aura. **Aura** is a warning or premonition of the attack that is always the same for a particular person. In the tonic phase, the person straightens out, becomes stiff, utters a cry and loses consciousness. If there is a tonic contraction of the respiratory muscles, the person becomes cyanotic. This phase rarely lasts more than 30 seconds. In the clonic phase, there is intermittent contraction and relaxation of the muscles. It lasts from a few seconds to several minutes. The tongue may be bitten as the jaws work up and down. The sphincters around the rectum and urinary tracts relax, causing the person to urinate or defecate. After a period of brief consciousness or semi-consciousness, during which the person complains of being very tired, he or she lapses into a sleep that may last several hours.

Complex partial (psychomotor; temporal lobe) epilepsy (**automatism**) usually starts with a blank stare, possibly chewing and then random activity. Persons appear unaware of their surroundings, may seem dazed, and may mumble. Undirected and clumsy actions such as picking at clothing may occur. There may even be an unprovoked 'flight or fight' response. Once a pattern is established, the same set of actions usually occurs with each seizure. The seizure lasts a few minutes, but post-seizure confusion can last substantially longer. There is no memory of what happened during the seizure period.

Simple partial (Jacksonian; partial sensory) seizures start with jerking in fingers or toes, which the person has awareness of, but cannot stop. Jerking may proceed to involve hands and arms. It sometimes spreads to the whole body and becomes a convulsive seizure.

Myoclonic seizures are brief, sudden, violent contractions of muscles in some part or the entire body. Often these are manifested by a sudden head jerk, followed by jerking of the arms and legs, and the trunk bending upon itself. The individual may lose consciousness, but the duration of a myoclonic seizure is much more brief than that of tonic-clonic, tonic-, or clonic-only types.

Atonic (akinetic) seizures are similar to absence seizures except that there is momentary diminution or abolition of postural tone. The individual tends to suddenly lose muscle tone and plummet to the ground, momentarily unconscious. A brief atonic seizure is known as a **drop attack**.

Infantile spasms involve quick, sudden movements that start between 3 months and 2 years of age. If a child is sitting up, the head will fall forward and the arms will flex forward. If lying down, the knees will be drawn up, with arms and head flexed forward as if the infant is reaching for support.

It has been estimated that about 10% of the population will have a seizure at some time during their lifetime. 20% of all persons with epilepsy have their first seizure before the age of 10 years. These are usually children with known or suspected neurological damage. 30% of persons with epilepsy have their first seizure in the second decade of life, 20% in the third decade, and 30% after the age of 40 years. Epilepsy affects 1.5 to 3.5 million Americans in any given year. 25 to 50% of the population with cerebral palsy has seizures. About one third of persons with mental retardation have seizures. About 20% to 35% of persons with autism have a seizure disorder.

Most individuals with epilepsy should be able to participate in sport. Risk factors include: excessive fatigue; sleep deprivation; hypoxia associated with high-altitude activities; hyponatremia associated with electrolyte loss; hypernatremia associated with dehydration; hyperthermia related to physical exhaustion and heat; and hypoglycemia associated with poor nutrition before activity. Contraindicated sports for all patients who have epilepsy include boxing and (unsupervised) scuba diving and mountain climbing. Patients with good seizure control can participate in both contact and noncontact sports without adversely affecting seizure frequency. Seizures during sports activity are rare, and exercise may have anti-epileptic effects (possibly because of increased attention and awareness). Seizures are more likely after than during exercise (15 minutes to 3 hours after exercise).

There are a number of factors, mostly relating to electrolyte balance in cellular fluids, which aggravate seizures. Laboratory-induced hyperventilation has been shown to provoke seizures. This does not imply however, that hyperventilation during exercise can do the same. This is because increased ventilation during exercise is a compensatory homeostatic mechanism and does not involve the respiratory alkalosis of induced hyperventilation.

Some anti-epileptic drugs may adversely affect sports performance, and exercise in turn may decrease serum drug levels by increasing circulating liver enzymes. *See also* HEAD INJURIES.

Bibliography

American Epilepsy Society. Http://www.aesnet.org

British Epilepsy Association. Http://www.epilepsy.org.uk

Dubow, J.S. and Kelly, J.P. (2003). Epilepsy in sports and recreation. *Sports Medicine* 33(7), 499-516.

Fountain, N.B. and May, A.C. (2003). Epilepsy and athletics. *Clinical Sports Medicine* 22(3), 605-616.

Gates, J.R. and Spiegel, R.H. (1993). Epilepsy, sports and exercise. *Sports Medicine* 15(1), 1-5.

Sirven, J.I. and Varrato, J. (1999). Physical activity and epilepsy. What are the rules? *The Physician and Sportsmedicine*, 27(3), 63-70.

EPIMER   *See under* CHEMICAL STRUCTURE.

EPINEPHRINE   Adrenaline. It is a catecholamine hormone secreted by the medulla of the adrenal gland. It produces effects similar to stimulation of the sympathetic nervous system. The release of epinephrine is stimulated by stress, hypotension and moderate-to-intense exercise. Target tissues are skeletal muscle and peripheral vascular smooth muscle.

Epinephrine has the following effects: i) blood pressure is increased; ii) blood flow is diverted to skeletal muscles, the brain and the heart, and away from the viscera; iii) metabolism is increased, resulting in an increase in blood glucose and free fatty acids, and an increase in muscle glycolysis; iv) muscle contraction is faster and stronger; v) the bronchioles expand to allow intake of more air; and vi) mental activity is sharper.

A motor neuron is **adrenergic** if it secretes epinephrine or norepinephrine when a nerve impulse reaches its ending. There are two types of adrenergic receptor: alpha and beta. Epinephrine combines with alpha and beta-receptors to about the same extent. Norepinephrine combines mainly with alpha-receptors, but is a less potent agonist than epinephrine and has little effect on beta-receptors. This accounts for the physiological differences between the actions of epinephrine and norepinephrine. *See* AUTONOMIC NERVOUS SYSTEM.

EPINEURIUM   *See under* PERIPHERAL NERVES.

EPIPHYSEAL GROWTH PLATE   Physis. A thin disc of cartilage found at the end of a long bone from where the bone grows in length. It separates the metaphysis from the epiphysis. The **metaphysis** is the growing part of a long bone between the diaphysis and the epiphysis. The **epiphysis** is the end portion of a long bone. It consists of a thin outer layer of compact bone enclosing spongy bone. The epiphysis ossifies separately from the **diaphysis** (shaft or central part of a long bone) to which it fuses when growth is complete.

Epiphyseal closure occurs at different ages. Bones of the upper limbs and scapulae become completely ossified at ages 17 to 20 years. Bones of the lower limbs become completely ossified at 18 to 23 years. Bones of the vertebrae, sternum and clavicle are the last to ossify at 23 to 25 years of age.

Epiphyseal injuries occur because children's muscles, tendons and ligaments are relatively stronger and more elastic compared to adults. Ligaments can be three times stronger than the soft cartilage of the growing end plate. This may cause tearing or separation from the end of the bone.

The following locations account for about 90% of epiphyseal injuries: distal radius (wrist), phalanges (finger), distal tibia (ankle), distal humerus (elbow), phalanges (toe), proximal humerus (shoulder), distal fibula (ankle), distal ulna (wrist), distal femur (knee) and metacarpal (hand). The distal radius is the most commonly injured, and this may result from a fall on the hand of an outstretched arm. An **epiphyseal fracture of the distal femoral epiphysis** is usually created by a shear force, commonly a valgus force applied to the thigh with the foot fixed and the knee hyperextended.

See also APOPHYSIS; AVULSION FRACTURE; OSTEOCHONDROSES; SLATER-HARRIS FRACTURES; SLIPPED CAPITAL FEMORAL EPIPHYSIS.

EPIPHYSIS   i) *See under* EPIPHYSEAL GROWTH PLATE. ii) A small endocrine gland in the brain.

EPISTAXIS   Nosebleed. A distinction can be made between lower and upper epistaxis. Most nosebleeds are lower, which means that they start in the lower part of the septum.

The **septum** is the semi-rigid wall that separates the two channels of the nose. It contains blood vessels that can be broken by a blow to the nose or the edge of a sharp fingernail. With lower-septum nosebleeds, bleeding can occur from one side of the nose or both. Upper nosebleeds are more rare. They start when bleeding begins high and deep within the nose. Blood flows down the back of the mouth and throat even when the patient is sitting up or standing. The most common cause of nosebleeds is a direct blow to the nose. The other main cause is dryness of the inside of the nose. They are more common during cold weather, when heating dries out nasal passages. Other causes of nosebleeds include colds, high altitude, allergies and medications. Occasionally, nosebleeds may indicate other disorders such as bleeding disorders, cancer, high blood pressure or disease of the arteries. They can also indicate **hereditary hemorrhagic telangiectasia (Osler-Weber-Rendu syndrome)**, which is a genetic disorder involving a vascular growth similar to a birthmark in the back of the nose. It affects 1 in 5,000 people, and is inherited as an autosomal dominant gene. It is caused by an abnormal gene on either chromosome 9 or 12. A person with hereditary hemorrhagic telangiectasia has a tendency to form blood vessels that lack the capillaries between an artery and vein. This means that arterial blood under high pressure flows directly into a vein without first having to squeeze through the small capillaries. The place where an artery is connected directly to a vein tends to be a fragile site that can rupture and result in bleeding. It is called a telangiectasis if it involves small blood vessels; and arteriovenous malformation if it involves larger blood vessels.

Lower-septum nosebleeds should be treated by the patient sitting up straight and pinching the nostrils together firmly for 10 minutes. An ice pack can also be applied to the nose and cheeks. If the nosebleed was caused by atmospheric dryness, the patient should breathe steamy air. After bleeding stops, petroleum jelly can be applied just inside the nose to prevent further bleeding.

Bibliography

Hereditary Hemorrhagic Telangiectasia Foundation International. Http://www.hht.org

EPITESTOSTERONE   *See* CHEMICAL STRUCTURE; TESTOSTERONE.

EPITHELIAL TISSUE   A category of tissues that is found in the skin, the alimentary canal and secretions of internal organs. A **simple epithelium** has only one layer; **stratified epithelium** has more than one layer. There are three basic shapes of epithelial tissue: squamous (flat), cuboidal and columnar. Epithelial tissues are named by the number of layers and the type of cell in its outermost layer. For example, the heart and blood vessels are lined by endothelium, which is a simple squamous epithelium. Epithelial tissue has different functions, depending on its location.

EPITHELIAL TISSUE MEMBRANES   The three primary types are mucous, serous and cutaneous membranes. **Mucous membranes** (**mucosa**) line body cavities that open directly to the outside of the body. These include the digestive, respiratory, urinary and reproductive tracts. Mucosa consists of various kinds of epithelial tissue over a layer of areolar connective tissue, and are moistened by mucus secreted by **goblet cells**. **Serous membranes** (**serosa**) line closed body cavities and cover the outside surface of organs in these cavities. Serosa consist of simple squamous epithelium over a thin layer of areolar connective tissue, and are kept moistened by serous fluid. The **cutaneous membrane** is the skin. It consists of the epidermis, which is stratified squamous epithelium; firmly attached to the **dermis**, which is mostly dense irregular connective tissue.

EPO   *See under* ERYTHROPOIETIN.

EPSTEIN-BARR VIRUS   *See under* CHRONIC FATIGUE SYNDROME; UPPER RESPIRATORY TRACT INFECTION.

EQUILIBRIUM   The state of a system, with respect to a given observable quantity, during the time for which there is no change in that quantity.
See also CHEMICAL REACTIONS; ENZYME; FORCE.

EQUILIBRIUM REFLEXES   Tilting reflexes. These are postural reflexes that appear between the ages of 5 and 18 months and remain the entire life in order to prevent falls. They are initiated primarily by vestibular input and can be elicited in any position the body assumes.

EQUINUS   A deformity in which the foot which has less than 10 degrees of ankle dorsal flexion when the subtalar joint is in a neutral position. The foot is then not able to function normally in propulsion. Compensation occurs with subtalar joint pronation,

which subsequently unlocks the midtarsal joint.
Clinical observations and symptoms of equinus include: severe hallux subluxation; bouncing gait; plantar callus 2,3,4; dorsal corns on toes; hammer toes; leg fatigue; talonavicular pain and severe postural symptoms.

Bibliography
Clinicians Corner. Http://www.footmaxx.com/clinicians

ERB'S PALSY   Erb-Duchenne paralysis. It is paralysis of the arm resulting from injury to the brachial plexus (usually during childbirth).

ERB'S POINT   The point on the side of the neck that lies 2 to 3 cm above the clavicle at the level of the transverse process of the 6th vertebra (C6). Pressure over this point elicits the Erb-Duchenne paralysis, and electrical stimulation over this area causes various arm muscles to contract. *See under* BRACHIAL PLEXUS INJURY.

ERGOGENIC AID   A substance or technique other than usual training that improves performance (or is believed by the user to improve performance). Ergogenic means 'work producing.' An **ergolytic** substance is one that has a detrimental effect on performance. Five classes of ergogenic aids can be distinguished: nutritional ergogenic aids (e.g. vitamins), physiological aids (e.g. blood doping), pharmacological aids (drugs), psychological aids (e.g. hypnosis) and mechanical or biomechanical aids (e.g. special clothing to decrease aerodynamic drag).

Bibliography
Williams, M.H. (1998). *The ergogenics edge*. Champaign, IL: Human Kinetics.

ERGOLYTIC   *See under* ERGOGENIC AID.

ERGOMETER   A device that measures work done. Examples are bicycle ergometer and treadmill.

ERYTHEMA   Redness of the skin due to capillary dilation.

ERYTHROCYTE *See* RED BLOOD CELL.

ERYTHROCYTHEMIA *See under* RED BLOOD CELL.

ERYTHROPOIESIS *See under* RED BLOOD CELL.

ERYTHROPOIETIN A hormone that is secreted mainly by the kidney and is the major stimulus for the production of erythrocytes in the bone marrow. **Human recombinant erythropoietin** is a drug that has the potential to produce erythrocythemia at least as great as blood doping. **Epoetin (EPO)** is the approved generic name for the drug, when referring to the recombinantly produced pharmaceutical product.

It has been shown to produce increases in hemoglobin and hematocrit with a resultant increase in maximal oxygen uptake and performance. EPO is on the World Anti-Doping Association (WADA) list of banned substances. The use of EPO has the potential to increase viscosity of the blood and cause thrombosis with potentially fatal results. Hypertension, congestive heart failure and stroke can be caused by erythrocythemia resulting from use of the drug.

Chronology

•1964 • At the Winter Olympics, Eero Mäntyranta of Finland won two gold medals in cross-country skiing. It was later found that he had a genetic mutation that increased the number of red blood cells in his body by 25 to 50%, and thus increased his aerobic capacity. His genes lacked a switch to turn off the production of erythropoietin.

•1989 • Biotech company, Amgen, began marketing Epogen, an injectable form of EPO produced by recombinant bacteria, as a treatment for severe anemia, a serious problem in patients with AIDS or kidney failure.

•1990 • The International Olympic Committee (IOC) banned the use of EPO, which had superseded blood doping as a way of increasing the number of red blood cells in the human body and thus as an ergogenic aid in endurance events. The deaths of 18 cyclists in the late 1980s and early 1990s in the Netherlands and Belgium was blamed on EPO. Subsequently, the role of EPO in these deaths has been disputed by some authors.

•1997 • Union Cycliste Internationale (UCI) introduced a 50% hematocrit measure and use of EPO became widespread. According to a report to the Italian Olympic Commission in 1998 that was never published, EPO was being used by a high percentage of professional cyclists.

•1998 • The 53-year-old Willy Voet, a soigneur (masseur-cum-trainer) with the Festina cycling team, was arrested while traveling to the Tour de France when police found that his car contained 400 different doping products including 250 vials of EPO. He later told *The Sunday Telegraph* (23 May 1999), "In cycling, doping is part of the job, it's so much the culture that you hardly realize it." Earlier in the year, another Festina soigneur was sacked after a French rider, Christophe Moreau, winner of five races in that year, tested positive for an anabolic steroid and accused one of the soigneurs of giving him the banned substance without his knowledge. Moreau and six other members of the team later admitted to using certain substances, including EPO. After the seventeenth stage of the Tour, five of the world's leading cycling teams pulled out of the race in protest at police raids on team hotels leaving only 14 of the 21 starting teams and 105 out of 189 riders remaining. Two rider demonstrations disrupted the Tour in protest at media coverage of drug matters and the harsh police treatment of the Festina team and a Dutch team. The UCI, cycling's world governing body, tested 143 riders at the Tour and all were below the allowed maximum of 50% hematocrit. The mean level analyzed was 45%. A normal person, living at sea level would have a reading of about 39%.

•1999 • While leading the Tour of Italy on the second last day, Marco Pantani, a 29-year-old Italian cyclist, was disqualified after failing a blood test that showed a hematocrit level of 52% against the permitted limit of 50%.

•2000 • A fully validated blood testing system for EPO was part of doping control at the Olympics. There were rumors that some athletes were using oxyglobin, a hemoglobin solution and drug, designed to treat health problems in animals such as cows, which has a similar effect as erythropoietin on red blood cell count.

Bibliography

Gaudard, A. et al. (2003). Drugs for increasing oxygen and their potential use in doping: A review. *Sports Medicine* 33(3), 187-212.

Mottram, D.R. (1999). Banned drugs in sport. Does the International Olympic Committee (IOC) list need updating? *Sports Medicine* 27(1), 1-10.

World Anti-Doping Agency. Http://www.wada-ama.org

ESOPHAGEAL SPHINCTER   It is the opening between the esophagus and the stomach that relaxes and opens to allow the bolus to travel into the stomach, and then closes behind it. It also acts as a barrier to prevent the reflux of gastric contents

ESOPHAGUS   The tube-like passage between the pharynx and the stomach. It carries materials such as food from the throat to the stomach.

Heart burn (pyrosis) is a burning sensation under the sternum (breastbone) or in the pit of the stomach. It is most commonly caused by an irritable digestive tract ('**acid indigestion**'). When the junction between the esophagus and stomach (**lower esophageal sphincter**) is relaxed, the acid gastric juice flows back into the esophagus and causes irritation of its surface (**esophagitis**). The term 'heartburn' refers to the fact that the esophagus lies just behind the heart and the acid produces a burning sensation. Heart burn may be a symptom of **gastroesophageal reflux disease**, which is tissue damage to the esophagus due to the reflux of gastric contents. Unlike the inner lining of the stomach, which produces large amounts of mucus that protect against corrosion from this acid, the lining of the esophagus does not have protection against the acid effects. About 10% of adults experience gastrointestinal reflux disease on a weekly or daily basis, and nearly a third of the US population is affected to some degree on a monthly basis. It is a risk factor for esophageal cancer.

ESTER   The product of a reaction of an organic acid with an alcohol; when hydrogen from the alcohol combines with the acid's hydrogen and oxygen, water is released and an ester linkage is formed. **Esterification** produces triglycerides, ditrigylcerides and monoglycerides (glycerol attached to one, two and three fatty acids, respectively).

ESTIMATED AVERAGE REQUIREMENT   *See under* DIETARY REFERENCE INTAKE.

ESTROGENS   Steroid hormones secreted by the ovaries. Gonadotropic hormones control the secretion of estrogens. The estrogen hormones of the ovary are estradiol and estrogen, and they are interconvertible. The most biologically active estrogen released by the ovary is estradiol-17b. Synthesis of estradiol-17b occurs mainly in the ovaries. Small amounts are also synthesized in the adrenal cortex, and this source accounts for the estrogen produced in men. Estradiol-17b increases the mobilization of free fatty acids from adipose tissue and inhibits glucose uptake by the peripheral tissues. Consequently, estradiol-17b has similar metabolic effects as growth hormone during exercise. Estrogens control the menstrual cycle, promote female sex characteristics, and increase the deposition of fat. Estrogens may also protect against peroxidative damage of membrane lipids and low-density lipoproteins.

Many women retain fluid as their estrogen levels rise during the menstrual cycle. This is because estrogens, being chemically similar to aldosterone, enhance sodium chloride reabsorption by the renal tubules. The edema experienced by many pregnant women is also largely due to the effect of estrogens. Menopause is associated with increased total serum cholesterol, triglycerides and fibrinogen, and a decrease in HDL cholesterol levels. These changes are thought to result from fluctuations in hormonal status, primarily a deficiency in estrogen. The addition of progestogen to estrogen may negate some of the beneficial changes of estrogen, most notably the increase in HDL cholesterol levels. However, progestogen has also been reported to offset the increase in triglycerides seen with unopposed estrogen replacement. Thus there are contradictory effects (both positive and negative) of hormone replacement therapy on risk factors of cardiovascular disease in women. Part of the increased incidence of cardiovascular disease in post-menopausal women may be attributable to increased central body fatness. The majority of interventional studies provide evidence that hormone replacement therapy attenuates the accumulation of central fat in postmenopausal women, compared with control or placebo-treated women.

For the World Anti-Doping Agency Prohibited List (2005), the category for agents with anti-estrogenic activity was divided into three subsections: aromatase inhibitors; selective estrogen receptor modulators; and other anti-estrogenic compounds. Substances that were previously prohibited "in men only" are now prohibited for all athletes. See also HYPOESTROGENISM.

Bibliography

Haddock, B.L., Marshak, H.P., Mason, J.J. and Blix, G. (2000). The effect of hormone replacement therapy and exercise on cardiovascular disease risk factors in postmenopausal women. *Sports Medicine* 29(1), 39-49.

Poehlman, E.T. and Tchernof, A. (1998). Traversing the menopause: Changes in energy expenditure and body composition. *Coronary Artery Disease* 9(12), 799-803.

Tchernof, A., Calles-Escandon, J., Sites, C.K. and Poehlman, E.T. (1998). Menopause, central body fatness, and insulin resistance: Effects of hormone-replacement therapy. *Coronary Artery Disease* 9(8), 503-511.

World Anti-Doping Agency. Http://www.wada-ama.org

ETHANOL   See ALCOHOL.

EUGLYCEMIA   The normal range for blood glucose (3.5 to 6 mmol/l).

EUHYDRATION   A normal state of body water content. See also DEHYDRATION.

EUKARYOTE   A cell characterized by membrane-bound organelles, including the nucleus in which cell division takes place by mitosis or meiosis. Animal and plant cells are both eukaryotes. In eukaryotes, a chromosome is a DNA molecule that contains genes in a linear order to which numerous proteins are bound and that has a telomere at each end and a centromere. In prokaryotes, a chromosome is a DNA molecule containing fewer proteins than chromosomes in eukaryotes, lacks telomeres and a centromere, and is often circular.

EUPNEA   See under RESPIRATION.

EVAPORATION   See under THERMO-REGULATION.

EVOLUTION   Cumulative changes in the genetic composition of a species through time, resulting in greater adaptation. **Microevolution** is the shifting of gene frequencies in a local population. **Macroevolution** refers to major transformations of organisms over geological time. **Genetic variation** refers to the genetic difference between members of a population. In the context of evolution, **fitness** is a measure of the average ability of organisms with a given genotype to survive and reproduce. A **species** is a group of organisms that generally bear a close resemblance in the more essential features of their organization. A **genus**, such as Homo, is a group of species sharing similarity in broad features, but distinguished by differences in detail. Humans are the only remaining species of hominids.

Bipedalism (the ability to walk upright on two legs) evolved in the *Australopithecus* genus at least 4.5 mya, while they also retained the ability to travel through trees. The *Homo* genus did not evolve for another 3 million or more years. Walking cannot explain most of the changes in body form that distinguish *Homo* from *Australopithecus*, according to Bramble and Lieberman (2004), and this implies that the ability to walk cannot explain the anatomy of the modern human body. Natural selection favored the survival of australopithecines that could run and, over time, favored the perpetuation of human anatomical features that made long-distance running possible. One theory to explain why natural selection favored human ancestors who could run long distances is that they could pursue predators long before the development of weapons, such as spears, decreased the need to run long distances. Another theory is that early humans ran to scavenge the carcasses of dead animals, maybe to beat hyenas or other scavengers.

Fossil evidence suggests that some of the anatomical features helping humans to run are: a tall body, with a narrow trunk, waist and pelvis, creating a greater skin surface area for dissipating heat during running; a more balanced head, including a flatter face, shifting the center of mass posteriorly so as to minimize bobbing up and down during running; a ligament that runs from the back of the skull and neck down to the thoracic vertebrae, helping the arms and shoulders counterbalance the head during running; larger vertebrae and intervertebral disks, providing greater shock absorption; larger gluteal muscles, for stabilization during running; decoupling of the shoulders from the head and neck, allowing the body to rotate while the head is kept in a neutral position during running; shorter forearms, making it easier for the upper body to counterbalance the lower body during running; long legs, to increase stride length; ligaments and tendons in the legs, such as the Achilles tendon, which act like springs that store and release mechanical energy during running; arch support in the feet, which make the foot more rigid and allow more efficient push off from the ground; and an enlarged heel bone for better shock absorption. *See also* HEREDITY.

Chronology

•33 - 22 mya • Hominoids (great apes) first appeared in the fossil record. Bipedal locomotion marked the origin of the hominoids.

•6.5 mya • The first hominids (apes closely related to human beings) appeared in the evolutionary record. *Sahelanthropus tchadensis*, for example, is a genus and species with a small, ape-like skull, but with some features associated with hominids. It is not known whether it was bipedal.

•5.8 – 4.0 mya • *Ardipithecus ramidus* appeared, as a species with more chimpanzee-like features than any other human ancestor.

•4.2 – 3.9 mya • *Australopithecus anamensis* appeared, with some chimpanzee-like characteristics, but with a humerus (upper-arm bone) that was quite human-like and a tibia (lower-leg bone) indicating the likelihood that this hominid species was bipedal.

•4.0 – 3.0 mya • *Australopithecus afarensis* was bipedal with human-like leg and pelvic bones, and ranged in height from three and a half feet to five feet. In 1999, a new species and genus of hominid, *Kenyanthropus platyops* was discovered in Eastern Africa. It may have co-existed with *Australopithecus afarensis* without direct competition for food resources. This discovery suggests that at least two lineages of early human relatives existed as far back as 3.5 mya and that the early stages of human evolution are more complex than previously thought.

•3.0 – 2.4 mya • *Australopithecus africanus* was similar in many ways to *Australopithecus afarensis*, but had a slightly larger brain, smaller canine teeth, and larger molars. Fossil evidence of the wear of the teeth suggests that this hominid species ate fruit and foliage.

•2.5 –1.6 mya • *Homo habilis* made and used primitive stone tools.

Hence this period is known as the Paleolithic (Old Stone) Age. About five feet tall and weighing 100 pounds, *Homo habilis* had a brain that was larger than any *Australopithecus* brain but smaller than the Homo erectus brain.

•2.2 – 1.0 mya • *Australopithecus robustus* was approximately the same size as *Australopithecus aranfensis*, but had a large, more robust (heavier, thicker) skull, as well as a jaw and large teeth that were well adapted to chewing.

•2.1 – 1.0 mya • *Australopithecus boisei* was similar to *Australopithecus robustus* except that its skull and teeth were even larger. Some experts consider these two hominid species were closely related, both branching from another species called *Australopithecus aethiopicus*. Others believe that *Australopithecus robustus* evolved from *Australopithecus africanus*. Like all of the other *Australopithecus* species, *Australopithecus boisei* walked upright. There is recent scientific evidence that some australopithecines were capable of a precision grip and thus capable of making stone tools.

•1.8 – 0.4 mya • *Homo erectus* had a skull with a primitive appearance, but the skeleton was very similar to that of modern humans, although more robust (heavier and thicker). *Homo erectus* was probably the first hominid species to use fire.

•400 – 200 kya • *Homo heidelbergensis*, also known as archaic *Homo sapiens*, had a brain that was larger than that of *Homo erectus* and smaller than that of a modern human. Cave shelters were first used 0.5 mya. Fossil remains of archaic *Homo sapiens* have been found in Africa and Europe.

•230 – 30 kya • *Homo neanderthalensis*, the immediate predecessor of *Homo sapiens* in Europe, Near East and Northern Africa had a body and brain that was larger than the modern human. They lived in small bands, controlled fire, erected shelters, and hunted cooperatively. Averaging five and a half feet in height and possessing short limbs, Neanderthals were well adapted to living in a cold climate; their short, heavy bodies conserved heat. Attached to their robust bones were powerful muscles. Around 0.8 mya, the Neanderthals invented new types of stone tools, such as blades and flints. During most of the glacial period, the Neanderthals were the only human inhabitants of Europe. In 1997, researchers extracted a portion of Neanderthal mitochondrial DNA. The fact that it was significantly different from modern human DNA lends support to the claim that Neanderhals were a different species.

•120 kya - • *Homo sapiens* (modern), also known as *Homo sapiens sapiens*, made elaborate tools out of bone, antler, ivory, stone and wood; and produced fine artwork in the form of carvings and cave paintings. There are two theories as to how *Homo sapiens* (modern) evolved from the local African populations of *Homo erectus*: Replacement theory and Multiregional Continuity theory. According to the Replacement ('Out of Africa') theory, *Homo neanderthalis* was a separate species; i.e. there was no gene flow or interbreeding. The Multiregional Continuity theory maintains that ancient regional populations maintained species continuity with *Homo sapiens* (modern) through gene flow; i.e. *Homo neanderthalis* was related to *Homo sapiens* (modern). Scientific data suggests that the Replacement theory better reflects the pattern of recent human evolution. It seems that the replacement of Neanderthals by moderns occurred with no clear evidence of an evolutionary step, i.e. the Neanderthal structure and culture became extinct. In 2003, three skulls found in Ethiopia, dated at 160 kya, were the oldest known modern human fossils yet found. The discoverers assigned them to a new species subspecies, *Homo sapiens idaltu*, on the basis that they are anatomically and chronologically intermediate between older archaic humans and more recent fully modern humans.

•9,000 BC • Neolithic (New Stone Age) farming communities were created in Near East (largest), Western Africa, northeastern China, Central and South America. Between 8,000 and 5,000 BC, some hunter-gathering groups developed more intensive techniques, which enabled them to establish more sedentary settlements. In what is now central Russia, for example, wooly mammoths were hunted and meat supplies were supplemented with intensive gathering.

•4,000 BC • The ox-drawn plow was invented in the Middle East.

Bibliography

Bramble, D.M. and Lieberman, D.E. (2004). Endurance running and the evolution of Homo. *Nature* 432 (7015), 345-352.

Stanford, C. (2003). *Upright: The evolutionary key to becoming human*. New York: Houghton Mifflin Company.

EXCESS POST-EXERCISE OXYGEN CONSUMPTION   *See under* OXYGEN DEBT.

EXCRETION   The removal of the waste products of metabolism.

EXERCISE   i) Generation of force by skeletal muscle. ii) Movement(s) performed to achieve a particular goal with respect to skill development or fitness training. iii) A subclass of physical activity, defined as planned, structured and repetitive bodily movement done to improve or maintain one or more components of physical fitness. *See also* KINESIOLOGY.

EXERCISE ADDICTION   *See* EXERCISE DEPENDENCE.

EXERCISE ADHERENCE   Persistence in exercise. People undertake exercise for a number of reasons. The Exercise Motivations Inventory – 2 (EMI-2) has the following scales: stress management, revitalization, enjoyment, challenge, social recognition, affiliation, competition, health pressures, ill-health avoidance, positive health, weight management, appearance, strength and endurance, and nimbleness.

Short-term drop out from exercise programs ranges from 35% to 80%. Long-term adherence to exercise is less than 10%. People drop out of aerobic exercise programs despite it being well known that participation must be maintained beyond the short term for health benefits to be obtained from exercise participation. Obesity, lack of motivation, blue-collar status and smoking are the most commonly identified personal characteristics directly related to decreased adherence to, and increased dropout from, exercise programs. Level of social support obtained by program participants, especially from family members, has been shown to be the environmental factor most highly correlated with exercise adherence. Also positively correlated are perceived convenience of the exercise setting and its proximity to the home or workplace. Lack of time is the most commonly reported reason for dropout from exercise programs, although the relationship of this factor to adherence remains unclear, as both adherents and non-adherents view time as a major barrier to participation. Increased participation and adherence often occur when moderate exercise is involved. Walking has a higher adherence than other aerobic activities. Women are more likely than men to participate in fitness activities such as walking, swimming or aerobic dance. Women often exercise with the goal of weight loss. In recent years, women have increased their activity levels to a greater extent than men. There is evidence that intervention strategies, such as goal setting, can improve exercise adherence.

A number of theories have been proposed to explain motivation for health-related exercise. Self-Efficacy theory has received support; the perceived ability to participate and to exercise regularly in a structured program seems to be the variable of prime importance. Theories transplanted from health psychology, such as the Health Belief model have received less support. The **Health Belief model** proposes that four types of beliefs influence health behaviors. Applied to physical activity, these health beliefs are as follows: i) the individual's perceived susceptibility to developing health problems because of inactivity; ii) the perceived impact of health problems on the individual's quality of life; iii) the individual's belief that adopting an active lifestyle will be of personal benefit; and iv) the extent to which the benefits of exercising exceed the costs of exercising for the individual. Research with the Health Belief model has found that people who perceive their health as poor, or who believe that exercise has limited health value, exercise less frequently.

The **Protection Motivation model** proposes that four cognitions are predictive of behavior: i) the perceived severity of the negative event; ii) the individual's perceived vulnerability to the negative event; iii) the perceived benefit of the alternative behavior; and iv) the individual's belief in his or her ability to engage in the behavior (self-efficacy). Regarding the first cognition, it has been found that the main function of perceived severity is to motivate people to think about starting an exercise program.

The **Theory of Reasoned Action** states that an individual's intention to perform a target behavior will predict whether that behavior is actually performed, and is a function of the perceived costs and benefit of the behavior, and social factors. If the individual believes physical activity has benefits such as improved mood, if they perceive minimal barriers (costs) to being active, and if they have a support system that encourages physical activity, they will intend to be active, which will cause them to be active.

The **Transtheoretical Model** postulates the following series of stages that an individual progresses through: pre-contemplation, contemplation, preparation, action and maintenance. Marcus et al. (1992) hypothesize that matching intervention strategies to the individual's stage should improve exercise adherence. In the preparation stages, for example, the use of cognitive processes should dominate, because planning is required.

Many exercisers experience relapse (stopping exercise for at least three months). Principles of relapse prevention include identifying high-risk situations (e.g. change in work hours) and problem-solving for those high-risk situations (e.g. change in location of exercise).

See also COGNITIVE DISSONANCE; SELF-EFFICACY; PEDOMETERS.

Bibliography

Bess, H.M. et al. (1996). Theories and techniques for promoting physical activity behaviours. *Sports Medicine* 22(5), 321-331.

Biddle, S. and Mutrie, N. (2001). *Psychology of physical activity: Determinants, well-being and interventions*. London: Routledge.

Biddle, S.J.H. and Nigg, C.R. (2000). Theories of exercise behavior. *International Journal of Sport Psychology* 31(2), 290-304.

Dishman, R.K. (1988, ed). *Exercise adherence*. Champaign, IL: Human Kinetics.

Dishman, R.K. (1994, ed). *Advances in exercise adherence*. Champaign, IL: Human Kinetics.

Leith, L.M. and Taylor, A.H. (1992). Behavior modification and exercise adherence: A literature review. *Journal of Sport Behavior* 15(1), 60-74.

Marcus, B.H. et al. (1992). Self-efficacy and the stages of exercise behavior change. *Research Quarterly for Exercise & Sport* 63, 60-66.

Marcus, B.H. et al. (1996). Exercise initiation, adoption, and maintenance. In: Raalte, J.L. and Brewer, B.W. (eds). *Exploring sport and exercise psychology*. pp133-158. Washington, DC: American Psychological Association.

Marcus, B.H. and Forsyth, L.H. (2003). *Motivating people to be physically active*. Champaign, IL: Human Kinetics.

Markland, D. and Ingledew, D.K (1997). The measurement of exercise motives: Factorial validity and invariance across gender of a revised Exercise Motivations Inventory. *British Journal of Health Psychology* 2, 361-376.

Roberts, G.C. (1992, ed). *Motivation in sport and exercise*. Champaign, IL: Human Kinetics.

Robison, J.I. and Rogers, M.A. (1994). Adherence to exercise programs. Recommendations. *Sports Medicine* 17(1), 39-52.

Willis, J.D. and Campbell, L.F. (1992). *Exercise psychology*. Champaign, IL: Human Kinetics.

EXERCISE-ASSOCIATED COLLAPSE *See under* HYPONATREMIA.

EXERCISE DEPENDENCE 'Exercise addiction.' It is a psychological and/or physiological dependence on a regular regimen of exercise that is characterized by withdrawal symptoms after 24 to 36 hours of abstinence. The Exercise Dependence Scale is based on the diagnostic criteria of the American Psychiatric Association for substance dependence: tolerance (either a need for increased amount of exercise to achieve the desired effect or diminished effect with continued use of the same amount of exercise); withdrawal (manifested by either the characteristic withdrawal symptoms for exercise such as anxiety or the same amount of exercise is taken to relieve or avoid withdrawal symptoms); intention effect (exercise is often taken in larger amounts or over a longer period than was intended); lack of control (there is a persistent desire or unsuccessful effort to cut down or control exercise); time (a great deal of time is spent in activities necessary to obtain exercise); reductions in other activities (social, occupational or recreational activities are given up or decreased because of exercise); and continuance (exercise is continued despite knowledge of having a persistent or recurrent physical or psychological problem that is likely to have been caused or exacerbated by the exercise).

Symptoms of exercise dependence include: heart palpitations, irregular heartbeat, chest pain, problem with appetite and digestion, sleep disorders, increased sweating, depression and (in some cases) emotional instability.

Persons with exercise dependence structure their lives around exercise to an extent that work and domestic responsibilities may be compromised. A genuine exercise addict would continue to exercise in the face of medical, vocational and social contraindications. There is evidence that some individuals may become dependent on exercise because of its effect on mood. Endorphins and other opioid peptides may be a factor in exercise dependence. A distinction can be made between a primary form of exercise dependence and a form that is secondary to an eating disorder. Davis (2000) argues that habitual, even excessive, exercise should not be termed an abuse or an addiction unless it satisfies the clinical criteria established for other addictions.

Yates et al. (1983) proposed that women who become anorexic and men who develop into compulsive exercisers have similar underlying psychological traits, such as introversion, depression and inhibition of anger. Gender differences in the expression of the two conditions can be attributed to the fact that culture values beauty for women and athleticism for men. Subsequent empirical research has failed to support the relationship between anorexia nervosa and compulsive exercise.

A distinction can be made between a committed and compulsive exercisers (Cockerill and Riddington, 1996): **compulsive exercisers** perceive exercise as work and no longer enjoy the pleasure that it once provided, but **committed exercisers** feel invigorated and strengthened by exercise. See also DRUG; SELF CONCEPT.

Chronology

•1976 • William Glaser's book *Positive Addiction* popularized the concept of beneficial addiction to exercise (especially running).

Bibliography

American Psychiatric Association. (1994). *Diagnostic and statistical manual of mental disorders*. 4th ed. Washington, DC: American Psychiatric Association.

Cockerill, I.M. and Riddington, M.E. (1996). Theory and practice: Exercise dependence and associated disorders: A review. *Counselling Psychology Quarterly* 9(2), 119-129.

Davis, C. (2000). Exercise abuse. *International Journal of Sport Psychology* 31(2), 278-289.

Eisler, I. and la Grange, D. (1990). Excessive exercise and anorexia nervosa. *International Journal of Eating Disorders* 9(4), 377-386.

Hausenblas, H.A. and Symons Downs, D.A. (2000). Exercise dependence: A systematic review. *Psychology of Sport and*

Exercise 3, 89-123.

Morgan, W.P. (1979). Negative addiction in runners. *The Physician and Sportsmedicine* 7(2), 57-70.

Yates, A., Leehey, K. and Shisslak, C.M. (1983). Running - An analog of anorexia? *New England Journal of Medicine* 308, 251-255.

EXERCISE-INDUCED ARTERIAL HYPO-XEMIA *See under* HYPOXEMIA.

EXERCISE-INDUCED BRONCHOCONSTRICTION This involves post-exercise constriction of the large and small airways. It is seen in nearly 90% of chronic asthmatics, 35 to 40% of allergic non-asthmatics and 3 to 4% in non-allergic people. The attack usually lasts 5 to 15 minutes and is followed by spontaneous resolution (some 20 to 60 minutes later). Symptoms include shortness of breath, chest tightening, wheezing and coughing. Some people undergo a second, 'late phase' response 4 to 6 hours after exercise. Usually this is of lesser intensity and is associated with airway inflammation.

Asthmatic patients do not exhibit exercise-induced bronchoconstriction until after exercise. In fact, there is bronchodilation while the individual is exercising. Bronchodilation during exercise is likely to be due to sympathetic stimulation with release of catecholamines, such as epinephrine.

One theory to explain exercise-induced bronchoconstriction is that inhalation of large volumes of dry, cold air during exercise leads to loss of heat and water from the bronchial mucosa, and airway cooling and drying. This increases the osmolality of the cells lining the airway, stimulating the release of mediators such as histamine from mast cells that then cause bronchocontriction. Evidence to support this theory is the effectiveness of mast cell stabilizers (sodium cromoglycate; nedocromil) and antileukotriene agents in preventing exercise-induced bronchoconstriction. Another theory to explain exercise-induced bronchoconstriction is that rapid rewarming triggers reactive hyperemia, with sudden blood flow and vascular permeability leading to edema and airway obstruction. The greater the difference in airway temperature during and after exercise, the greater is the severity of obstruction. Evidence to support this theory is the observation that, after exercise, inhaling warm air worsens the bronchoconstriction while inhaling cold air lessens it.

The prevalence of bronchial asthma is higher among skiers exposed to cold and dry air than among non-skiers. The upper-airway passages are responsible for warming and humidifying inhaled air. During exercise in cold and dry air, warming and humidifying of the inhaled air continues in the bronchial tree. Under these conditions, both the nasal and bronchial mucosa are cooled by inhaled air and remain cooled throughout the respiratory cycle.

Asthma is more common among swimmers than among other athletes, because many children were encouraged to begin swimming as exercise treatment for their breathing problems. Exercising in a warm, humid environment and breathing slowly through the nose help to control exercise-induced bronchoconstriction. Swimming induces less severe bronchoconstriction than other sports. A possible explanation for this is the high humidity of the inspired air at water level, which decreases respiratory heat loss. There is no conclusive evidence, however, that swim training causes a decrease in the severity or frequency of exercise-induced bronchoconstriction. Two potentially negative effects of swimming for asthmatic patients are as follows: i) exaggerated parasympathetic tone due to the mammalian diving reflex has been shown to trigger bronchoconstriction; and ii) chemicals in the water such as chlorine can cause irritation. Chloramines, which give the characteristic smell of indoor swimming pools, are produced when chlorine reacts with polluting proteins that enter the water from the urine and sweat of swimmers. Chloramines can trigger asthma.

Fitness training does not eliminate, but can minimize, the effect of exercise-induced bronchoconstriction by improving baseline pulmonary function and aerobic capacity. It is best treated and pre-treated by inhalation of beta-2 agonists. Preventative (and management) programs, however, are likely to be ineffective when allergic responses are compounded by exposure to air pollution. *See* SODIUM CHROMOGLYCATE.

Bibliography

Afraiabi, R. and Spector, S.L. (1991). Exercise-induced asthma. *The Physician and Sportsmedicine* 19(5), 49-62.

Bar-Or, O. and Inbar, O. (1992). Swimming and asthma. Benefits and deleterious effects. *Sports Medicine* 14(6), 397-405.

Bundgaard, A. (1985). Exercise and the asthmatic. *Sports Medicine* 2, 254-266.

Cummiskey, J. (2001). Exercise-induced asthma: An overview. *American Journal of Medical Science* 322(4), 200-203.

Fitch, K.D. (1986). The use of anti-asthmatic drugs. Do they affect sports performance? *Sports Medicine* 3, 136-150.

Hough, D.O. and Dec, K.L. (1994). Exercise-induced asthma and anaphylaxis. *Sports Medicine* 18(3), 162-172.

Langdeau, J.B. and Boulet, L.P. (2001). Prevalence and mechanisms of development of asthma and airway hyperresponsiveness in athletes. *Sports Medicine* 31(8), 601-616.

Latvala, J.J. et al (1995). Cold-induced responses in the upper respiratory tract. *Arctic Medical Research* 54(1), 4-9.

McCarthy, P. (1989). Wheezing or breezing through exercise-induced asthma. *The Physician and Sportsmedicine* 17(7), 125-130.

Roberts, J.A. (1988). Exercise-induced asthma in athletes. *Sports Medicine* 6, 193-196.

Rundell, K., Wilber, R. and Lemanske, R. (2002, eds). *Exercise-induced asthma*. Champaign, IL: Human Kinetics.

Spooner, C.H. et al. (2004). Mast-cell stabilizing agents to prevent exercise-induced bronchoconstriction (Cochrane Review). In: *The Cochrane Library*, Issue 3. Chichester, UK: John Wiley & Sons.

Stamford, B. (1991). Exercise-induced asthma. *The Physician and Sportsmedicine* 19(8), 139-140.

Tan, R.A. and Spector, S.L. (1998). Exercise-induced asthma. *Sports Medicine* 25(1), 1-6.

Thickett, K.M. et al. (2002). Occupational asthma caused by chloramines in indoor swimming pool air. *European Respiratory Journal* 19(5), 827-832.

Virant, F.S. (1992). Exercise-induced bronchospasm: Epidemiology, pathophysiology, and therapy. *Medicine and Science in Sports and Exercise* 24, 851-855.

Voy, R.O. (1986). The US Olympic Committee experience with exercise-induced bronchospasm, 1984. *Medicine and Science in Sports and Exercise* 18, 328-330.

EXERCISE-INDUCED MUSCLE DAMAGE *See under* MUSCLE SORENESS.

EXERCISE INTENSITY   *See under* AEROBIC TRAINING; STEADY STATE.

EXERCISE PHYSIOLOGY   The description and explanation of functional changes in the body brought about by single exercise sessions, or repeated exercise sessions (training). It is concerned with exercise testing and exercise prescription in both sport and health-related contexts. *See also* PHYSIOLOGY.

Chronology

•1843 • Edinburgh physician Andrew Combe's *The Principles of Physiology Applied to the Preservation of Health and to the Improvement of Physical and Mental Education* endorsed physical activity for growing children and that active sports were superior to walking.

•1888 • Fernand Lagrange's *The Physiology of Bodily Exercise* was published.

•1892 • The first formal exercise physiology laboratory was established in the USA at Harvard University. It was housed in the newly created Department of Anatomy, Physiology and Physical Training at the Lawrence Scientific School.

•1964 • The National Institutes of Health established the Applied Physiology Study Section to evaluate the increasing number of applications for federal funding for projects that related to exercise.

•1997 • The American Society of Exercise Physiologists was founded to provide a forum for leadership and exchange of scientific information and to stimulate discussion and collaboration among exercise physiologists.

Bibliography

American College of Sports Medicine (2001). *ACSM's resource manual for Guidelines for Exercise Testing & Prescription*. 4th ed. Philadelphia, PA: Lippincott Williams & Wilkins.

Åstrand, P.O. et al. (2003). *Textbook of work physiology: Physiological bases of exercise*. 4th ed. Champaign, IL: Human Kinetics.

Bowers, R.W. and Fox, E.L. (1992). *Sports physiology*. Dubuque, IA: WC Brown.

Brodie, D. (1996, ed). *A reference manual for human performance in the field of physical education and sport sciences*. Lewiston, NY: The Edwin Mellin Press.

Buskirk, E.R. and Tipton, C.M. (1997). Exercise physiology. In: Massengale, J.D. and Swanson, R.A. (eds.). *The history of exercise and sport science*. pp367-438. Champaign, IL: Human Kinetics.

Cerny, F.J. and Burton, H.W. (2001). *Exercise physiology for health care professionals*. Champaign, IL: Human Kinetics.

Ehrman, J.K. et al. (2003, eds). *Clinical exercise physiology*. Champaign, IL: Human Kinetics.

Froelicher, V.F. and Quaglietti, S. (1996). *Handbook of exercise testing*. Boston, MA: Little Brown.

Gore, C.J. (2000, ed). *Physiological tests for elite athletes*. Champaign, IL: Human Kinetics.

Hasson, S.M. (1994, ed). *Clinical exercise physiology*. St Louis, MI: Mosby.

Heyward, V.H. (1998). *Advanced fitness assessment and exercise prescription*. 3rd ed. Champaign, IL: Human Kinetics.

Johnson, E.P (2001, ed). *ACSM's resource manual for Guidelines for Exercise Testing & Prescription*. 4th ed. Philadelphia, PA: Lippincott Williams & Wilkins.

LeMura, L. and von Duvillard, S. (2003). *Clinical exercise physiology. Application and physiological principles*. Philadelphia, PA: Lippincott Williams & Wilkins.

McArdle, W.D., Katch, F.I. and Katch, V.L. (2000). *Essentials of exercise physiology*. 2nd ed. Philadelphia, PA: Lippincott Williams& Wilkins.

McArdle, W.D, Katch, F.I. and Katch, V.L. (2004). *Exercise physiology. Energy, nutrition, and human performance*. 5th ed. Philadelphia, PA: Lippincott Williams & Wilkins.

Newsholme, E., Leech, A. and Duester, G. (1994). *Keep on running. The science of training and performance*. Chichester, W. Sussex: John Wiley.

Plowman, S.A. and Smith, D.L. (2003). *Exercise physiology for health, fitness and performance*. 2nd ed. San Francisco, CA: Benjamin Cummings.

Powers, S.K. and Howley, E.T. (2004). *Exercise physiology. Theory and application to fitness and performance*. 5th ed. Boston, MA: McGraw-Hill.

Robergs, R.A. and Roberts, S.O. (2000). *Fundamental principles of exercise physiology*. Boston, MA: McGraw-Hill.

Skinner, J.S. (1993). *Exercise testing and exercise prescription for special cases*. 2nd ed. Philadelphia, PA: Lippincott Williams & Wilkins.

Wasserman, K. et al. (2004). *Principles of exercise testing and interpretation. Including pathophysiology and clinical applications*. 4th ed. Philadelphia, PA: Lippincott Williams & Wilkins.

Wilmore, J.H. and Costill, D.L. (2004). *Physiology of sport and exercise*. 3rd ed. Champaign, IL: Human Kinetics.

EXERCISE PRESCRIPTION   See under PHYSICAL FITNESS.

EXERCISE PSYCHOLOGY   An outgrowth of sport psychology that is focused on two areas: (i) participation in exercise motivated by reasons of health; and (ii) effects of exercise on mental health. The emergence of exercise psychology is largely due to the increased attention given to health-related fitness in sports medicine and physical education. *See* EXERCISE ADHERENCE; MENTAL HEALTH.

Bibliography

Biddle, S. and Mutrie, N. (2001). *Psychology of physical activity: Determinants, well-being and interventions*. London: Routledge.

Carron, A.V., Hausenblas, H.A. and Estabrooks, P.A. (2003). *The psychology of physical activity*. Boston, MA: McGraw-Hill.

Buckworth, J. and Dishman, R.H. (2002). *Exercise psychology*. Champaign, IL: Human Kinetics.

Willis, J.D. and Campbell, L.F. (1992). *Exercise psychology*. Champaign, IL: Human Kinetics.

EXERCISE SCIENCE   *See under* KINESIOLOGY.

EXERGONIC   *See under* THERMODYNAMICS.

EXHAUSTION   Complete inability of muscle(s) or the individual to maintain exercise. *See also* FATIGUE.

EXOCRINE GLAND   *See under* GLAND.

EXOCYTOSIS   *See under* ACTIVE TRANSPORT.

EXOGENOUS   Derived or originating externally.

EXOSTOSIS   A bony projection capped by cartilage that arises from any bone, which develops from cartilage. *See* BUNION; HALLUX VALGUS; TACKLER'S EXOSTOSIS.

EXOTHERMIC   *See under* THERMO-DYNAMICS.

EXPERIENCE   Factors within the environment that may alter the appearance of various developmental characteristics through the process of learning.

EXPERTISE   Highly developed knowledge, understanding and skill. Since it was first discussed by Simon and Chase (1973), it has been widely suggested that elite performers require more than 10 years practice to acquire the necessary skills and experience to perform at an international level.

Ericsson et al.'s (1993) **Deliberate Practice theory** proposes that expertise is developed via deliberate practice. In contrast to play, deliberate practice is a highly structured activity, the goal of which is to improve performance. Specific tasks are devised to overcome weaknesses, and performance is carefully monitored to provide cues for ways to improve it further. It is predicted that the amount of time an individual is engaged in deliberate practice activities will be related to that individual's acquired performance. In soccer, a positive linear relationship has been found between accumulated individual plus team practice and skill.

Based on data from young men and women from a number of domains (e.g. Olympic swimmers and mathematicians) in the USA, Bloom (1985) identified three phases in the development of expert performers: i) early years – the child receives instruction from a local teacher and parents play a major role in motivation of the child; ii) middle development years – typically between ages of 10 and 13 years when the child become strongly committed to their pre-performance goals and works with a more advanced coach who is regarded as one of the best within a larger geographical area; and iii) latter years – during which the child works with an expert coach of whom there are only a small number in the country, and great sacrifices are required from the family.

In a longitudinal study of more than 200 high school students in a number of domains including athletes, Csikszentmihalyi, Rathunde and Whalen (1993) found the following three characteristics to be common to coaches and teachers who helped cultivate the talent of their students: i) the coaches were effective because they enjoyed what they were doing, were devoted to the domain and encouraged their athletes to excel beyond their current level of talent; ii) the coaches created optimal learning conditions so that athletes were not bored or overly

frustrated; and iii) the coaches had an ability to understand the needs of athletes and a genuine concern for the overall development of the athletes. *See also* PERCEPTION.

Bibliography

Bloom, G.A., Salmela, J.H. and Schinke, R.J. (1995). Expert coaches' views on the training of developing coaches. In R. Van Fraechan-Raway and Y. Vanden Auweele (eds.). *Proceedings of the 9th European Congress on Sport Psychology*. pp 401-408. Brussels, Belgium: Free University of Brussels.

Côté, J. (1999). The influence of the family in the development of talent in sport. *The Sport Psychologist* 13, 395-417.

Côté, J. and Salmela, J.H. (1996). The organizational tasks of high-performance gymnastic coaches. *The Sport Psychologist* 10, 247-260.

Csikszentmihalyi, M., Rathunde, K. and Whalen, S. (1993). *Talented teenagers: The roots of success and failure*. New York: Cambridge.

Ericsson, K.A., Krampe, R.T. and Tesch-Römer, C. (1993). The role of deliberate practice in the acquisition of expert performance. *Psychological Review* 100(3), 363-406.

Ericsson, K.A. (1996, ed.). *The road to excellence: The acquisition of expert performance in the arts and sciences, sports and games*. Hillsdale, NJ: Erlbaum.

Helsen, W.F., Starkes, J.L. and Hodges, N.J. (1998). Team sports and the theory of deliberate practice. *Journal of Sport & Exercise Psychology* 20, 12-34.

Helsen, W.F. et al. (2000). The roles of talent, physical precocity and practice in the development of soccer expertise. *Journal of Sports Sciences* 18(9), 727-736.

Simon, H.A. and Chase, W.G. (1973). Skill in chess. *American Scientist* 61, 394-403.

Starkes, J.L. and Anderson, K.A. (2003, eds). *Expert performance in sports: Advances in research on sport expertise*. Champaign, IL: Human Kinetics.

EXPIRATORY RESERVE VOLUME   The maximum amount of gas that can be expired from the end- expiratory position. *See also* VITAL CAPACITY.

EXTENSOR THRUST REFLEX   A primitive reflex that may be classified as either exteroceptive or proprioceptive. Pressure against the sole of the foot stimulates the Pacinian corpuscles in the subcutaneous tissue and elicits the reflex contraction of the extensor muscles of the lower extremity, making the leg into a rigid segment. When foot leaves the floor, the reflex response ceases, and the limb is free to move again. It is normal in infants from birth to 3 months and it strengthens the extensors, thereby promoting balance between flexor and extensor postural tone. In the first two months, it is sometimes mistaken for early standing ability.

Failure of the extensor thrust reflex to become integrated includes an inability to maintain a proper sitting position. It is a common problem in nonambulatory persons with cerebral palsy, who tend to slide out of a wheelchair unless it is specially designed.

EXTEROCEPTORS Receptors that are located at or near the external surface of the body and are sensitive to stimuli originating outside the body and provide information about the external environment. Sensations for hearing, vision, smell, taste, touch, pressure, vibration, temperature and pain are conveyed by exteroceptors.

See also INTEROCEPTORS; MECHANO-RECEPTORS; PROPRIOCEPTORS.

EXTRACELLULAR Located outside one or more cells.

EXTRAPYRAMIDAL MOTOR SYSTEM *See under* BRAIN.

EXTRAVASTATION Movement of a fluid (e.g. blood, lymph, urine) out of a vessel into the tissues.

EXTRINSIC MOTIVATION *See under* INTRINSIC MOTIVATION.

EXUBERANT Excessive proliferation or growth.

EXUDATE A fluid with a high content of protein and cellular debris that has escaped from blood vessels and has been deposited in tissue or on tissue surfaces, usually as a result of inflammation.

EYE DOMINANCE The ability of one eye to lead the other in task involving visual tracking or visual fixation. About 75% of children will develop a dominant eye by 3 years of age and about 95% by 5 years. **Unilateral dominance** refers to right eyed and right handed, or left eyed and left handed. **Crossed lateral dominance** refers to right eyed and left handed, or left eyed and right handed. There may be a relationship between eye dominance and baseball hitting, because crossed-lateral dominance seems to be higher in baseball players than in the general population.

The dominant eye can be found as follows. Extend your arms forward at shoulder height and form a small triangular hole between the thumbs and index finger. Pick a distant object and center it in the hole formed by your hands. Without moving your head or hands, close one eye at a time. The eye that has the object lined up with the hole is the dominant eye.

Bibliography

Payne, V.G. and Isaacs, L.D. (2004). *Human motor development. A lifespan approach.* 6th ed. Boston, MA: McGraw-Hill.

EYE INJURIES Abrasion may occur when a foreign body scratches the cornea. Lacerations are caused by sharp objects, such as a finger nail.

An **orbital fracture** is a blowout fracture caused by impact from a blunt object, usually larger than the eye orbit. A sudden increase in intraorbital pressure is released in the area of least resistance, typically the orbital floor. It is common in soccer. Signs and symptoms consistent with orbital fracture include gross bony deformity, limitation of gaze, diplopia and malposition of the globe. The majority of patients who sustain orbital fractures are able to return to sport, but persistent diplopia is not uncommon.

The frequency of eye injuries in soccer has contributed to the recommendation by the American Academy of Pediatrics' Committee on Sports Medicine and Fitness, and the American Academy of Ophthalmology Committee on Eye Safety and Sports Ophthalmology that protective sports eye equipment using polycarbonate lenses be worn during soccer practice and competition.

In the USA, more than 42,000 sports-related and recreational eye injuries were treated in hospital emergency departments in 2000. 72% of the injuries occurred in individuals younger than 25 years, 41% occurred in individuals younger than 15 years and 8% occurred in children younger than 5 years. Baseball and basketball are associated with the most eye injuries in athletes from 5 to 24 years old. Baseball is the leading cause of sports-related eye injuries in children, and the highest incidence occurs in children aged 5 to 15 years. Approximately one third of baseball-related eye injuries occur as a result of being struck by a pitched ball.

See also CATASTROPHIC INJURIES; RETINA.

Bibliography

American Academy of Pediatrics (2001). Protective eyewear for young athletes. *Pediatrics* 98(2), 311-313.

American Academy of Pediatrics (2001). Risk of injury from baseball and softball in children. *Pediatrics* 107(4), 782-784.

American Academy of Pediatrics and American Association of Ophthalmology (2004). Injuries in youth soccer. A subject review. *Ophthalmology* 111(3), 600-603.

Petrigliano, F.A. and Williams, R.J. 3rd (2003). Orbital fractures in sport: A review. *Sports Medicine* 33(4), 317-322.

EYE MOVEMENTS **Binocular tracking** involves directing the eyes from one line of sight to another. It involves smooth pursuit (slow velocity) and saccadic (high velocity) eye movements. The **smooth pursuit** eye movements can match eye-movement speed with the speed of the projectile to maintain a stable retinal image. **Saccadic** eye movements are fast, jerky movements aimed at fixating an object onto the fovea, the most acute area of the eye for vision. The saccadic eye movement system detects and corrects differences between projectile location and eye fixation. It is primarily used when objects are traveling greater than 24 to 33 m/s. Saccadic eye movement ability tends to decrease with aging, increasing the chance of a visual tracking error.

Nystagmus is used to direct the fovea towards the oncoming visual scene during self-rotation.

Optokinetic movements are used to hold images of the seen world steadily on the retina during sustained head rotation. **Vestibular movements** are used to hold the image of the seen world steady on the retina during brief head rotation. **Vergence** (version) is used to move the eyes in opposite directions so that he image of a single object is placed on both fovae.

F

FABELLA A sesamoid bone, present in 10 to 18% of the normal population, located in the tendinous portion of the lateral *gastrocnemius* muscle. The anterior surface of the fabella articulates with the posterior portion of the lateral femoral condyle. The fabella may become inflamed, especially during late adolescence, causing pain in the posterolateral knee.

FACET DYSFUNCTION *See under* NECK INJURIES.

FACET JOINTS *See under* SPINE.

FACIAL FRACTURES These occur in 2% of all athletes. Sports that are at higher risk of facial fractures are those that involve small objects projected at high velocity (e.g. baseball) and also sports with high levels of physical contact and collision (e.g. football).

Over 100,000 sport-related injuries could be prevented annually in the USA by the use of appropriate head and face protection. Facemasks, with throat protection, are required for fencing, baseball/softball catchers, and for goalkeepers in field hockey, ice hockey, and lacrosse.

See also DENTAL INJURIES; EAR INJURIES; EYE INJURIES; NASAL INJURIES; TEMPORO-MANDIBULAR JOINT.

Bibliography

Laskin, D.M. (2000). Protecting the faces of America. *Journal of Oral & Maxillofacial Surgery* 58(4), 363.

Rupp, T.J. and Bednar, M. (2002). Facial fractures. Http://www.emedicine.com

FAD Flavin adenine dinucleotide. It contains riboflavin. A co-enzyme involved in oxidation-reduction reactions. It can accept two electrons and two protons from hydrogen atoms. The reduced form is expressed as $FADH_2$.

See also under ELECTRON TRANSPORT CHAIN.

FAMILIAL Tending to be present in more members of the same family than can be accounted for by chance.

FARTLEK TRAINING *See under* INTERVAL TRAINING.

FASCIA Dense, fibrous, unorganized connective tissue. Connective tissue that is not bone, tendon, cartilage or ligament. The skin is separated from the muscles and bones by two layers of adipose tissue: the superficial and deep fascia. The **superficial fascia** is a fat-filled fibrous mesh that connects the skin to the underlying sheet of deep fascia. The **deep fascia** that envelopes the muscle is known as the **epimysium**. Within the muscle, deep fascia can be found in the perimysium, endomysium and sarcolemma.

FASCICLE *See under* TENDON.

FASCICULATION Abnormal, spontaneous twitch of all skeletal muscle fibers in one motor unit that is visible at the skin surface. It is not associated with movement of the affected muscle. It is found in progressive diseases of motor neurons, e.g. polio.

FASCICULI *See under* MUSCLE; PERIPHERAL NERVES.

FASCIOTOMY A surgical procedure that cuts away fascia in order to relieve tension or pressure. The most common condition for which fasciotomy is performed is plantar fasciitis.

FAT Any substance extractable in fat solvents (e.g. alcohol) and, besides those containing fatty acids, includes sterols (which often occur chemically combined with fatty acids), steroids, carotene and, in plants, terpenes.

Adipose tissue is connective tissue that contains fat. **White adipose tissue** is found in subcutaneous fat, intra-abdominal fat and other locations (e.g. fat pads in the soles of the feet) and its adipocytes contain a single large lipid droplet. **Yellow fat** is so named because of the accumulation of dietary carotenoids (yellow pigments). **Neutral fat** is composed of fatty acids and glycerol. **Triglyceride (triacylglycerol)** is neutral fat composed of three molecules of fatty acid and one of glycerol. It is the most abundant lipid found in humans. In humans, total body fat consists of essential fat and storage fat. **Essential fat** is required for normal functioning of the body. It is found in the bone marrow, heart, lungs, liver, spleen, kidneys, muscles and many tissues of the central nervous system. In females, **sex-specific fat** (as in the breasts) is also classed as essential fat. In order to maintain good health, it seems that a person should not decrease fat below the essential fat level. Fats are much better adapted than glycogen to serve as a storage form of energy. The fat stored in adipose tissue is often referred to as **storage fat**. It includes the adipose tissue that protects internal organs and the subcutaneous adipose tissue (found in the superficial fascia). Essential fat values for men and women are on average 3% and 12%, respectively, of body mass. Storage fat values for men and women are on average 12% and 15%, respectively, of body mass. About 50,000 to 60,000 kcal of energy is stored as triglycerides in the entire mass of all of the adipocytes throughout the body. Excess energy from fat, alcohol and protein is converted to fat and stored in the body's fat cells.

The **High-Fat Diet theory** is based on the premise that raised levels of free fatty acids (FFA) in the blood may be associated with an increase in the rate of fat oxidation. A high-fat diet has not been shown to improve performance either in the short term (i.e. less than six days) or the longer term. An increased fat intake does not stimulate its own oxidation, but rather stimulates oxidation of the fat stored in the human body. There is evidence that adaptation to a fat-rich diet leads to an increased capacity of the fat oxidative system and an enhancement of the fat supply and subsequently the amount of fat oxidized during exercise. In most cases, however, muscle glycogen storage is compromised and muscle glycogen breakdown is diminished to a certain extent. This is probably part of the explanation for the lack of performance enhancement after adaptation to a fat-rich diet. Chronic high-fat diets may provoke adaptive responses preventing the detrimental effects on exercise performance. A disadvantage of high fat diets is that high blood fat levels are associated with cardiovascular disease. High-fat diets, due to their high energy density, also stimulate voluntary energy intake. The only practical way to significantly elevate plasma triglyceride is by ingesting triglycerides. It is not possible to ingest free fatty acids, because they are too acidic and because they need a protein carrier for intestinal absorption.

See also ABDOMINAL OBESITY; BROWN FAT; CARNITINE; CELLULITE; ENERGY SUBSTRATE UTILIZATION; FATTY ACIDS; LIPIDS; MEDIUM-CHAIN TRIGLYCERIDES; OBESITY.

Bibliography

Hawley, J.A., Brouns, F. and Jeukendrup, A. (1998). Strategies to enhance fat utilization during exercise. *Sports Medicine* 25(4), 241-257.

Helge, J.W. (2000). Adaptation to a fat-rich diet: Effects on endurance performance in humans. *Sports Medicine* 30(5), 347-357.

Jeukendrup, A.E., Saris, W.H. and Wagenmakers, A.J. (1998). Fat metabolism during exercise: A review. Part III: Effects of nutritional interventions. *International Journal of Sports Medicine* 19(6), 371-379.

Ranallo, R.F. and Rhodes, E.C. (1998). Lipid metabolism during exercise. *Sports Medicine* 26(1), 29-42.

Schrauwen, P. and Westerterp, K.R. (2000). The role of high-fat diets and physical activity in the regulation of body weight. *British Journal of Nutrition* 84(4), 417-427.

FATIGUE   This is the failure of muscle(s) to maintain force (or power output) during sustained or repeated contractions. It is a self-protective mechanism against damage to the contractile mechanisms of muscle. The Catastrophe theory used in engineering has been used to explain abrupt changes in the function of individual muscle cells. For the muscle as a whole, fatigue may be manifested as a more gradual loss of force.

Both central nervous system and peripheral mechanisms are likely to contribute to fatigue. Central causes of fatigue include motivation, impaired neural transmission down the spinal cord, and impaired recruitment of motor neurons. Peripheral causes of fatigue may involve impairment of the function of peripheral nerves, neuromuscular junction transmission, electrical activity of muscle fibers or the processes of activation within the muscle fiber. It seems that the primary sites of fatigue are within the muscle and do not generally involve peripheral nerves or the neuromuscular junction. Muscle glycogen depletion and accumulation of hydrogen ions are also factors that likely contribute to fatigue during high-intensity exercise.

In well-motivated, normal people, the decrease in force during a sustained muscular contraction is most likely due to peripheral factors. This can be demonstrated by the electrical stimulation of a peripheral nerve and by showing failure (independent of motivation or voluntary effort) of muscle contractile force.

The following factors are each involved in endurance exercise and fatigue (to a varying degree, depending on the environmental conditions and the nature of the activity): depletion of muscle and liver glycogen; decrease in blood glucose; dehydration; and increase in body temperature. Despite adequate free fatty acids, a certain level of muscle glycogen metabolism may be essential for the maintenance of essential Krebs cycle intermediates. Other factors must be involved, because muscle glycogen depletion can exist without fatigue. Muscle organelles, especially the sarcoplasmic reticulum, are probably involved in the fatigue process.

Following short-duration, high intensity exercise, recovery in force production usually displays two components likely caused by separate mechanisms. First, hydrogen ions interfere with the excitation-coupling process by inhibiting the release of calcium ions from the sarcoplasmic reticulum and inhibiting the binding of calcium ions to troponin, thus decreasing the amount of interacting cross-bridges. Hydrogen ions also inhibit the activity of phosphofructokinase. Second, there is a slower change involving several sites and steps in muscle

contraction that are mediated at least in part by hydrogen ions and inorganic phosphate ions.

Bibliography

Appell, H.J., Soares, J.M.C. and Duarte, J.A.R. (1992). Exercise, muscle damage and fatigue. *Sports Medicine* 13(2), 108-115.

Brooks, G.A. (2001). Lactate doesn't necessarily cause fatigue: Why are we surprised? *Journal of Physiology* 536(1), 1.

Davis, J.M. (1995). Central and peripheral factors in fatigue. *Journal of Sports Sciences* 13, S49-S53.

Davis, J.M. and Fitts, R. (2001). Mechanisms of muscular fatigue. In: American College of Sports Medicine. *ACSM's resource manual for Guidelines for exercise testing and prescription.* 4th ed. pp184-197. Philadelphia, PA: Lippincott Williams & Wilkins.

Fitts, R.H. (2004). Mechanisms of muscular fatigue. In: Poortmans, J.R. (ed). *Principles of exercise biochemistry.* 3rd rev ed. pp279-300. Basel, Switzerland: Karger.

Gandevia, S.C. (1992). Some central and peripheral factors affecting human motoneuronal output in neuromuscular fatigue. *Sports Medicine* 13(2), 93-98.

Gibson, H. and Edwards, R.H.T. (1985). Muscular exercise and fatigue. *Sports Medicine* 2, 121-132.

McKenna, M.J. (1992). The roles of ionic processes in muscular fatigue during intense exercise. *Sports Medicine* 13(2), 134-145.

Roberts, D. and Smith, D.J. (1989). Biochemical aspects of peripheral muscle fatigue. *Sports Medicine* 7, 125-138.

St. Clair Gibson, A., Lambert, M.L. and Noakes, T.D. (2001). Neural control of force output during maximal and submaximal exercise. *Sports Medicine* 31(9), 637-650.

FAT PAD Specialized soft tissue structure for bearing weight and absorbing impact.

See FLAT FEET; HEEL FAT PAD; HOFFA'S DISEASE.

FATTY ACID A component of fats. Fatty acids may be saturated or unsaturated. Fats from animal sources are rich in saturated fatty acids, whereas fats from plant sources (vegetable oils) are rich in unsaturated fatty acids. **Saturated fatty acids** are fatty acids completely filled by hydrogen with all carbons in the chain linked by single bonds. **Unsaturated fatty acids** have at least one double bond between two of their carbons. In **monounsaturated fatty acids**, the carbon chain contains one double bond. The major fatty acid of olive oil is 18-carbon monounsaturated oleic acid. In **polyunsaturated fatty acids**, the carbon chain contains two or more double bonds.

Oxidative rancidity occurs when unsaturated fatty acids come into contact with air, and oxygen atoms can attach to its double bond sites. Oxidation of fatty acids is likely to be much lower in fresh than processed foods. The more unsaturated a fatty acid is, the more that it is vulnerable to oxidation.

Hydrogenation involves adding hydrogen atoms to double bonds, converting them to single bonds. Hydrogenation of monounsaturated and polyunsaturated fatty acids decreases the number of double bonds they contain, thereby making them more saturated.

In **cis fatty acids**, the hydrogens surrounding a double bond are both on the same side of the carbon chain, causing a bend in the chain. Most naturally occurring fatty acids are cis fatty acids. In **trans fatty acids**, the hydrogens surrounding a double bond are on the opposite sides of the carbon chain; the bent carbon chain straightens out, and the fatty acid becomes more solid at room temperature. There is evidence that trans fatty acids may raise blood levels of LDL cholesterol. They are even more destructive than saturated fat, because they also lower the HDL cholesterol.

Long-chain fatty acids contain 12 to 22 carbon atoms. **Medium-chain fatty acids** contain 6 to 10 carbon atoms. **Short-chain fatty acids** contain less than 6 carbons. As chain length increases, fatty acids become solid at room temperature. Shorter fatty acids are also more water soluble, a property that affects their absorption in the digestive tract. Most fatty acids in the body contain 14 to 22 carbons, with 16 (palmitic), 18 (oleic) and 18 (stearic) being most common. Generally 18-carbon polyunsaturated fatty acids are found in plant foods. Stearic acid and palmitic acid are two of the most abundant saturated fatty acids in the diet.

Essential fatty acids are those required for growth and health that cannot be synthesized by the body. They must therefore be obtained from the diet. In humans, linoleic acid and gamma-linoleic acids are the only essential fatty acids. They are required for cell membrane synthesis and fat metabolism.

Omega-3 fatty acids are polyunsaturated fatty acids in which the first double bond starting from the methyl end of the molecule lies between the 3rd and 4th carbon atoms. They are found primarily in fish oils and may be metabolized in the body to eicosanoids. Research shows that omega-3 fatty acids can modestly lower blood pressure and can help decrease blood triglycerides. The Inuits (Greenland Eskimos) have a high dietary intake of omega-3 fatty acids from marine mammals and fish, but low incidence of atherosclerosis. **Alpha-linolenic acid** is an essential omega-3 fatty acid that contains 18 carbon atoms and 3 double bonds. Through the processes of elongation and desaturation, alpha-linolenic acid can ultimately be converted to **eicosapentaenoic acid** with 20 carbons and 5 double bonds and docohexanoic acid with 22 carbons and 6 double bonds. **Elongation** is the process by which the liver adds carbons to build storage and structural fats, to manufacture the fat in breast milk, or to make fatty acids for use in other compounds. **Desaturation** is the insertion of double bonds into fatty acids to change them into new fatty acids. For these reactions to occur, however, they may have to compete with the omega-6 fatty acids and trans fatty acids for the same enzymes, so only a proportion of alpha-linolenic acid is actually converted to eicosapentaenoic acid and docohexanoic acid.

Omega-6 fatty acids are polyunsaturated fatty acids in which the first double bond starting from the methyl end of the molecule lies between the 6th and 7th carbon atoms. Linoleic acid is an essential omega-6 fatty acid that contains 18 carbons and two double bonds, and is an important precursor of eicosanoids. Another omega-6 fatty acid, **arachidonic acid**, it is sometimes considered a semi-essential fatty acid in that it can be synthesized only from the essential fatty acid linoleic acid after linoleic acid needs are met.

Omega-9 fatty acids, such oleic acid, are polyunsaturated fatty acids in which the first double bond starting from the methyl end of the molecule lies between the 9th and 10th carbon atoms.

See also under DIET; GLUCOSE; LIPOLYSIS.

FATTY ACID DEGRADATION The breakdown of fatty acids; it involves activation of fatty acids followed by beta-oxidation. Activation of fatty acids occurs in the cytosol. The activated fatty acid is transported from the cytosol across the mitochondrial membrane to the inside of the mitochondrion where beta-oxidation takes place.

Activation involves linking a molecule of coenzyme A to the carboxyl end of the fatty acid. This initial step is accompanied by the breakdown of ATP to AMP and two inorganic phosphates. Since the terminal phosphates of both ATP and ADP are high-energy bonds, the energy released in this reaction is equivalent to that released when 2 ATP are hydrolyzed to 2 ADP and two inorganic phosphates. Thus, although only 1 ATP is used in the reaction, the energy cost is equivalent to 2 ATP. Using stearic acid (18-carbon) as an example, the formation of stearyl CoA costs 2 ATP.

The inner mitochondrial membrane is impermeable to acyl CoA (where acyl is a long chain fatty acid) so a transport system that uses carnitine is required. (Short and medium-chain free fatty acids do not require carnitine to enter the mitochondrial matrix.) Acyl CoA is converted (esterified) to acyl carnitine by the enzyme carnitine acyltransferase I on the inner surface of the outer mitochondrial membrane. Acyl carnitine is transported across the inner mitochondrial membrane by the enzyme carnitine-acylcarnitine translocase in exchange for carnitine. Once in the mitochondrial matrix, acyl carnitine is converted back to acyl CoA by the enzyme carnitine acyltransferase II that is located on the inner aspect of the inner mitochondrial membrane. The free carnitine can be exchanged for another incoming molecule of acyl carnitine.

Beta-oxidation is the breakdown of a fatty acid into numerous 2-carbon acetyl CoA molecules. Enzymes clip a 2-carbon link from the beta end of the fatty acid by breaking the bond between the alpha carbon (C2) and beta carbon (C3). This 2-carbon link is converted to one acetyl CoA, while also forming 1 $FADH_2$ and 1 NADH. These coenzymes enter the oxidative phosphorylation pathway, with NADH + H^+ forming 2.5 ATP; and $FADH_2$ forming 1.5 ATP, for a total of 4 ATP. Each passage through

this sequence shortens the fatty acid chain by two carbon atoms until all the carbon atoms have been transferred to coenzyme A (CoA). The final 2-carbon link becomes one acetyl CoA, without producing $FADH_2$ and NADH. The acetyl CoA molecules then enter the Krebs cycle, each 2-carbon fragment producing 2 molecules of CO_2, and ultimately 10 ATP via the Krebs cycle and oxidative phosphorylation. When the terminal acetyl CoA is split from the fatty acid, another CoA is added (ATP is not required for this step) and the sequence is repeated. Formation of 9 acetyl CoA from one stearyl CoA, using the sequence of beta-oxidation reaction, yields 8 $FADH_2$ + 8 NADH + H^+ (i.e. 8 cycles of beta-oxidation) in the oxidative phosphorylation pathway, i.e. (8 x 2.5 ATP) + (8 x 1.5 ATP) = 32 ATP. Transfer of electrons from 8 $FADH_2$ and 8 NADH to oxygen in the electron transfer chain yields 9 x 10 ATP = 90 ATP. The total yield of ATP from one molecule of stearic acid is 90 + 32 − 2 = 120 ATP.

Beta-oxidation is regulated largely by the concentration of free fatty acids available, but also hormonal control by lipases (increased glucagons and epinephrine) and decreased malonyl CoA. **Malonyl CoA** is an intermediate of fatty acid synthesis. Malonyl CoA inhibits carnitine transferase, thus inhibiting entry of acyl CoA into the mitochondria. Fatty acid degradation and synthesis do not occur together.

A certain level of carbohydrate breakdown is required for lipids to be continually metabolized for energy. The degradation of fatty acids via the Krebs cycle continues only if sufficient oxaloacetate is available to combine with the acetyl CoA formed during beta-oxidation. Fatty acids cannot be converted into pyruvate or oxaloacetate to synthesize glucose, because the conversion of acetyl CoA is not reversible. Acetyl CoA enters the Krebs cycle by combining with oxaloacetate to form citrate. This oxaloacetate is generated from pyruvate during carbohydrate breakdown under the control of pyruvate carboxylase. Pyruvate formation during glucose metabolism plays an important role in maintaining a proper level of this oxaloacetate intermediate. When the carbohydrate level decreases, the oxaloacetate level may become inadequate. To this extent, therefore, 'lipids burn in a carbohydrate flame.'

The mechanisms controlling fatty acid uptake and oxidation during various exercise modes are still not completely elucidated. Changes in malonyl CoA concentration in skeletal muscle do not seem to play a major regulatory role in controlling long-chain fatty acid oxidation during exercise in humans. Kiens and Roepstorff (2003) suggest that the availability of free carnitine may play a major regulatory role in oxidation of long-chain fatty acids during exercise.

Bibliography

Insel, P., Turner, R.E. and Ross, D. (2004). *Nutrition.* 2nd ed. Sudbury, MA: Jones and Bartlett.

Kiens, B. and Roepstorff, C. (2003). Utilization of long-chain fatty acids in human skeletal muscle during exercise. *Acta Physiologica Scandanavia.* 178(4), 391-396.

Roberts, R.A. and Roberts, S.O. (2000). *Fundamental principles of exercise physiology.* Boston, MA: McGraw-Hill.

FATTY ACID SYNTHESIS Lipogenesis. It occurs in the cytosol from excess acetyl CoA. Acetyl CoA is successively attached in 2-carbon increments until the long chain fatty acid chain is completed. Lipogenesis is not simply the reverse of fatty acid degradation. There is a different set of enzymes, the reactions take place in a different location (beta oxidation occurs inside mitochondria), and nicotinamide dinucleotide phosphate ($NADP^+$) is used as a coenzyme rather than nicotinamide dinucleotide (NAD^+). Important sites of fatty acid synthesis include the liver, adipose tissue and lactating mammary gland.

Excess fatty acids and proteins are converted to fat and stored. Excess carbohydrate does not significantly increase fat storage, but the body burns more carbohydrate and less fat, thus more fat is stored. ***De novo* lipogenesis** is making fat from carbohydrate. Net *de novo* lipogenesis is absent or very low in humans under most dietary conditions. In humans, *de novo* lipogenesis from excess glucose occurs only to a negligible degree in the liver. A high rate of *de novo* lipogenesis has been documented in humans only under conditions of massive carbohydrate overfeeding, e.g. 5,000 to 6,000 kcal carbohydrate per day for more than a week, and also with insulin resistance. *See also* FUTILE CYCLING.

FEBRILE Pertaining to, or characterized by, fever.

FECES The residue of food that is either undigested or unabsorbed.

FEEDBACK i) Any process in which the output in some way controls the input (see under HOMEOSTASIS). ii) The effect of the consequences of behavior on future behavior. In motor learning, feedback is important for motivation, reinforcement/punishment, and error correction information. A distinction can be made between internal and external (augmented feedback). **Internal feedback** is sensory feedback (visual, proprioceptive, etc). **Augmented feedback** is information provided to a learner from an external source that describes the outcome of a performance and/or the quality of the performance itself. It may be knowledge of results, knowledge of performance or augmented sensory feedback (biofeedback). Both knowledge of results and knowledge of performance can be valuable in skill learning situations. **Knowledge of results** is concerned with task outcome and will be beneficial for skill learning: learners use knowledge of results to confirm their own assessments of task-intrinsic feedback, even though it may be redundant with task-intrinsic feedback; learners may need knowledge of results because they cannot determine the outcome of performing a skill on the basis of the available task-intrinsic feedback; learners often use knowledge of results to motivate themselves to continue practicing the skill; and teachers may want to provide only knowledge of results in order to establish a 'discovery learning' practice environment in which learners are encouraged to engage in trial and error as the primary means of learning to perform a skill.

Knowledge of performance is concerned with the quality of the performance and can be beneficial for skill learning when: skills must be performed according to specified movement characteristics, such as springboard dives; specific movement components of skills that require complex coordination must be improved or corrected; the goal of the action is a kinematic, kinetic, or specific muscle activity; and knowledge of results is redundant with the task intrinsic feedback. Augmented feedback can take many different forms and may involve the use of technology. For example, researchers have developed swimming paddles containing force sensors and sound generators that transmitted an audible signal to transmitters in a swimmer's cap. The sensors were set at a desired water-propulsion force threshold, so that when the swimmer reached this threshold, a sound signal would be produced. This would provide highly skilled swimmers with information to maintain their optimal velocity and number of arm cycles in a training session.

Augmented feedback should not be given after every trial. According to the Guidance hypothesis, if the learner receives augmented feedback on every trial, then it will effectively 'guide' the learner to perform the movement correctly. The flipside, however, is that the learner becomes dependent on its availability and performs poorly when it is not available. Receiving augmented feedback less frequently during practice encourages the learner to engage in more beneficial learning strategies during practice.

Visual feedback is not always beneficial. For example, the more that athletes train using feedback from mirrors, the more they become dependent on that feedback. When powerlifters who practiced their squat with a mirror for 100 trials were asked to perform the lift without the mirror, they increased the amount of error of their knee joint angle by 50%.

See also BIOFEEDBACK.

Bibliography

Anderson, D.I. and Sidaway, B. (1994). Coordination changes associated with practice of a soccer kick. *Research Quarterly for Exercise and Sport* 65, 93-99.

Chollet, D., Micallef, J.P. and Rabischong, P. (1988). Biomechanical signals for external feedback to improve swimming techniques. In Ungerechts, B.E., Wilke, K. and Reichle, K. (Eds). *Swimming science V*. pp389-396. Champaign,

IL: Human Kinetics.

Liebermann, D.G. et al. (2002). Advances in the application of information technology to sport performance. *Journal of Sports Sciences* 20(10), 755-769.

Magill, R.A. (2004). *Motor learning and control. Concepts and applications.* 7th ed. Boston: MA: McGraw-Hill.

Salmoni, A.W., Schmidt, R.A. and Walter, C.B. (1984). Knowledge of results and motor learning: A review and reappraisal. *Psychological Bulletin* 95, 355-386.

Southard, D. and Higgins, T. (1987). Changing movement patterns: Effects of demonstration and practice. *Research Quarterly for Exercise and Sport* 58, 77-80.

Tremblay, L. and Proteau, L. (1998). Specificity of practice: The case of powerlifting. *Research Quarterly for Exercise and Sport* 69, 284-289.

FEMALE ATHLETE TRIAD   A triad of related disorders: eating disorders, menstrual dysfunction and bone mineral disorders such as osteoporosis. It is clear that secondary amenorrhea is associated with malnutrition and eating disorders. Furthermore, bone mineral disorders are related to menstrual dysfunction. Eating disorders, or disordered eating, may represent the initiating factor of this triad.

Bibliography

Nattiv, A. and Lynch, L. (1994). The female athlete triad. *The Physician and Sportsmedicine* 22(1), 60-68.

West, R.V. (1998). The female athlete. The triad of disordered eating, amenorrhea and osteoporosis. *Sports Medicine* 26(2), 63-71.

Yeager, K.K. et al (1993). The female athlete triad: Disordered eating, amenorrhea, osteoporosis (commentary). *Medicine and Science in Sports and Exercise* 25(7), 775-777.

FEMINISM   *See under* GENDER.

FEMORAL NECK   The femoral neck has two angular relationships with the femoral shaft that are important for hip joint function: the neck-to-shaft angle and femoral version.

The **neck-to-shaft angle** is the angle of inclination of the neck to the shaft in the frontal plane.. It facilitates freedom of motion of the hip joint. It offsets the femoral shaft from the pelvis laterally. The neck-to-shaft angle is normally 125 degrees, but it can vary from 90 to 135 degrees. Deviation of the femoral shaft in either way alters the force relationships about the hip joint. **Coxa valga** is a neck-to-shaft angle that is greater than 125 degrees. With such an angle, the leg length is increased, the abductor muscles are less effective, there is increased load on the femoral head, and decreased load on the femoral neck. In normal children, it is associated with upward, anterior dislocations of the hip. The condition is nearly always congenital and is often called **congenital dislocation of the hip**. It is the fourth most common orthopedic birth defect. Many nonambulatory persons with severe disability develop coxa valga between ages of 2 and 10 years. In this condition, the head of the femur is usually displaced upward and posteriorly. Casting, bracing and surgery are used for correction.

Coxa vara is a neck-to-shaft angle that is less than 125 degrees. With such an angle, leg length is shortened, the abductor muscles are more effective, there is a lesser load on the femoral head, but more load on the femoral neck. It is more common than coxa valga, and can be either congenital or acquired. In the acquired form, the epiphysis of the femoral head slips down and backward, making the angulation of the femoral neck more horizontal. It may be called either **slipped capital femoral epiphysis** or **adolescent coxa vara**, and is more common in males than females. It is the most common hip disorder in adolescents. It is usually an overuse injury that probably occurs secondary to chronic microtrauma to the physis (from shear forces) during the adolescent growth spurt. Avascular necrosis and chondrolysis may ensue with risk of secondary osteoarthritis. The causation may be a combination of genetic, biomechanical and hormonal influences. If identified early, this condition is usually treated by several weeks of abstention from weight bearing. If the condition is allowed to progress, bracing and surgery may be required to correct it.

Femoral version is the angle between the femoral neck and a line between the two femoral condyles in the transverse plane. This angle usually projects anteriorly, thus is referred to as **femoral anteversion (angle of anteversion)**. In an adult, the femoral neck is typically rotated anteriorly by 10 to 15 degrees with respect to the femur. Excessive femoral anteversion is associated with a tendency toward internal rotation of the leg during gait to keep the femoral head in the acetabular cavity. Children with anteversion tend to sit with their feet outside them ('W' sitting) and walk with their toes turned in, but they would find it difficult to sit cross-legged. Other adjustments to excessive femoral anteversion include: an increase in Q-angle, patellar problems, greater pronation at the subtalar joint, and lumbar lordosis. **Femoral retroversion** occurs when femoral version projects posteriorly; there is a tendency toward external rotation of the leg during gait. Children with retroversion can sit with their legs crossed and walk with their toes turned. Femoral version is common in children, but is usually outgrown.

See also under AGING; HIP JOINT, DISLOCATION.

Bibliography

Ask Dr. Chris. Http://guardian.curtin.edu.au:16080/cga/faq/torsion.html

Levangie, P.K. and Norkin, C.C. (2001). *Joint structure and function: A comprehensive analysis.* 3rd ed. Philadelphia, PA: F.A. Davis Co.

Merck Manual of Diagnosis and Therapy. Http://www.merck.com

FEMORAL NECK STRESS FRACTURES   An injury that occurs secondary to repetitive microtrauma and is often seen in runners with persistent groin pain. There are two types of stress fractures of the femoral neck: distraction and compression. The **distraction type** occurs as a transverse fracture and involves the superior part of the femoral neck. This area is under tension and displacement may occur. The **compression type** involves the inferomedial femoral neck. This area is under compression and displacement may occur. Femoral neck stress fractures occur more frequently in the thin, amenorrheic athlete involved in running or endurance sport.

FEMORAL NERVE   Formed from the posterior portions of the ventral rami of L2, L3 and L4, the femoral nerve passes between the *iliopsoas* muscles. It enters the thigh deep to the inguinal ligament, which is the upper border of the **femoral triangle**. The other boundaries of the femoral triangle are (laterally) the *sartorius* muscle and (medially) the *adductor longus* muscle. In the triangle, the femoral nerve divides into 5 motor branches to the four muscles of the *quadriceps femoris* muscles and also the *sartorius* muscle. It also divides into 2 sensory branches, the saphenous (supplying the skin of the medial leg) and the lateral femoral cutaneous nerves (supplying the skin of the anterolateral thigh). The femoral nerve is not commonly entrapped at any particular site along its course, and is rarely injured in sports.

FEMORAL TORSION   A femur that is anterverted will also be subjected to torsion at the knee joint. *See under* FEMORAL NECK.

FEMORAL VALGUS   A misalignment in which the femur tends outwards from its proximal to distal end. There is tensile stress on the medial side of the hip joint and the lateral side of the knee joint. It thus manifests as a bow-legged posture. It is usually congenital rather than mechanically induced, and therefore little can be done to correct it by strength or flexibility training. Rear-foot valgus may arise in order to compensate for femoral valgus with the result that a tensile stress is placed on the medial side of the ankle and subtalar joints. Athletes with bowed legs are predisposed to injuries in the patellar region and also to iliotibial band friction syndrome. Femoral valgus is often found with tibial varus.

FEMORAL VARUS   A misalignment in which the femur tends inwards from its proximal to distal end. There is tensile stress on the lateral side of the hip joint and on the medial side of the knee joint. It thus manifests as a knock-kneed posture. It tends to occur in females more frequently than males, and is possibly related to the wider pelvis of females. Femoral varus affects the Q-angle. A tibial valgus may arise to help compensate for a femoral varus.

FEMUR   The longest and strongest bone in the body. The medial slant of the femur serves to place the center of the knee joint more closely under the center of motion of the hip joint. Hence the mechanical axis of the femur (a line connecting the center of the femoral head with the center of the knee joint) is almost vertical. *See also* EPIPHYSEAL GROWTH PLATE; EPIPHYSIS.

FERRITIN   *See under* IRON.

FETAL ALCOHOL SYNDROME   A condition caused by alcohol in the mother's blood being passed directly through the placenta to the fetus. The fetus does not have any ethanol oxidizing or alcohol dehydrogenase capacities. More than 80% of children with fetal alcohol syndrome demonstrate prenatal and postnatal growth deficiency, mild to moderate mental retardation, microcephaly, infantile irritability, and characteristic facial features. 50% of affected individuals also have poor coordination, hypotonia, attention-deficit disorders with hyperactivity, decreased adipose tissue, and other identifiable facial features. 20 to 50% of affected children demonstrate a variety of other birth defects, including cardiac abnormalities, hemangiomas, and eye and ear anomalies.

Up to 10 times the number of babies who are born with fetal alcohol syndrome are born with lesser degrees of alcohol-related damage. This condition is termed **fetal alcohol effects**. Many of the same symptoms are observed in children with fetal alcohol effects, but less severely so than fetal alcohol syndrome.

Alcohol is the leading known cause of birth defects and mental retardation in the USA. The rate of children born with fetal alcohol syndrome increased from 1 per 10,000 births in 1979 to 6.7 per 10,000 births in 1993. Worldwide incidence of fetal alcohol syndrome is 1.9 per 1,000 live births. However, when children with less severe manifestations of the syndrome (fetal alcohol effects) are included, the estimated incidence may be as great as 1 in 300 live births. Fetal alcohol syndrome occurs in up to 40% of the babies born to women who are alcoholics or chronic alcohol abusers; this includes binge drinking (five or more drinks on one occasion). The American Academy of Pediatrics recommends abstinence from all alcohol consumption for women who are pregnant or who are planning a pregnancy. Fetal alcohol syndrome is also associated with paternal alcoholism. Prenatal alcohol exposure does not always result in fetal alcohol syndrome, but there is no known safe level of alcohol consumption during pregnancy. It has been found that mothers of children with fully expressed fetal alcohol syndrome drink alcohol more, and drink earlier in gestation, than those with infants without fully expressed clinical features. Mothers who only drink later in gestation have an increased frequency of premature deliveries and deliveries of babies small for gestational age.

See also under COCAINE.

Bibliography

American Academy of Pediatrics. Http://www.aap.org

American Academy of Pediatrics (1993). Fetal alcohol syndrome and fetal alcohol effects. *Pediatrics* 91(5), 1004-1006.

National Organization on Fetal Alcohol Syndrome. Http://www.nofas.org

FETUS   The developing human from 3 months to birth.

FEVER   Any body temperature above normal body temperature. **Normal body temperature** is 37 degrees Celsius. **Hyperthermic fever** involves a body temperature of at least 42 degrees Celsius. It often results from infection, but it may be caused by other conditions such as allergic reactions or cancer.

White blood cells, injured tissue cells and macrophages release pyrogens (cytokines; most notably interleukin-1) that act on the hypothalamus, causing the release of prostaglandins. The prostaglandins, in turn, reset the hypothalamus thermoregulatory set point to a higher temperature, causing the body to initiate its heat-raising mechanisms. Due to vasoconstriction, heat loss from the body surface declines, the skin cools and shivering begins to generate heat. The temperature increases until it reaches the new setting, and then body temperature is maintained at the 'fever setting'

until immune systems overcome the disease process. The set point is then reset to a lower (or normal) level that triggers the heat loss mechanisms. Sweating begins and the skin becomes flushed and warm.

Fever, by increasing the metabolic rate, helps speed the various healing processes, and it also appears to inhibit bacterial growth. But fever may be dangerous, because if body temperature remains or rises above a certain point, proteins may be denatured and permanent brain damage may occur.

FIBER   Dietary fiber. *See under* CARBOHYDRATE.

FIBERGLASS   *See under* COMPOSITES.

FIBRIN   *See under* BLOOD CLOTTING.

FIBRINOGEN   *See under* BLOOD CLOTTING.

FIBROBLAST   *See under* CONNECTIVE TISSUE.

FIBROCYTE   *See under* CONNECTIVE TISSUE.

FIBROMYALGIA SYNDROME   It is a chronic pain syndrome with musculoskeletal stiffness and soft tissue tender points. It is associated with fatigue, sleep disturbance, and many other problems such as irritable bowel, headaches and cognitive impairments. It affects an estimated 2 to 4% of the general population, with most patients aged between 40 and 60 years and about 90% being women.

Diagnostically characterized a non-articular form of rheumatism, fibromyalgia syndrome is now considered a separate syndrome from chronic fatigue syndrome. However, there appears to be considerable overlap between chronic fatigue syndrome and the fibromyalgia syndrome in terms of diagnostic criteria.

There are many theories of the etiology of fibromyalgia syndrome, but no conclusive support for any one theory. Light aerobic exercise on a daily basis may be of benefit, but excess, or the wrong kind, of exercise may exacerbate symptoms.

Bibliography

The American Fibromyalgia Syndrome Association. Http://www.afsafund.org

The National Fibromyalgia Research Association. Http://www.nfra.net

FIBROSIS   Formation of fibrous tissue as a reparative or reactive process, as opposed to formation of fibrous tissue as a normal constituent of an organ or tissue. *See* CYSTIC FIBROSIS.

FIBULA   *See under* LOWER LEG.

FICK PRINCIPLE   *See under* CARDIAC OUTPUT; OXYGEN UPTAKE.

FICK'S LAW   *See under* GAS DIFFUSION.

FIGHT OR FLIGHT RESPONSE   *See under* AUTONOMIC NERVOUS SYSTEM.

FIGURE-GROUND PERCEPTION   The ability to separate an object of visual regard from its surroundings.

FILTRATION   Movement of solutes due to a pressure gradient. It is the process by which water and solutes are forced through a membrane or capillary wall by hydrostatic pressure.   Blood pressure moves solutes from the high pressure in plasma to the lower pressure in interstitial fluid or the kidney nephron. This separates small and large molecules.

FINITE-ELEMENT MODELLING   An engineering/mathematical method that makes use of simple shapes, which are assembled to form complex geometrical structures. In a model, a finite number of elements are connected at nodes to form mathematical representations of a structure such as bone. In a computer simulation, equations derived from the model can be used to predict the stress and strain responses to loading.

Bibliography

Nahum, A.M. and Melvin, J.W. (1993, eds). *Accidental injury:*

Biomechanics and prevention. New York: Springer Verlag.

FITNESS   *See* EVOLUTION; PHYSICAL FIT-NESS.

FIXATOR   *See under* MUSCLE ACTION.

FLAIL CHEST   Paradoxical movement of a segment of the chest wall caused by a significant force diffused over a large area that results in fractures of three or more ribs anteriorly and posteriorly within each rib. The actual motion of the flail segment is usually limited by the surrounding structural components, the intercostals and the surrounding musculature. Respiratory insufficiency in flail chest is much more likely to result from the underlying severity of pulmonary contusion and ventilation-perfusion mismatch than the actual structural defect to the chest wall.

FLAT FEET   Pes planus. **True flat feet** is the most serious of foot defects in which the longitudinal arch is flat and the foot pronated. It may be acquired or congenital, and is common in children with visual impairments (probably due to their shuffling gait) and children who are obese.

Such a foot may have lax ligaments and poor muscle support, resulting in excessive medial movement of the talonavicular joint. This causes many problems arising from excessive and prolonged pronation and a loose foot (instead of a rigid foot) during the take-off phase of running. True flat feet is diagnosed as first, second or third degree depending on whether the navicular is 1, 2 or 3 inches from its correct position. Treatment can involve strengthening exercise (especially supination and inversion), stretching (of muscles and connective tissues on the lateral aspect of the foot) and orthotics.

Functional (physiologic) flat feet is a defect caused by weakened and stretched muscles, ligaments and fascia in the foot. 97% of children younger than 2 years have varying degrees of flat foot, but only 4% of 10-year old children are flat footed. Thus there is considerable spontaneous correction of flat feet. Physiologic pes planus does not need any treatment; orthotics have no role. **Flexible (postural) flat feet** is characterized by a loss of the arches during weight bearing only. **False flat feet** is a condition resulting from the presence of a fat pad on the plantar surface of the feet.

FLATUS   Intestinal gas that is a natural by-product of digestion. Most people pass between 200 and 2000 ml of gas per day, mainly through the anus. People with hemorrhoids and hence tight sphincters have louder flatus than those with lax sphincters. **Flatulence** refers to the presence of gas in the gut as a result of swallowing air (**aerophagia**) while eating or drinking, decreased intestinal transit time and excessive bacterial fermentation. Most swallowed air is subsequently belched, and only a small amount passes into the small bowel. Flatus arises from decreased transit, because there is not sufficient time for the absorption of gases by the colon. Foods that produce flatus contain nutrients that are incompletely digested by human intestinal enzymes. Insoluble fiber found in wheat bran and some vegetables passes essentially unchanged through the intestines and produces little gas. Fats and proteins cause little gas. Soluble fiber, found in oat bran, beans, peas and most fruit, is not broken down until it reaches the large intestine where digestion causes gas. They pass into the colon where they produce flatus from bacterial fermentations. The composition of flatus depends on the origin. The presence of oxygen and nitrogen in flatus indicates aerophagia; hydrogen, ammonia, carbon dioxide and methane indicate bacterial fermentation. Nitrogen usually predominates and most of it is accounted for by diffusion from the blood to bowel. It is unclear whether carbon dioxide is a direct or indirect product of bacterial metabolism. A more important source is the reaction of bicarbonate and hydrogen ions. Carbon dioxide can account for up to 50 to 60% of the gas in flatus, usually in association with hydrogen. Large amounts of disaccharides, such as lactose, are passed to the colon and fermented to hydrogen. Methane is produced by bacterial fermentation of endogenous substances in the colon. The rate at which methane is produced depends only minimally on food ingestion. The tendency to produce large quantities of methane appears to be familial, appearing during infancy and persisting through the lifespan.

FLAVIN ADENINE DINUCLEOTIDE   *See* FAD.

FLAVIN MONONUCLEOTIDE   FMN. It is a coenzyme synthesized from riboflavin, and acts as a component of Complex I of the electron transport chain.

FLAVONOIDS   *See under* PHYTOCHEMICALS.

FLEXIBILITY   The range of movement possible around a joint or a series of joints. Flexibility is determined by the shape and size of the bones, the strength and insertion of muscles and the elasticity of ligaments, tendons and other connective tissues. Flexibility can be improved (or maintained) by stretching the muscles and connective tissues that surround the joint. Tissue with low stiffness has a high ability to be stretched easily. Tissue with a low damping ratio has a poor ability to absorb tensile shocks. Tissue with low tissue stiffness and low damping ratio is at risk of overload injury.

Passive flexibility is the degree to which a joint can be moved as a result of passive movement. Static flexibility should not be confused with joint laxity that is a function of the joint capsule and ligaments. **Active flexibility** is the degree to which a joint can be moved as a result of active movement. Active flexibility is more strongly related to sporting performance than passive flexibility. Passive flexibility provides a protective reserve if a joint is unexpectedly stressed beyond its normal operational limits. Combined strength and stretching exercises are more effective in developing dynamic flexibility.

While increased flexibility is important for performance in some sports that rely on extremes of motion for movement, decreased flexibility may actually increase economy of movement in sports that emphasize use of the mid-portion of the range of movement.

In the 1940s and 1950s, many athletes refrained from weightlifting, because it was believed that such resistance training would slow them down and increase muscle size to the point that they became 'muscle bound.' This myth was dispelled by research over the next decade that showed that weight training did not have negative effects on speed or flexibility. In fact, most athletes who perform exercises correctly, through the full range of movement, have exceptional flexibility and strength gains, which are associated with significant gains in speed of movement.

Flexibility may be measured directly or indirectly. Direct methods include use of a goniometer, Leighton flexometer, electrogoniometer or radiography. The **goniometer** consists of a 180-degree protractor. The center of the goniometer is positioned at the axis of rotation of the joint and the arms of the goniometer are aligned with the long axis of the two bones of the joint being measured. Problems with goniometry include identifying the axis of movement and positioning of the goniometer arms. The **Leighton Flexometer** consists of a gravity needle and a strap attachment for the limb. It overcomes the problems associated with the goniometer, because neither the axis of rotation of the joint nor the long axis of the bones needs to be identified. It is a reliable instrument, but it does not adequately distinguish between hip and back flexibility. An **electrogoniometer** is a goniometer with a potentiometer located at its axis of rotation so that as the angle between the goniometer arms changes, the amount of electrical current output to a recorder changes. An electrogoniometer records displacement and velocity during movement, and can thus be used to measure dynamic flexibility. **Radiography**, possibly the most valid technique, has practical problems such as radioactive exposure. Indirect methods usually involve linear measures of distances between two bones or from an external object. An example is the 'sit and reach test' used to measure flexibility of the back and hamstring muscles. Such tests are useful for comparing the flexibility of the same person over time, but not for comparing the flexibility of different people. This is because the measures are affected by anthropometric variables such as limb length.

See also HYPERFLEXIBILITY; HYPO-FLEXIBILITY; STRETCHING.

Bibliography

Alter, M.J. (2004). *Science of flexibility*. 3ʳᵈ ed. Champaign, IL: Human Kinetics.

Gleim, G. and McHugh, M.P. (1997). Flexibility and its effect on sports injury and performance. *Sports Medicine* 24(5), 289-299.

Hubley-Kozey, C.L. (1991). Testing flexibility. In: MacDougall, J.D., Wenger, H.A. and Green, H.J. (eds). *Physiological testing of the high performance athlete*. 2ⁿᵈ ed. pp309-359. Champaign, IL: Human Kinetics.

Siff, M.C. (2000). Biomechanical foundations of strength and power training. In Zatsiorsky, V. (ed). *Biomechanics in sport. Performance enhancement and injury prevention. Vol. IX of the Encyclopedia of Sports Medicine*. pp103-139. Oxford: Blackwell Science.

FLEXION   It is anterior movement for the head, trunk, upper extremity and hip, but it is a posterior movement for the knee, ankle (plantar flexion) and toes.

FLEXION RELAXATION RESPONSE   *See under* LUMBAR-PELVIC RHYTHM.

FLEXOR REFLEX   Withdrawal reflex. It is a reflex that is triggered by a variety of receptors, especially in response to pain and is a means of self-protection. Afferent neurons from nociceptors transmit information to the spinal cord, where they have excitatory synapses or interneurons, which then excite efferent neurons that innervate skeletal muscles that cause withdrawal of limb or other body part. Activity in flexor reflex afferents results in activation of all flexors in the limb to withdraw it from the potentially damaging stimulus. During the flexor reflex, extensor muscles of the opposite limb are activated via glutaminergic excitatory interneurons. This gives rise to the **crossed extensor reflex**, which ensures support of the body during withdrawal. The flexor reflex can be suppressed by descending activity if the affected limb must be used for support at the same time.

FLOW   i) In fluid mechanics, it is the forward continuous movement of a fluid through closed or open channels or conduits. *See* BLOOD VISCOSITY. ii) In psychology, an altered state of consciousness that typically occurs when there is a balance between the perceived challenges of a situation and a person's perceived skills or capabilities. The nine scales of the Flow State Scale are: challenge-skill balance, action-awareness merging, clear goals, unambiguous feedback, concentration on the task at hand, sense of control, loss of self consciousness, transformation of time and autotelic (intrinsically-rewarding) experience. Following Csikszentmihalyi's (1990) discussion of enjoyment and flow as an optimal experience that is intrinsically rewarding and autotelic (i.e. doing the activity is the reward), Kimieck and Harris (1996) defined enjoyment as an optimal psychological state that leads to performing an activity primarily for its own sake and is associated with positive feeling states. *See also under* PEAK EXPERIENCE; STRESS.

Bibliography

Csikszentmihalyi, M. (1990). *Flow: The psychology of optimal experience*. New York: Harper and Row.

Jackson, S.A. and Marsh, H.W. (1996). Development and validation of a scale to measure optimal experience: The Flow State Scale. *Journal of Sport & Exercise Psychology* 18, 17-35.

Jackson, S.A. and Csikszentmihalyi, M. (1999). *Flow in sports*. Champaign, IL: Human Kinetics.

Kimiecik, J.C. and Stein, G.L. (1992). Examining flow experiences in sport contexts: conceptual issues and methodological concerns. *Journal of Applied Sport Psychology* 4, 144-160.

Kimiecik, J.C and Harris, A.T. (1996). What is enjoyment? A conceptual/definitional analysis with implications for sport and exercise psychology. *Journal of Sport & Exercise Psychology* 18, 247-263.

FLUID Any substance that can flow, i.e. liquids and gases. Fluidity is the reciprocal of viscosity.

FLUID FRICTION Friction appertaining to the relative movement of a solid over a fluid. It is proportional to the speed of motion and the area of the surface of contact.

FLUID REPLACEMENT This is necessary during exercise to counteract dehydration. The American College of Sports Medicine (1996) recommends that athletes ingest about 500 mL of fluid 2 hours before exercise to ensure adequate hydration. It is wise for athletes to drink an additional 250 to 500 mL of fluid on particularly hot days. During exercise, athletes should start drinking early, and at regular intervals, in an attempt to consume fluids at a rate that is sufficient to replace all the water that is lost through sweating.

Obligatory urine losses persist after exercise, even in the dehydrated state, because of the need for elimination of metabolic waste products. Respiratory and transcutaneous losses also contribute to an ongoing loss of water from the body. The volume of fluid consumed after exercise-induced or thermal sweating must therefore be greater than the volume of sweat lost if effective rehydration is to be achieved (Shirreffs et al, 2004). This contradicts the earlier recommendation that after exercise athletes should match fluid intake exactly to the measured body mass loss.

The temperature of the ingested fluid should be between 15 and 22 degrees Celsius. According to Maughan and Rehrer (1993), starting with a large fluid bolus, and repeatedly ingesting additional amounts so as to maintain a high volume of liquid in the stomach, will lead to a greater water and carbohydrate delivery to the small intestine. There are individual differences in tolerance of large volumes of water in the stomach, but there may be a training effect that allows larger volumes to be consumed without problems. Ingestion of increased volumes of drinks immediately prior to and during exercise should therefore be practiced during training.

Carbohydrate-electrolyte beverages ('sports drinks') are formulated to provide fluid, carbohydrates and electrolytes before, during and after exercise. The ideal fluid replacement beverage for exercise in the heat is one that can simultaneously deliver an optimal combination of carbohydrate and fluid. There are four situations in which consuming sports drinks appears to be superior to water: i) if a carbohydrate deficiency exists in blood, liver or muscle (this most often occurs during single exercise sessions lasting longer than one hour); ii) when exercise is strenuous (greater than 70% maximal oxygen uptake) and lasts longer than 50 to 60 minutes (there is very little evidence that carbohydrates in fluids affect performance when exercise lasts less than 50 to 60 minutes, regardless of intensity); iii) if a sodium or sodium chloride deficiency exists; and iv) if it is necessary to rapidly replace lost plasma water after exercise, at a rate faster than can be provided by normal meals.

Variables that can be manipulated to alter the functional characteristics of a sports drink include: carbohydrate content (concentration and type); osmolality; electrolyte composition; and concentration, flavoring components and other active ingredients (e.g. caffeine).

Increasing the carbohydrate content of drinks will increase the amount of fuel that can be supplied, but it will tend to decrease the rate at which water can be made available. The choice of beverage composition will thus be influenced by the relative importance of the need to supply fuel and water. This in turn depends on the intensity and duration of the exercise task, on the ambient temperature and humidity, and on the physiological and biochemical characteristics of the individual athlete. During a slow cross-country ski tour, sweat losses will be small and fluid replacement will be secondary to carbohydrate supply. Carbohydrate content can be as high as 10 to 15%. On a hot and humid day, fluid replacement takes priority. A hypotonic or isotonic solution should be used and carbohydrate content should not exceed 5 to 6%.

Gastric emptying rate refers to the rate at which fluid empties from the stomach. The maximum amount of fluid that empties from the stomach during exercise is 0.8 to 1.2 l/h in most athletes. In exercise of up to 70% of maximal oxygen uptake, gastric emptying rate is controlled by normal nutritional and physiological factors. Even at higher intensities, there is little evidence to suggest that the decrease is sufficient reason to avoid fluid ingestion during exercise. In exhausting endurance exercise, 30 to 50% of participants may suffer gastrointestinal symptom(s) such as a stomach ache, vomiting and heartburn. Such symptoms may be caused by pre-exercise ingestion of foods rich in dietary fiber, protein and fat and strongly hypertonic drinks. A

significant disruption of acid-base balance leads to a decreased gastric emptying rate. Stress and anxiety, leading to the secretion of catecholamines, beta-endorphins and some gastrointestinal hormones, cause a decreased gastric emptying rate. Dehydration leads to decreased gastric emptying rate and increased risk of gastrointestinal distress.

The primary determinant of gastric emptying rate is the volume of the drink. The volume of ingested fluid is critical for both rapid gastric emptying and complete rehydration. In the 1980s, the observation that the addition of carbohydrate to water temporarily slowed gastric emptying rate was interpreted to suggest that fluid replacement solutions should not contain much carbohydrate. It is now understood that the slight slowing of gastric emptying caused by solutions containing up to 8% carbohydrate is a relatively minor factor in fluid replacement rate compared with the large influence of increased fluid volume for increasing gastric emptying and fluid replacement rate.

Carbonation and temperature of ingested drinks do not have a major influence on gastric emptying.

The osmolality of ingested fluids is important as this can influence the rates of both gastric emptying and intestinal water flux and thus determine the effectiveness of fluids at delivering water for rehydration. Increasing the osmolality of the gastric contents will tend to delay gastric emptying. Increasing the carbohydrate or electrolyte content of sports drinks will generally result in an increased osmolality. The composition of the drinks and the nature of the solutes are, however, of greater importance than the osmolality itself. Although most of the popular sports drinks are formulated to have an osmolality close to that of body fluids, and are promoted as 'isotonic' drinks, there is evidence that hypotonic solutions are more effective when rapid rehydration is required. Although it is argued that a higher osmolality is inevitable when adequate amounts of carbohydrate are to be included in sports drinks, the optimum amount of carbohydrate necessary to improve exercise performance has not been clearly established. Hypertonic beverages may inhibit diffusion of water out of the intestinal lumen, leading to discomfort or diarrhea.

Beverages containing 4 to 8% solutions of glucose polymers (maltodextrins), glucose and other simple sugars seem to have suitable gastric emptying characteristics for optimizing fluid and energy delivery during prolonged exercise, with no adverse effects. There is some evidence that substitution of glucose polymers for free glucose results in a decreased osmolality for the same carbohydrate content and may increase the volume of fluid and the amount of substrate delivered to the intestine. This has led to the inclusion of glucose polymers of varying chain lengths in the formulation of sports drinks.

Small amounts (i.e. 2 to 3%) of fructose in beverages seem to speed up the gastric emptying rate more than the same (calorific) amount of glucose. High concentrations (at least 10%) of fructose, however, can cause gastrointestinal problems both at rest and during exercise.

60% of fluid absorption occurs in the small intestine. An optimal concentration of carbohydrate, especially in the form of glucose in conjunction with sodium, will stimulate absorption. Sodium will stimulate sugar and water uptake in the small intestine, and will help to maintain the volume of extracellular fluid. High sodium content, although it may stimulate jejunal absorption of glucose and water, tends to make drinks unpalatable. Sodium should be included in fluids consumed during exercise lasting longer than 2 hours of by individuals during any event that stimulates heavy sodium loss (more than 3 to 4 g of sodium). In terms of replacing the sodium lost in sweat as well as the water, it might be suggested that rehydration drinks should have a sodium concentration similar to that of sweat. The sodium content of sweat varies widely, however. No single formulation will meet this requirement for all individuals in all situations. Sports drinks commonly contain 10 to 25 mmol/l; oral rehydration solutions intended for use in the treatment of diarrhea-induced dehydration, which may be fatal, have higher sodium concentrations, in the range of 30 to 90 mmol/l. Most soft drinks, such as cola, contain virtually no sodium (1 to 2 mmol/l).

Potassium is also included in sports drinks in concentrations similar to those in sweat, but unlike sodium there is no strong scientific evidence for its inclusion. There is no evidence for the inclusion of any other electrolytes. There is insufficient theoretical rationale or data to recommend inclusion of protein in solutions ingested during exercise.

Oxygenated waters have become commercially available. It is doubtful whether 'superoxygenated water' can add oxygen to the blood or muscle.

See also GLYCEROL; HYPONATREMIA.

Chronology

•1934 • The drink "Barley Water" was available for players during the world's foremost tennis championship at Wimbledon.

•1967 • Stokeley-Van Camp acquired the rights to sell Gatorade in the USA. It became the global leader in the sports drink sector. It was named after an American College Football team, the Florida Gators who used a carbohydrate-electrolyte drink designed by Robert Cade from the University of Florida, during half-time of the Miami Orange Bowl playoff. The Gators came from behind to win the playoff against the number one team, Georgia Tech. In 1983, Gatorade was bought by Quaker Oats Co, now a wholly owned subsidiary of Pepsi Co, Inc.

•1985 • World champion decathlete Daley Thompson of the UK promoted Smith Kline Beecham's Lucozade as a beverage for everyday energy replacement. Shortly after the emergence of pioneering sports drinks, such as Dexters in 1986, Lucozade was promoted as a sports drink. Lucozade was launched as Glucozade in 1927. Formulated by a pharmacist in Newcastle (UK), it was promoted as a source of glucose energy for sick children.

•1997 • A survey by the Food Commission of 22 popular sports and energy drinks marketed in the UK found that nearly all the products were high in sugar (up to fifteen level teaspoons per serving) yet only 5 out of 22 stated how much sugar they contained. SmithKline Beecham, manufacturers of Lucozade products, told the researchers that this information was 'confidential.' (*The Food Magazine*, November 1997)

•1998 • An analysis of the sports nutrition market, excluding sports drinks, revealed that six manufacturing companies, representing 56% of the market, had annual sales of $10 to $80 million, with the rest of the market comprised of 94 other companies. The sports drink market was dominated by Gatorade (85%), while Pepsi's All Sport and Coca-Cola's Powerade each had 12% of the sales.

Bibliography

American College of Sports Medicine (1996). Position stand on exercise and fluid replacement. *Medicine and Science in Sports and Exercise* 28(1), i-vii.

Armstrong, L.E. (2000). *Performing in extreme environments*. Champaign, IL: Human Kinetics.

Coyle, E. (2004). Fluid and fuel intake during exercise. *Journal of Sports Sciences* 22, 39-55.

Gisolfi, C.V. and Duchman, S.M. (1992). Guidelines for optimal replacement beverages for different athletic events. *Medicine and Science in Sports and Exercise* 24(6), 679-87.

Hawley, J.A., Dennis, S.C. and Noakes, T.D. (1992). Oxidation of carbohydrate ingested during prolonged endurance exercise. *Sports Medicine* 14(1), 27-42.

Maughan, R.J. and Rehrer, N.J. (1993). Gastric emptying during exercise. *Gatorade Sports Science Exchange* 46(6).

Maughan, R.J. (1998). The sports drink as a functional food: Formulations for successful performance. *Proceedings of the Nutrition Society* 57, 15-23.

Maughan, R.J. and Noakes, T.D. (1991). Fluid replacement and exercise stress: A brief review of studies on fluid replacement and some guidelines for the athlete. *Sports Medicine* 12(1), 16-31.

Maughan, R. et al (1993). Fluid replacement in sport and exercise. A consensus statement. *British Journal of Sports Medicine* 27(1), 345.

Millard-Stafford, M. (1992). Fluid replacement during exercise in the heat. Review and recommendations. *Sports Medicine* 13(4), 223-233.

Murray, R. (1987). The effects of consuming carbohydrate-electrolyte beverages on gastric emptying and fluid absorption during and following exercise. *Sports Medicine* 4, 322-351.

Noakes, T.D. (1993). Fluid replacement during exercise. *Exercise and Sport Sciences Reviews* 21, 297-330.

Porcari, J.P. et al. (2002). Effects of superoxygenated water on exercise performance and recovery. *Medicine and Science in Sports and Exercise* 34, S295.

Shi, X. and Gisolfi, C.V. (1998). Fluid and carbohydrate replacement during intermittent exercise. *Sports Medicine* 25(3), 157-172.

Shirreffs, S.M., Armstrong, L.E. and Cheuvront, S.M. (2004). Fluid and electrolyte needs for preparation and recovery from training and competition. *Journal of Sports Sciences* 22, 57-63.

FLUORINE An element, which, as a 'trace element' in its ionized form (fluoride), is primarily deposited in the skeletal system, especially the teeth, where its major function is the prevention of dental caries. Bones and teeth contain 99% of the body fluoride. **Dental caries** is evidence of tooth decay on any surface of a tooth. Tooth decay can cause pain and lead to infections in surrounding tissues. Periodontal diseases include **gingivitis** and **periodontitis**, which are both inflammatory conditions of the **gingival tissues** (gum tissues around the teeth). In severe forms, periodontitis includes loss of supporting bone tissue, which can lead to tooth loss. Regular teeth cleaning by a dentist or dental hygienist helps prevent periodontal diseases.

The main dietary source of fluoride is water. **Fluoridation status** refers to the status of a community water system with regard to water fluoridation level. Most water contains some amount of fluoride. The recommended amount of fluoride in water systems is 0.7 to 1.2 ppm, which is equivalent to 0.7 to 1.2 mg/L. Water systems are considered to be naturally fluoridated if they contain naturally occurring fluoride at least 0.7 ppm. The majority of municipal water supplies in the USA are artificially fluoridated. Excess fluoride can cause **fluoresis**, however; and severe fluoresis can weaken teeth. An adult male residing in a community with fluoridated water has an intake range from 1 to 3 mg/day.

The fluoride content of most foods is low (less than 0.05 mg/100 g). Rich sources of fluoride include tea and marine fish such as sardines that are consumed with their bones. Tea contains 0.1 to 0.6 mg of fluoride per 100 ml (3.5 fluid oz) serving. Sardines contain 0.2 to 0.4 mg of fluoride per 100 g (3.5 ounces).

Adequate intake levels are based on estimated intakes (0.05 mg/kg body weight), which have been shown to decrease the occurrence of dental caries most effectively without causing the unwanted side effect of tooth enamel mottling (dental fluorosis). The adequate intake for adults is 4 mg (males) and 3 mg (females).

Bibliography

Centers for Disease Control and Prevention. Http://www.cdc.gov

Oregon State University. The Linus Pauling Institute. Micronutrient Information Center. Http://lpi.oregonstate.edu/infocenter

FLUX   The flow of physical entities (e.g. a gas) across a given area or in a given direction. It may refer to the number of molecules crossing a membrane per unit time. ii) Discharge of a fluid material in large amount from a cavity or surface of the body. iii) Become liquid or fluid when heated.

FMN   *See* FLAVIN MONONUCLEOTIDE.

FOLIC ACID   *See under* VITAMIN B$_2$.

FOLLICLE-STIMULATING HORMONES   *See under* GONADOTROPIC HORMONES.

FOOD   Material containing nutritional substances. *See under* DIET; NUTRITION.

FOOT   The function of the two feet is to absorb shock, adapt to the underlying surface, keep the body balanced and enable locomotion. Shock absorption occurs through the flexion present in the hip and knee joints, in addition to the dorsal flexion at the ankle joint and pronation at the subtalar joint.
The foot can be divided into three parts; front (fore-foot), middle (mid-foot) and back (hind-foot; rear-foot). The **forefoot** comprises the five metatarsal bones and the fourteen phalanges. The big toe (hallux) has only two phalanges, one less than the other toes. The **midfoot** is composed of five of the seven tarsal bones: the navicular, cuboid and three cuneiform bones. The boundary between the midfoot and forefoot consists of five tarsometatarsal joints. **The hind-foot** consists of the talus (ankle bone) and the calcaneus (heel bone). The talus links the tibia and the fibula to the foot.
Ligaments and fascia of the foot include the **calcaneonavicular ('spring') ligament**, which is the bifurcated ligament that runs between the calcaneus, the navicular and cuboid bones and the plantar fascia. *See also under* OSSICLES.

FOOT, ARCHES   There are three arches formed by the tarsals and metatarsals: the lateral and medial longitudinal arches, and the transverse arch.
The **lateral longitudinal arch** is lower and flatter than the medial arch. It is composed of the calcaneus, cuboid and the fourth and fifth metatarsals, with the cuboid as the keystone. It provides support during weight bearing.
The **medial longitudinal arch** contributes dynamically to shock absorption. It runs across the calcaneus to the talus, navicular, cuneiform and first three metatarsals. It is much more mobile than the lateral arch. The **peroneal tendons** lie behind the lateral malleolus and contribute to dorsal flexion and pronation of the ankle joint. The **peroneus longus tendon** is one of the structures that create a dynamic sling supporting the longitudinal arches of the foot.
The **transverse arch** is at right angles to the longitudinal arches. It is composed of the cuneiforms, the cuboid and the five metatarsal bases. The wedge shapes of the cuneiforms help hold the transverse arch together. The transverse arch can support a significant portion of body weight during weight bearing. The bones act as beams for support of this arch, which flatten with weight bearing. The flattening of this arch causes the forefoot to spread out a considerable distance in a shoe, and thus it is important that a shoe can accommodate this spread.
The most common cause of **transverse arch collapse** is associated with stretching of the calcaneonavicular ('spring') ligament. This is caused by hyperpronation as a result of inadequate functioning of the supporting *tibialis posterior* muscle. This mechanism may also give rise to entrapment of the medial calcaneal nerve that passes from a deep connective tissue layer to a more superficial level at the inner edge of the heel where the thick heel skin meets the thinner skin on the medial side of the foot. Increased pressure from the shoes over this area is another cause of medial calcaneal nerve entrapment.

FOOT, COMPARTMENT SYNDROME   Exertional compartment syndrome. Foot compartment syndrome is a serious potential complication of foot crush injury, fractures, surgery, and vascular injury. Fasciotomy is indicated when compartment pressure exceeds 30 mmHg, or if compartment pressure is greater than 10 to 30 mmHg below diastolic pressure. There are nine compartments of the foot that can be classified into intrinsic, medial, central and lateral compartments.

Bibliography

Fulkerson, E., Razi, A. and Tejwani, N. (2003). Review: Acute compartment syndrome of the foot. *Foot and Ankle International* 24(2), 180-187.

FOOT DEFORMITIES *See* CLAW TOE; EQUINUS; FLAT FOOT; FOOT DROP; FOOT PRONATION; FOREFOOT VALGUS; FORE-FOOT VARUS; HALLUX RIGIDUS; HALLUX VALGUS; HAMMER TOE; MALLET TOE; MORTON'S NEUROMA; PES CAVUS; PLANTAR FLEXED FIRST RAY; REARFOOT VARUS; SYNDACTYLISM; TALIPES.

FOOT DROP Drop foot. *See under* GAIT.

FOOT, FRACTURES *See* ANKLE JOINT, INJURIES; FRIEBERG'S DISEASE; SEVER'S DISEASE; TARSAL FRACTURE; TIBIAL-FIBULAR FRACTURE.

FOOT GRASP REFLEX *See* BABINSKI REFLEX.

FOOT, MOVEMENTS The movement of **pronation**, when the foot is off the ground (i.e. non-weight bearing; open kinetic chain), consists of eversion, abduction and dorsal flexion. Since the talus is locked in the mortise, the calcaneus moves with respect to the talus. When the foot is on the ground (i.e. weight bearing; closed kinetic chain), pronation consists of eversion, adduction and plantar flexion. The talus moves on the calcaneus. The movement of **supination** is just the opposite, with inversion, adduction and plantar flexion in the non-weight bearing position, and inversion, abduction and dorsal flexion in the weight bearing position.

Eversion (movement of the sole of the foot outward so that the soles face away from each other) is the movement in the frontal plane in which the lateral border of the foot moves toward the leg in non-weight bearing, or the leg moves toward the foot in weight bearing as the calcaneus lies on its medial surface. Muscles that produce eversion are: *extensor digitorum longus, peroneus tertius, peroneus longus* and *peroneus brevis*. **Inversion** (movement of the sole of the foot inward so that the soles face toward each other) is the frontal plane movement, which occurs as the medial border of the foot moves toward the medial leg in non-weight bearing, or as the medial aspect of the leg moves toward the medial foot in weight bearing as the calcaneus lies on the lateral surface. Muscles that produce inversion are: *tibialis anterior, tibialis posterior, flexor digitorum longus, flexor hallucis longus* and *extensor hallucis longus*.

Abduction is the transverse plane movement, with the toes pointing out, which occurs with external rotation of the foot on the leg and lateral movement of the calcaneus in the non-weight bearing position, or internal rotation of the leg with respect to the calcaneus and medial movement of the talus in weight bearing. Muscles that produce abduction are: *peroneus longus* and *peroneus brevis*. **Adduction** is the transverse plane movement, with the toes pointing in, which occurs as the foot internally rotates on the leg in non-weight bearing and the calcaneus moves medially, or the leg externally rotates on the foot in weight bearing and the talus moves laterally. Muscles that produce adduction are: *flexor hallucis longus* and *extensor hallucis longus*.

Dorsal flexion (pulling the foot up towards the knee) is the sagittal plane movement that occurs as the calcaneus moves up on the talus in non-weight bearing, or as the talus moves down on the calcaneus in weight bearing. Muscles that produce dorsal flexion are: *tibialis anterior, extensor digitorum longus, peroneus tertius* and *extensor hallucis longus*. **Plantar flexion** (pointing the foot down) is the sagittal plane movement that occurs as the calcaneus moves distally while non-weight bearing, or as the talus moves proximally while weight bearing. Muscles that produce plantar flexion are: *tibialis posterior, gastrocnemius, plantaris, soleus, peroneus longus, peroneus brevis, flexor digitorum longus* and *flexor hallucis longus*.

See also ANKLE JOINT; FOOT, PRONATION; SUBTALAR JOINT.

FOOT PRONATION Pronation makes the foot more flexible and allows for irregularities in the running or walking surface and positional variations in the trunk. It is also an important factor in enabling the foot and leg to absorb and dissipate the force of impact while running. Excessive pronation (hyperpronation), however, is harmful and is often induced when a person runs in a toe-out position. The toe-out position may be caused by lateral rotation of the hip, tibial torsion or forefoot abduction. It causes the body's line of gravity to move from the initial contact point of the foot with the ground to the medial side of the foot as the person transfers weight forward. This causes a collapse of the medial side of the foot and puts undue stress on the muscles that support the arches of the foot. Excessive pronation that is not associated with the toed-out position may be caused by weakness in the structures supporting the medial arch, by an abnormally flat foot with little natural arch or (most commonly) by forefoot varus. Excessive pronation will have secondary effects on the lower extremities, such as an increased compensatory internal rotation of the tibia resulting in lower leg and knee problems. The degree of eversion, and therefore pronation, determines the degree of compensatory internal tibia rotation.

If excessive pronation continues for too long during the mid-support and take-off phases of running, overuse injury can develop. Training errors include running on cambered surfaces, running around a track in one direction, running on very hard surfaces, running on bumpy terrain, changing shoes, increasing distance too soon, increasing training speed too soon and excessive hill running. Increased pronation is associated with injuries such as medial tibial stress syndrome, tibialis posterior tendon injury, Achilles bursitis or tendon injury, patellofemoral disorders, iliotibial friction syndrome, lower extremity stress fractures, plantar fasciitis, posterior tibial tendon dysfunction, metatarsalgia and hallux valgus. Specific anatomic abnormalities and abnormal biomechanics of the lower extremity are not correlated with specific injuries on a predictable basis.

If excessive or prolonged pronation occurs in an athlete experiencing pain in the lower extremity, then orthotic shoe inserts may be indicated. There are three categories of **orthotic shoe inserts**: rigid, semi-rigid, and flexible or soft. Rigid inserts are designed primarily to control motion, whereas

flexible inserts provide relatively more cushioning. Semi-rigid inserts are typically used for athletes and offer both control of foot motion and shock-absorbing capacity.

Researchers in the running shoe business now recognize that some pronation is natural, and even necessary, in normal walking and running to transfer weight from the outside edge of the foot, where most people land, toward the foot's midline. Use of rigid devices, such as 'dual-density midsoles,' may do more harm than good.

As a foot deformity, pronation is usually acquired and can be cured, if identified early, through corrective shoes and exercises.

See also ANKLE JOINT; FLAT FEET; RUNNING INJURIES; SUBTALAR JOINT.

Bibliography

Gross, M.L. and Napoli, R.C. (1993). Treatment of lower extremity injuries with orthotic shoe inserts. An overview. *Sports Medicine* 15(1), 66-70.

Hintermann, B. and Nigg, B.M. (1998). Pronation in runners. Implications for injuries. *Sports Medicine* 26(3), 169-176.

Wright, K. (2000). Watching your steps. *Building the Elite Athlete (Scientific American, special issue)*, 52-57.

Stovitz, S.D. and Coetzee, J.C. (2004). Hyperpronation and foot pain. Steps toward pain-free feet. *The Physician and Sportsmedicine* 32(8). Http://www.physssportsmed.com

FOOTBALLER'S ANKLE Chronic periostitis or paratenonitis with calcification, and exostoses. It may occur on the anterior margin of the lower end of the tibia and over the talus as a result of repeated trauma, such as a football making contact with the dorsal and medial aspects of the foot.

FORCE The push or pull exerted upon a body or object. A force may set a body into motion, change the acceleration of a moving body or produce distortion, such as contraction of muscle to move bones. **An internal force** is a force that is developed from within the body, especially those produced by muscle contraction. An **external force (load)** is a force that is developed from outside the body. External forces of relevance to the biomechanics of sport are mainly gravity, friction and drag. Loads applied to the skeletal system in different directions may produce the following forces: compression, tension, bending, shear and torsion.

The Standard International unit is the newton. One newton (N) is a force that accelerates a 1 kg mass at a rate of 1 m/s². The US Customary unit is the pound force (lbf). 1 N = 0.225 lbf. 1 lbf = 4.448 N.

The measurement of muscle force in humans can be accomplished only with invasive techniques under appropriate medical conditions, involving either the attachment of a force transducer to a tendon or the insertion of an optic fiber through a tendon.

Stable equilibrium occurs if an object is displaced as a result of work done by a force and returns to its original position. **Unstable equilibrium** occurs if an object is displaced and tends to increase its displacement. **Neutral equilibrium** occurs if the object is displaced by a force and moves to a new position. In order for a body to be in **static equilibrium**, there must be no net force acting in any direction and there must be no net force about any point in the body (i.e. the sum of the moments of force in a clockwise direction about any point must equal the sum of moments in a counter-clockwise direction about that point). This is known as the **principle of moments**.

In solving equilibrium problems, a **free body diagram** is used to identify all the possible forces that could be acting on a body. The name refers to the fact that the body is 'freed' from its external contacts that are replaced by reaction forces. The **principle of transmissibility** states that, although the external effects of a force on a rigid body depend upon the magnitude and line of action of the force, it is independent of the point of application of the force. A **space diagram** is a simplified scale drawing of the part of the body of interest, used to estimate the relative position or orientation of the forces acting on the body. A **force diagram** is a scaled diagram in which forces, represented by vectors, may be added or subtracted. **Resolution of forces** is the separation of force into two or more components of force, which produce the same result as the single force. When the two components are at

90 degrees to each other they are called **rectangular components**. **Composition of forces** is the method of determining the single resultant force that would produce the same external effect as a number of separate forces. **Resultant (net) force** is the sum of all forces acting on the body. It is expressed as a single force that produces the same result or external effect on a body as a number of separate forces. **Equilibrium** is the condition when the resultant force and moment acting on a body are zero. **Equilibrium force** is the single force that would maintain the static equilibrium of a body. It is equal, but opposite, to the resultant force. When two forces act on a body at the same point, the resultant force will be the diagonal of a parallelogram drawn from the point of application and of which the two force vectors are sides. This is known as the **parallelogram of forces**. When, as the result of the action of a number of forces, a body is in equilibrium, the resultant of all the forces must be zero. When three non-parallel forces act upon a body in equilibrium their lines of action must intersect at a common point (the **point of concurrency**). There is no net turning effect at this point. When there are three forces that are not concurrent (i.e. only two of the forces intersect at a common point), the third force would produce a moment of force about this point. This would violate the conditions for equilibrium.

See also CENTRIPETAL FORCE; DRAG; ECCENTRIC FORCE; FORCE PLATE; FRICTION; IMPACT; NEWTON'S LAWS; STRENGTH; TORQUE; WORK.

Bibliography
Enoka, R.M. (2002). *Neuromechanics of human movement*. 3rd ed. Champaign, IL: Human Kinetics.

FORCED EXPIRED VOLUME See under VITAL CAPACITY.

FORCE PLATE Force platform. A device used to measure the force exerted on it by a subject. In accordance to Newton's 3rd law, this force has the same magnitude as, but is opposite in direction from, the reaction force exerted on the subject by the platform. It is most commonly used in sports biomechanics to measure the contact forces between a sports performer and the ground (**ground reaction force**; **ground contact force**).

A force plate is usually bolted to a base plate that is set in concrete. The force plate produced by Advanced Mechanical Technology, Inc (AMTI) is of the strain-gauge type. Electrical resistance strain gauges are made of a material of which the resistance changes with its deformation (strain). The strain gauges are mounted on a sensor, such as an axially loaded cylinder, which deforms slightly when a force is applied to it. Kistler's force plate is piezo-electric. It relies on the development of an electrical change in certain crystals (e.g. quartz) when subject to an applied force.

A force plate provides inputs for joint moment and force calculations. It provides whole body measurements, but does not show how the applied force is distributed over the contact surface (e.g. shoe/foot). Force plates measure the position of the point of application of the force (**center of pressure**) on the platform. This is the point at which the force can be considered to act, although the pressure is distributed over the platform (and foot). There may actually be no pressure acting at the center of pressure, e.g. when it is below the arch of the foot or between the feet during a double stance. When pressure exists under both the heel and ball of the foot, the center of pressure will be in the mid-foot region, which in itself is not bearing much pressure. A **force line** is the line representing the ground reaction force vector drawn starting at the center of pressure and with magnitude and direction determined by the measured components of the ground reaction force vector.

The most commonly used convention for measurement is: F_z as the vertical (up-down) component, F_y as the anteroposterior (forward-backward) component and F_x as the mediolateral (side-to-side) component. F_y and F_x are shear components because they act parallel to the surface of the ground. Since ground reaction force relates to the motion of the total body center of mass, the anteroposterior force profile can be related to the acceleration profile of the center of mass during support.

Pressure platforms, pads or insoles are required to see how the applied force is distributed over the contact surface. *See* PRESSURE PAD.

Chronology

•1969 • The Kistler company constructed the first commercially available piezo-electric force plate for gait analysis for the biomechanics laboratory of the ETH Zurich.

•1976 • Advanced Mechanical Technology, Inc. (AMTI) constructed the first commercially available strain gauge force plate for gait analysis at the biomechanics laboratory of the Boston Children's Hospital.

FORCE-VELOCITY RELATIONSHIP In concentric muscle action, force decreases with increased velocity of shortening. In eccentric muscle action, force increases with increased velocity of lengthening. *See also* POWER-VELOCITY RELATIONSHIP.

FOREARM MUSCLES *See under* ELBOW JOINT COMPLEX.

FOREFOOT ADDUCTUS A single (transverse) plane, fixed position where the angle formed by the longitudinal bisection of the rearfoot and the metatarsals is angled toward the midline of the body away from the longitudinal bisection of the rearfoot.

FOREFOOT EQUINUS A forefoot fixed in a position it would assume if plantar flexed. The condition must not be confused with metatarsus equinus in which there is a plantar flexion at the midtarsal joints.

FOREFOOT SUPINATUS A forefoot fixed in an inverted position about the longitudinal axis of the midtarsal joint, when the rest of the foot is in the subtalar neutral position. It mimics forefoot varus. Long-term compensatory calcaneal eversion can eventually twist the forefoot into a soft tissue or positional varus position of the forefoot relative to the rearfoot. It is not an osseous abnormality. Tonic spasm of the *tibialis anterior* muscle simultaneously dorsal flexes the 1st ray and temporarily inverts the forefoot around the longitudinal axis of the midtarsal joint. Forefoot supinatus disappears with the use of foot orthotics in the form of forefoot wedging.

FOREFOOT VALGUS   A fixed structural abnormality in which the plantar aspect of the forefoot is everted, on the frontal plane, relative to the plantar aspect of the rearfoot, when the calcaneum is vertical and the midtarsal joints are locked and fully pronated. It is not as common as forefoot varus. It may be caused by a bony deformity in which the plantar surface of the metatarsals evert relative to the calcaneus with the subtalar joint in the neutral position. It is typically seen in a high-arched foot. Forefoot valgus may be flexible or rigid. With **flexible forefoot valgus**, there is sufficient range-of-movement in the midtarsal joint to bring the entire forefoot to the ground. It requires inversion to make the foot plantigrade. Inversion occurs around the longitudinal axis of the midtarsal joint. With **rigid forefoot valgus**, range of motion in the midtarsal joint is not enough to allow the lateral column of the foot to touch the ground, thus compensatory supination from the subtalar joint is required. This is rarely seen clinically.

Bibliography
Clinicians Corner. Http://www.footmaxx.com/clinicians

FOREFOOT VARUS   Metatarsus adductus. Metatarsus varus. A misalignment in which the plantar surface of the forefoot is inverted relative to the plantar surface of the rear foot when the subtalar joint is in a neutral position and the forefoot is maximally pronated at the metatarsal axis on the sagittal plane. There is medial displacement of the metatarsals on the cuneiform. It is the most common congenital foot deformity, and the most common cause of excessive pronation.

True forefoot varus is an intrauterine positional deformity that resolves in 90% of cases by the age of 4 years. Treatment is necessary only if the deformity is rigid or persisting. It is usually noticed at around 6 months when the child begins to pull itself upright. It affects about 1 out of every 1,000 to 2,000 live births. Risk factors include a condition called **oligohydramnios**, where the mother does not produce enough amniotic fluid in the uterus.

With **uncompensated** forefoot varus, the rearfoot is rigid and cannot compensate. Instead of subtalar joint compensation, it will have to try to take place in the midtarsal joint. With **partially compensated** forefoot varus, the degree of forefoot varus is greater than the available degree of calcaneal eversion. With **compensated** forefoot varus, the degree of forefoot varus is equal to or less than the degree of calcaneal eversion. The person compensates by pronating the subtalar joint during midstance and terminal stance to allow the 1st metatarsal to contact the ground.

Bibliography
Clinicians Corner. Http://www.footmaxx.com/clinicians

FORWARD HEAD   A deformity in which the neck is flexed and the head is held forward and downward, usually with the chin dropped; the earlobe is no longer in alignment with the acromion. It creates a constant flexion moment of the head over the spine. When the head and chin are not dropped, it is known as **cervical lordosis** ('poke neck'). It is common in persons with nearsightedness.

In severe cases of forward head, usually accompanied by round back (kyphosis), the cervical spine hyperextends to compensate for forward droop of the head and the increasing dorsal convexity of the thoracic spine. This results in overstretching and sagging of the neck flexor muscles. The neck extensor muscles (mainly the upper *trapezius*, *splenius capitis* and *splenius cervicis*) are shortened and tightened. This tightness is accentuated in the area of the seventh cervical vertebra, where a layer of fat tends to accumulate. The combined prominence of the seventh cervical vertebra and excess adipose tissue is called a **dowager's hump**.

FRACTURE   A break in the continuity of bone. Damage to bone may occur from direct or indirect injury. When the fracture is at the specific site of force application it is a **direct injury**. When the fracture is remote from the location of force application it is an **indirect injury**.

The application of relatively small forces over a small area causes transverse fracture, whereas application of large forces over a large area causes extensive comminuted fracture and large forces over a small area causes penetrating comminuted fracture. A **transverse fracture** occurs when the fracture line is perpendicular to the long axis of the bone. It is usually the result of a bending injury. A **comminuted fracture** occurs when bone is broken into more than two fragments. A **fissured fracture** is an incomplete longitudinal break.

Tensile loading results in either transverse fracture or avulsion fracture. Compressive (axial) loading causes oblique fracture. An **oblique fracture** occurs when the fracture line is diagonally across the shaft of the bone. Bending can result in a **butterfly fracture**, which is a type of comminuted fracture in which the middle fragment is triangulated. A combination of bending with compression produces a combination of transverse fracture and oblique fracture.

Fractures resulting from torsional force may occur in the lower extremity when the foot is planted and the body is changing direction, as might occur in football or skiing. Torsional loading results in spiral fracture. A **spiral fracture** occurs when the fracture line spirals around the shaft of the bone. A combination of bending with torsion and compression results in complex fracture pattern.

A **simple (closed) fracture** is one in which the skin is undamaged. A **compound (open) fracture** is one in which the fractured ends of the bone pierce the skin. Compound fractures are associated with a high risk of infection in the bone. An **articular surface fracture** involves an adjacent joint surface. A **pathologic fracture** occurs through weak or diseased bone and is produced by minimum force.

An **osteochondral fracture** is a fracture that is through the articular cartilage as well as bone. It may be caused by a direct blow to the knee or by a shearing force of twisting and weight bearing such as when cutting sharply to the opposite side.

An **epiphyseal fracture** occurs in growing children and involves injury to the growth plate of a long bone. A **metaphyseal fracture** involves the area adjacent to the growth plate, but removed from the adjacent joint. A **diaphyseal fracture** involves the zone between the two growth plates.

A **greenstick fracture** is an incomplete fracture that passes only part way through the shaft of the bone. It occurs only in children because of the increased elasticity of young bones. A **buckle fracture** (**torus fracture**) is a type of greenstick fracture that occurs when a compressive force is applied on a child's bone, e.g. as a result of falling on the outstretched hand. Because immature bone is more ductile, it may fail first in compression and a buckle fracture may result on the compressive side.

The risk of fracture depends on a number of factors, including the material properties of the bone and the nature of loading. Most bones are designed to resist axial (compressive) forces, thus excessive loads applied in other directions are more likely to cause fracture. Cortical (compact) bone is generally more fracture resistant than trabecular (cancellous) bone. This is because cortical bone is denser than trabecular bone. Cortical bone can withstand greater stress in compression than tension and greater stress in tension than shear. Clinically, shear fractures are most often seen in cancellous bone. *See also* AVULSION FRACTURE; BENDING; EYE INJURIES; METATARSAL FRACTURES; OSTEO-CHRONDRAL FRACTURES; STRESS FRAC-TURE.

FRACTURE ENERGY *See* TOUGHNESS.

FRAGILE X SYNDROME A disorder that results from a defect on a person's X chromosome. 'Fragile' refers to a gap or break in the long arm of the X chromosome. Fragile X is caused by a defect in the FMR1 gene, which is located on the long arm of the X chromosome. Within this gene lies a region of DNA that varies in length from one person to another. When this DNA is longer than normal, the gene change is called a **premutation**. A person with a premutation does not typically have symptoms of fragile X, but the stretch of DNA is prone to further expansion when it is passed from a woman to her children. When the length of this DNA exceeds a certain point, the gene is switched off and does not produce the protein that it normally makes. This gene change is called a **full mutation**. A male who inherits a full mutation exhibits characteristics of fragile X syndrome because his only X chromosome contains the mutated gene. A female may not be as severely affected as a male because each cell of her body needs to use only one of its two X chromosomes and randomly inactivates the other. Carrier men pass the premutation (a small defect in FMR1) to all their daughters, but none of their sons. Each child of a carrier woman has a 50% chance of inheriting the gene. The fragile X permutation can be passed silently down through generations in a family before a child manifests the syndrome.

Physical indicators of fragile X syndrome include a long narrow face and prominent ears, flat feet and hyperflexibility. It is the single most common inherited cause of mental impairment. It occurs in 1 of 2,000 males and 1 of 4,000 females, but frequently goes undiagnosed. Males are more severely handicapped than females with mental retardation, severe communicative problems and repetitive behaviors involving stereotypies. Females are generally socially withdrawn and have borderline intelligence, performing poorly in mathematics and are subject to disorders of mood. Seizures affect about 25% of people with fragile X syndrome.

See also SENSORY INTEGRATION DISORDER.

Chronology

•2002 • In three years on the Northwest High School football team, in McDermott (Ohio), Jake Porter, a 17-year old who was born with Fragile-X syndrome, had barely ever stepped on the field. He had never run with the ball or made a tackle. In their match against Waverly High School, it was agreed beforehand by the coaches of each team that Jake would come into play at the end of the game. With 5 seconds left, Northwest was losing 42-0 and Jake trotted out to the huddle. Northwest's coach and Jake's best friend, Dave Frantz had a talk with the opposing coach, Derek Dewitt. On resumption of play Jake got the ball and ran, initially in the wrong direction, but toward the line of scrimmage once rerouted by the back judge. He completed a 48-yard run for a touch down. Before the play, Coach Dewitt had called over his defense and said, "They're going to give the ball to number 45. Do not touch him! Open up a hole and let him score! Understand?" As a result of Jake's play, people in the two towns seemed to treat one another better. Coach Dewitt said, "I have this bully in one of my [phys-ed] classes. He's a rough, out-for-himself type kid. The other day I saw him helping a couple of special-needs kids play basketball. I about fell over."

Bibliography
FRAXA Research Association. Http://www.fraxa.org

Reilly, R. (2002). The play of the year. Http://sportsillustrated.cnn.com/inside_game/rick_reilly/news/2002/11/12/life_of_reilly/

FRAME OF REFERENCE *See under* INERTIA.

FRANKFORT PLANE *See under* VERTEX.

FRANK-STARLING LAW *See under* CARDIAC CYCLE.

FREE ENERGY ΔG. Energy that is available to do work. *See under* THERMODYNAMICS.

FREE NERVE ENDINGS *See under* MECHANO-RECEPTORS.

FREE RADICALS Radicals. Reactive species. These are highly reactive atoms or molecules that possess at least one unpaired electron in their outermost shell of electrons. This is an extremely unstable configuration, and free radicals quickly react with other molecules or radicals to achieve the stable configuration of four pairs of electrons in their outermost shell (one pair for hydrogen). **Reactive nitrogen species** and **reactive oxygen species** are highly reactive chemicals containing nitrogen and oxygen, respectively.

Reactive oxygen species are formed by several different mechanisms: the interaction of ionizing radiation with biological molecules; as an unavoidable byproduct of cellular respiration; and the synthesis by dedicated enzymes in phagocytic cells, such as neutrophils and macrophages. Reactive oxygen species also have important functions in cells. For example, the cells of the thyroid gland must make hydrogen peroxide in order to attach iodine atoms to thyroglobulin in the synthesis of thyroxine; macrophages and neutrophils must generate reactive oxygen species in order to kill some types of bacteria that they engulf by phagocytosis; and bacteria are engulfed into a phagosome. Examples of reactive oxygen species are hydrogen peroxide, hypochlorite ions, hydroxyl radical (the most reactive) and superoxide (the most common free radical in biology).

Primary sources of free radical production in skeletal muscle are the mitochondria, xanthine oxidase, NAD(P)H oxidase, and the production of nitric oxide by nitric oxide synthase. Secondary sources for free radical production during exercise include: auto-oxidation of catecholamines; radical generation by phagocytic white cells; and radical formation due to the disruption of iron-containing proteins. Free radical production in the mitochondria is the primary source of radical production in contracting skeletal muscles. While 95 to 98% of the oxygen consumption of skeletal muscle results in the formation of ATP and water, the remaining 2 to 5% of this oxygen undergoes one electron reduction to produce superoxide radicals.

Two major classes of endogenous protective mechanisms work together to decrease the harmful effects of oxidants in the cell: non-enzymatic and enzymatic. Some of the important non-enzymatic defences are: glutathione, vitamin E, vitamin C, lipoic acid, carotenoids, uric acid, bilirubin and ubiquinone. As the majority of free radicals are formed in lipid layers, the first line of defence is provided by lipophilic antioxidants such as vitamin E and ubiquinone.

Lipid peroxidation is a harmful biochemistry initiated by oxygen-derived free radicals and is produced in the intermediate metabolism during exercise. Consequences of lipid peroxidation taking place in the polyunsaturated fatty acids part of membranes include alterations in enzyme function and changes in the fluidity of membranes. There is evidence that vitamin E acts as an antioxidant to prevent lipid peroxidation. Hydrophilic antioxidants such as vitamin C provide a later line of defense. Vitamin C is the predominant plasma antioxidant that scavenges free radicals and prevents their entry into LDL cholesterol. Vitamin C regenerates oxidized vitamin E and increases cholesterol excretion.

There are three primary antioxidant enzymes in cells: superoxide dismutase, glutathione peroxidase and catalase. Each of these enzymes is capable of producing other less reactive species or neutralizing reactive oxygen metabolites.

Superoxide is formed in the body either deliberately by white blood cells to kill invading bacteria and viruses, or as a leakage of energy during metabolism (some electrons passing down the electron transport chain leak away from the main path – especially as they pass through ubiquinone and go directly to reduce oxygen molecules to the superoxide anion). In both situations, it appears that the superoxide formed can cause molecular changes that can result in various types of damage. A major source of superoxide is macrophages and neutrophils. An enzyme, **NADPH oxidase**, found on the surface of these cells, is activated when the macrophages and neutrophils encounter a foreign invading molecule like a bacterium. The enzyme adds an electron to the oxygen molecules around it creating superoxide. **Superoxide dismutase** is the first defense against superoxide radicals. Found in all cells, superoxide dismutase promotes the dismutation of superoxide radical, and forms hydrogen peroxide and oxygen. Hydrogen peroxide is toxic to cells and must therefore be removed. This occurs by reduction, using catalase and glutathione peroxidase as enzymes. The majority of the hydrogen peroxide is broken down to oxygen and water by the catalase. **Hydrogen peroxide** destroys bacteria by oxidizing various metabolic control molecules (possibly thiol groups) and generates further radicals within the bacteria by reacting with copper and iron. Neutrophils can enhance the destructive power of hydrogen peroxide by reacting with the salt in the body using an enzyme called myeloperoxidase.

Glutathione peroxidase is located in both the cytosol and mitochondria of cells, and is responsible for removing hydrogen peroxide and other organic hydroperoxides from the cell. It utilizes reduced glutathione as a reducing equivalent to reduce hydrogen peroxide to form oxidized glutathione and water. Concentration of glutathione in skeletal muscle varies depending on muscle fiber types. **Glutathione** is the most abundant non-protein thiol source in muscle cells. It is primarily synthesized in the liver and is transported to tissues via the circulation. Glutathione directly scavenges a variety of radicals, including hydroxyl and carbon-centered radicals, by donating a hydrogen atom. It has been postulated that glutathione can reduce vitamin E radicals that are formed in the chain-breaking reactions with alkoxyl or lipid peroxyl radicals. Glutathione can also reduce the semi-dehydroascorbate radical (vitamin C radical) derived from the recycling of vitamin E and to reduce alpha-lipoic acid to dihydrolipoate.

Similar to superoxide dismutase and glutathione, **catalase** activity is highest in highly oxidative muscles and lowest in muscle with a large percentage of fast-twitch fibers. Catalase is found primarily in peroxisomes, organelles involved in nonmito-chondrial oxidation of fatty acids and amino acids, and they generate hydrogen peroxide. Iron is an essential co-factor in the antioxidant enzyme catalase.

During normal conditions, free radicals are generated at a low rate and are subsequently dealt with by antioxidant systems. Excess free-radical formation has been hypothesized to contribute to cancer, atherosclerosis, aging, and exercise-associated muscle damage. During high-intensity exercise, the flow of oxygen through skeletal muscle cells is greatly increased at the same time as the rate of ATP breakdown exceeds the rate of ATP synthesis. The oxidation of cellular components (**oxidative stress**) can occur when an imbalance exists between oxidants and antioxidants. Oxidative stress occurs under conditions when local antioxidant defenses are depleted because of oxidants, or when the rate constants of the free radical reactions are greater than the rate constants of the antioxidant defense mechanisms. A paradox of free radicals is that exercise is associated with increased production of free radicals, but the more trained an individual is, the more likely that individual is able to counteract an increase in free radicals generated by exercise.

Endurance training promotes an increase in both total superoxide dismutase and glutathione peroxidase activity in skeletal muscles. The training-induced increase of antioxidant enzymes is limited to highly oxidative skeletal muscles. Training does not result in an increase in muscle catalase activity. Glutathione plays a pivotal role in the maintenance of the intracellular redox status and antioxidant enzyme function during acute and chronic exercise. Regular endurance training improves the glutathione antioxidant reserve in active skeletal muscles by increasing glutathione levels. The mechanism responsible for this is unknown.

The low incidence of vitamin deficiencies among athletes indicates that antioxidant deficiencies are not common. High doses of antioxidants may shift the intracellular redox balance towards a reduced state and impair skeletal muscle contractile function and exercise performance. Thus, supplementing the diet with antioxidants cannot be recommended at the present time.

See also AGING; ALPHA-LIPOIC ACID; CAROTENOIDS; COPPER; IRON; MANGAN-ESE; MUSCLE SORENESS; NITRIC OXIDE; NUTRITION; PHYTOCHEMICALS; SELENIUM; UBIQUINONE; VITAMIN C; VITAMIN E.

Bibliography

Adams, A.K. and Best, T.M. (2002). The role of antioxidants in exercise and disease prevention. The *Physician and Sportsmedicine* 30(5), 37-44.

Jenkins, R.R. (1988). Free radical chemistry. Relationship to exercise. *Sports Medicine* 5, 156-170.

Maughan, R.J., King, D.S. and Lea, T. (2004). Dietary supplements. *Journal of Sports Sciences* 22, 95-113.

Powers, S.K. and Leeuwenburgh, C. (1999). Exercise training-induced alterations in skeletal muscle antioxidant capacity: A brief review. *Medicine and Science in Sports and Exercise* 31(7), 987-997.

Powers, S.K. et al. (2004). Dietary antioxidants and exercise. *Journal of Sports Sciences* 22, 81-94.

Radák, Z. (2000). *Free radicals in exercise and aging*. Champaign, IL: Human Kinetics.

Spriet, L.L. and Gibala, M.J. (2004). Nutritional strategies to influence adaptations to training. *Journal of Sports Sciences* 22, 127-141.

FRENCH PARADOX The French have the lowest mortality rate from ischemic heart disease and cardiovascular diseases in Western industrialized nations (35% and 39% lower than the USA and UK, respectively), yet their diet is high in saturated fat. This has recently been attributed to their regular consumption of food and beverages (especially red wine) that are rich in phytochemicals such as polyphenols. Resveratrol is an important component of grape polyphenols and is found mainly in grape skin. Non-grape sources of resveratrol include peanuts. There is evidence, mainly from *in vitro* research, that resveratrol is an effective antioxidant and anti-platelet agent. It inhibits lipid peroxidation of LDL cholesterol. Proanthocyanidin is present in the seeds. Red wine extract as well as resveratrol and proanthocyanidin are equally effective in decreasing myocardial ischemic reperfusion injury (Das et al, 1999). Epidemiological studies have not convincingly shown a superiority of red wine versus alcohol or other alcoholic beverages. There is evidence that moderate alcohol intake may prevent certain cardiovascular conditions, especially heart attacks and ischemic strokes. Animal research has shown that grape juice is much more effective than red wine or dealcoholized red wine at the same polyphenol dose for inhibiting atherosclerosis and improving lipids and antioxidant parameters.

The French paradox might be explained in terms of the French consuming wine with their meal, possibly preventing blood clotting triggered by fat; or eating their biggest meal in the middle of the day rather than in the evening, enabling more efficient metabolism of fat and less likelihood of blood clots forming.

Bibliography

Das, D.K., Sato, M. et al. (1999). Cardioprotection of red wine: The role of polphenolic antioxidants. *Drugs and Experimental Clinical Research* 25(2-3), 115-120.

Klatsky, A.L. (2003). Drink to your health? *Scientific American* 288(2), 74-81.

Sun, A.Y., Simonyi, A. and Sun, G.Y. (2002). The 'French paradox' and beyond: Neuroprotective effects of polyphenols. *Free Radical Biology and Medicine* 32(4), 314-318.

Vinson, J.A., Teufel, K. and Wu, N. (2001). Red wine, dealcoholized red wine, and especially grape juice, inhibit atherosclerosis in a hamster model. *Atherosclerosis* 156(1), 67-72.

FRENZEL MANEUVER See under HYPER-BARIC PHYSIOLOGY.

FREQUENCY The number of cycles per second. 1 hertz (Hz) is equal to 1 cycle/s.

FRICTION A force that opposes the relative motion of two bodies in contact. It acts in a direction tangential to the surface of contact. It is the resultant of the two horizontal (shear) components of the ground reaction force (F_y and F_x), i.e. it is the reaction of the ground to the forces exerted in the horizontal plane by the person or object. The Standard International (SI) unit is the newton (N). The US Customary unit is pound force (lbf).

Friction is equal to the normal force multiplied by the coefficient of friction. The normal force is exerted by either body on the other, perpendicular to their mutual interface. In many situations, the normal force is just the weight of the object that is sitting on some surface. If an object is on an incline or has components of applied force perpendicular to the surface, then it is not equal to the weight.

If the two bodies are at rest, then the frictional forces are called **static friction**. Static friction is increased if the force pressing the two surfaces together is increased and/or the textures of the surfaces are rough. The maximum force of static friction between any pair of dry unlubricated surfaces is: i) independent of the contact area; and ii) proportional to the normal force. If there is relative motion between the two bodies, then the force acting between the surfaces is called **dynamic friction**. It has been found experimentally that the dynamic coefficient of friction is less than the static coefficient of friction, and that dynamic coefficient of friction depends on the relative speed of the object.

The coefficient of friction depends on the nature of the interacting surfaces. The greater the magnitude of the coefficient of friction, the greater is the interaction between the molecules of the interfacing surfaces. The magnitude of the coefficient of friction between shoes and surfaces may be calculated by the ratio of friction to ground reaction force at the pointing time just before the shoe moves relative to the ground.

Sliding friction refers to two bodies sliding. **Rolling friction** refers to one body rolling on another. For sliding or rolling, the coefficient of friction is the ratio of the following two forces: i) the force parallel to the surface of contact between two bodies, which opposes the motion of a body that is sliding or rolling over another; and ii) the force perpendicular to the surface of contact between the two bodies. A ball and a puck have similar coefficients of friction, but the rolling ball is hindered much less by friction than a sliding puck. A puck of the same size and weight as a ball will slide at the same speed as the ball until the ball starts rolling, whereupon the ball will move quickly away from the puck.

Treaded tires in vehicles allow water to be removed from the contact area between the tire and road surface minimizing loss of friction. Cleated shoes increase the coefficient of friction and provide better traction against the ground. In certain sports, the tangential (usually horizontal) force is transmitted by interlocking surfaces (traction) rather than by friction, such as when spikes or studs penetrate or substantially deform a surface. During a sprint start in track athletics, the coefficient of friction limits performance. A larger value on a synthetic track compared with a cinders track allows the runner a greater forward inclination of the trunk and a more horizontally directed leg drive and horizontal impulse. On tracks with lower values of coefficient of friction, the runner must use shorter strides. The static coefficient of friction (shoe stationary relative to the ground) has been reported to range from 0.3 to 2.0, with 0.6 for a cinder track and 1.5 for grass. Running tracks used for international competitions must have a minimum coefficient of sliding friction of 0.5 under wet conditions (when the surface is most slippery).

Fluid friction is a type of friction concerned with the relative movement of a solid and a fluid. It is proportional to the speed of motion and the surface area of contact.

Surface friction is a type of friction that exists at the surface of a solid body immersed in a much larger volume of fluid that is in motion relative to the body. It is a component of drag in swimming.

In speed skating, sharpened blades minimize friction in the direction parallel to the blade length. The high pressures involved cause localized melting of the ice, which, along with the smooth blade surface, decreases friction. Fresh ice has a lower coefficient of friction. If there were no friction, the skater would continue gliding forever. Very cold ice is not as slippery as warmer ice.

In skiing, many turns require side-slipping, in which the skis are somewhat parallel to the fall line of the slope. The skier changes the effective ski-snow coefficient of friction by changing the angle base of the ski and the snow surface. When the uphill edges of the skis dig into the snow, they create considerable resistance to motion as they sideslip down the slope. When the skis are flattened against the surface, side-slipping becomes easier. A combination of flattening and edging the ski against the snow to sideslip down the slope is the easiest way to turn.

In tennis, rebound is greater on a higher-friction (slow) court, like clay, than a low-friction (fast) court, like grass. On clay the ball can lose as much as 40% of its forward speed, whereas on grass the ball only loses a small amount of its forward speed. Therefore, clay-court specialists are usually baseline-predominant players whereas grass-court specialists are powerful servers and volleyers.

Bibliography

Zumerchik, J. (1997, ed). *Encyclopedia of sports science*. New York: Macmillan Library Reference.

FRIEBERG'S INFARCTION Frieberg's disease. Avascular necrosis of the metatarsal head. It results from repetitive stress with microfractures at the junction of the metaphysis and growth plate. It is typically seen in teenage females and most commonly afflicts the second metatarsal.

FRIEDREICH'S ATAXIA *See under* ATAXIA.

FRONTAL PLANE Coronal plane. The plane that runs at right angles to the sagittal plane and divides the body into front and back halves.

FRUCTOSE A monosaccharide found in honey and

fruit. The liver is the major organ involved in fructose metabolism. Excessive use of fructose can cause osmotic diarrhea and high blood triglyceride levels.

The utilization of fructose differs in muscle and liver. In muscle, hexokinase can phosphorylate fructose to fructose 6-phosphate, which is a direct glycolytic intermediate. Hepatic fructose is phosphorylated by fructokinase yielding fructose 1-phosphate. A form of aldolase converts fructose 1-phosphate to dihydroxyacetone and glyceraldehyde. The dihydroxyacetone is converted by triose phosphate isomerase to glucose 3-phosphate and enters glycolysis.

Heriditary fructose intolerance (fructose 1-phosphate aldolase deficiency) is a disorder usually found in children, in which the body is unable to metabolize fructose. It is inherited as an autosomal recessive trait, and has an incidence of 1 in 20,000. Symptoms range from vomiting and hypoglycemia to severe metabolic acidosis and coma. It is treated by administration of glucose and elimination of fructose from the diet.

See under CARBOHYDRATE; FLUID REPLACEMENT; GLYCOLYSIS.

FUNCTIONAL ANATOMY *See under* ANATOMY.

FUNCTIONAL RESIDUAL CAPACITY The volume of gas left in the lungs at the resting end expiratory position.

FUNDAMENTAL POSITION *See under* ANATOMICAL POSITION.

FUNNEL CHEST *See* PECTUS EXCAVATUM.

FUNNY BONE *See under* ULNAR NERVE.

FURUNCLE *See under* SKIN.

FUTILE CYCLING *See under* THERMO-GENESIS.

G

GABA   *See* GAMMA AMINOBUTYRATE.

GAIT   The pattern of how a person walks. A child develops adult patterns of gait around the age of 3 years. The normal gait cycle begins with heel strike, and then very brief supination with force moving forward. This action is followed by pronation of the foot, whereby the weight becomes distributed over the midfoot, and finally a toe-off (which is associated with a brief supination).

Scissors gait is associated with quadriplegic spastic cerebral palsy. The legs are flexed, inwardly rotated and adducted at the hip joint, causing them to cross alternately in front of each other. There is excessive knee flexion. Toe walking causes a narrow base. Scissors gait may be caused by the positive supporting reflex. If the arms are involved, they are flexed and pronated, carried close to the body, with a fisted hand.

Hemiplegic gait is a limp caused by asymmetry in extension. It is associated with hemiplegic spastic cerebral palsy and stroke. It tends to occur with any disorder producing an immobile hip or knee. The individual leans to the affected side, and the arm on that side is held in a rigid, semi-flexed position.

Ataxic (cerebellar) gait is associated with ataxic cerebral palsy, Friedreich's ataxia and similar *les autres* conditions. The individual walks with a wide base of support, there is irregularity of steps, unsteadiness, and a tendency to reel to one side. The individual seems to experience difficulty in judging how high to lift the legs when climbing stairs.

Shuffling (slouch) gait is associated with immaturity of the central nervous system and probably retention of tonic labyrinthine reflex-prone and symmetrical tonic neck reflex. The lower body is not able to move independently of the upper body. It is seen in severe mental retardation. There is excessive flexion at the hip, knee and ankle joints; contact with the ground is flat footed. There is usually forward inclination of the trunk, and no opposition of arms and legs.

Propulsion (festination) gait is associated with Parkinson's disease. The individual walks with a forward leaning posture and short, shuffling steps that begin slowly and become progressively more rapid. This gait is seen also in very old persons with low fitness.

Steppage (foot-drop) gait is associated with flopping of the foot on the floor. Knee action is higher than normal, but the toes still tend to drag on the floor. It is caused by paralysis or weakness of the ankle dorsal flexors. It results in excessive hip and knee flexor work.

Waddling gait is characterized by rolling movement from side to side. This is usually caused by structural problems, such as genu varus, hip problems and dislocations, genu valgus or leg length discrepancy.

Muscular dystrophy gait is an awkward side-to-side waddle, swayback, arms held in backward position, and frequent falling.

Gluteus maximus lurch is characterized by alternate sticking out of the chest (salutation) and pulling back of the shoulders. It is associated with polio and other spinal paralysis conditions in which the paralyzed limb cannot shift the bodyweight forward onto the normal limb. To compensate, the trunk is thrust forward.

Trendelenburg gait involves a limp caused by paralysis or weakness of the *gluteus medius* muscle, a hip abductor. The pelvis is lower on the unaffected side. Each time the weight is transferred during walking, to compensate for weakness of the *gluteus medius*, the body leans slightly in the direction of the weight transfer.

Antalgic gait, seen in most patients with osteoarthritis, is a 'pain-relieving gait.' The weight is moved off the painful limb as quickly as possible, thus shortening the stance phase on the side of the painful limb. To maintain balance, the arm is thrown out laterally on the side opposite the painful limb. The arm is thrown out while the patient is in the stance phase on the good limb.

See also INFANT WALKERS; WALKING.

GALACTOSE A monosaccharide. When bonded to glucose, galactose forms the disaccharide lactose, the carbohydrate of milk. Galactose is readily converted to glucose in the liver. Galactose enters glycolysis by its conversion to glucose 1-phosphate.

GALACTOSEMIA An inborn error in carbohydrate metabolism; the infant cannot metabolize galactose.

GALEAZZI FRACTURE *See under* ELBOW FRACTURES.

GALL BLADDER A muscular sac in which bile from the liver is stored until its release into the intestine.

GALLOPING A form of locomotion that is a front-facing movement; a step is taken onto the forward leg followed by a leap onto the rear foot, with the same leg always leading. Motor milestones are as follows: galloping in a basic, but inefficient manner (4 years) and galloping skillfully (6 years). Sliding is similar to galloping, but it is performed sideways.

Bibliography

Payne, V.G. and Isaacs, L.D. (2004). *Human motor development. A lifespan approach.* 6th ed. Boston, MA: McGraw-Hill.

GALVANIC SKIN RESPONSE A method to detect, amplify and record electrical activity on the surface of the skin using electrodes. It is often taken from the palm of the hand.

GAMEKEEPER'S THUMB *See under* META-CARPOPHALANGEAL JOINT.

GAMES *See under* SPORT.

GAMETE A mature reproductive cell, such as sperm or egg in animals. **Homogametic** means producing only one kind of gamete with respect to the sex chromosomes. **Heterogametic** refers to the production of dissimilar gametes with respect to the sex chromosomes. In most animals, including humans, the male is the heterogametic sex.

GAMMA AMINOBUTYRATE GABA. It is the ionized form of gamma aminobutyric acid. A neurotransmitter that inhibits directly the firing of neurons containing receptors for GABA and indirectly the release of other brain transmitters including acetylcholine, norepinephrine, dopamine and serotonin. *See under* DEPRESSANTS.

GAMMA HYDROXYBUTYRATE It is a powerful, rapidly acting central nervous system depressant that results from the metabolism of gamma aminobutyrate (GABA). In the USA, over-the-counter sales of gamma-hydroxybutyrate were banned in 1990 and became a Schedule I Controlled Substance in 2000. It produces euphoric and hallucinogenic states and it can become addictive with sustained use. It has been used as an ergogenic aid in sport, because of the belief that it is a growth hormone releaser. Side effects of gamma hydroxybutyrate can be severe and include loss of consciousness.

GAMMA INTERFERON *See under* IMMUNITY.

GAMMA MOTOR NERVE *See under* MUSCLE SPINDLE; NEURONS.

GANGLION i) Any group of nerve cell bodies in the central or peripheral nervous system. ii) A cyst containing fluid rich in mucopolysaccharide within fibrous tissue, muscle, bone or cartilage. The plural of ganglion is ganglia. *See under* CARPAL TUNNEL SYNDROME.

GANGRENE Necrosis caused by a lack of blood supply. It is a complication resulting from infectious or inflammatory processes, injury or degenerative changes associated with chronic diseases, such as diabetes mellitus. The incidence of gangrene from trauma has decreased due to prompt surgical management of wounds with the removal of dead tissue.

GAS   A state of matter in which the molecules are virtually unrestricted by cohesive forces. The volume of gas varies inversely with the pressure, if the temperature is kept constant; i.e. when volume increases, pressure decreases (and vice versa). This is called **Boyle's law**. The volume of a gas is directly proportional to its absolute temperature if the pressure is kept constant; i.e. volume increases as temperature increases, if the pressure is kept constant. This is called **Charles's law**.

The total pressure exerted by a mixture of gases is equal to the sum of the partial pressures of the various gases. This is called **Dalton's law**. The **partial pressure** of a gas in a mixture is the pressure the gas would exert if it were alone in a container. If the temperature is constant, the quantity of a gas that will go into solution is proportional to the partial pressure of the gas. This is called **Henry's law**. The greater the partial pressure, the greater is the amount of gas that will go into solution. The movement of gases by diffusion from alveolar air into the capillary blood in the lungs, and vice versa, can be explained in terms of pressure differences and pressure gradients.

GAS ANALYSIS   *See under* OXYGEN UPTAKE, MEASUREMENT OF.

GAS DIFFUSION   The diffusion of gas is governed by **Fick's Law**, which states that the rate of gas transfer through a sheet of tissue is proportional to the tissue area, a diffusion constant and the difference between the pressure of the gas on each side of the membrane and is inversely proportional to the thickness of the tissue. The diffusion constant is proportional to the gas solubility and inversely proportional to the square root of the molecular weight of the gas. On a per-molecule basis, carbon dioxide (molecular weight = 44) diffuses about 20-times as fast through thin membranous tissues as oxygen (molecular weight = 32) because carbon dioxide has a higher solubility (even though the molecular weight of carbon dioxide is relatively close to that of oxygen).

GAS EXCHANGE RATIO   *See* RESPIRATORY EXCHANGE RATIO.

GASTRIC   Relating to the stomach.

GASTRIC EMPTYING RATE   *See under* FLUID REPLACEMENT.

GASTRIN   *See under* GASTROINTESTINAL SYSTEM; NEUROTRANSMITTER.

GASTROCNEMIUS   The medial head of the *gastrocnemius* muscle has its origin on the posterior of the medial femoral condyle. It merges with the lateral head and then the Achilles tendon, and inserts into the calcaneus. The medial head (or sometimes the lateral head) may incur a strain at the musculotendinous junction. This injury, known as '**tennis leg**,' is common in middle-aged tennis players (after degeneration of the muscle-tendon junction) and is typically caused by vigorous muscle contraction while the knee is extended and the ankle is in dorsal flexion.

GASTROESOPHAGEAL REFLUX DISEASE *See under* ESOPHAGUS.

GASTROINTESTINAL SYSTEM   Gastro-intestinal tract. It is comprised of the mouth, esophagus, stomach, small intestine, large intestine and rectum. The **stomach** is the enlarged, muscular, sac-like portion of the digestion tract between the esophagus and the small intestine. The **small intestine** extends from the stomach to the cecum and consists of the duodenum, jejunum and ileum. The **large intestine** extends from the ileocecal valve to the anus and is comprised of the cecum, colon, rectum and anal canal.

The **enteric nervous system** is a local system of nerves in the gastrointestinal wall that is stimulated by both the chemical composition of chyme and by the stretching of the gastrointestinal lumen that results from food in the gastrointestinal tract. **Chyme** is the semi-fluid mass of partly digested food passed from the stomach into the duodenum. The enteric nervous system plays an essential role in the control of gastrointestinal motility, blood flow, transport of water and electrolytes, and acid secretion in the gastrointestinal tract.

The stomach usually empties completely within 4 hours after a meal. The larger the meal, the greater the stomach distension and the more liquid its contents, the faster the stomach empties. The rate of gastric emptying depends also on the contents of the duodenum. As chyme enters the duodenum, receptors in its wall respond to chemical signals and to stretch. As a consequence, there is triggering of **enterogastric reflexes** and hormonal mechanisms, which inhibit gastric secretory activity and prevent further duodenal filling by decreasing the force of pyloric contractions. A meal that is rich in carbohydrates moves through the duodenum rapidly, but fats form an oily layer at the top of the chyme and are digested more slowly by enzymes acting in the intestine. When chyme entering the duodenum is fatty, food may remain in the stomach for six hours or more.

Pepsin is a protein-digesting enzyme produced by the stomach. **Pepsinogen** is an inactive form of pepsin. **Gastrin** is a polypeptide hormone released from the walls of the stomach mucosa and duodenum that stimulates gastric secretions and motility.

About 30 to 65% of long distance runners experience gastrointestinal symptoms related to exercise. Gastrointestinal hormones, and especially prostaglandins, may be of crucial importance for the production of symptoms. Intestinal absorption, secretion and permeability may also be altered during exercise, provoking intestinal dysfunction.

The most common complaint is the urge to defecate while running, affecting 36 to 63% of runners. Diarrhea is experienced by 8 to 54% of runners. Abdominal cramps are experienced by about one third of runners. Other common complaints include the need to stop to move the bowels, rectal bleeding and incontinence. Sports drinks with carbohydrate concentrations greater than 6 to 10% can cause diarrhea. Lower gastrointestinal symptoms (such as incontinence) are more commonly experienced than upper gastrointestinal symptoms (such as heart burn).

Although the gastrointestinal system does not adapt to increased exercise-induced physiological stress, adequate training leads to a less dramatic decrease of gastrointestinal blood flow at sub-maximal exercise intensities and is important in the prevention of gastrointestinal symptoms. Exercise of high intensity decreases the absorption of water and nutrients. This decrease, however, is not of such magnitude that it may explain the diarrhea in athletes. **Diarrhea** is water stools caused by digestion products moving through the large intestine too rapidly for sufficient water to be reabsorbed. It is a symptom of many disorders (including stress), which cause increased peristalsis. **'Runner's diarrhea'** is common because running appears to cause a greater degree of gastrointestinal disturbance than other activities involving high-energy output. Although intrinsic gastrointestinal motility is probably decreased during exercise (because parasympathetic efferent signals are decreased and sympathetic efferent signals are increased), the entire body is bouncing up and down with each stride. This mechanical explanation is supported by the observation that gastrointestinal disturbances are experienced mainly during the running part of triathlon events. Mechanical vibration is more than doubled in running compared with cycling. Hypertrophy of the *psoas* muscles, pressing on the gastrointestinal tract, has also been postulated as a cause of gastrointestinal symptoms due to running.

Constipation involves infrequent and difficult bowel movements followed by a sensation of incomplete evacuation. A diet that is low in fiber and high in fats is the most common cause of constipation.

See also APPENDIX; FLATULENCE; FLUID REPLACEMENT; GALL BLADDER; GASTRIC EMPTYING RATE; PANCREAS.

Bibliography

Brouns, F. and Beckers, E. (1993). Is the gut an athletic organ? Digestion, absorption and exercise. *Sports Medicine* 15(4), 242-257.

Gil, S.M., Yazaki, E. and Evans, D.F. (1998). Aetiology of running-related gastrointestinal dysfunction. How far is the finishing line? *Sports Medicine* 26(6), 365-378.

Putukian, M. and Potera, C. (1997). Don't miss gastrointestinal disorders in athletes. *The Physician and Sportsmedicine* 25(11), 80-94.

GEARS *See under* EFFICIENCY.

GENDER A distinction can be made between sex and gender. **Sex** concerns biological differences. **Gender** is what culture makes out of the 'raw material' of biological sex.

Feminism is a social/cultural movement motivated towards ending sexist oppression. There are a number of different schools of thought in feminism, including Marxist, Radical, Liberal, and Socialist. **Marxist feminism** believes that equality between the sexes can never be achieved under capitalism. Sexism in sport is a component of bourgeois ideology that underpins division of labor between the sexes. Such a division is regarded as essential to the stability of capitalism. **Radical feminism** believes that male domination and female subordination are universal because sexism has its roots in biological differences and not in capitalism. **Liberal feminism** is concerned with 'equal rights for women.' Radical feminism criticizes liberal feminism for its emphasis on individual equal rights and for ignoring the patriarchal nature of the social system. **Patriarchy** is defined as a system of power relations in which men dominate women. Radical feminism advocates the destruction of patriarchal ideologies and structures, rather than 'equal opportunity' for women within these oppressive structures. Drawing upon both Radical and Marxist feminism, **Socialist feminism** attempts to understand the relationships between capitalist and gender relations. **Men's Studies** regards feminism as a critique that has potential for liberating men, as well as women, from the limitations of sexism.

The role of the media is emphasised in sport feminism. Analyses of newspaper accounts have shown that men receive more attention and more favourable portrayals than women in the sports news. Partial and selective media portrayals of women's athletic achievements have reinforced traditional, stereotypical female body images. A content analysis of nearly 4,000 feature articles in *Sports Illustrated* from 1954 through 1987 found that males were featured in nearly 91% of these articles, nearly 92% were written by male authors, and most dealt with exclusively male sports. The sporting achievements and lives of males were acclaimed in 90.8% of 3,723 articles.

Feminist authors argue that notions of gender have underpinned the development of modern sport. The **Victorian ideals of femininity** (submissiveness, grace, beauty and passivity) were said to conflict with the ideal images of sporting life (strength, toughness, power, aggressiveness and achievement). The elite sports woman may be faced with a conflict between being a sportsperson and being a woman. Palzkill (1990) views lesbianism in elite sport in terms of coping with this conflict of roles. On the other hand, Allison (1991) argues that despite the popular notion that female athletes constantly struggle with their femininity, most of the research has shown that this role conflict seems to be relatively low among female athletes.

The Bem Sex Role Inventory, which is made up of 20 masculine, 20 feminine, and 20 neutral statements, is based on the premise that personality characteristics of masculinity and femininity are linked to biological sex. According to Bem (1974), individuals classified as androgenous (high on both masculine and feminine characteristics) were better adjusted, more adaptable and more flexible than their sex-typed (male/female) peers. **Psychological androgyny** involves a combination of assertiveness and competence with compassion, warmth and emotional expressiveness. It has subsequently been found that both male and female team athletes were more likely to score highly on masculinity or androgeny than on femininity. Female athletes who participated in individual sports scored high on femininity, while their male counterparts were distributed evenly across the three groups.

Since at least the 1940s, sport has provided psychological and social space for lesbians to gather and build a subculture. According to Cahn (1994), lesbians could not publicly claim their identity without risking expulsion, ostracism and loss of athletic activities and social networks that had become crucial to their sense of well-being. Krane (1996) argues that lesbians are socialized within a homonegative and heterosexist society and they develop homonegative attitudes. The sport environment further promotes and sustains homonegative attitudes and behaviors. **Heterosexism** is an ideological system that denies, denigrates and stigmatizes any non-heterosexual form of behavior, identity, relationship or community. **Homophobia** is irrational fear and intolerance of lesbians and gay men. **Homonegativism** is intentional, rather than irrational, negative attitudes and behaviors toward non-heterosexuals. Griffin (1992) argued that homophobia serves not only to reinforce compulsory heterosexuality in the single-sex sporting subcultures, but also to keep heterosexual people of both sexes within the boundaries of traditional masculinity and femininity. According to Griffin (1992), lesbian and feminist sport participation is a threat to male domination. Manifestations of homophobia in women's sport can be divided into six categories: a) silence; b) denial; c) apology; d) promotion of heterosexy image; e) attacks on lesbians; and f) preference for male coaches.

A major reason why many males enter into bodybuilding is low self-esteem, which for many triggers a need to compensate by building their physiques. In the subculture of Southern California bodybuilding, there is a prevalent practice of 'hustling' - the widespread selling of sexual favours by bodybuilders to homosexual men. Klein (1990) argues that hustling supports the comic-book notion of masculinity so prevalent in bodybuilding, fulfils some bodybuilders' needs for admiration, is for many a temporary solution to an economic crisis in the competitive bodybuilders' pursuit of success, and is crisis for those who must maintain heterosexual self perceptions while engaging in homosexual practices.

The popularity of professional wrestling in the late 1990s, according to Coakley (2004), was grounded in the heroic orientations built into the storylines and the personas portrayed in the events. Storylines were based on hypermasculine, heterosexual and homophobic men with personas that were consistently staged and promoted.

Cheerleading when it emerged in the late 1800s was an exclusively male activity. When females started to participate in cheerleading during World War I, they were seen as treading on the male territory of sport and as being in danger of becoming masculinized. In the 1940s and 1950s cheerleading came to be dominated by females as males dropped out of the activity in large numbers. By 1970, cheerleading was regarded as a naturally feminine activity. In the late 1970s males began to re-enter cheerleading at the collegiate level. Cheerleaders now symbolize dominant values about how females should look and act in American society. However, the male cheerleader has become increasingly accepted because the image he has constructed does not challenge traditional gender notions or power relations, but reinforces them. This is because the most crucial activity in cheerleading is stunts, with which the demonstration of strength is interpreted as proof of masculinity.

With respect to female boxing, the position of the Women's Sports Foundation is that, "boxing is a dangerous sport in which sport governing bodies should continue to develop new safety measures to protect male and female participants. As long as competing athletes are matched by ability, muscle mass and other standardized physical variables critical to success in sport, competition between males and females should be permitted."

Chronology

•380 BC • Plato wrote, "I assert without fear of contradiction that gymnastics and horsemanship are as suitable to women as to men." (*Laws VII, 804*)

•90 AD • In Rome, Emperor Domitian provided the spectacle of dwarves in combat against women. Women were gladiators until the 3rd century AD when they were specifically out-lawed by Emperor Septimus Severus.

•1823 • Catherine Beecher founded the Hartford Female Seminary at which she promoted the need for programs of daily exercise for women. Beecher was a strong advocate of exercise for women and she rejected the German system of gymnastics as too strenuous for ladies. Her system included a system of light exercise she called calisthenics (from "the two Greek words *kalos*, signifying beautiful, and *sthenos*, signifying strength"). The most influential of Beecher's books was *A Manual of Physiology and Calisthenics for Schools and Families* (1856).

•1836 • Mary Lyon founded Mount Holyoke Female Seminary in South Hadley, Massachusetts. In 1893, it became Mount Holyoke College. Lyon was a strong advocate of daily exercise for women and a program of useful exercise through domestic duties was developed. Although copied by many schools, it had no appeal to many educators as a real physical education program for girls.

•1866 • In a letter to her brother, Vassar College student Annie Gliddens wrote: "They are getting up various clubs now for outdoor exercise. They have a floral society, boat-clubs, and base-ball. I belong to one of the latter, and enjoy it hugely I can assure you." This is the earliest documented reference to women playing baseball in the USA.

•1869 • A.G. Drachmann, a Danish physician, published a handbook of gymnastics that questioned whether women should do the same exercises as men.

•1883 • Eliza M. Mosher was appointed resident physician at Vassar College. She introduced the divided skirt, a forerunner of the Bloomers of the 1890s. In 1896, she went to the University of Michigan as its first Dean of Women and the first Director of Physical Education for Women.

•1888 • The safety cycle was invented by the Amateur Athletic Union. Its drop bar made it easier for women to cycle. Also, Amelia Bloomer's full, loose trousers gathered at the knee, allowed women to cycle with more freedom. In 1850, Bloomer began publicizing a new style of women's dress, first introduced by Fanny Kemble. In 1896, Susan B. Anthony said that the bicycle "has done more to emancipate women than anything else in the world."

•1901 • British physical educator Constance Applebee introduced field hockey to American college women. In the same year, Vassar College became the first college to offer varsity field hockey. In 1922, the US Field Hockey Association was founded. Unlike basketball, from the beginning field hockey was designated as an exclusively female sport. Because of its British roots and its associations with elite institutions, it assumed an upper-class aura.

•1903 • Luther Gulick, who had left the Springfield YMCA to become director of physical education for New York City's schools, established the Public Schools Athletic League. It was designed to provide all school children in New York City with an opportunity to participate in highly organized sport, but interschool athletic competitions were forbidden. There were different forms of competition geared toward children of various age levels and athletic ability. Girls were provided with a program that emphasized less strenuous group activities.

•1912 • The *Ladies Home Journal* published an article by Dudley Sargent entitled, "Are athletics making girls masculine?" At the time, Sargent was director of Harvard University's Hemenway Gymnasium.

•1914 • In *The Special Theory of Gymnastics*, J. Lindhart of the

Central Gymnastic Institute in Copenhagen attacked the Ling gymnastics because they did not give sufficient consideration to the physical and psychical differences between men and women.

•1917 • The Committee on Women's Athletics was established by the American Physical Education Association (APEA). It set standards for women's physical education programs and discouraged intercollegiate athletics. It drafted separate rules for women's collegiate field hockey, swimming, track and field, and soccer.

•1920 • At the meeting of the Conference of College Directors of Physical Education, members justified their opposition to intercollegiate athletics for women using a number of reasons including that it is "unsocial."

•1928 • Women were first admitted to the Olympic Games as track and field competitors. American Elizabeth Robinson became the world's first woman Olympic athletics gold medalist when she won the 100 meters in 12.2 seconds. Britain declined to send a team because the women were resentful that only five events were being held, but finally relented in 1932 when the program expanded.

•1932 • At the Olympic Games, Mildred Ella "Babe" Didrikson Zaharias became the first woman to win medals in three Olympic events - two gold medals (javelin and 80 meter hurdles) and a silver medal (high jump). Didrikson was penalized in the high jump, because she 'dived' over the bar. The no-diving rule was eliminated the following year. Named by the Associated Press as the top female athlete of the first half of the twentieth century, she pitched spring training for major league men's teams (it was even reported that she once struck out Joe DiMaggio); was a three-time All-American (1930-1932) in basketball; played on two city championship softball teams in Dallas; won every major golf tournament that she competed in between 1940 and 1950, and was leading money winner on the LPGA tour 1948-1951. She died of cancer at the age of 45 in 1956. Her sexual identity was scrutinized until she married wrestler George Zaharias in 1939. In 1952, *Pat and Mike* portrays a character, acted by Katharine Hepburn, modeled after Babe Didrikson Zaharias. Not until the publication of her biography by Susan Cayleff (1995) was Didrikson's intimate relationship with another woman, Betty Dodd, revealed publicly.

•1942 • The All American Girls Baseball League was formed by Philip K. Wrigley, who was owner of Chicago Cubs National League baseball team. Wrigley sold his interest in the league to Arthur Myerhoff, who administered the league form 1944 to 1950. It was originally called the All American Girls Softball League, but was changed to baseball before play started in 1943.

It was later changed to All American Girls Professional Baseball League. In 1943, it was actually fast-pitch softball using an underhand delivery. The uniform was designed by a poster artist and described in *Time* magazine (14 June 1943) "as dignified as the field hockey costume of New England's fashionable boarding schools, it still had the provocativeness of a skating skirt." In 1943, there were four teams and 176,000 fans were attracted. At its zenith, 1948, there were ten teams and 910,000 fans were attracted. In 1943 a 12" diameter ball was used and, by the league's final season in 1954, a 9" regulation baseball. A "femininity principle" was strictly applied and Black women were prohibited. All players attended classes where they learned 'ladylike' behavior. Pastel skirted uniforms, makeup, long hair and stringent controls on athletes' public appearance. They went to great lengths to show that the baseball players were unquestionably normal, feminine women who happened to play baseball. A movie about the All American Girls Professional Baseball League was released in 1992, *A League of Their Own*, and starred Geena Davis and Madonna.

•1953 • Hugh Hefner published the first issue of *Playboy*, featuring Marilyn Monroe. Complete nudity was not shown until 1972. Many sports women have featured in *Playboy*, including skater Katarina Witt, boxer Mia St. John, and professional wrestlers Chyna and Sable.

•1956 • At a conference for directors of college women's physical education, Dr Josephine Renshaw warned educators about the danger of same-sex attachments among college female athletes.

•1964 • The year of the first official swimsuit issue of *Sports Illustrated*, and the approximate time, according to Davis (1997), that the magazine "began to encourage the view that the ideal consumers are men rather than women and men, which would suggest a shift in purpose, away from a primary focus on the display of fashion toward a primary focus on the display of women's bodies."

•1965 • Donna de Varona became the first female sports broadcaster on national television in the USA.

•1969 • Johnell Hoss of South Bend Riley High School sued the Indiana High School Athletic Association (IHSAA) after discovering she could not play golf because there were no girls teams. The Court ruled in favor of the IHSAA, but Hoss appealed to the Indiana Supreme Court and won. In 1973, golf and track were added to the IHSAA girls' sports schedule.

•1972 • In the USA, the Equal Opportunity Act empowered enforcement of Title VII of the Civil Rights Act of 1964 and the enactment and enforcement of the Title IX Educational Assistance Act heralded an expansion of opportunities for women in sports.

Title IX is considered the most important influence on US women's sport in the twentieth century. It stated; "No person in the United States shall on the basis of sex, be excluded from participation in, be denied the benefits of, or be subjected to discrimination under any educational program or activity receiving Federal financial assistance." Under the Title IX Compliance Test (1979), an institution must meet one of the following three criteria: i) the number of male and female athletes at a school must be in proportion to the overall student body. If women are half the school's population, then half of its athletes should be women; ii) a school must demonstrate that it has increased opportunities for women, mostly by adding women's sports; iii) a school must continue to show that its existing athletic programs meet the interests of women on campus. Most schools have chosen to match the ratio of men and women athletes to the ratio of men and women in the student body. As budgets have decreased, men's programs (typically those that do not generate revenue) have been eliminated. Football has presented a problem because in Division I football the maximum of 85 scholarships needs to be offset by five women's sports that offer 17 scholarships each.

•1974 • The Women's Sports Foundation was founded by Billie Jean King. Donna de Varona was a founding member and the first president. Other champion female athletes joined to become a collective voice for women and girls in sport.

•1981 • The Association for Intercollegiate Athletics for Women (AIAW) was dissolved. In conjunction with the effects of Title IX, this led to a dramatic decrease in the number of women coaches and administrators in sport. Before Title IX in 1972, female administrators ran more than 90% of women's collegiate athletics programs and coached 90 to 100% of teams. In 2000, only 18.5% of women's programs were administered by women and coaches had decreased to 45.6%.

•1981 • Billie Jean King held a press conference to reveal that a former lesbian lover was suing her for palimony. With her husband by her side, King called her seven-year relationship with Marilyn Barnett a "mistake."

•1981 • The New York Post 'outed' Martina Navratilova by disclosing her relationship with writer and lesbian activist Rita Mae Brown.

•1982 • The Supreme Court upheld that Title IX does cover employees (coaches etc.) as well as students.

•1984 • The US Supreme Court ruled in Grove City College versus Bell that the Title IX language applied only to a specific program or department that received federal funds. In effect the court's decision said that women could be denied equality in sports. Immediately after the Grove City decision various women's groups began to lobby Congress to pass legislation restoring the weakened civil rights.

•1987 • Pat Griffin proposed a program for the American Alliance for Health, Physical Education, Recreation and Dance (AAHPERD) annual conference entitled, "Doing Research on Controversial Topics: Homosexuality and Homophobia in Physical Education and Sport."

•1988 • The Civil Rights Restoration Act of 1987 reversed Grove City, restoring Title IX's institution-wide coverage. One of its implications was the restoration of the original broad interpretation of Title IX.

•1989 • The LPGA developed promotional material featuring photographs of women golfers posing pin-up style in swimsuits.

•1990 • Former Wimbledon tennis champion, Margaret Court, a born-again Christian, publicly called Martina Navratilova a poor role model after Navratilova won her record-breaking ninth Wimbledon championship. Apparently Court's outburst was provoked by Navratilova post-victory public display of affection for her lover in the stands.

•1992 • The Supreme Court ruled that monetary damages are available under Title IX in the Franklin versus Gwinnett County Public School case.

•1995 • CBS golf commentator Ben Wright was quoted in a newspaper article as saying that lesbians ruin the LPGA Tour.

•1996 • The number of female athletes participating in the modern Summer Olympic Games rose from 0 in 1896 to 11 (0.01%) in 1900 to 385 (9.4%) in 1948 to 3,684 (34%) in 1996. 7,059 men competed in the 1996 Summer Olympics.

•1999 • In ESPN's list of the top 100 athletes of the 20th century, only eight women were included. The highest placed were Jackie Joyner-Kersee (#23), Martina Navratilova (#17) and Babe Didrikson Zaharias (#10).

•2001 • Of the 20 "Outstanding Sports Personality" nominees for the Sports Emmy Awards, none were women.

•2001 • In a position statement of the Women's Sports Foundation, Donna Lopiano stated that whenever a men's sport is eliminated from a NCAA Division I athletic program, the educational institutions blame Title IX and women's sports. Lopiano argued: "The problem is not Title IX. The problem is college presidents not putting a stop to the embarrassing waste of money in football and men's basketball programs."

•2001 • The 1st Women's Amateur World Boxing Championships were held in Scranton, PA. There were more than 150 competitors from 35 nations.

•2001 • Gabriella Reece, a 6 foot 3 inch beach volleyball player,

was featured in *Playboy*. She said; "I don't think of the images as sexual. They're more a statement that women can be really powerful, really feminine, really natural and really confident and just put it out there. No big deal. I'm trying to say, check me out."

•2002 • The US Secretary of State announced the establishment of a Commission on Opportunities in Athletics. The stated purpose of the Commission was "to collect information, analyze issues and obtain broad public input directed at improving the application of current Federal standards for measuring equal opportunity for men and women and boys and girls to participate in athletics under Title IX."

•2003 • Annika Sorenstam, who won 13 out of 25 LPGA tournaments the previous year, accepted a sponsor's exemption to play in the Bank of America Colonial tournament, a PGA Tour event, in Fort Worth and became the first woman to play in a PGA tournament since Babe Zaharias competed in the 1945 Los Angeles Open. In response to a criticism of Sorenstam's entry, Billie Jean King, Founder and Chair of the Women's Sports Foundation, stated, "The Women's Sports Foundation is disappointed by the views of PGA professional Vijay Singh. By saying he will withdraw from competition if paired with Sorenstam for next week's Colonial is a step back for both men's and women's sports. Sorenstam is not playing on a gender mission; she is playing to compete with the best and to challenge herself as a professional athlete."

Bibliography

Allison, M.T. (1991). Role conflict and the female athlete: Preoccupations with little grounding. *Journal of Applied Sport Psychology* 3, 49-60.

Bem, S.L. (1974). The measurement of psychological androgyny. *Journal of Consulting and Clinical Psychology* 42, 155-162.

Birrell, S. and Cole, C.L. (1994, eds). *Women, sport and culture*. Champaign, IL: Human Kinetics.

Cahn, S.K. (1994). *Coming on strong. Gender and sexuality in twentieth-century women's sport*. New York: The Free Press.

Cayleff, S.E. (1995). *The life and legend of Babe Didrikson Zaharias*. Champaign, IL: University of Illinois Press.

Coakley, J. (2004). *Sports in society. Issues and controversies*. 8th ed. Boston, MA: McGraw-Hill.

Davis, L.R. (1990). Male cheerleaders and the naturalization of gender. In: Messner, M.A. and Sabo, D.F. (eds.). *Sport, men, and the gender order: Critical feminist perspectives*. pp153-161. Champaign, IL: Human Kinetics.

Davis, L. (1997). *The swimsuit issue and sport: Hegemonic masculinity in Sports Illustrated*. Albany, NY: State University of New York

Press.

Dunning, E.(1986). Sport as a male preserve: Notes on the social sources of masculinity and its transformations. *Theory, Culture and Society* 3(1), 79-90.

Griffin, P. (1992). Changing the game: Homophobia, sexism and lesbianism in sport. *Quest* 44, 251-265.

Griffin, P. (1998). *Strong women, deep closets. Lesbians and homophobia in sport*. Champaign, IL: Human Kinetics.

Griffin, P. and Genasci, J. (1990). Addressing homophobia in physical education: Responsibilities for teachers and researchers. In: Messner, M.A. and Sabo, D.F. (eds.). *Sport, men, and the gender order: Critical feminist perspectives*. pp211-222. Champaign, IL: Human Kinetics.

Hargreaves, J.A. (1990). Gender on the sports agenda. *International Review for the Sociology of Sport* 25(4), 287-308.

Hargreaves, J.A. (1994). *Sporting females. Critical issues in the history and sociology of women's sports*. London: Routledge.

Klein, A.M. (1990). Little big man: Hustling, gender narcissism, and bodybuilding subculture. In: Messner, M.A. and Sabo, D.F. (eds.). *Sport, men, and the gender order: Critical feminist perspectives*. pp127-139. Champaign, IL: Human Kinetics.

Krane, V. (1996). Lesbianism in sport. Toward acknowledgement, understanding and theory. *Journal of Sport and Exercise Psychology* 18, 237-246.

Lee, J. (1992). Media portrayals of male and female Olympic athletes: Analyses of newspaper accounts of the 1984 and the 1988 Summer Games. *International Review for the Sociology of Sport* 27(3), 197-222.

Lumpkin, A. and Williams, L.D. (1991). An analysis of Sports Illustrated feature articles, 1954-1987. *Sociology of Sport Journal* 8(1), 16-32.

Messner, M.A. and Sabo, D.F. (1990, eds). *Sport, men, and the gender order: Critical feminist perspectives*. Champaign, IL: Human Kinetics.

Messner, M.A. (2002). *Taking the field: Women, men and sports*. Minneapolis: University of Minnesota Press.

Nelson, M.B. (1991). *Are we winning yet? How women are changing sports and sports are changing women*. New York: Random House.

Nelson, M.B. (1994). *The stronger women get, the more men love football: Sexism and the American culture of sports*. New York: Harcourt Brace.

Palzkill, B. (1990). Between gym shoes and high-heels - The development of a lesbian identity and existence in top class sport. *International Review for the Sociology of Sport* 25(3), 221-234.

Tomlinson, A. (1999). *The game's up: Essays in the cultural analysis of sport, leisure and popular culture*. Aldershot, England: Ashgate Publishing Ltd.

Wigmore, S. (1996). Gender and sport: The last 5 years. *Sport Science Review* 5(2), 53-71.

Women's Sports Foundation. Http://www.womensports foundation.org

Wrisberg, C.A., Draper, M.V. and Everett, J.J. (1988). Sex role orientation of male and female collegiate athletes from selected individual and sport teams. *Sex Roles* 19, 81-90.

GENDER DIFFERENCES   Based upon the average physical dimensions obtained from measurement of thousands of subjects from anthropometric surveys (Behnke and Wilmore, 1974), men and women can be compared:

Reference Man:
Age: 20-24, height: 68.5 in., weight: 154 lb, total fat: 23.1 lb (15%), storage fat: 18.5 lb (12%), essential fat: 4.6 lb (3%), muscle: 69 lb (44.8%), bone: 23 lb (14.9%), remainder: 38.9 lb (25.3%)

Reference Woman:
Age: 20-24, height: 64.5 in., weight: 125 lb, total fat: 33.8 lb (27%), storage fat: 18.8 lb (15%), essential fat: 15 lb (12%), muscle: 45 lb (36%), bone: 15 lb (12%), remainder: 31.2 lb (25%).

Men have wider shoulders, whereas women have wider hips. Women tend to have smaller bodies than men, lower bone strength and a higher proportion of fat mass to fat-free mass. Absolute skinfold measurements for a given relative fatness are smaller in women than for men. Women not only carry more of their fat on the outside, they also distribute more of it to the extremities than men, and this is reflected in higher triceps and thigh skinfold thicknesses relative to trunk measures such as the subscapular skinfold. Women have an obligatory deposition of fat in gender-specific sites, most importantly the breasts, hips and thighs. In swimming, the distribution of body fat in women is such that their legs float high in water. This makes them more horizontal in the water with the result that body drag is decreased. The distribution of fat-free mass in men is such that their legs tend to swing down and float lower in the water with the result that body drag is increased. Females tend to have a lower resting metabolic rate because they have less muscle mass, which is more metabolically active than fat. With less absolute muscle mass and smaller muscle fibers, women display approximately two-thirds of the absolute overall strength and power of men. Women possess about 40 to 60% of the upper body strength, and 70 to 75% of the lower body strength of men. The distribution of muscle fiber types is similar in men and women. Women who follow the same well-designed strength training programs as men benefit from bone and soft-tissue modeling, increased lean body mass, decreased fat, and enhanced self esteem and self confidence. Men have superior absolute strength due to size and body structural differences, rather than hormonal differences. Men typically have a taller, wider frame that supports more muscle, and broader shoulders that provide a greater mechanical advantage. Women have about one tenth the testosterone of men, but the level of testosterone varies greatly among women and influences women's strength development more than that of men. Women who have higher testosterone levels may have a greater potential for strength and power development than other women. Strength training helps decrease body fat and increase lean weight, but only women with a high genetic predisposition for hypertrophy, who participate in high-volume, high-intensity training will see substantial increases in limb circumference. There is little gender difference in other measures of strength such as relative strength.

Women typically have smaller lung volumes and maximal expiratory flow rates even when corrected for height relative to men. Differences in resting and exercising ventilation across the menstrual cycle and relative to men have also been reported, but the functional significance remains unclear. Expiratory flow limitation and a high work of breathing are seen in women.

Although injuries are more sport specific than gender specific, the following injuries have been found to occur commonly in women: ankle ligament injuries, anterior cruciate ligament (ACL) injuries, iliotibial band tendon injury, pes anserinus tendon injury, rotator cuff injuries, stress fractures and spondylolysis. Females are at increased risk for certain sports injuries, especially those involving the knee joint, due to gender differences in coaching, fitness training, anatomy, hormones, biomechanics and the contact nature of some sports. Women sustain two to eight times more ACL injuries for the same sport than men. Female athletes tend to have greater ligamentous laxity and flexibility than males. This laxity may contribute to the increased incidence of patellar subluxations and ligament sprains seen in female athletes. The effect of the menstrual cycle on soft tissues is not well understood. One theory is that hormones such as estrogen, which can relax soft tissue, may predispose female athletes to ACL tears. Estrogen, a hormone with receptors on the human ACL, decreases collagen synthesis and fibroblast proliferation. It has been postulated that any rise in estrogen, such as during the midcycle of the menstrual period, may diminish the tensile strength of the ACL. In addition, estrogen has been reported to decrease fine motor skills by acting on the central and peripheral nervous systems. Motor skill deficits may diminish the normal neuromuscular protective mechanisms of the knee. The effect of relaxin increases the risk of ligamentous injuries during pregnancy. Other anatomical risk factors include increased width of pelvis, increased femoral anteversion, less muscular development (especially of the *vastus medialis obliquus*), greater knee hyperextension, lower center of gravity, shorter legs, narrower femoral notch and external tibial torsion, and greater genu valgus than males. In females with a decreased femoral notch-to-width ratio, a smaller anterior cruciate ligament and smaller notch-space available for the ACL combine to increase risk of injury. The patellofemoral joint is the most common compartment of the knee injured. The *vastus medialis obliquus* is a primary compensating factor for lateral patellar instability. It is the only structure that provides an active medial vector to counterbalance the valgus force. The factors of genu valgus, weak *vastus medialis obliquus* and femoral anteversion increase the laterally directed forces on the patellofemoral joint and increase stresses on the medial compartment and the medial collateral ligament. Females tend to have an increased Q-angle, which imposes excessive laterally directed forces on the *quadriceps femoris* muscle. The higher incidence of overuse injuries among females may be partly explained by the fact that repetitive impact of loads of the body weight will be absorbed by a weaker musculoskeletal system in females compared to that of men of equal body weight. There is evidence from video analysis that women tend to play sports in a more erect position. A more upright position amplifies ground reaction forces that increase the load transmitted to the knee and maximizes anterior shear forces from the *quadriceps femoris*. Improvement of jumping and landing technique seem to decrease the incidence of ACL injuries in female athletes.

Performance-matched groups of males and females are found to have very similar physiological profiles. Conversely, males and females with comparable physiological traits should be expected to perform at the same level. The inter-gender differences in cardiorespiratory endurance vary from 9% at the age of 6 years to 48% at the age of 16. This gender difference in cardiorespiratory endurance is apparently related to gender-related variance in maximal oxygen uptake and work efficiency. Differences in percentage of fat account for most of the superior levels of cardiorespiratory endurance in males. Differences in hemoglobin concentration and maximal stroke volume probably explain most of the variance not accounted for by the percentage of fat mass.

The pace for the world record time in the men's marathon during the early 1990s (333 meters per minute) was faster than the pace for the world record of the 10,000 meters run in the late 1930s. Furthermore, the world record in the marathon for women during the early 1990s was faster than the men's best was until 1952. The following physiological factors appear to act as determinants of distance running performance: maximal oxygen uptake, lactate threshold and running economy. The improvement in performance by men in distance running probably resulted from progressive increases in maximal oxygen uptake as a result of changes in training from the late 1800s to the 1930s. From the 1930s to the 1960s, performance improved because training programs changed in a manner that allowed the top athletes to sustain a

greater fraction of their maximal oxygen uptake in competition. The improvement since the 1960s is likely due to a combination of better tracks and equipment along with enhanced competition opportunities for a larger fraction of the world's population. The rapid improvement in performance by women since the early 1970s seems to have resulted from the rapid emergence of improved opportunities for competition and harder training regimes. Lactate threshold seems to be a more significant limiting factor in elite female distance running than maximal oxygen uptake and running economy.

Seiler and Sailer (1997) analyzed the results of 182 championship finals (91 men, 91 women) from 12 Olympics and five IAAF world championships held between 1952 and 1996, collecting a total of 1091 data points. If the marathon is excluded, the mean performance gap for the other running events increased from 11% in the mid 1980s to 12% in the mid 1990s. In the marathon, males slowed from a mean time of 2:11.30 in the 1980s to 2:14.21 in the 1990s. Female times in the marathon were unchanged in the 1990s (2:30.02 vs. 2:30.17).

Chronology

•1894 • Michael Breal, a classical philologist, wrote to his friend Baron Pierre de Coubertin, suggesting a new race for the 1896 Olympic Games. With a view to making a link to the Ancient Greek Games, he proposed a long endurance run. It was the marathon.

•1896 • The first woman known to have run the marathon was Stamatis Rovithi who ran the proposed course of the marathon a month before the first modern Olympic Games. Another Greek woman, Melpomene, tried to enter the Olympic marathon, but was refused. She ran along the side of the course when the race began and eventually joined the male runners. She completed a distance that only 8 of the 15 male starters could accomplish. Melpomene finished in 4 hours 30 minutes.

•1920 • After the death of a marathon runner in the 1912 Olympic Games, all marathon runners had to undergo a physical examination before the next Games in Antwerp, the first such medical requirement in the history of the Olympics.

•1926 • Violet Percy ran the first recorded women's marathon in London in 3 hours 40 minutes and 22 seconds. Official records of women's times in the marathon did not begin until 1964.

•1927 • The first official list of women's world athletics records was issued by the Féderation Sportive Feminine Internationalè (FSFI).

•1928 • Three women collapsed during the 800 meters run at the Olympic Games. As a consequence, no races beyond 200 meters were run at the Olympics for women until 1960 when the 800 meters was restored.

•1967 • Roberta Gibb and Kathy Switzer defied the rules to sneak into the Boston Marathon. Switzer had actually registered as "K. Switzer." Gibb, who had also sneaked in the previous year, was forced off the course by officials shortly before she reached the finishing line. Switzer, protected by male friends, was able to cross the finishing line. Following adverse publicity, Boston Marathon officials decided that they would not prevent women from running in the 1968 race, but they still were not allowed to enter the race officially. The Boston Marathon added a women's division in 1972, after the New York Marathon had done so the previous year.

•1972 • Six women competed in the New York Marathon and staged a protest of the ruling that they must start the race 10 minutes ahead of the men. When the time elapsed, the women ran with the men. After the Amateur Athletic Union added 10 minutes to their finishing times, the women sued and simultaneous starting times soon became the rule.

•1973 • The first all-women's marathon was held at Waldniel in Germany.

•1981 • The first official women's world record in the 5,000 meters was 15:14.51 by British runner Paula Fudge (GB). In 1997, the world record was 14:28.09 (Jiang Bo, China).

•1982 • Judy Mable Lutter founded the Melpomene Institute, named in honor of the Greek marathon runner in the 1896 Olympic Games, to foster a greater awareness of women's issues both inside and outside of sport.

•1984 • For women, the 3,000 meters, marathon and synchronized swimming were introduced to the Olympic Games.

•2002 • Taylor Davison, a 10-year old and the only girl on her football team, left practice complaining of a headache and collapsed as she walked off the field with her coach. Three days later she died. It was reported that she had taken a hard hit during a full-contact practice three days earlier, sat out three plays with a headache, returned to the field, and did not complain of head pain until her collapse three days later. The Women's Sports Foundation stated that what happened to Taylor Davison was a tragedy and an accident that had nothing to do with gender. "Pre-puberty, girls and boys do not differ significantly in height, weight, fat-free mass, girth, bone width, and skinfold thickness. … Once boys reach puberty, in general, it is unfair for boys to compete against girls on equal terms. … Girls who desire to compete on boys' teams should be permitted to do so if they have the size, strength and skill to match up to the boys they are playing with and against and can therefore do so safely. Physiological differences within the sexes are greater than the differences between the sexes. … Prior to puberty, there are no gender-based physiological reasons to separate males and females in sports competition. However, sex separate programs may be appropriate because of non-gender differences in skill or experience. … Post-puberty, there is no reason for girls not to participate in contact sports with and against other girls."

•2003 • Paul Tergat won the Real Berlin marathon, in a time of 2:04.55, beating Khalid Khannouchi's world record by 43 seconds.

•2003 • Paula Radcliffe set a new women's world record when she finished the London Marathon in 2:15.25. She beat her own record from the 2002 Chicago Marathon by 1 minute 53 seconds.

Bibliography

Behnke, A.R. and Wilmore, J.M. (1974). *Evaluation and regulation of body build and composition*. Englewood Cliffs, NJ: Prentice Hall.

Boden, B.P., Griffin, L.Y. and Garrett, W.E. (2000). Etiology and prevention of noncontact ACL injury. *The Physician and Sportsmedicine* 28(4), 53-60.

Ebben, W.P. and Jensen, R.L. (1998). Strength training for women: Debunking myths that block opportunity. *The Physician and Sportsmedicine*, 26(5), 86-97.

Holloway, J.B. and Baechle, T.R. (1990). Strength training for female athletes: A review of selected aspects. *Sports Medicine* 9 (4), 216-228.

Hutchinson, M.R. and Ireland, M.L. (1995). Knee injuries in female athletes. *Sports Medicine* 19(4), 288-302.

Joyner, M.J. (1993). Physiological limiting factors and distance running: Influence of gender and age on record performances. *Exercise and Sport Sciences Reviews* 21, 103-133.

Junge, A. and Dvorak, J. (2004). Soccer injuries: A review on incidence and prevention. *Sports Medicine* 34(13), 929-938.

Lewis, D.A., Kamon, E. and Hodgson, J.L. (1986). Physiological differences between genders. Implications for sports conditioning. *Sports Medicine* 1, 357-369.

Martin, D.E. and Gynn, R.W.H. (2000). *The Olympic marathon*. Champaign, IL: Human Kinetics.

Pate, R.R. and Kriska, A. (1984). Physiological basis of the sex difference in cardiorespiratory endurance. *Sports Medicine* 1,

87-98.

Sanborn, C.F. and Jankowski, C.M. (1994). Physiologic considerations for women in sport. *Clinics in Sports Medicine* 13(2), 315-327.

Seiler, S. and Sailer, S. (1997). The gender gap: Elite women are running further behind. *Sports Science News* (May-June). Http://www.sportsci.org

Sheel, A.W. et al. (2004). Sex differences in respiratory exercise physiology. *Sports Medicine* 34(9), 567-579.

Sport Research Review Mar/Apr 1990. Women in Sports. Nike, Inc. *The Physician and Sportsmedicine* 18(3), 157-160.

Wells, C.L. (1991). *Women, sport and performance: A physiological perspective.* 2nd ed. Champaign, IL: Human Kinetics.

Whipp, B. and Ward, S. (1992). Will women soon outrun men? *Nature* 355, 25.

Women's Sports Foundation. Http://www.womensports foundation.org

GENDER VERIFICATION

GENDER VERIFICATION   Until the mid-1970s, when it was deemed unreliable, the **sex chromatin test** (**buccal smear test**) was used to establish the gender of athletes in international competition. It consists of microscopic examination of epithelial cells scraped from the inside of the cheek. The cells are stained to reveal the presence or absence of the **Barr body**, which is caused by inactivation of one of the two X chromosomes in female cells and which appears in 20 to 30% of nuclei. If the cells had two X chromosomes, the mark of a genetic female, then a dark spot (the Barr body) would be seen inside the cell's nucleus. Male cells do not show this Barr body as they have only one active X chromosome. The test therefore indicates the number of X chromosomes in the cell nucleus and thus reflects sex chromosome constitution. The sex chromatin test provoked much controversy, because there are a number of genetic disorders that can interfere with the process of sex development and lead to paradoxical findings between anatomical sex and chromosomal sex. It would have permitted recognized males with an XXY karyotype, or Klinefelter's syndrome, and XX males, who have a portion of the testicular determining gene transposed onto the X chromosome.

The sex chromatin test was replaced by an updated DNA test. At the 1992 Olympic Games, women athletes were tested using the polymerase chain reaction to amplify DNA sequences on the Y chromosome that identifies genetic sex only. The **polymerase chain reaction** is a quick, easy method for generating multiple copies of any fragment of DNA, without using a living organism such as E. coli bacteria. It is a chemical reaction that uses the polymerase enzyme to carry out *in vitro* replication of DNA. A **polymerase** is a naturally occurring enzyme that catalyzes the formation and repair of DNA (and RNA). A double stranded DNA is heated to a temperature at which the strands separate. Then, short single strands of DNA (**primers**) with sequences complimentary to the ends of the regions that one wishes to amplify are allowed to assemble into the larger template molecules. The polymerase catalyzes the template-directed synthesis of new double-stranded DNA molecules that are identical in sequence to the starting material.

Some individuals with an apparently normal male chromosome constitution develop to adulthood as females and are referred to as **XY females**. The two most common types of XY female are those with **gonadal dysgenesis**, in which only vestiges of the gonads remain and no male hormones are produced, and those with the **androgen insensitivity syndrome** (or **testicular feminization syndrome**).

Approximately 1 in 20,000 genetic males has a defect in his androgen receptors that results in androgen insensitivity. People with androgen insensitivity syndrome have a functioning Y sex chromosome (and therefore no female internal organs), but an abnormality of the X sex chromosome that renders the body completely or partially incapable of recognizing the androgens produced. In the case of complete androgen insensitivity, the external genital development takes a female form. In the case of partial androgen insensitivity, the external genital appearance may lie anywhere along the spectrum from male to female. Androgen insensitivity syndrome is inherited as a genetic condition in the family known as X-linked recessive inheritance pattern, or partly recessive gene or male-limited autosomal dominant. In about two thirds of all cases, androgen insensitivity syndrome is inherited from the mother. In the other third, there is a spontaneous mutation in the egg. The XY fetus develops testes around the eighth week of gestation. The fetus develops mainly in a female direction. The testes still produce Mullerian inhibiting factor, thus the Mullerian ducts atrophy. The fetus is unable to develop a uterus, fallopian tubes or the upper part of the vagina. At birth the child looks like a girl, except for the presence of the testes, either in the labia or in the lower part of the groin. At puberty, the girl develops breasts and a woman's body. With no ovaries to produce female sex hormones, the body converts some of the testosterone and androstenedione produced by the testes into the female sex hormone estradiol. If the testes are found by a physician, they are usually removed because they could turn cancerous. Estrogen replacement is then prescribed to substitute for the hormones that had been produced by the testes. Without a uterus, she does not menstruate. If the vagina is too short for comfortable sexual intercourse, it can be stretched. XY females are likely to be tall with long legs, well-developed breasts, and clear skin.

There is increased frequency of XY females among athletes in comparison with the general population. Ferguson-Smith (1998) argues that this is because XY females are selected on the basis of their stature. Clinical research has shown that XY female patients with either androgen insensitivity or pure gonadal dysgenesis have a mean adult height on average 10 cm greater than female controls (and patients with XX gonadal dysgenesis) and only 2 cm less than normal male controls. This effect is largely, if not entirely, due to determinants for stature carried by the differential region of the Y chromosome.

Gender dysphoria is a general term for persons who have confusion or discomfort about their birth gender. Milder forms of gender dysphoria cause incomplete or occasional feelings of being the opposite sex. The most intense form of the condition, with complete gender reversal is called transsexualism. A **transsexual** is a male or female who has a lifelong feeling of being trapped in the wrong body. Hermaphrodites and others with ambiguous sex characteristics at birth may or may not develop gender dysphoria. The vast majority of transsexuals, however, have no identifiable physical abnormality. With hormonal treatment and surgery, most transsexuals can achieve satisfactory physical appearance and sexual function. For a male becoming a female, treatment with female hormones is required for at least a year before irreversible surgical steps are taken. This produces changes in secondary sex characteristics, such as decrease in body hair, breast development, and feminization of body shape and skin texture. An artificial vagina is created and lined with the skin of the penis, the nerves and blood vessels of which remain largely intact. Scrotal tissue is used to create labia, and the urethra is shortened and positioned in the female position. The female to male conversion involves use of testosterone, mastectomy, and surgical removal of the ovaries and uterus. Some patients may even have a penis constructed and artificial testes implanted, with construction of a male urethra and relocation of the clitoris to the head of the penis. *See also* CHROMATIN.

Chronology

•1930 • Zdena Koublova of Czechoslavakia won the 800 m run at the 3rd World Women's Games. Later Czech officials admitted that Koublova is male. This eventually led to the introduction of gender testing in sport.

•1932 • Stella Walsh (Stanislawa Walasiewiczowna) of Poland won the gold medal in the Women's 100 m in the Olympic Games. She became a US citizen in 1947. She was caught in the crossfire during an armed robbery and killed in Cleveland in 1980. An autopsy following her death found that she was actually a man. Walsh had mosaicism; being neither male nor female, having male sex organs (non-functioning) and both male and female chromosomes.

•1938 • The German high jumper Dora Ratjen, who set of world record of 5ft 6 in, was exposed as an imposter who had male sex organs. She was banned and subsequently changed her name to Hermann. Hermann Ratjen posed as a woman 'Dora' and came 4th in the 1936 Olympics. In 1957, Ratjen confessed that he was a man.

•1966 • At the European Athletics Championships in Budapest, the genitalia of female competitors were inspected by a panel of doctors and officials. After a visual inspection, the panel would issue a certificate of femininity. Immediately before the first parade, five women record-holders dropped out with unexpected illnesses and the Olympic gold-winning Russian sisters Irina and Tamara Press suddenly announced their retirement.

•1967 • The International Amateur Athletics Federation (IAAF) introduced "femininity control," the sex chromatin test.

•1967 • At the European Cup Finals, Ewa Klobukowska of Poland became the first athlete to fail the sex chromatin test and it was it was declared that she had "one chromosome too many to be declared a woman for the purposes of athletic competition." She was barred from international competition, stripped of all her past medals and world records.

•1968 • The International Olympic Committee (IOC) Medical Commission introduced sex testing.

•1976 • Richard Raskind had a sex change operation and adopted the name Renee Richards. The US Tennis Association attempted to ban Richards, but the New York Supreme Court ruled there was "overwhelming medical evidence that [Richards] is now a female." Richards was never accepted as a competitor outside the USA, but worked on a part-time basis as a traveling consultant for Martina Navratilova from 1981 to 1988.

•1985 • Spanish hurdler Maria Patino failed the sex chromatin test, but was convinced that she was just as female as the other competitors, despite having one X chromosome and one Y chromosome. After a three year legal campaign, she was reinstated.

•1992 • Following a workshop on "femininity verification" it organized in 1990, the International Amateur Athletic Federation (IAAF) defied the International Olympic Committee (IOC) and stopped gender testing. After recognizing the complaints of the IAAF, the American Medical Association (AMA) and the American Board of Obstetrics and Gynecology (ABOG), the IOC discontinued sex testing for athletes.

•1996 • At the Olympic Games, 8 out of 3,387 female athletes had positive results from DNA screening for gender verification. 7 had androgen insensitivity, 4 incomplete and 3 complete; the other athlete had previously undergone gonadectomy and was presumed to have 5-alpha-steroid reductase deficiency, which is an autosomal recessive sex-limited condition resulting in the inability to convert testosterone to the more physiologically active dihydrotestosterone. Because dihydrotestosterone is required for the normal masculinization of the external genitalia *in utero*, genetic males with 5-alpha-reductase type 2 deficiency are born with ambiguous genitalia (i.e. male pseudohermaphroditism). The eight women were subject to further scrutiny and discussion before being allowed to compete.

•1999 • The International Olympic Committee (IOC) ratified the abandonment of on-site genetic screening of female athletes. Testing was suspended on a trial basis for the Olympic Games at Sydney in 2000 and the Winter Olympic Games at Salt Lake City in 2002, but the IOC has reserved the right to reapply testing in any individual case that is brought to their attention.

•2004 • By competing in the Women's Australian Open, 37 year-old Mianne Bagger became the first transsexual to play in a professional golf tournament. Bagger was a 4-handicap golfer, but then stopped playing in order to undergo transformation to a female with hormone therapy in 1992. Three years later Bagger had a sex-change operation and then resumed playing in 1998. Women's Golf Australia removed their "female at birth" clause in 1998 and gave Bagger an exemption to the tournament.

Bibliography

Birrell, S. and Cole, C. (1990). Double fault: Renee Richards and the construction and naturalization of difference. *Sociology of Sport Journal* 7, 1-21.

Bouchard, C., Dionne, F.T., Simoneau, J.A. and Boulay, M.R. (1992). Genetics of aerobic and anaerobic performance. *Exercise and Sport Sciences Reviews* 20, 27-58.

Elsas, L.J. et al. (2000). Gender verification of female athletes. *Genetic Medicine* 2(4), 249-254.

Ferguson-Smith, M.A. (1998). Gender verification and the place of XY females in sport. In Harries, M. et al. (eds). *Oxford textbook of sports medicine*. 2nd ed. pp355-365. Oxford: Oxford University Press.

Ferguson-Smith, M.A. and Ferris, E.A. (1991). Gender verification in sport: The need for change? *British Journal of Sports Medicine* 25(1) 17-20.

Ferris, E.A. (1992). Gender verification testing in sport. *British Medical Bulletin* 48(3), 683-697.

Peel, R. (1994). *Eve's rib. Searching for the biological roots of sex differences*. New York: Crown Publishers.

Simpson, J.L. et al. (2000). Gender verification in the Olympics. *Journal of the American Medical Association* 284(12), 1568-1569.

The Zenith Foundation. Http://www.genderweb.org

Wilson, B.E. (2004). 5-alpha-reductase deficiency. Http://www.emedicine.com

GENE   A unit of the material of inheritance. *See* HEREDITY.

GENE THERAPY   A technique in which a

functioning gene is inserted into a cell to correct a genetic error or to introduce a new function to the cell for therapeutic purposes. Adenoviruses are often used as a delivery system for gene therapy because they are relatively large and can carry big genes. Gene therapy could be particularly useful in initiating and accelerating the repair of connective tissue such as cartilage.

Svensson et al. (1997) used an adenovirus to deliver the gene for erythropoietin to mice and monkeys. Mouse hematocrit was increased from 49% to 81%, while monkey hematocrit increased from 40% to 70% or more. A single injection elevated hematocrit for over a year in the mice and for 12 weeks in the monkeys. Successful gene therapy could lead to problems, however, mainly because there is no way to turn the gene off once it has been inserted. Some of the monkeys in Svensson et al's study produced too much erythropoietin and had to be bled in order to thin their blood and keep them alive.

Barton-Davis et al. (1998) used an adenovirus to deliver the insulin-like growth factor-1 (IGF-1) gene into the leg muscles of mice. After 3 months, the leg muscles of the mice injected with IGF-1 gene had grown by 15%, and increased in strength by 14%, even though the animals had not taken any special exercise. It was proposed that these effects are primarily due to stimulation of muscle regeneration via the activation of satellite cells by IGF-I. In effect, the mice expressed IGF-1 as if they had been engaging in strenuous exercise. This supports the hypothesis that the primary cause of aging-related impairment of muscle function is a cumulative failure to repair damage sustained during muscle utilization. Gene transfer of IGF-1 into muscle could form the basis of a human gene therapy for preventing the loss of muscle associated with aging and may be of benefit in diseases where the rate of damage to skeletal muscle is accelerated. It is possible that some people naturally produce more IGF-1. One of the unknowns about gene therapy in humans, however, is whether or not a second dose will have the same effect as the first one. It is possible that the body will build antibodies against the virus that inserts the gene into the cells so that a repeated injection with the same virus may not work.

Bibliography

Anderson, J.L., Schjerling, P. and Saltin, B. (2000). Muscle, genes and athletic performance. *Scientific American* 283(3), 48-55.

Barton-Davis, E.R. et al. (1998). Viral mediated expression of insulin-like growth factor 1 blocks the aging-related loss of skeletal muscle function. *Proceedings of the National Academy of Science* 95(26), 15603-15607.

Lamsam, C., Fu, F.H. et al. (1997). Gene therapy in sports medicine. *Sports Medicine* 25(2), 73-77.

Svensson, E.C. et al. (1997). Long-term erythropoietin expression in rodents and non-human primates following intramuscular injection of a replication-defective adenoviral vector. *Human Gene Therapy* 8(15), 1797-1806.

GENITO-URINARY INJURIES The **vulva** is the external genitalia of the female that consists of the mons pubis, the labia majora and minoris, the clitoris, the vestibule of the vagina and its glands, and the opening of the urethra and the vagina. The vagina may be injured by contact with water at high speed, especially during water skiing, or water may be forced through the fallopian tubes (resulting in localized pelvic peritonitis). A neoprene™ wet suit serves as a preventative measure. **Vulvar hematomas** may occur as a result of straddle injuries, often in gymnastics. In severe cases, laceration may occur.

Injuries to the penis are rare because of its mobility in the non-erect state. The scrota are at risk of injury in ball sports such as cricket. Athletic supports (jock straps) and boxes (protective cups) offer some protection against scrotal trauma. Protective cups are required for baseball catchers and ice hockey goalkeepers. Blunt scrotal trauma, such as occurs from a knee to the groin, can cause a contusion, hematoma, torsion, dislocation or rupture of the testicle. If the tunica vaginalis ruptures, the vascular and tubercle components of the testes can be seriously damaged. Congenital variations in testicular suspension make certain individuals susceptible to torsion of the spermatic cord ('**testicular torsion**'), which is a surgical emergency because it causes strangulation of gonadal blood supply with subsequent testicular necrosis and atrophy. Occasionally, blunt trauma leads to swelling in the tunica vaginalis resulting in a traumatic

hydrocele, a disorder in which serous fluid accumulates in a body sac (especially in the scrotum. In 9 to 18% of men, there may the occurrence of a **variocele**, a dilation of the veins along the spermatic cord (vas deferens) in the scrotum (caused by incompetent or inadequate valves within these veins). The incidence of varioceles is higher in men between 15 and 25 years old. Varioceles are found in approximately 15 to 20% of all males and in 40% of infertile males.

See also PRIAPISM; RUNNER'S BLADDER.

Chronology

•1874 • The Bike Web Manufacturing Company invented the Athletic Supporter in response to a request from the Boston Athletic Club to design apparel that would provide comfort and support for bicycle jockeys riding the cobblestone streets of Boston. Originally known as the "bicycle jockey strap," the jock strap was patented in 1897. The first mass marketing of the jock strap came in the 1902 edition of the Sears and Roebuck Catalog that described the athletic supporter as being "medically indicated" for all males who engage in sports or strenuous activity.

Bibliography

Kim, E.D. (2001). Variocele. Http://emedicine.com/topic2757.htm

GENOME The total complement of genes contained in a cell or virus.

GENOTYPE See under HEREDITY.

GENU RECURVATUS Back knees. Hyper-extended knees. It is the tendency of the knees to hyperextend. Hyperextension of the knees tends to tilt the pelvis forward and contributes to lordosis. It may be caused by knee extensor weakness, tight calf muscles, Achilles tendon contractures and bony abnormalities. In cerebral palsy, genu recurvatus often results from surgical overcorrection of knee flexion deformities. Severe cases of genu recurvatus are usually treated by prescription of a knee-ankle brace that holds the foot in slight dorsal flexion and the knee in flexion.

GENU VALGUS Knocked knees. It is a condition in which the legs are bowed inwards in the standing position. It exists when the medial tibiofemoral angle is greater than 195 degrees. The inward bowing usually occurs at or around the knees. Standing with the knees together, the feet are far apart. This condition will increase the compressive force on the lateral condyle, while increasing the tensile stresses on the medial structures. Pronation and weakness in the longitudinal arch of the feet usually accompany genu valgus.

No treatment or exercises are recommended for genu valgus in children younger than age of 7 years because, developmentally, this is a normal condition. Severe cases that persist are treated with surgery (osteotomy). Genu valgus is common in obese children. Poor alignment of the knee results in a disproportionate amount of weight being borne by its medial aspect and predisposes the joint to injury.

GENU VARUS Bowed legs. It is a condition in which the legs are bowed outwards in the standing position, resulting in the knees being separated when the ankles are touching. It exists when the medial tibiofemoral angle is 180 degrees or less (exceeding 180 degrees as measured laterally). One or both legs can be affected. The bowing can occur in either the femur or the tibia, but is more common in the tibia. In this condition, the compressive stresses on the medial tibial condyle are increased, whereas the tensile stresses are increased laterally. Genu varus is frequently accompanied by compensatory deformities in the feet.

The legs of infants often bow during the first few months of walking because of imbalance of strength between the peroneal and tibial muscle groups. By the age 2 or 3 years, this problem resolves itself in most children. Most children become knock-kneed until the age of 4 years, and finally straighten up by the age of 6 or 7 years. There are pathological causes of genu varus, e.g. Blount's disease (tibia varus).

GESTALT PSYCHOLOGY A school of thought in psychology based on the premise that behavior cannot be explained by decreasing it to its simplest units. 'Gestalt' is a German word meaning a form or configuration with properties that are more than just the sum of the parts. With its emphasis on the perception and experience of the world by a particular person at a particular moment in time, Gestalt psychology is related to phenomenology.

Gestalt therapy is a form of psychotherapy based on the premise that an individual acts out a variety of roles that are not necessarily consistent, but that are situation specific and derive meaning from their configurations in the particular situation. Role-playing involves acting out the personality of oneself or someone else, and is one of the techniques used in Gestalt therapy.

Bibliography

Riet, V., Van De Korb, M. and Gorrell, J.J. (1980). *Gestalt therapy*. New York: Pergamon Press.

Syer, J. and Connolly, C. (1998). *Sporting body, sporting mind: Athlete's guide to mental training*. Rev. ed. London: Simon & Schuster.

GESTATIONAL DIABETES *See under* PREGNANCY.

GILBERT'S SYNDROME A relatively common and benign, congenital (probably hereditary) liver disorder. It is characterized by a mild, fluctuating increase in serum bilirubin, a breakdown product of hemoglobin that is a yellow pigment excreted by the liver into bile, due to a slight deficiency in the enzyme UDB glucuronyl transferase. Occasionally mild jaundice may appear, and the white of the eye becomes yellow. It is estimated that 3 to 7% of the adult population has Gilbert's syndrome, and it is more common in males. Onset of Gilbert's syndrome usually occurs in the teenage years or early adulthood.

Bibliography

British Liver Trust. Http://www.britishlivertrust.org.uk

GINSENG The root of the plant *Panax ginseng* has been used for many centuries in the Orient as a tonic to decrease fatigue. The main active constituents of the Panax species are triterpenoid glycosides (saponins; ginsenosides; panaxosides), which are steroid substances. American ginseng and red ginseng are not comparable in ginsenosides to Panax ginseng. Pharmacological research has found that ginseng has the potential to increase non-specific resistance to various stressors. In America, ginseng is not included in the Generally Recognized as Safe (GRAS) list, nor has the US government set guidelines for the manufacture and quality control of commercial ginseng preparations. The Food and Drug Administration (FDA) in the USA regards ginseng as a food. Ginseng is comprised of approximately 70% carbohydrate, 12% protein; and contains a range of vitamins, minerals and other substances (e.g. ephedrine). There is no convincing scientific evidence that ginseng enhances performance in humans. Side effects associated with chronic intake of ginseng include hypertension, insomnia, nervousness and depression.

Bibliography

Bahrke, M.S. and Morgan, W.P. (1994). Evaluation of the ergogenic properties of ginseng. *Sports Medicine* 18(4), 229-248.

Bahrke, M.S. and Morgan, W.P. (2000). Evaluation of the ergogenic properties of ginseng: An update. *Sports Medicine* 29(2), 113-133.

GIRTH Circumference (of a body segment, for example). The standard girth sites in humans include: abdomen (at the level of the umbilicus); arm (midway between the acromion and olecranon processes, with arm to the side of the body); calf (at the maximum girth between the knee and ankle joint); forearm (maximum girth, with the arms hanging down, but slightly away from the trunk and palms facing forward); hips (at the maximal girth of the hips or buttocks region, above the gluteal fold, whichever is larger); thigh (at the maximal girth of the thigh, below the gluteal fold, with the legs slightly apart); and waist (at the narrowest part of the torso, above the umbilicus and below the xiphoid process).

GLAND A type of effector organ. There are two types of gland: endocrine and exocrine. **Endocrine glands** have no secretory ducts and secrete hormones directly into the extracellular spaces around the gland before the hormones diffuse into the blood for transport throughout the body. **Exocrine glands**, such as the eccrine glands, have secretory ducts that lead directly to the body compartment or surface where the secreted substance is required.

GLASSES   Sport-specific features of glasses include the spring hinges in the temples of shooting glasses, which allow the frame to flex without breaking during recoil. In basketball and soccer, prescription polycarbonate goggles with a wrap-around strap can be used. Polycarbonate is approximately 10 times more impact resistant than other plastics. Tinted lenses may be of benefit in some sports, e.g. lenses that enhance yellow may be advantageous in tennis where the balls are usually yellow. Polarized lenses filter out glare and reflected light, thus may be helpful in skiing, shooting, golf and many other outdoor sports. Glare is a visual condition in which the observer feels discomfort and/or exhibits a lower performance in visual tasks. It is produced by a relatively bright source of light within the visual field. All lenses used outdoors should provide protection from harmful ultraviolet light (UVA and UVB).

Bibliography

All About Vision. Http://www.allaboutvision.com

D & J Brower Opticians. Http://www.brower.co.uk

GLAUCOMA   An eye disease in which the fluid pressure inside the eyeball rises to a point at which it damages the optic nerve, first affecting peripheral vision and later causing central vision blindness. In the USA, nearly 3 million people have glaucoma. Glaucoma is five times more likely to occur in African Americans than in Caucasians.

Bibliography

National Eye Institute. Http://nei.nih.gov

GLENO-HUMERAL JOINT   *See* SHOULDER JOINT.

GLENOID LABRUM   *See under* SHOULDER JOINT.

GLIAL CELLS   *See under* NERVOUS SYSTEM.

GLOBAL POSITIONING SYSTEM   GPS. It is a navigation system that uses 27 operational satellites in orbit around the earth. It is funded by the US Department of Defense for navigation, but is increasingly used for aviation, marine and outdoor-recreational purposes. Each satellite is equipped with an atomic clock. The satellites first set the clock in the GPS receiver by synchronizing it with the atomic clock in the satellite. The satellites then constantly send information (at the speed of light) about the exact time to the GPS receiver.

By comparing the time given by a satellite and the time within the GPS receiver, the signal time is calculated. The distance to the satellite is then calculated by multiplying the signal distance time with the speed of light. By calculating the distance to at least four satellites, the exact position can be trigonometrically determined. The signal from the satellites is influenced by the atmosphere and also by the bouncing off various local obstructions before reaching the receiver.

The technique of the differential global positioning system has been proposed as a way to monitor the position and speed of an athlete during outdoor activities with acceptable precision, thus controlling inclination and speed.

Chronology

•2002 • In the 148th University Boat Race, rowed between Putney and Mortlake on the River Thames in London (UK), both the Oxford and Cambridge boats carried a small, strengthened waterproof box that contained a Global Positioning System device that sent out readings every second for the position and speed of the boat. It also measured the stroke rates.

Bibliography

Larsson, P. (2003). Global positioning system and sport-specific testing. *Sports Medicine* 33(15), 1093-1101.

GLOBIN   The protein of hemoglobin. It is a globular polypeptide chain.

GLOBULAR PROTEINS   Any protein that is readily soluble in aqueous solvents.

GLOBULIN   A type of protein found in serum. Globulins function as antibodies.

GLOMERULONEPHRITIS   *See under* NEPHRITIS.

GLOTTIS   An elongated, narrow opening where the cavity of the larynx divides into two parts by two folds of mucous membrane stretching from front to back. It is the narrowest section of the air passages. *See also* EPIGLOTTIS.

GLUCAGON   A protein hormone secreted by the alpha cells of the islets of Langerhans in the pancreas. It promotes the release of glucose from the liver to the blood by stimulating both glycogenolysis and gluconeogenesis in the liver. It thus has the opposite effect to that of insulin. Glucagon also increases lipolysis in adipose tissue. Its secretion is controlled by plasma glucose level at the pancreas. Secretion of glucagon is minimal during mild-to-moderate intensity exercise, but increases with prolonged exercise.

GLUCOCORTICOIDS   *See under* CORTICO-STEROIDS.

GLUCONEOGENESIS   The process of making new glucose from amino acids and other non-carbohydrate substances, such as lactate, glycerol and pyruvate. About 90% of gluconeogenesis takes place in the liver; the remainder takes place in the kidneys. Gluconeogenesis is preceded by the glucose-alanine cycle. Gluconeogenesis is not simply the reversal of glycolysis; there are additional enzymes that are not involved in glycolysis. *See* AMINO ACID DEGRADATION.

GLUCOSE   A carbohydrate and the major nutrient from which the body obtains energy. **Blood glucose (blood sugar)** is glucose that is dissolved in blood plasma. The liver stores glucose as glycogen. When the liver converts glycogen back to glucose, it feeds glucose into the blood. The breakdown of glycogen to glucose is called glycogenolysis. Normal blood glucose levels are between 70 and 120 mg/dL.

Post-prandial levels are typically 90 to 150 mg/dL (one hour after meals) and 80 to 140 mg/dL (two hours after meals). An adequate blood glucose level is necessary for normal functioning of the central nervous system. Glucose is the only sugar that can pass the blood-brain barrier. An adult brain uses about 120 g per day, whereas only about another 40 g are required for the rest of the body. Working muscles take up an average of only 4% of the glucose circulated to it. This is probably a protective mechanism to ensure availability for the brain. The maintenance of blood glucose level depends on the amount of glycogen stored in the liver and the activity of the enzymes involved in glycogenolysis and gluconeogenesis.

Blood glucose level is mainly controlled by the following hormones: insulin, glucagon, epinephrine, norepinephrine and the glucocorticoids. The production of glucose in the liver during exercise is stimulated by glucagon, epinephrine and norepinephrine. It is suppressed by insulin or an increase in blood glucose concentration. It appears that a decrease in insulin and an increase in glucagon are both required for glucose production in the liver to increase normally during exercise of moderate intensity (60 to 70% maximal oxygen uptake) and moderate duration (40 to 60 minutes).

Consuming large amounts of simple carbohydrates before exercise can have profound effects on blood glucose and insulin during exercise. The high glucose absorption causes an exaggerated insulin response, such that blood glucose, after rising, actually falls lower than the level it was before the intake of simple carbohydrate. A greater dependence is placed on muscle glycogen as a fuel. The low blood glucose level (hypoglycemia) and increased glycogen utilization can be detrimental to both aerobic and anaerobic exercise. This effect of pre-exercise glucose feeding does not occur during exercise partly because of increased alpha-adrenergic stimulation of the beta cells of the pancreas.

'Hitting the wall' and **'bonking'** are terms used in association with glycogen depletion during marathon running. However, the significant decrease in exercise intensity after 3 hours of strenuous endurance exercise has also been associated with damage to the fibrous connective tissue that surrounds the muscles, as a result of the repeated stretching and tearing of the leg muscle fibers each time the feet hit the ground. Cyclists, after two hours of hard racing, do not 'hit the wall' because their muscles are subjected to the smooth rotary motion of pedaling rather than the constant shocks of the foot hitting the ground.

It is accepted that there is a relationship between glucose and fatty acids, but there is controversy as to whether this relationship is regulated by glucose or by fatty acids. According to Randle et al. (1963), the balance between glucose and fat oxidation is determined by the intracellular availability of fatty acids. Increasing fatty acid availability attenuates carbohydrate oxidation during exercise, mainly via sparing of intramuscular glycogen. Sidossis (1998) argues that it is the intracellular availability of glucose, rather than fatty acids, that regulates substrate interaction during exercise. According to Randle (1998), the evidence for the inhibitory effects of fatty acids on whole body glucose utilization and oxidation (predominantly muscles) is decisive and enzyme mechanisms mediating these effects are well established.

See also DIET; GLUT-4; HYPERGLYCEMIA; HYPOGLYCEMIA.

Bibliography

Randle, P.J., Garland, P.B., Hales, C.N., and Newsholme, E.A. (1963). The glucose-fatty acid cycle: Its role in insulin sensitivity and the metabolic disturbances of diabetes mellitus. *Lancet* 1, 785-789.

Randle, P.J. (1998). Regulatory interactions between lipids and carbohydrates: The glucose fatty acid cycle after 35 years. *Diabetes Metabolism Review* 14(4), 263-283.

Sidossis, L.S. (1998). The role of glucose in the regulation of substrate interaction during exercise. *Canadian Journal of Applied Physiology* 23(6), 558-569.

Stamford, B. (1991). How exercise affects your blood sugar. *The Physician and Sportsmedicine* 19(2), 139-140.

GLUCOSE-ALANINE CYCLE Felig cycle. Amino acids in muscle are converted to glutamate and then to alanine. The alanine released from the exercising muscle is transported to the liver where it undergoes deamination. The remaining carbon skeleton is converted to glucose (gluconeogenesis) and then released into the blood and delivered to the working muscles. After 4 hours of continuous light exercise, the liver's output of alanine-derived glucose can account for 45% of the total glucose released from the liver. With more intense exercise, precursors of gluconeogenesis could account for 60% of the glucose output.

GLUCOSE POLYMERS *See* MALTODEXTRINS.

GLUCOSE TOLERANCE *See under* INSULIN RESISTANCE.

GLUT-4 Glucose transporter 4. A glucose transport protein. When glucose and insulin levels are high, or during exercise, most of the glucose enters skeletal muscle cells by GLUT-4. In resting skeletal muscle, most glucose enters by the GLUT-1 carriers. *See also under* INSULIN RESISTANCE.

GLUTAMATE *See* GLUTAMIC ACID.

GLUTAMIC ACID A five-carbon, nonessential, glycogenic (glucogenic) amino acid. It is ionized at the pH of the cell, and is thus in the form of glutamate. It is a precursor of the neurotransmitter GABA and of the two non-essential amino acids glutamine and proline. Glutamate is responsible for gathering both the ammonia molecules from the amino acids incorporated into urea. If the carbon skeleton of glutamate were to be used for energy, all five carbons (like those of glutamine and proline) would enter the Krebs cycle at alpha ketoglutarate by the action of glutamate dehydrogenase. These carbons can exit the Krebs cycle at oxaloacetate and be converted to glucose via phosphoenolpyruvate.

Monosodium glutamate (MSG), sodium bound to glutamic acid, is a flavor enhancer added to many foods. Some people may react to MSG and develop MSG symptom complex. In MSG-intolerant people with asthma, this may cause bronchospasm. *See also* GLUTAMINE.

GLUTAMINE A five-carbon, non-essential amino

acid that is formed from glutamic acid by the addition of ammonia. It is the most abundant amino acid in human muscle and plasma, contributing 50 to 60% of the total free amino acid pool. It is one of the few substances that can readily pass through the blood-brain barrier, and is taken up by the brain in greater quantities than any other amino acid.

Glutamine is an important fuel for some key cells of the immune system. Both the plasma concentration of glutamine and the functional ability of immune cells of the blood are decreased after prolonged, exhaustive exercise. Glutamine feeding has had beneficial effects in clinical situations, and the provision of glutamine after intensive exercise has decreased the incidence of infections (particularly of upper respiratory tract infection). There is no firm evidence as to precisely which aspect of the immune system is affected by glutamine feeding during the transient immunodepression that occurs after prolonged, strenuous exercise. However, there is increasing evidence that neutrophils may be implicated. Since injury, infection, nutritional status and acute exercise can all influence plasma glutamine level, these factors must be controlled and/or taken into consideration if plasma glutamine is to prove a useful marker of immunodepression and impending overtraining.

Bibliography

Castell, L. (2003). Glutamine supplementation in vitro and in vivo, in exercise and in immunodepression. *Sports Medicine* 33(5), 323-345.

Castell, L.M. and Newsholme, E.A. (2001). The relation between glutamine and the immunodepression observed in exercise. *Amino Acids* 20(1), 49-61.

Walsh, N.P., Blannin, A.K., Robson, P.J. and Gleeson, M. (1998). Glutamine, exercise and immune function. Links and possible mechanisms. *Sports Medicine* 26(3), 177-191.

GLUTATHIONE   A tripeptide coenzyme of glutathione reductase involved in metabolism. It is composed of glutamic acid, cysteine and glycine. In its reduced state, glutathione helps maintain the iron in hemoglobin in the ferrous state. Red blood cells that are deficient in glutathione are more susceptible to hemolysis. Glutathione in the red blood cells is reduced by NADPH. *See under* FREE RADICALS.

GLUTEALE   Midgluteal arch. An anatomical landmark that is the point at the sacrococcygeal fusion in the midsagittal plane.

GLUTEUS MEDIUS SYNDROME   A tendon injury at the insertion of the *gluteus medius* muscle that may be due to tilting of the pelvis during running and is aggravated by the effects of fatigue and any leg length inequality.

GLYCEMIC INDEX   It is a standardized rating of the increase in blood glucose after ingestion of a standard amount of carbohydrate. It is a percentage value based on the area under the blood glucose response curve of a food containing 50 g of available carbohydrate divided by the area of the blood glucose response of 50 g of carbohydrate in a reference food. Originally, the reference food used for calculating the glycemic index was glucose, but now it is usually white bread containing 50 g of carbohydrate. Bread is preferred to glucose, because it is more palatable and avoids the possibility of delayed gastric emptying from the high osmolality of a glucose solution. It thus greatly decreases variability among individuals.

The higher the glycemic index, the faster the increase in blood glucose and the more rapid the energy supply. The glycemic index was originally used for the design of therapeutic diets such as for diabetics. A low glycemic index is associated with improved insulin sensitivity. Compared to normal persons, Type-2 diabetics have a much greater and more prolonged increase in blood glucose. Thus, to avoid large increases in blood glucose, individuals with diabetes should avoid foods with a high glycemic index. The development of the glycemic index countered the view that the glucose response of carbohydrates could be categorized according to complex and simple carbohydrates. Some complex carbohydrates have a very low post-prandial glycemic index, whereas others induce higher glycemic responses. It can vary greatly within the same class of food. Basmati rice is rich in amylose, which is harder to break down, and it has a glycemic index of 58, whereas instant-cook rice has a glycemic index of 87. The glycemic index is higher when the carbohydrate meal is easily soluble and cooked rather than raw. It is lower when lipids and proteins are co-ingested and when there is a large quantity of dietary fiber. A limitation of the glycemic index is that it only gives a value for a single food and not meals. It has been shown, however, that the glycemic index for individual foods can be used to predict the glycemic index for a mixed meal.

The glycemic index compares the potential of foods containing the same amount of carbohydrate to raise blood glucose. However, the amount of carbohydrate consumed also affects blood glucose levels and insulin responses. **Glycemic load** corrects glycemic index for serving size. It is calculated by multiplying the glycemic index by the amount in grams provided by a food and dividing the total by 100.

Raisins (60 g serving, 42.7 g carbohydrate) have a glycemic index of 64 and glycemic load of 27.3. Crunch Nut cornflakes (30 g serving, 22.9 g carbohydrate) have a glycemic index of 72 and a glycemic load of 16.5. Yellow box honey (25 g serving, 20.5 g carbohydrate), with 46% fructose, has a glycemic index of 35 and glycemic load of 7.2. Yapunya honey from Australia (25 g serving, 20.5 g carbohydrate), with 42% fructose, has a glycemic index of 52 and glycemic load of 10.7. White rice (boiled) from India, type not specified (150 g serving, 42 g carbohydrate) has a glycemic index of 48 and glycemic load of 20.2. White rice (boiled) from Pakistan, type not specified (150 g serving, 42 g carbohydrate) has a glycemic index of 69 and glycemic load of 29. Spaghetti, white, durum wheat (USA), boiled 20 minutes (180 g serving, 44.3 g carbohydrate) has a glycemic index of 64 and glycemic load of 28.3. Spaghetti, white (Australia), boiled (180 g serving, carbohydrate 44.3 g) has a glycemic index of 38 and glycemic load of 16.8. Potato, Russet Burbank (USA), baked without fat (200 g serving, 29 g carbohydrate) has a glycemic index of 94 and glycemic load of 27.3. Potato, Russet Burbank (Canada), baked without fat (150 g serving, 21.8 g carbohydrate) has a glycemic index of 56 and glycemic load of 12.2.

Strategies for lowering dietary glycemic load include: increasing the consumption of fruits, vegetables, legumes (peas and beans), nuts and whole grains; decreasing the consumption of starchy high glycemic index foods such as potatoes, white rice and white bread; decreasing the consumption of sugary foods like cookies, candy, cakes and soft drinks.

There is insufficient evidence that athletes who consume a low glycemic index carbohydrate-rich meal prior to a prolonged event will gain clear performance benefits. However, athletes wishing to consume carbohydrates 30 to 60 minutes before exercise should be encouraged to ingest low glycemic index foods. Consuming these types of foods will decrease the likelihood of creating hyperglycemia and hyperinsulinemia at the onset of exercise, while providing exogenous carbohydrate throughout exercise. It is recommended that high glycemic index foods be consumed during exercise. These foods will ensure rapid digestion and absorption, which will lead to elevated blood glucose levels during exercise. The glycemic index has also been used to determine the best type of carbohydrate for promoting increases in muscle glycogen during the hours immediately after exercise. Foods with a higher glycemic index seem to be better for optimizing muscle glycogen synthesis in the first two hours after exercise. The reason for this is not clear. *See also* DIET.

Bibliography

Burke, L.M., Collier, G.R. and Hargreaves, M. (1998). Glycemic index: A new tool in sport nutrition? *International Journal of Sport Nutrition* 8(4), 401-415.

Sydney University Glycemic Index Research Service. Http://www.glycemicindex.com

Walton, P. and Rhodes, E.C. (1997). Glycaemic index and optimal performance. *Sports Medicine* 23(3), 164-172

GLYCEROL A three-carbon alcohol that is produced in the human body and distributed within and between all cells at low concentrations. Biochemically, the most important form of glycerol is glycerol 3-phosphate, a substrate in triglyceride synthesis that reacts with two fatty acyl CoA molecules to form phosphatidate.

Clinically, glycerol infusion and ingestion have been used in the treatment of cerebral edema resulting from acute ischemic stroke, intraocular hypertension (glaucoma), intracranial hypertension, postural syncope and improved rehydration during acute gastrointestinal disease. Glycerol is effective in decreasing excess accumulation of fluid (edema) in the brain and eye. An osmotic effect occurs because concentrated extracellular glycerol enters brain tissues, cerebrospinal fluid and the eye's aqueous humor at a slow rate, which draws fluid from these tissues.

Glycerol hyperhydration is glycerol ingestion with added fluid. Hyperhydration or increasing body water content above normal (euhydration) level was thought to have some benefit during exercise heat stress. Attempts to overdrink, however, have been minimized by a rapid diuretic response. Recent research has found that hyperhydration (water or glycerol) does not alter core temperature, skin temperature, whole body sweating rate, local sweating rate, sweating threshold temperature, sweating sensitivity or heart rate responses compared to euhydration. If euhydration is maintained during exercise-heat stress, then hyperhydration appears to have no meaningful advantage. The use of glycerol is banned by the World Anti-Doping Agency (WADA).

Bibliography

Latzka, W.A. and Sawka, M.N. (2000). Hyperhydration and glycerol: Thermoregulatory effects during exercise in hot climates. *Canadian Journal of Applied Physiology* 25(6), 536-545.

Maughan, R.J. (1998). The sports drink as a functional food: Formulations for successful performance. *Proceedings of the Nutrition Society* 57, 15-23.

Robergs, R.A. and Griffin, S.E. (1998). Glycerol. Biochemistry, pharmacokinetics and clinical and practical applications. *Sports Medicine* 26(3), 145-167.

Shirreffs, S.M., Armstrong, L.E. and Cheuvront, S.M. (2004). Fluid and electrolyte needs for preparation and recovery from training and competition. *Journal of Sports Sciences* 22, 57-63.

World Anti-Doping Agency. Http://www.wada-ama.org

GLYCEROL PHOSPHATE SHUTTLE

See under MITOCHODRIAL MEMBRANE SHUTTLES.

GLYCINE A two-carbon, non-essential, glycogenic (glucogenic) amino acid. It is the simplest of the amino acids, having only a hydrogen atom as its side-chain. Glycine is derived from the amino acid serine.

GLYCOGEN It is the storage form of glucose in humans. Glycogen is not a significant food source of carbohydrate, but technically it is a complex carbohydrate. It is stored in the liver and skeletal muscle. In an average 80 kg male, there is 400 g of muscle glycogen, 100 g of liver glycogen and 3 g of blood glucose. Muscle glycogen does not contribute to blood glucose supply; it is available only to the specific muscle in which it is contained. The amount of muscle glycogen is an important factor in determining endurance performance. During prolonged sub-maximal exercise, muscle glycogen can contribute three times or more fuel than blood glucose.

Liver glycogen must be replenished every day by dietary carbohydrate, because muscle glycogen stores are not available to the brain. Since skeletal muscle has access to liver glycogen stores, it competes directly against the brain for all available carbohydrate. In a marathon race, working muscle consumes as much glucose in 2 hours as the brain requires in a week.

Glycogen synthesis is catalyzed by **glycogen synthetase**, an enzyme that is regulated by an epinephrine-cAMP mechanism, as well as intracellular metabolic conditions that favor phosphorylase activation during contractions and synthetase activation during rest, low glycogen concentrations, and increased blood glucose and insulin concentrations. Glycogen synthesis is actually dependent on a series of reactions in which glucose 6-phosphate is converted to glucose 1-phosphate, which is activated by its addition to a nucleotide, uridine monophosphate, to form uridine diphosphate-glucose. Finally, uridine diphosphate is removed and the remaining glucose molecule is added to a glucose polymer chain within the large glycogen molecule.

There are two glycogen pools within muscle, proglycogen and macroglycogen. **Proglycogen** storage is most prominent during the first phase of recovery and is sensitive to the provision of dietary carbohydrate. During the second phase of glycogen recovery, glycogen storage occurs mainly in the pool of **macroglycogen**, which is a glycogen molecule with greater amounts of glucose relative to the glycogenin core. **Glycogenin** is a protein that primes glycogen synthesis. The amount of glycogenin will influence how much glycogen the cell can store. An increase in macroglycogen pool appears to account for glycogen supercompensation in the muscle after 2 to 3 days of high carbohydrate intake.

The main differences between liver and skeletal muscle glycogen synthesis are in the predominant substrates used. Muscle glycogen synthesis occurs predominantly from glucose conversion to glucose 6-phosphate and then to uridine disphospate-glucose. In the liver, glucose is only a substrate for glycogen synthesis in the post-absorptive state after a high carbohydrate meal when blood glucose concentrations are sufficiently elevated for glucokinase activity to exceed rates of the reverse reaction catalyzed by the enzyme glucose-6 phosphorylase. **Glucokinase** is an enzyme of the transferase class that is highly specific for glucose. The main substrates for liver glycogen synthesis are lactate, fructose, alanine, glutamine and glycerol. This phenomenon has been termed the '**glucose paradox**,' or the indirect pathway of glycogen synthesis. About 60% of liver glycogen synthesis is direct. 40% is indirect (paradoxical), but it depends on pre- and post-prandial conditions.

The highest rates of muscle glycogen storage occur during the first hour after exercise, due to activation of glycogen synthetase by glycogen depletion, and exercise-induced increases in insulin sensitivity, and permeability of the muscle cell membrane to glucose. Supplements composed of glucose or glucose polymers are more effective for the replenishment of muscle glycogen stores after exercise than those composed of predominantly fructose. Some fructose is recommended, however, as it is more effective than glucose in the replenishment of liver glycogen. There is strong evidence that co-ingestion of protein with carbohydrate will increase the efficiency of muscle glycogen storage when the amount of carbohydrate ingested is below the threshold for maximal glycogen synthesis or when feedings are more than one hour apart. Feeding a high amount of carbohydrate at frequent intervals, however, negates the benefits of added protein. Nevertheless, intake of protein in recovery meals is recommended to enhance net protein balance, tissue repair and adaptations involving synthesis of new proteins. It seems that alcohol interferes with muscle glycogen synthesis.

For optimal training performance, muscle glycogen stores must be replenished on a daily basis. Following the cessation of exercise and with adequate carbohydrate consumption, muscle glycogen is rapidly resynthesized to near pre-exercise levels within 24 hours. Muscle glycogen then increases very gradually to above-normal levels over the next few days.

There is evidence that the ability to increase muscle glycogen in the trained state may be due not only to an increase in the enzyme glycogen synthetase, but also to increased GLUT-4. Glucose is transported across the muscle cell membrane down a concentration gradient by specific glucose transporter proteins such as GLUT-4 (which is the major transporter protein in muscle).

See also CARBOHYDRATE LOADING.

Bibliography

Adamo, K.B. and Graham, T.E. (1998). Comparison of traditional measurements with macroglycogen and proglycogen analysis of muscle glycogen. *Journal of Applied Physiology* 84, 908-913.

Burke, L.M., Kiens, B. and Ivy, J.L. (2004). Carbohydrates and fat for training and recovery. *Journal of Sports Sciences* 22, 15-30.

Friedman, J.E., Neufer, P.D. and Dohm, G.L. (1991). Regulation of glycogen resynthesis following exercise: dietary considerations. *Sports Medicine* 11(4), 232-243.

Ivy, J.L. (1991). Muscle glycogen synthesis before and after exercise. *Sports Medicine* 11(1), 6-19.

Katz, A. and Sahlin, K. (1990). Role of oxygen in regulation of glycolysis and lactate production in human skeletal muscle. *Exercise and Sport Sciences Reviews* 18, 1-28.

Loucks, A.B. (2004). Energy balance and body composition in sports and exercise. *Journal of Sports Sciences* 22, 1-14.

Nielsen, J.N. and Richter, E.A. (2003). Regulation of glycogen synthase in skeletal muscle during exercise. *Acta Physiologica Scandanavia* 178(4), 309-319.

GLYCOGENOLYSIS   The breakdown of glycogen to glucose. A glycosyl (glucose) molecule is split off the glycogen, an inorganic phosphate is added and glucose-6 phosphate is formed. During high-intensity exercise, glycogen supplies most of the glucose units. The breakdown of muscle glycogen is controlled by the enzyme phosphorylase through a series of events initiated by calcium ions and increased inorganic phosphate. See under LIVER.

GLYCOGEN STORAGE DISEASES   Glyco-genosis. A set of diseases that have an inherited absence or deficiency of any of the enzymes responsible for forming or releasing glycogen. These enzyme defects lead to abnormal tissue concentrations of glycogen or to structurally abnormal forms of glycogen.

See ACID MALTASE DEFICIENCY; DEBRANCHER ENZYME DEFICIENCY; PHOSPHORYLASE DEFICIENCY; PHOSPHO-FRUCTOKINASE DEFICIENCY; PHOSPHO-GLYCERATE KINASE; PHOSPHOGLYCERATE MUTASE DEFICIENCY.

Bibliography

Association for Glycogen Storage Diseases. Http://www.agsdus.org

Muscular Dystrophy Association. Http://mdausa.org

GLYCOGEN SUPERCOMPENSATION   *See* CARBOHYDRATE LOADING.

GLYCOLIPID   A compound consisting of both fatty acids and carbohydrates, but also containing nitrogen. Glycolipids are found in the myelin sheath that covers and protects the nerves.

GLYCOLYSIS   A series of chemical reactions that take place in the watery medium outside of the mitochondria in which glucose is broken down to pyruvic acid. There are two forms of glycolysis; neither involves oxygen, but one is associated with the aerobic energy systems ('**aerobic glycolysis**;' '**slow glycolysis**'), and the other is associated with one of the anaerobic energy systems ('**anaerobic glycolysis**;' '**lactic acid system**;' '**lactacid system**;' '**fast glycolysis**'). The latter, known as the **Embden-Myerhof pathway**, is more rapid and involves the additional step of the conversion of pyruvic acid to lactic acid. There is a greater amount of energy released in 'aerobic glycolysis,' because of mitochondrial respiration. The predominant fuel for 'aerobic glycolysis' is glucose; for 'anaerobic glycolysis' it is glycogen.

The amount of ATP produced from anaerobic glycolysis is small compared with that liberated in the Krebs cycle of the aerobic energy system, but it can be provided quickly due to the high concentration of glycolytic enzymes. In exercise of maximal intensity that lasts longer than a few seconds, increasingly more energy is produced from glycolysis, but the capacity of glycolysis is no greater than about 2 minutes. The aerobic energy system provides a small proportion of the total energy in maximal exercise of short duration, but the proportion of the total energy provided by the aerobic system increases as the duration of maximal exercise increases.

Glycolysis yields 2 molecules of ATP directly and 2 molecules of NADH. This occurs in the cytoplasm. Each glucose molecule yields 2 ATP, because each glucose molecule generates two 3-carbon units (e.g. pyruvate) and 2 acetyl CoA. The NADH molecules cannot cross the inner mitochondrial membrane, and the electrons they carry must be 'shuttled across' the mitochondrial membrane. During anaerobic glycolysis, these hydrogens are transferred to pyruvate to form lactate and regenerate the hydrogen-free form of the coenzyme (NAD^+). Under aerobic conditions, however, these hydrogens are transferred to an intermediate in the cytosol that is able to cross the mitochondrial membrane. Once within the mitochondria, the hydrogens are transferred from this intermediate either to NAD^+ or FAD, depending on the enzymes present in the mitochondria of different tissues (*see* MITOCHONDRIAL MEMBRANE SHUTTLES).

The conversion of pyruvic acid to acetyl CoA,

which occurs inside the mitochondrion, yields 2 molecules of NADH for each molecule of glucose and so produces 2 x 2.5 molecules of ATP. The Krebs cycle, which also occurs inside the mitochondria, yields 2 molecules of ATP, 6 NADH and 2 $FADH_2$, or a total of 20 ATP, for each molecule of glucose. If the substrate is glycogen, only 1 ATP is used and the net gain is 3 ATP rather than 2 ATP. The hydrogen atoms operated on in the Krebs cycle pass through the electron transport chain by means of co-enzymes and are oxidized.

In terms of each reaction stage, the number of ATP molecules formed from the oxidation of one molecule of glucose are as follows: phosphoglycerate kinase reaction (1 ATP x 2), pyruvate kinase reaction (1 ATP x 2), oxidation of cytoplasmic NADH via glycerol phosphate shuttle (1.5 ATP x 2) or malate-aspartate shuttle (2.5 ATP x 2), pyruvate dehydrogenase reaction (3 ATP x 2), oxidation of acetyl CoA, including electron transfer chain (10 ATP x 2). The hexokinase reaction and phosphofructokinase reaction each costs 1 ATP. Therefore the total number of ATP formed is 31 (when the glycerol phosphate shuttle is used) or 33 (when the malate-aspartate shuttle is used).

In detail, the reactions of glycolysis are as follows. In the **hexokinase reaction**, one inorganic phosphate is transferred from ATP to glucose, producing glucose 6-phosphate. In the **phospho-glucoisomerase reaction**, the atoms that make up glucose 6-phosphate are rearranged to form fructose 6-phosphate. In the **phospho-fructokinase (PFK) reaction**, one phosphate is transferred from ATP to fructose 6-phosphate producing 1,6-diphosphate. In the **aldolase reaction**, the 6-carbon 1,6-diphosphate is split into two 3-carbon sugars (dihydroxyacetone phosphate and glyceraldehyde 3-phosphate) that are identical except for a different arrangement of their component atoms. In the **triosephosphate isomerase reaction**, the atoms of dihydroxy-acetone phosphate (DHAP) are rearranged to form glyceraldehyde 3-phosphate.

The following reactions occur twice, so that two molecules of pyruvate are formed. In the **glyceraldehyde-phosphate dehydrogenase reaction**, a pair of hydrogen atoms is transferred from glyceraldehyde 3-phosphate to NAD^+, thus forming NADH. This reaction releases enough energy for a phosphate to be added from the phosphate pool in the cytoplasm so that the product becomes 1,3 diphosphoglycerate. In the **phosphoglycerate kinase reaction**, a phosphate is transferred to ADP to form ATP and the product becomes 3-phosphoglycerate. In the **phospho-glyceromutase reaction**, the atoms of 3-phosphoglycerate are rearranged (the phosphate is moved from C3 to C2) so that the product becomes 2-phosphoglycerate. In the **enolase reaction**, a water molecule is removed, which weakens the bond between the remaining phosphate groups and the rest of the atoms; 2-phosphoglycerate becomes phosphoenolpyruvate. In the **pyruvate kinase reaction**, the remaining phosphate is transferred from phosphoenolpyruvate to ADP so that ATP and pyruvate are formed.

There are 4 fewer hydrogen atoms in 2 pyruvic acid molecules ($2C_3H_4O_3$) than one glucose molecule ($C_6H_{12}O_6$). These are the hydrogen atoms that are carried by NAD^+. If the hydrogen atoms carried by NAD^+ as NADH are unable to enter the electron transport chain, they are transferred to pyruvate, forming lactate, which regenerates the NAD^+. If the endpoint is lactic acid ($2C_3H_6O_3$), all of the hydrogen atoms are accounted for. When there is sufficient oxygen, pyruvate is converted to acetyl CoA in a reaction (the 'link reaction') that takes place in the mitochondrial matrix and is catalyzed by pyruvate dehydrogenase. Pyruvate is transported across the mitochondrial membranes by a specific carrier. There is neither use, nor production, of ATP in the link reaction. Two hydrogen atoms (because two pyruvate molecules are formed from one molecule of glucose) are removed and picked up by NAD^+ to be transferred to the electron transport chain. Pyruvate is converted to acetic acid with one molecule of carbon dioxide being removed. Acetic acid is then combined with coenzyme A to form acetyl CoA.

Primary stimulators of glycolysis include ADP, phosphate ions, AMP, ammonium ions and increased temperature. Primary inhibitors of glycolysis include

ATP, creatine phosphate, protons and citrate. See also under GROWTH.

Bibliography

Curtis, H. and Barnes, N.S. (1989). *Biology*. 5th ed. New York: Worth Publishers.

Houston, M.E. (2001). *Biochemistry primer for exercise science*. 2nd ed. Champaign, IL: Human Kinetics.

Insel, P., Turner, R.E. and Ross, D. (2004). *Nutrition*. 2nd ed. Sudbury, MA: Jones and Bartlett.

Vander, A., Sherman, J. and Luciano, D. (2001). *Human physiology. The mechanisms of body function*. 8th edition. Boston, MA: McGraw-Hill.

GLYCOPROTEIN A compound consisting of both protein and oligosaccharides. Glycoproteins include structural molecules, lubricants, and transport molecules for vitamins, lipids, hormones and enzymes. **Proteoglycans** are a subclass of glycoproteins that contain a protein to which is attached one or more specialized carbohydrate side chains, called **glycosaminoglycans**. Proteoglycans are matrix macromolecules that possess great water-binding capacity. *See under* CARTILAGE.

GLYCOSURIA Presence of sugar in the urine.

GNATHION An anatomical landmark that is the most inferior border of the mandible in the mid-sagittal plane.

GOAL An outcome or target that an individual or group may strive for. Goal theory is based on the premise that behavior is determined by intentions to attain various goals. It proposes that a person's performance will be maximized when he or she holds specific, difficult goals. Such goals will be accepted when the individual understands what behaviors will lead to goal achievement, and when he or she feels competent to do those behaviors.

Goal setting is a motivational technique that involves the assigning or choosing of goals to be attained. It had been used widely and effectively in the organizational domain before its use became widespread in sport. The acronym **SMART** is often used to describe the principles of goal setting; goals should be **S**pecific, **M**easurable, **A**chieveable, **R**ealistic and **T**ime bound. Achievable refers to whether or not the person has the talents and resources. Realistic refers to whether or not the goal is practical and rewarding in the context of the rest of the person's life.

On the basis that an individual's performance is typically more objective in sports than in organizational settings, Locke and Latham (1985) argued that goal setting could work even better in sport than in organizations. In sport psychology, only some of the studies have supported the hypothesis that specific, difficult goals would produce higher levels of performance than no goals or 'do your best goals.' Unlike in the organizational domain, there has not been support in the sporting domain for the hypothesis that performers should be encouraged to strive for goals that are 'difficult, but realistic' (i.e. challenging). Furthermore, no support has been found for the notion that performance would decrease if goals were set unrealistically high. A potential explanation for the lack of differences between goal difficulty conditions is the fact that many participants in sport psychology research seem to spontaneously set goals on their own, despite being provided specific goals by the experimenter. Many coaches subscribe to the value of short-term goals. Locke and Latham (1985) hypothesized that using both short-term and long-term goals will lead to better performance than using long-term goals alone. This hypothesis is based on the premise that long-term goals are often too vague and future oriented to have significant motivational impact in the present. Research results from testing this hypothesis have been equivocal.

Weinberg's (1996) guidelines for effective goal setting are: set specific goals; set realistic, but challenging goals; set both short- and long-term goals; set goals for both practice and competition; write down goals; develop goal-achievement strategies; set goals that focus on performance rather than outcomes; set individual and team goals; provide social support for goals; and evaluate goals in light of feedback.

Common goal-setting problems include: failure to monitor goal progress and readjust goals; failure to recognize individual differences in terms of goal orientation; failure to set specific measurable goals; and setting too many goals. *See also* MOTIVATION; PERFECTIONISM.

Bibliography

Burton, D. (1993). Goal setting in sport. In: Singer, R. Murphy, M. and Tennant, L.K. (eds). *Handbook of research on sport psychology*. pp467-491. New York: MacMillan.

Dweck, C.S. (1992). The study of goals in psychology. *Psychological Science* 3(3), 165-167.

Locke, E.A. and Latham, G.P. (1985). The application of goal setting to sport. *Journal of Sport Psychology* 7, 205-222.

Locke, E.A. and Latham, G.P. (1990). *A theory of goal setting and task performance*. Englewood Cliffs, NJ: Prentice Hall.

Weinberg, R.S. (1994). Goal setting and performance in sport and exercise settings: A review and critique. *Medicine and Science in Sports and Exercise* 26(4), 449-477.

Weinberg, R. (1996). Goal setting in sport and exercise: Research to practice. In Van Raalte, J.L. and Brewer, B.W. (eds). *Exploring sport and exercise psychology*. pp3-24. Washington, DC: American Psychological Association.

GOAL ORIENTATION

Goal perspective. This is concerned with the 'higher-level classes' of goals that are behind outcomes individuals strive for. Roberts (1984) used the theory of Maehr and Nicholls (1980) to propose that three goals may be relevant to sport: to seek 'social approval' from significant others; to demonstrate 'competitive ability' (how one's ability compares to that of another person's ability); and to demonstrate 'sport mastery' (emphasis on improving skill rather than winning). Individuals who drop out from sport may often be those who have the desire to demonstrate competitive ability. An emphasis on sport mastery and a focus on specific, rather than general abilities may help decrease the negative impact of unfavorable perceptions of ability. More recently, sport psychologists have used Nicholls' (1984) distinction between task-oriented and ego-oriented motivation. **Task-orientation** implies an emphasis on the process of the activity and basing success on self-referenced improvement. **Ego-orientation** implies an emphasis on outcomes and success based on doing better than others. There is research evidence that task-oriented individuals typically experience greater interest in sports tasks, persist longer and are more likely to be performing the task for its own sake. This has led to a tendency at the practical level to emphasize task orientation in goal setting in sport and physical education at the expense of ego-orientation. Hardy (1998) recommends that coaches encourage athletes to maintain a balanced perspective by reinforcing the use of multiple sources of competence information, and encourage them to set outcome (ego-oriented), performance (task-oriented) and process goals by which to judge their personal development. **Process goals** are concerned with particular elements of a task, such as specific aspects of technique. Furthermore, theories of goal orientation assume that all individuals conceive their ability on the basis of their primary reasons or goals for activity participation (Pringle, 2000).

Bibliography

Duda, J.L. (1992). Motivation in sport settings: A goal perspective approach. In: Roberts, G.C. (ed). *Motivation in sport and exercise*. pp57-91. Champaign, IL: Human Kinetics.

Duda, J.L. (1997). Perpetuating myths: A response to Hardy's 1996 Coleman Griffith Address. *Journal of Applied Sport Psychology* 9, 303-309.

Hardy, L. (1998). Responses to reactants on three myths in applied consultancy work. *Journal of Applied Sport Psychology* 10, 212-219.

Maehr, M.L. and Nicholls, J.G. (1980). Culture and achievement motivation. In: Warren, N. (ed). *Studies in cross cultural psychology* (vol 3). pp221-267. New York: Academic Press.

Nicholls, J.G. (1984). Achievement motivation: Conceptions of ability, subjective experience, task choice and performance. *Psychological Review* 91, 328-346.

Pringle, R. (2000). Physical education, positivism, and optimistic claims from achievement goal theorists. *Quest* 52, 18-31.

Roberts, G.C. (1984). Toward a new theory of motivation in sport: The role of perceived ability. In: Silva, J.M. and Weinberg, R.S. (eds). *Psychological foundations of sport*. pp214-228. Champaign, IL: Human Kinetics.

Roberts, G.C. (2001). *Advances in motivation in sport and exercise*. Champaign, IL: Human Kinetics.

GOLFER'S ELBOW

See MEDIAL EPICON-DYLITIS.

GOLGI APPARATUS   *See under* ENDOPLASMIC RETICULUM.

GOLGI TENDON ORGANS   Sense organs found at the junction of muscle fibers and tendons. Golgi tendon organs are sensitive to the amount of tension developed in the tendon and fire maximally when the muscle spindle is inactive and minimally when the muscle spindle is active. Golgi tendon organs generate an inhibitory local-graded potential in the spinal cord known as the **inverse stretch reflex**. If the graded potential is sufficient, relaxation, or **autogenic inhibition**, will be produced in the muscle fibers connected with the Golgi tendon organ that is stimulated. The alpha motor neuron output to muscles that are either undergoing a high-velocity stretch or producing a high-resistance output is decreased. Even at low levels of tension, Golgi tendon organs provide sensory feedback to the spinal cord, thereby providing fine-tuned feedback information that can potentially assist in continuous control throughout a movement. Golgi tendon organs are most sensitive to tension generated by muscle contraction (i.e. active rather than passive tension), and during stretching require a high tension in order to be activated. Furthermore, Golgi tendon organ discharge rarely persists through sustained muscle stretch.

It is thought that Golgi tendon organs impair the ability of muscle to achieve its full contractile potential, thus hindering the muscle's full expression of force output. Resistance training may lead to a decrease in the sensitivity of Golgi tendon organs. This decreased sensitivity results in the disinhibition of the muscle, which in turn, leads to a greater force production by the involved muscle. Golgi tendon organ response can be inhibited in extreme and exceptional circumstances, such as if a mother had to lift a heavy object off her child.

See also under MECHANORECEPTORS; STRETCHING.

Bibliography

Alter, M.J. (1996). *Science of stretching*. 2nd ed. Champaign, IL: Human Kinetics.

GONAD   The undifferentiated organ that will later become either a testis or an ovary. There are two primordial systems of ducts, one female (**Mullerian ducts**) and one male (**Wolffian ducts**). A human embryo is neither male nor female for the first 7 weeks after conception. At 7 weeks, the fetus has an embryonic reproductive system consisting of a pair of gonads, which can grow into either ovaries or testes, plus a mass of tissue called the **genital ridge**, which can develop into either a clitoris and labia, or a penis and scrotum. During the 8th week, the fetus chooses between 2 paths. If the fetus is genetically male - if it has a Y chromosome - then a 'master switch' on the Y chromosome clicks on at this time. This switch, which is a single gene called the **testes-determining factor**, triggers a whole series of events that will point the fetus in the male direction. The testes-determining factor signals the embryonic gonads to form into testes, which then begin to produce male hormones. The major hormone produced by the testes is testosterone, which stimulates the Wolffian ducts to start developing into the male duct system. At the same time, some of the testosterone is converted by the body into dihydrotestosterone, which prompts the genital ridge to begin forming into male genitals. The testes also produces **Mullerian-inhibiting factor**, which causes the (female) Mullerian ducts to atrophy and eventually be absorbed by the body. For a female fetus, nothing happens in the 8th week. Instead the fetus continues to grow and develop, before the gonads transform into ovaries in the 13th week. The genital ridge evolves into the clitoris and labia, and the Mullerian ducts mature into the uterus, fallopian tubes and upper one-third of the vagina. The Wolffian ducts shrivel up.

The penis of the male and the much smaller clitoris of the female both come from the embryonic genital tubercle or phallus. Men have a vestigal uterus, the utriculus masculinus in the prostate; and women have a homologue prostate in the glands at the lower end of the urethra.

It is the hormonal environment of the womb, not the chromosomes, which directly determines the sex of the fetus. The Y chromosome holds relatively few genes, and most of them are duplicates of genes that lie on the X chromosome. Only a small number of genes are unique to the Y chromosome. These include the testes-determining factor, a gene involved with male fertility and sperm production, and the H-Y antigen gene (which does not seem to be involved in sexual differentiation).

Bibliography

Peel, R. (1994). *Eve's rib – Searching for the biological roots of sex differences.* New York: Crown Publishers.

GONADOTROPIC HORMONES Gonadotrophic hormones. **Follicle-stimulating hormone** and **luteinizing hormone**. Both are secreted by the anterior pituitary gland, and stimulate the sex organs to grow and secrete their hormones at a faster rate. Luteinizing hormone works with follicle-stimulating hormone to stimulate production of estrogen and progesterone by the ovaries and testosterone by the testes. The secretion is controlled by hypothalamic follicle-stimulating hormone-releasing factor and luteinizing hormone-releasing factor, in addition to estrogen and progesterone (in females) and testosterone (in males).

Luteinizing hormone and follicle-stimulating hormone are necessary to initiate the maturation of the egg, stimulate ovulation and support the corpus luteum after ovulation. The levels of follicle-stimulating hormone and luteinizing hormone change relative to each other throughout the cycle. Estrogen stimulates the endometrium to develop, and the withdrawal of both estrogen and progesterone results in menstrual shedding. When estrogen is present without progesterone, the endometrium will build up and usually bleed erratically and infrequently.

In the testes, testosterone works with follicle-stimulating hormone to promote spermatogenesis. The effects of exercise on luteinizing hormone and follicle-stimulating hormone are not clearly understood, but chronic training can alter levels of both hormones in females and may also affect the menstrual cycle.

GONADOTROPIN-RELEASING HORMONE

Gonadotrophin-releasing hormone. It is a hormone that must be secreted by the hypothalamus in a regular, pulsatile pattern. It is released into the portal vessels, and then travels to the pituitary gland. In the pituitary gland, the gonadotropin-releasing hormone affects the cells that produce gonadotropic hormones. The cells that produce gonadotropin-releasing hormone in the hypothalamus can be congenitally deficient or the pituitary stalk can be damaged, decreasing the gonadotropin-releasing hormone pulses that reach the pituitary gland. These decreased pulses can result in amenorrhea.

See also HUMAN CHORIONIC GONADOTROPIN.

GONIOMETER *See under* FLEXIBILITY.

GOUT *See under* ARTHRITIS; PROTEIN.

GRACILIS SYNDROME An overuse injury that is most commonly caused by repetitive microtrauma to the *gracilis* muscle at its point of origin on the pubic symphysis.

GRAFT Any tissue that is unattached and can be used for transplantation.

GRANULATION Proliferation of immature connective tissue (fibroblasts) and capillaries (angioblasts) in the chronic stages of inflammation.

GRANULOCYTES *See under* LEUKOCYTES.

GRAPHITE *See under* COMPOSITES.

GRASPING *See* PREHENSION.

GRASS BURN A form of friction burn due to abrasion of the skin on grass.

GRAVES' DISEASE Diffuse toxic goiter. It is 'diffuse' because the whole thyroid gland is involved; 'toxic' due to the feverish, flushed symptoms; and 'goiter' for the enlargement of the thyroid gland, which swells in the neck. It is the most common form of overt hyperthyroidism, but it is not the most common thyroid disease. **Hyperthyroidism** is a set of symptoms resulting from elevated levels of thyroid hormones. These excess hormones affect many organ systems and cause varying degrees of a spectrum of illnesses. In Graves' disease, an autoimmune disease, the cells of the immune system attack thyroid cells, stimulating them to make too much thyroid hormone. It affects less than 0.5% of men, but more than 3% of women.

Bibliography

National Graves' Disease Foundation. Http://www.ngdf.org

Thyroid Foundation of America. Http://www.tsh.org

GRAVITY   Gravitational force. It is the gravitational attraction at the surface of a planet or some other celestial body. On earth, it is the force imparted by the earth to a mass that is at rest relative to the earth (viewed from a frame of reference fixed in the earth). The magnitude of gravity at sea level decreases from the poles (where the centrifugal force is zero) to the equator (where the centrifugal force is maximum, but is directed opposite to gravity).

Gravitational acceleration is the acceleration of a body (of negligible mass compared to the earth) towards the center of mass of the earth. It has an international standard value, g, equal to 9.80665 m/s^2 (32.2 ft/s^2), which is the value measure in Paris (France), but it varies slightly with latitude and altitude.

In a giant swing on the high bar, a gymnast exploits gravitational acceleration and changes in moment of inertia. Like a child on a swing, the gymnast extends her legs at the point of highest velocity and curls them up at the point of zero velocity. To gain even greater height, gymnasts exploit the elasticity of the bar by timing their dismount with the flexing of the bar.

See also MICROGRAVITY.

GRAY MATTER   *See under* BRAIN; CENTRAL NERVOUS SYSTEM.

GROIN   An ill-defined anatomical area lying between the abdomen and thigh. Musculoskeletal causes of groin injury include adductor muscle strain, osteitis pubis and psoas tendon injury. Abdominal/genital causes include sports hernia. Gynecological causes may be ovarian in origin.

GROSS MOTOR SKILL DISORDER   A disorder where an affected individual has a problem with those skills carried out by large muscle groups.

GROUND REACTION FORCE   *See under* FORCE PLATE.

GROUP   *See under* TEAM.

GROWTH   Increase in size of the body or parts of the body. It involves an increase in the quantity of metabolically active protoplasm accompanied by hypertrophy and/or hyperplasia. A **distance curve** plots accumulative growth obtained over time. A **velocity curve** plots rate of change in growth per unit of time.

Development is progress over time towards the mature adult state and refers to both growth (structural changes) and maturation (functional changes). It is a continuous process; being only arbitrarily separated into 'stages' or 'age periods.' **Adulthood** can arbitrarily be subdivided into early adulthood (20 to 40 years), middle adulthood (40 to 60 years) and late adulthood (60 years to death). **Maturation** refers to qualitative changes that enable one to progress to higher levels of functioning. The term growth is often used interchangeably with development, and is often used to refer to the totality of physical change.

The **prenatal period** is from conception to birth. The **embryonic period** is the first eight weeks. The **fetal period** is 8 weeks after conception to birth, and is the point at which the individual becomes recognizable as a human. The **neonatal period** is the first 22 days after birth. **Infancy** is the period from birth throughout the first year of life to the onset of independent walking when an infant thus becomes a **toddler** and remains so, arbitrarily, until 4 years of age. The following periods are also arbitrary and involve gradual transformation: **early childhood** (4 to 7 years), **middle childhood** (7 to 9 years) and **late childhood** (9 to 12 years).

Adolescence is the time between the onset of puberty and attainment of adult status. **Puberty** is the time of sexual maturation; it is a succession of anatomic and physiologic changes in early adolescence that culminate in fertility. When puberty ends, the adolescent has achieved full sexual maturity. The events of puberty, which are triggered by secretion of hormones from the hypothalamus, pituitary gland and gonads, also produce a number of changes indirectly related to sexual functions. These include the adolescent growth spurt, a set of physical features collectively termed secondary sexual characteristics (including facial hair and deepening of the voice in males; and breast development in females) and alterations in body composition (in particular, augmented muscle mass in males and increased deposition of body fat in females). The most commonly used rating system for sexual maturation is that devised by Tanner (1969), which describes features of breast development, pubic hair and genitalia separately for boys and girls in five stages. Stage 1 represents the immature, pre-pubertal state, while the adolescent with stage 5 findings is fully mature. The average child progresses through these pubertal stages over a period of about 4 years. The process begins sooner in girls, usually with breast development (**thelarche**) starting at the age of 10.5 to 11 years. Puberty is initiated in boys with genital enlargement at the age of 11 to 12.5 years. The initiation of menses (**menarche**) in girls typically occurs at the age of 12.6 years in the USA. It is a relatively late event in the course of puberty, occurring usually at stage 4. Girls usually do not become fertile until 1 to 2 years after menarche. The total duration of puberty may be as short as 18 months or as long as 8 years. It seems that no more than 60% of children can be expected to follow the standard progression outlined by Tanner (1969), and developmental stages are not necessarily followed in the prescribed order. Breast development, for example, reaches stage 2 or 3 in 75% of girls before the appearance of pubic hair, but in 10%, pubic hair is at stage 2 or 3 before the breasts reach stage 2.

The **adolescent growth spurt** (**circum-pubertal period**) is a period of accelerated growth that lasts about 4_ years. **Peak height velocity** is the maximum rate of growth in height. Males begin their growth spurts around the age of 11 to 14 years, reach peak height velocity by age 14 years and taper off by age 15 years. Females begin their growth spurts around the age of 9 to 11 years, reach peak height velocity by age 11 years and taper off by age 13 years. Males appear to reach their mature adult heights around the age of 18 years; whereas females appear to reach their mature adults heights at around age 16 years. **Adolescent awkwardness** is a period of time during the growth spurt that is associated with peak height velocity and is accompanied by a temporary disruption in motor performance. It is found primarily in boys. **Peak weight velocity** is the period during the adolescent growth spurt when weight gain is the greatest. It is generally greater in boys than in girls. Peak weight velocity occurs closer to peak height velocity in boys than in girls. In adolescent males, weight gain is primarily due to increased height and muscle mass. Fat mass tends to remain relatively stable at this time. Weight gain in adolescent girls is due largely to increases in fat mass, height and, to a lesser degree, to increases in muscle mass.

Growth is more rapid in infancy than in early childhood. It slows down after the first 2 years, but maintains a constant rate until puberty. The term 'catch-up' is often used in the context of growth. It refers to a return to a predetermined behavior or growth pattern after being thrown off course by deprivation, for example. Relatively minor deviations in the growth pattern can be compensated, but major deviations, especially during infancy and childhood, may not be subject to 'catch up.'

With regard to sports training and growth delay, there are two schools of thought among growth researchers. One is that no viable evidence supports an adverse effect of sports training on growth; the other argues that observations of 'catch-up' growth, observed after decreasing or ceasing training, provide compelling evidence that growth is affected.

Skeletal age is the **biological age** of the developing skeleton and refers to an individual's maturational status. **Morphological age** is a comparison of one's attained size (height and weight) to normative standards. It is assessed by X-ray analysis of the carpal bones in the hand and wrist. As a child matures, primary and secondary centers of bone ossify, rendering them opaque to X-rays. Progressive enlargement of these ossified bone centers can be compared with a set of standard films in which each film in a series represents bone development of children of a similar age.

The early maturing child has an advanced biological age relative to chronological age. Chronological age is not a reliable indicator of biological maturity. Use of morphological markers, such as height and weight, has limited value because of the large inter-individual variability at maturity. Age of the peak height velocity is useful for comparison of biological maturity levels between individuals. Secondary sexual characteristics help define level of sexual maturity, but these are useful markers only in the adolescent age group. There appear to be two separate periods of biological growth: the pre-pubertal years, when growth is controlled by growth hormone; and the pubertal years, when the influence of reproductive hormones becomes superimposed on the actions of growth hormone.

A study on baseball found that 71% of the participants had advanced skeletal ages relative to their chronological ages and 29% were delayed in their skeletal age. In general, motor performance is negatively related to biological maturity in girls, but positively related to maturity status in boys.

Youth competition based on chronological age may give an advantage not only to individuals who mature early, but also to individuals born during the earliest part of the selection year. It has therefore been hypothesized that those born at the start of the selection year may be older not only chronologically, but also biologically. There is empirical evidence to support this hypothesis. For example, a study of a Swedish Under-17 male soccer squad found that there was a significant bias in selection towards birth dates in the early part of the selection year. These youths were also found to have significantly greater body mass and body height values than predicted for their chronological age, suggesting an advanced biological age.

Changes in physique tend to appear between 3 and 8 years of age. There is a redistribution of subcutaneous fat, development of muscle and a lengthening of the legs relative to stature.

Most of the body's fat cells are created during embryogenesis and the first decade of life. From birth to age of 6 years, the number and size of fat cells increases three-fold in both boys and girls. After about 8 years of age, girls begin gaining fat mass at a greater rate than boys do (probably because of a lower rate of fat oxidation that occurs as a result of an increase in the size of fat cells). In nonobese children, there is little or no increase in the number of fat cells between the age of 6 years and adolescence. The rate of fat increase in girls almost doubles that of boys during adolescence, due mainly to changes in female hormone levels. There is an increase in both the size and number of fat cells (mostly in the area of the pelvis, buttocks and thighs).

Children have a lower concentration and rate of utilization of muscle glycogen. Glycolysis is limited because of a low level of the enzyme phosphofructokinase. Thus the ability of children to perform intense anaerobic tasks that last 10 to 90 seconds is significantly lower than that of adults. Children have lower maximal blood lactate values, but stores and breakdown of ATP and creatine phosphate are the same. Children reach the steady state faster than adults. Thus children contract a lower oxygen deficit and recover faster. This makes children well suited to intermittent physical activity.

By all the different methods of laboratory assessment, peak and mean anaerobic power rise with chronological age, whether expressed in absolute or mass-relative terms. Maximal and sub-maximal exercise lactate levels rise virtually linearly with age during childhood. Excess post-exercise oxygen consumption increases throughout the course of childhood. Little is known about the factors that might trigger the development of anaerobic fitness in children. In general, speed improves until about the age of 13 years in both boys and girls. Girls then level off or even regress, but boys tend to continue improving throughout the adolescent years.

Cardiac output increases during exercise in the child as in the adult, but at a given power output the heart rate in the child is greater and the stroke volume is smaller. Maximal cardiac output is lower in children because of size difference. Maximal stroke volume is lower due to size and heart volume difference. Resting ventricular size and stroke volume increase during the course of childhood in direct relationship to body dimensions. Resting heart rate falls as a consequence of intrinsic sinus node maturation, while myocardial contractility is unchanged. Changes in resting cardiac output parallel those of oxygen uptake, increasing in absolute value, but declining relative to body mass.

Blood volume, hemoglobin concentration and total hemoglobin are lower in children. There is a potential deficiency of peripheral blood supply during maximal exertion in hot climates. During childhood, there is no change in blood volume relative to body mass. Blood hemoglobin concentration rises slowly during childhood, without gender differences. At puberty, significant increases are observed in males secondary to bone marrow stimulation by testosterone. Athletic training does not influence hemoglobin concentration in children. The arterial-mixed venous oxygen difference at rest and maximal exercise appears to be independent of age. There is also a smaller increase in blood pressure during exercise in the child than in the adult. Maximal systolic and diastolic blood pressures are lower in children. Maximal minute ventilation is smaller. In children, respiratory frequency is increased and tidal volume is shallower. Alveolar ventilation is sufficient for gas exchange, because children's physiologic dead space is smaller than that of adults. The regulation of ventilation is less efficient in the child than in the adult. This may explain the relatively higher metabolic cost of sub-maximal exercise. Resting lung tidal volume increases with age in childhood, but declines slowly relative to body size. Respiratory frequency at rest also progressively falls. Therefore, resting ventilation relative to body mass falls as children age. During sub-maximal work, children breathe more rapidly than adults. A progressive decline in maximal breathing rate is also observed during childhood. Children hyperventilate

during exercise in comparison to adults, showing lower alveolar partial pressure of carbon dioxide and higher ratio of pulmonary ventilation to oxygen uptake. Maximal exercise ventilation rises with age in close proportion to body height. Maximal tidal volume per unit body mass is stable throughout childhood. There is no evidence that the aerobic training response of children is inferior to that of adults; the main basis for the increase in oxygen uptake seems to be an increase in stroke volume. The improvements in maximal aerobic power that occur as a child develops seem to be due to both increased body size and improved function. Absolute maximal oxygen uptake increases during the childhood years in both girls and boys. Average maximal oxygen uptake related to bodyweight, however, remains stable in boys of all ages, while values for girls decline progressively as they grow. Relative maximal oxygen uptake is a valid index of endurance performance only for comparison of children of similar biological age. The influence of body fat can render relative maximal oxygen uptake useless as a marker of cardiovascular fitness. Absolute values of maximal oxygen uptake progressively rise during the course of childhood. Resting metabolic rate (oxygen uptake) increases with age during childhood. Expressed relative to either body mass or surface area, however, total energy expenditure decreases. Mean gender differences in maximal oxygen uptake are very small before puberty, but values in males are consistently greater than in females. Maximal oxygen uptake relative to body mass changes little during childhood in boys and declines in girls. During the same time, dramatic improvements are observed in endurance fitness (1-mile times, for example). There is no strong relationship between the level of habitual physical activity and aerobic fitness (maximal oxygen uptake) in children. Daily activities of children are typically short-burst and non-sustained activities that would not be expected to improve maximal oxygen uptake. Improvements in maximal oxygen uptake occur in children after a period of endurance training. These increases are less than those expected in adults. *See also* COLD STRESS; HEAT STRESS; RESISTANCE TRAINING; RUNNING ECONOMY.

Chronology

•1992 • The Council on Physical Education for Children released a document entitled "Developmentally Appropriate Physical Education Practices for Children." It made the point that children are not miniature adults, but rather have different needs and interests from those of adults.

•1992 • In *A Matter of Time: Risk and Opportunity in the Nonschool Hours*, the Carnegie Council on Adolescent Development reported that boys and girls from low income neighborhoods in the USA were seriously underserved in all forms of childhood and youth services including those for sport.

•1997 • The Fédération Internationale de Gymnastique raised the age eligibility for international gymnastics competitions by one year, so female gymnasts must turn 16 years of age the year they compete at the senior international level. In 1976, the six US Olympic team gymnasts were on average 17.5 years old, 5 feet 3 inches tall and 106 pounds. By the 1992 Olympics, the average US gymnast was 16 years old, 4 feet 9 inches tall and 83 pounds.

Bibliography

Armstrong, N. and Welsman, J. (1997). *Young people and physical activity*. Oxford: Oxford University Press.

Bale, P. (1992). The functional performance of children in relation to growth, maturation and exercise. *Sports Medicine* 13(3), 151-159.

Baxter-Jones, A.D.G. (1995). Growth and development of young athletes. Should competition levels be age-related? *Sports Medicine* 20(2), 59-64.

Beunen, G. and Malina, R.M. (1988). Growth and physical performance relative to the timing of the adolescent spurt. In K.B. Pandolf (ed.). *Exercise and Sport Sciences Reviews* 16, 503-540.

Birrer, R.B. and Levine, R. (1987). Performance parameters in children and adolescent athletes. *Sports Medicine* 4, 211-227.

Brewer, J., Balsom, P. and Davis, J. (1995). Seasonal birth distribution among European soccer players. *Sports, Exercise and Injury* 1(3), 154-157.

Cahill, B.R. and Pearl, A.J. (1993, ed). *Intensive participation in children's sport*. Champaign, IL: Human Kinetics.

Chan, K-M and Micheli, L.J. (1998, eds). *Sport and children*. Hong Kong: Williams and Wilkins Asia-Pacific Ltd.

Cheung, L.W.Y. (1995). *Child, health, nutrition and physical activity*. Champaign, IL: Human Kinetics.

Dalton, S.E. (1992). Overuse injuries in adolescent athletes. *Sports Medicine* 13(1), 58-70.

Krogman, W.M. (1959). Maturation age of 55 boys in the Little League World Series. *Research Quarterly* 30, 54-56.

Malina, R.M. and Bouchard, C. (1991). *Growth, maturation and physical activity*. Champaign, IL: Human Kinetics.

News Brief. Sports training and growth delay. Is there a connection? *The Physician and Sportsmedicine* 29(2).

Rowland, T.W. (1990). Developmental aspects of physiological function relating to aerobic exercise in children. *Sports Medicine* 10(4), 255-266.

Rowland, T.W. (1996). *Developmental exercise physiology*. Champaign, IL: Human Kinetics.

Rowley, S. (1986). *The effect of intensive training on young athletes: A review of the research literature*. London: Sports Council.

Shephard, R.J. (1982). *Physical activity and growth*. Chicago: Year Book Medical Publishers.

Smoll, F.L. and Smith, R.E. (1996). *Children and youth in sport. A biopsychological perspective*. Madison, WI: Brown and Benchmark.

Tanner, J.M. (1969). Growth and endocrinology of the adolescent. In: Gardner, L.I. (ed) *Endocrine and genetic diseases of childhood*. pp14-64. Philadelphia: W.B. Saunders.

Turley, K.R. (1997). Cardiovascular responses to exercise in children. *Sports Medicine* 26(4), 241-257.

Van Praagh, E. (1998, ed). *Pediatric anaerobic performance*. Champaign, IL: Human Kinetics.

Zauner, C.W., Maksud, M.G. and Melichna, J. (1989). Physiological considerations in training young athletes. *Sports Medicine* 8(1), 15-31.

GROWTH FACTOR A protein that is involved in cell differentiation and growth.

GROWTH HORMONE Somatotropin. A hormone secreted by the anterior pituitary gland. Growth hormone release is stimulated by a variety of substances, including growth hormone releasing factor, norepinephrine, epinephrine, levodopa, arginine and insulin; and by sleep. The growth hormone receptor is widely distributed throughout the body and has been identified on the cell-surface membranes of hepatocytes, adipocytes, fibroblasts, lymphocytes and chondrocytes. Growth hormone stimulates tissue growth, mobilizes fatty acids for energy and inhibits carbohydrate metabolism. It is secreted more during exercise, but this effect is not so great in trained individuals. The exact mechanism of the exercise-induced growth hormone response is not known, but possible mechanisms include neural input (afferent stimulation) or direct stimulation by nitric oxide and lactate. Exercise intensities above the lactate threshold and durations of at least 10 minutes appear to elicit the greatest stimulus to the secretion of growth hormone.

Resistance training results in a significant exercise-induced growth hormone response, with the load and frequency of training being key determinants. Many of the effects of growth hormone on protein synthesis, however, are mediated through insulin-like growth factors (somatomedins).

Endurance training seems to result in decreased resting growth hormone and a blunted exercise-induced growth hormone response, which may be associated with increased tissue sensitivity to growth hormone.

Until recombinant growth hormone became available in 1986, the only source was the pituitary glands of human cadavers. Recombinant growth hormone does not carry the risk of diseases such as **Creutzfeldt-Jakob disease** (a slowly progressive fatal disease caused by a prion).

There has been limited use of growth hormone supplementation by athletes, but no benefits of this hormone as an ergogenic aid have been clearly demonstrated. There is no evidence that supplemental growth hormone produces effects of the same magnitude in normal individuals as in those who are deficient in their own production of growth hormone. Animal experiments have shown that growth hormone causes muscle growth, but with no increase in strength.

Intravenous infusion of the amino acids arginine or ornithine produces a relatively consistent increase in growth hormone secretion in normal individuals and is used by endocrinologists to test a patient for normal growth hormone response. This is used as the basis for the marketing of dietary supplements containing these amino acids as 'growth hormone releasers.' There is no scientific evidence, however, that oral administration of these amino acids produces a similar rise in growth hormone, or that any such rise would be sufficient to produce improvement in performance. The rise in growth hormone levels that occurs during high-intensity resistance training is actually as large as the rise obtained with intravenous arginine.

It is not known whether growth hormone abuse causes adverse effects in healthy adults, although **acromegaly** (enlargement of the hands, head and feet) as a result of growth hormone abuse has been suspected. Clinical experience with acromegalics suggests that prolonged exposure to elevated doses of growth hormone has a detrimental effect on the neuromuscular system.

Use of growth hormone is banned by the World Anti-Doping Agency (WADA).

See also ORYZANOL; SLEEP.

Chronology

•1984 • Robert Kerr told *People* magazine that human growth hormone was the "fad anabolic drug" of the 1984 Olympic Games.

•1985 • Genentech, a pharmaceutical company based in California, announced that it had received approval from the Food and Drug Administration (FDA) to begin the manufacture of biosynthetic human growth hormone, marketed under the name Protropin.

•1996 • A Latvian company was harvesting growth hormone from human cadavers and selling it for use in sport.

•1996 • A research project called GH2000 was established using joint funding from the European Union, the International Olympic Committee (IOC) and the pharmaceutical industry. The main objectives of GH2000 were to define the limits of acceptable physiological ranges for human growth hormone in the population as a whole and in elite athletes, and to establish an acceptable testing procedure for the 2000 Olympic Games. Peter Sonksen, the scientist who was head of GH2000, has claimed that his team's findings – delivered six months before the 2000 Olympic Games, were advanced as any subsequent work on growth hormone. Wu (1999) reported an approach with the rationale that human growth hormone, as secreted by the pituitary gland, consists of several different isoforms, whereas recombinant growth hormone is a purified form with a distinct molecular weight.

•2003 • Tim Montgomery, the world record holder in the 100 meters, reportedly testified under oath that he had used growth hormone. The *San Francisco Chronicle* (24 June, 2004) reported Montgomery's testimony that Victor Conte of BALCO gave him doses of growth hormone and a drug known as "the clear" (now known to be tetrahydrogestrinone) over an 8-month period ending in the summer of 2001.

Bibliography

Drugs in Sport. Http://www.drugsinsport.net

Godfrey, R., Madgwick, Z. and Whyte, G. (2003). The exercise-induced growth hormone response in athletes. *Sports Medicine* 33(8), 599-613.

Jenkins, P.J. (2001). Growth hormone and exercise: Physiology, use and abuse. *Growth Hormone and IGF Research* 11, S71-S77.

Macintyre, J.G. (1987). Growth hormone and athletes. *Sports Medicine* 4, 129-142.

Mackay, D. (2004). IOC 'four years late' catching cheats. *The Observer* (UK), 8 August.

Todd, J. and Todd, T. (2001). Significant events in the history of drug testing and the Olympic movement 1960-1999. In: Wilson, W. and Derse, E. (eds). *Doping in elite sport. The politics of drugs in the Olympic movement*. pp65-128. Champaign, IL: Human Kinetics.

World Anti-Doping Agency. Http://www.wada-ama.org

Wu et al. (1999). Detection of doping with growth hormone. *The Lancet* 353, 895.

GROWTH PLATE   *See* PHYSIS.

GDP   *See* GUANOSINE DIPHOSPHATE.

GTP   *See* GUANOSINE TRIPHOSPHATE.

GUANINE   A nitrogenous purine base found in DNA and RNA.

GUANOSINE   A nucleoside containing guanine and ribose.

GUANOSINE DIPHOSPHATE   GDP. It is a nucleotide that contains guanine, ribose and two phosphates. It is required for the oxidation of alpha ketoglutaric acid in the Krebs cycle.

GUANOSINE TRIPHOSPHATE   GTP. It is a high-energy phosphate compound that is equivalent in energy to ATP and is vital for vision, gluconeogenesis and protein synthesis.

GUANYLATE CYCLASE   Guanyl cyclase. A family of enzymes that catalyze the formation of the second messenger cyclic GMP from GTP. Guanylate cyclases are either soluble (activated by nitric oxide) or membrane-bound and linked to a receptor (activated by peptide hormones).

GUIDANCE   *See under* LEARNING.

GULLAIN-BARRÉ SYNDROME   A transient condition of progressive muscle weakness caused by inflammation of the spinal and cranial nerves (**polyneuritis**). Weakness, sometimes followed by paralysis, first affects the feet and lower legs, then the upper legs and trunk, and eventually the facial muscles. Most patients make a full recovery, but rehabilitation may require many months of bracing and therapy. The incidence of the condition is 1 per 100,000, with equal numbers of males and females affected.

Those who make a complete recovery do not need to restrict their physical activity, but those who do not make a complete recovery need to maintain or improve their physical fitness.

Bibliography

The GBS Foundation International. Http://www.gullain-barre.com

Winnick, J.P. (2000, ed). *Adapted physical education and sport*. 3rd ed. Champaign, IL: Human Kinetics.

GUT   Intestine. *See under* GASTROINTESTINAL SYSTEM.

GUYTON'S CANAL SYNDROME   Cyclist's palsy. Handlebar palsy. It is the ulnar nerve analogue of median nerve compression at the wrist. It presents with paresthesias throughout all five fingers as the ulnar nerve innervates most of the intrinsic muscles of the hand. It results from repeated irritation of the deep branch of the ulnar nerve just distal to **Guyton's canal**, which is a fibro-osseous tunnel formed by the volar ligament (roof), the hamate (lateral wall), and the pisiform and pisohamate (medial wall). The ulnar nerve runs between the pisiform and hook of hamate through Guyton's canal. The ulnar nerve may be compressed in Guyton's canal in cyclists as a result of wrist hyperextension and direct pressure from the handlebars. Preventative measures include handlebar padding, padded gloves, modified handlebars and changing the position of the hands at frequent intervals. It can be seen in conjunction with carpal tunnel syndrome.

GYMNAST'S WRIST An overuse injury that is typically caused by high compression across the distal radial physis, but which may also involve the distal ulnar physis. During floor routines and vaulting, the wrist is subject to significant compression that may be as much as 5 to 11 times body weight.

Bibliography
Cervoni, T. et al. (1997). Stress lesions of the upper extremity in athletes. *The Physician and Sportsmedicine* 25, 50-55.

GYNECOMASTIA Benign enlargement of the male breast resulting from proliferation of the glandular component of the breast. It results from altered estrogen-androgen balance, in favor of estrogen, or increased breast sensitivity to normal circulating estrogen level. **Physiologic gynecomastia** occurs primarily in the newborns and in adolescents at puberty. In newborns, the neonatal breast tissue results from the action of maternal estrogens, placental estrogens or both in concert. The increased breast tissue usually disappears in a few weeks. In **adolescent gynecomastia**, the breast tissue growth is often asymmetric. Incidence may be as high as 60 to 70%. It is typically a firm, tender and painful subareolar mass anywhere from 1 to 5 cm in diameter. In 90% of cases, symptoms disappear within a period of a month to a few years. It usually regresses by 20 years of age, but residual gynecomastia may be present in one or both breasts. **Pathologic gynecomastia** is caused by testosterone deficiency, increased estrogen production or increased conversion of androgens to estrogen. Estrogen in males is mainly from peripheral conversion of androgens (testosterone and androstenedione) through the action of the enzyme aromatase, mainly in adipose tissue, muscle and skin. The normal ratio of testosterone to estrogen production is about 100 to 1. The normal ratio of testosterone to estrogen in circulation is about 300 to 1. Pathological conditions associated with gynecomastia include Klinefelter syndrome, testicular feminization, hermaphroditism, adrenal carcinoma, liver disorders and malnutrition. There are many drugs that cause gynecomastia, including drugs that inhibit testosterone synthesis and action (e.g. metronidazole) and by other (unknown) mechanisms (e.g. tricyclic anti-depressants, heroin, marijuana, anabolic steroids). 90% of physiologic gynecomastia involutes spontaneously within 2 years. In drug-induced gynecomastia, withdrawal leads to regression in 60% of patients.

Drug treatment includes anti-estrogens such as tamoxifen. In a liposuction-assisted mastectomy, the surgeon primarily targets the glandular breast tissue and the deep layers of subcutaneous fat. Complications include hematoma, breast asymmetry, nipple or areola necrosis, and nipple or areola inversion. Gynecomastia is a risk factor for male breast cancer.

Bibliography
Ali, F. and Bain, J. (2003). Gynecomastia. Http:///www.emedicine.

Segu, V.B. (2002). Gynecomastia. Http://www.emedicine.com

H

H$^+$ *See* HYDROGEN ION.

HABITUATION A decrease in a response to a stimulus seen with repeated presentation of the stimulus.

HAGLUND'S DISEASE *See under* ACHILLES TENDON.

HALDANE EFFECT *See under* CARBON DIOXIDE.

HALDANE TRANSFORMATION *See under* OXYGEN UPTAKE.

HALF LIFE The time required for half of a substance to disappear from a system. This disappearance could be either loss of a radioisotope as it decays to become another radioisotope (or to become a stable element) or loss of molecules that were formerly present in tissues, but have been degraded into other metabolites.

HALLUX Big toe. It is the 1st metatarsophalangeal joint.

HALLUX RIGIDUS A stiff and painful 1st hallux arising from microtrauma, osteonecrosis or osteoarthritis. An osteophyte may develop on top of the joint, as a natural response of the body to the worn joint. It occurs most commonly in young males. Etiological factors include a flattened metatarsal head, long 1st hallux, *pes planus* and excessive pronation. It is seen more commonly in athletes, especially runners, than in the sedentary population because of repetitive stress. Sport postures that require squatting, such as baseball catching, cause repetitive stress on the 1st metatarsophalangeal joint.

HALLUX VALGUS A complex forefoot deformity involving adduction and varus rotation of the 1st metatarsal, abduction and valgus rotation of the hallux, and prominence of the medial aspect of the joint. Adduction of the great toe at the 1st metatarsophalangeal joint by greater than the normal 10 degrees causes shoes to exert undue pressure against the medial aspect of the head of the 1st metatarsal. An exostosis forms on the medial side of the foot where the angle is greatest. The exostosis is covered by a bursa that can sometimes become inflamed as a result of being exposed to pressure (a bunion) and eventually a calcium deposit builds up on the head of the 1st metatarsal. This phenomenon occurs so frequently that the terms bunion and hallux valgus are used as synonyms. Risk factors include a depressed anterior arch, excessive pronation, ill-fitting shoes, tight lacing and a displacement of the 1st metatarsal bone. Treatment involves removing the bunion and calcium deposit. Shoes should be properly fitted, with low heels and stiff soles; wide, square-shaped toe box; toe portion stretched to accommodate a bunion; extra depth in the shoe to accommodate a dorsal flexed 2nd toe; and no inseam where the shoe contacts with the medial metatarsal head. Bunions are less common in cultures in which shoes are not worn.

Hallux valgus can give rise to metatarsalgia, because the other toes have to take more of the weight of the body during walking. With moderate to severe hallux valgus deformities, there can be disorders of the 2nd hallux, such as hammer toe and claw toe.

Juvenile hallux valgus involves the equivalent resultant deformity, with a general absence of chronic tissue reaction, painful symptoms and degenerative joint disease, and a few adaptive changes of the 1st metatarsophalangeal joint.

HAMATE BONE Hamatum. Unciform. It is one of the carpal bones and it projects anteriorly on the lateral side of the palm. Fracture of the hamate may result from repetitive compressive stresses with a bat, racquet or club impinging on the hypothenar eminence in baseball players, tennis players and golfers, respectively. It accounts for 2% of carpal fractures. It is less likely to occur in a cricket batsman, because the handle of a cricket bat is sprung to absorb impact. *See also under* GUYTON'S TUNNEL SYNDROME.

HAMMER TOE   A flexion contracture of the proximal interphalangeal (PIP) joint in one of the lesser four toes, caused by insufficiency of the anterior transverse arch or by tight-fitting shoes.

HAMSTRINGS   A group of muscles comprising the *biceps femoris, semimembranosus and semitendinosus.* All the hamstring muscles, except the short head of the *biceps femoris* cross both the hip joint and knee joint. In the late swing phase of the gait cycle, the hamstrings decelerate the leg. With sudden acceleration from the stabilizing flexion to active extension, the hamstrings may incur a strain injury. Other actions that may cause hamstring strain include the sprint start, and the take-off in high jump and long jump. The hamstrings are the most commonly strained muscles of the thigh, and the risk of such injury is increased when athletes are cold or have performed an inadequate warm up. The short head of the biceps is most commonly affected, especially where it inserts as a tendon into the head of the fibula.

Hamstring syndrome occurs when the sciatic nerve becomes entrapped by a fibrous band between the *biceps femoris* and *semitendinosus* muscles. Risk factors of hamstring syndrome include: lack of flexibility in the hamstrings; strength or power imbalances between the quadriceps and hamstrings; bilateral differences between the hamstrings in terms of strength or power; and the fact that the *biceps femoris* receives two nerve supplies (one to the short head and one to the long head).

Hamstring pain is frequently associated with spondylolisthesis as a result of a postural reflex to stabilize the body's center of gravity that is displaced anteriorly as a result of the spondylolisthesis. Otherwise undiagnosed low back pain has been attributed to tightness of the hamstrings. *See also under* LOW BACK PAIN; PELVIC GIRDLE.

HAND   The bones of the hand are arranged in three arches, two transverse and one longitudinal. The **proximal transverse arch** is at the level of the carpometacarpal joints with the keystone being the capitate. It is a relatively fixed arch, remaining arched even when the hand is open. The **distal transverse arch** is at the level of the metacarpophalangeal joints with the keystone being the 2nd and 3rd metacarpals. It is relatively mobile. The 1st, 4th and 5th metacarpals rotate around the 2nd and 3rd metacarpals to either flatten or increase its arc.

The two transverse arches are connected by the rigid portion of the **longitudinal arch**, which is made up of the four digital rays and the proximal carpus. The 2nd and 3rd metacarpal bones form the central pillar of this arch. The **longitidunal arch** is completed by the individual digital rays and the mobility of the thumb. It allows the palm to flatten or cup itself to accommodate objects of various sizes and shapes. *See also* CARPOMETACARPAL JOINTS; INTERPHALANGEAL JOINTS; METACARPOPHALANGEAL JOINTS.

HANDEDNESS   Most children display a consistent preference for one hand by the age of 5 years, but some children begin to rely on the use of one hand as young as 6 months. In general, the earlier a child shows a specific dominance for a hand, the more strongly dominant the handedness will be.

Approximately 13% of the population is currently left-handed. This may be higher than in the past, due to increased social acceptability of left-handedness. A distinction can be made between 'forced' left-handedness, which occurs because of pathology such as injury to the left hemisphere; and 'natural' left-handedness, which may have a genetic basis. McManus (2002) believes that there is a gene for right-handedness and a 'maverick' gene, which, if inherited, give an equal chance of making a person right or left handed.

The advantage of being left-handed in some sports comes from the fact that left-handers are less common than right-handers. There is little evidence that left-handers have superior motor skills. Left-handers know more about their right-handed opponents than vice versa. If the proportion of left-handers becomes too high, the advantage would disappear. In tennis, for example, left-handers would have an advantage if around 20% of the top players are left-handed, but not if 50% were left-handed. In group matches at the World Cup in cricket, it was found that of the 177 players who went to the crease, 42 (24%) were left handed. The left-handers were found to score an average of 20 runs per innings compared with 11 for right-handers. They also had longer innings: 25 versus 15 balls. It is often said in cricket that a combination of a left-hander and a right-hander at the crease is the most difficult to bowl at. The rationale is that such a partnership breaks up the bowler's ability to bowl at particular line and length. From all the partnerships at the World Cup, there was no evidence that this particular combination is any more successful.

Some sports disadvantage the left-handers because of the rules. In polo, mainly on the grounds of safety, the mallet must be held in the right hand on the right side of the horse.

Bibliography

Anything Left Handed. Http://www.anythingleft-handed.co.uk

Brooks, R et al. (2003). Sinister strategies succeed at cricket World Cup. *Proceedings of the Royal Society Series B (Supplement, Biology Letters)* 271, 564-566.

McManus, C. (2002). *Right hand, left hand. The origins of asymmetry in brains, bodies, atoms and cultures.* London: Weidenfeld and Nicholson.

HAND GRASP REFLEX   *See* PALMAR GRASP REFLEX.

HAND MUSCLES   The **intrinsic muscles of the hands** consist of the muscles of the hypothenar and thenar eminences, the interosseus muscles and the lumbrical muscles.

The **hypothenar eminence** is a group of muscles that act on the fifth (little) finger and comprises the *abductor digiti minimi, flexor digiti minimi brevis* and *opponens digiti minimi*. It is less prominent than the thenar eminence and the fifth finger cannot oppose the other digits. The **thenar eminence** is a group of muscles that acts on the

thumb and is comprised of the *abductor pollicis brevis, flexor pollicis brevis* and *opponens pollicis*. Acting together, these muscles oppose the thumb to the other fingers.

Muscles that flex one or more fingers are: *Flexor digitorum superficialis, flexor digitorum profundus, flexor pollicis longus, flexor pollicis brevis, flexor digiti minimi brevis, opponens digiti minimi, lumbricales, palmar interossei* and *dorsal interossei*. Muscles that extend one or more fingers are: *Extensor digitorum communis, extensor digiti minimi, abductor pollicis longus, extensor pollicis brevis, extensor pollicis longus, extensor indicis* and *lumbricales*. Muscles that produce abduction of one or more fingers are: *Abductor pollicis longus, abductor pollici brevis, flexor pollicis brevis, abductor digiti minimi* and *dorsal interossei*. Muscles that produce adduction of one or more fingers are: *Adductor pollicis* and *palmar interossei*.

Most tendons in the hand are restrained to some extent by sheaths and retinaculae that keep them close to the skeletal plane, so that they maintain a relatively constant moment arm, rather than bowstringing across the joints. The pulley system of the flexor tendon sheath in the finger is the most highly developed of these restraints. The digital flexor tendon sheath is comprised of 5 strong annular pulleys, which are important in assuring efficient digital motion by opposing the tendons to the phalanges.

HANGMAN'S FRACTURE   Bilateral pars interarticularis fracture of the 2nd cervical vertebra (C2) is known as 'hangman's fracture.' It may be caused by a severe extension injury, such as where the face forcibly hits dashboard or from hanging.

HAPTIC PERCEPTION   The combined use of tactile perception through the skin and kinesthetic perception of the position and movement of the joints and muscles.

HAPTOGLOBIN   *See under* HEMOGLOBIN.

HARDNESS   A measure of the resistance of a material to scratching or indentation. It is a mechanical property that is relevant both to the strength of a structure and to its surface wear.

HAY FEVER   *See under* RHINITIS.

HEAD   The skull is covered by the scalp on the outside and protects the brain on the inside. Between the skull and the brain are three layers of tissue: the dura mater, the arachnoid and the pia mater. The **dura mater** is a thick fibrous membrane that encloses the various venous sinuses. Between the dura mater and the arachnoid is a potential space called the **subdural space**. Between the pia mater and the arachnoid is the **subarachnoid space** in which flows the cerebro-spinal fluid. It also contains the major arterial blood vessels and the bridging cerebral veins.

HEADACHE   There are many different types of headache. **Tension-type headaches** are the most common, affecting more than 75% of headache sufferers. Tension-type headaches are typically a steady ache rather than a throbbing one and affect both sides of the head. Causes include stressful events.

 Migraine is an idiopathic, recurring headache disorder manifesting in attacks lasting 4 to 72 hours with symptoms such as nausea, vomiting and photophobia. A **'classic' migraine** is characterized by the occurrence of an aura 10 to 30 minutes before the migraine attack and involves disturbed vision; a **'common' migraine** is not preceded by an aura. Most migraine sufferers report a family history of migraines. It is thought that the migraine is due to distortion and spasm of cerebral blood vessels. Serotonin is released, closing the arteries, and contributing to decreased blood flow to the brain. Other arteries in the brain try to vasodilate, increasing the production of chemicals that cause inflammation and sensitivity to pain. Prevalence of migraine in the general population is 15 to 30%, being higher in women. About 60% of female migraine patients report a relationship between the menstrual cycle and their acute headaches. Any form of exertion, including coughing and orgasm, can trigger migraine. Hypoglycemia *per se*, is not responsible for the precipitation of migraine attacks as a result of hunger. The lowest blood glucose levels recorded during fasting in subjects experiencing an attack are not different from those in subjects who do not develop headache. Increased turnover of brain serotonin, as a consequence of a chronic stress reaction with heightened activity of the sympathetic nervous system, may be involved in producing headache provoked by fasting. Migraine patients who are physically active may find that exercise provokes a migraine attack or that regular exercise helps to reduce the severity of their headaches. Other triggers for migraine include: certain foods (e.g. chocolate) or food additives (e.g. monosodium glutamate), changes in barometric pressure (e.g. before a storm), exposure to certain scents (e.g. perfume), blinking lights (e.g. headlights at night on a freeway) and changes in daily routine (e.g. sleeping more or less than normal). Drug therapy for migraine headaches includes the combination of ergotamine and caffeine. **Ergotamine** is a class of medication called ergot alkaloids. It works together with caffeine by preventing the vasodilation in the head that causes headaches.

 Rebound headache may occur among people with tension-type headaches as well as those with migraines. It appears to be the result of taking prescription or nonprescription pain relievers daily or almost every day, contrary to directions on the package label.

 Cluster headache is a debilitating neuronal headache with pain usually beginning in, around or above the eye or the temple. Occasionally the face, neck, ear or hemicranium may be affected. It is always unilateral, and generally affects the same side in subsequent attacks. Attacks last from 30 minutes to 2 hours in about 75% of cases. Attacks range in frequency from six per 24 hours to one per week, with a mean of one to two per day. Cluster headache occurs in 1 in 200 men and in 1 in 1,000 women in any year. Lacrimation from the eye on the affected side is the most associated symptom. A blocked nasal passage, rhinorrhea, red eye, and sweating and pallor of the forehead and cheek are often found. Sensitivity to alcohol during the cluster headache attack occurs in at least half the patients. Patients who are sensitive to alcohol note that attacks are triggered within 5 to 45 minutes after the ingestion of modest amounts of alcohol. Vigorous physical activity at the earliest sign of an attack can, in some patients, decrease or even aborting an attack. Cluster headaches are clinically different from migraines. Propranolol is effective in treating migraine, but has not been shown to be effective in cluster headache. Lithium is beneficial for cluster headaches, but ineffectual in migraine. In most patients with cluster headaches as a chronic syndrome, lithium therapy prevents attacks that are provoked by alcohol. The drugs effective in the treatment of the cluster headache syndrome enhance serotonergic neurotransmission, as also occurs in the treatment of migraine. This suggests that unstable serotonergic neurotransmission, at different loci, may be common to both disorders.

Exertional headache is migrainous in nature. Straining or Valsalva-type maneuvers precipitate the acute onset of severe throbbing pain, usually occipital, for a few seconds to a few minutes. This severe pain is then followed by a dull, aching pain that may last for hours. One theory of exertional headaches is that exertion increases cerebral arterial pressure, causing the pain-sensitive venous sinuses at the base of the brain to dilate. With maximal lifts, systolic blood pressure of weightlifters may reach levels above 400 mm Hg and diastolic pressure may exceed 300 mm Hg. Exertional headaches tend to recur over weeks to months when the activity is repeated.

Effort headaches are the most common type of headache in athletes and are associated with a variety of sports. They are not necessarily benign. Migrainous in nature, these vascular headaches are more frequent in hot weather and tend to recur with exercise.

Sexual headache (coital cephalgia) may occur before, during or after orgasm. The 'active partner' seems to be more likely to experience sexual headache than the 'passive partner.' Men are affected by sexual headache four times more than women. Headaches are more frequent during attempts to have several orgasms during one sexual encounter. It is not only sexual intercourse (coitus) that causes sexual headache, but also masturbation or even getting in the position for intercourse. **Preorgasmic tension-type headache** is a dull, tight, cramping headache that is usually bilateral and occipital/cervical in location. **Orgasmic headache** has an abrupt or explosive onset, in the occipital region, behind the eyes, or generalized. **Postorgasmic headache** upon standing occurs as a result of low cerebrospinal fluid pressure. It can result from a dural tear as a result of physiologic stress during coitus. Most sexual headaches are benign, but some are malignant. Bleeding associated with subarachnoid hemorrhage may occur at the time of sexual intercourse. Risk factors associated with sexual headaches include: hypertension, obesity, lack of exercise, psychosexual stress (e.g. extramarital affairs), the degree of sexual excitement, kneeling position during sexual intercourse, history of migraine or exertional headache, family history of headache, and occlusive arterial disease. 40% of patients with sexual headaches also experience benign exertional headache. Many patients with sexual headache have a history of migraine. In some people, however, sexual intercourse may provide migraine relief.

Trauma to the head and neck in sport may lead to headaches. At least six distinct forms of **posttraumatic headache** exist: **chronic muscle contraction headache**; **mixed headache** (episodic migraine superimposed on chronic muscle contraction headache); **trauma-triggered migraine** (clinically indistinguishable from migraine and seen in sports such as soccer, which have repetitive heading of the ball); **traumatic dysautonomic cephalgia** (due to blows on the anterior neck that trigger autonomic symptoms); **second-impact catastrophic headache** (a usually fatal consequence of brain injury thought to be due to diffuse cerebral edema after repeated brain injury) and superficial pain at the site of head or skull trauma.

Cervicogenic headaches are caused by abnormalities of the joints, muscles, fascia and neural structures of the cervical spine. Sharing many of the clinical features of chronic tension headache, the pain at onset is usually occipital and may radiate to the anterior aspect of the skull and face. They may be related to scuba diving, rock climbing or tennis, in which repeated cervical extension is common.

Cervical injury in collision or contact sports may also cause a cervicogenic headache.

Goggle headache (supraorbital neuralgia), commonly seen in swimmers and scuba divers, is pain in the face and temporal area caused by wearing a mask or goggles that are too tight. In divers, 'mask squeeze' occurs on descent to depth as increased pressure decreases the air space inside the mask. Better fitting goggles can help alleviate symptoms in swimmers, but not in scuba divers. **Swimmer's headache** occurs from jumping into cold water.

Diver's headache is a vascular-type headache in scuba divers thought to be due to carbon dioxide accumulation during skip breathing, which is holding the breath (on inhalation or exhalation) in order to conserve air. This is, in effect, hypoventilation and there is a risk of pulmonary barotrauma (especially if near the surface). Divers are also prone to headaches from other causes such as cold exposure, muscle or temporomandibular joint pain from gripping the mouthpiece too tightly, middle ear and sinus barotraumas, cerebral decompression illness, and tank gas impurities (e.g. low levels of carbon monoxide).

Altitude headache is a type of vascular headache that often accompanies acute mountain sickness in unacclimatized individuals who ascend above 8,000 feet.

Bibliography

Cheshire, W.P. and Ott, M.C. (2001). Headache in divers. *Headache* 41, 235-247.

Diamond, S. (1996). Managing migraines in active people. *The Physician and Sportsmedicine* 24(12), 41-53.

Evans, R.W. and Couch, J.R. (2001). Orgasm and migraine. *Headache* 41(5), 512-514.

McCrory, P. (1997). Recognizing exercise-related headache. *The Physician and Sportsmedicine* 25(2), 41-48.

Sami, H.R. and Couch, J.R. (2004). Primary headache associated with sexual activity. Http://www.drsami.com/neuroblog/

Worldwide Cluster Headache Support Group. Http://www.clusterheadaches.com

HEAD INJURIES   Prevention of head injuries is important, because the nerve cells of the brain and spinal cord, unlike most other cells in the body, are not capable of regeneration.

Force applied through the center of mass of the head causes linear translation of the head. Force applied off-center, such an upper-cut punch to a boxer's chin, causes rotation of the head. Direct compressive forces, such as a forceful blow to the resting head, are generally well tolerated unless they cause focal pathology such as fractures and hematomas.

Rotational acceleration and/or deceleration creates tensile and shearing forces between the brain and its surrounding attachments, resulting in more serious injury that often occurs in another area other than the anatomical site of impact. Rotational forces are more likely to cause loss of consciousness associated with deep shearing injuries of nerve fibers (diffuse axonal injury), whereas translational forces are more likely to cause skull fractures, intracranial hematomas and cerebral contusions.

There are about 300,000 sports-related brain concussions per year in the USA. **Concussion** is a clinical syndrome characterized by immediate and transient impairment of neurologic function (e.g. disturbance of vision, confusion and amnesia) due to mechanical acceleration/deceleration forces acting on the brain. The site of maximum injury is usually at the point of impact (**coup injury**). An example of a deceleration force is when an athlete's head strikes the ground. The site of maximum injury is opposite the point of impact (**contrecoup injury**). Concussion may also result indirectly from a sharp blow to the athlete's torso or pelvis (e.g. falling on ice). In sports, milder forms of head injury are common and often do not involve loss of consciousness, reflecting preservation of the reticular activating system, a network of neurons that functions to stimulate the cerebral cortex. The distinction between '**mild brain trauma**' and more serious head injuries is based on the presence or absence of loss of consciousness, the presence and duration of post-traumatic amnesia, and other post-traumatic historical and physical findings. There is evidence that mouthguards are effective in protecting against concussion and injuries to the cervical spine. **Concussive convulsions** are nonepileptic phenomena that are immediate sequelae of concussive brain injury, with an approximate incidence of 1 case in 70 concussions.

Structurally, head injuries may be classed as either closed head or penetrating injuries. **Closed head injuries**, such as concussion, result from rapid translational or rotational acceleration of the head with concomitant damage to the brain or its surrounding structures, but with no exposure to the external environment. Closed-head injuries occur most frequently in boxing and American football. **Penetrating injuries** occur when an object directly penetrates the skull and its neurovascular contents. Tissue damage may be restricted to a limited area (**focal injury**) or pervade a large region of neural tissue (**diffuse injury**).

Head injuries are often **insidious**, in that evidence at the time of primary injury may not reveal associated secondary injuries that will subsequently develop. Extensive brain injury may occur in the absence of superficial damage; but evidence of extensive superficial damage, such as copious bleeding, does not always predict brain injury.

Fractures of the cranium usually result from blunt trauma such as from a fall or from a direct blow to the head. Cranial fractures are commonly associated with injury to the brain and meninges. These injuries include cerebral contusions and intra-cranial hemorrhage. With regard to intracranial hemorrhage, bleeding may occur in the epidural space, the subdural space or the subarachnoid space. Contusions can occur directly beneath the site of impact (**coup injury**) or opposite to the site of impact (**contrecoup injury**). Contrecoup contusions result from the impact of a moving head against an unyielding surface and occur most commonly in the temporal and frontal regions. Blunt force applied to a resting (but unfixed) head results in coup injury and only rarely causes contrecoup injury.

Second impact syndrome is the rapid development of diffuse brain swelling in the setting of a recent head injury, usually concussion, followed by a second impact to the head. It is often a fatal condition, and is one reason why conservative guidelines should be followed in permitting athletes to return to sport after a head injury.

An **epidural (extradural) hematoma** is an accumulation of blood between the cranium and the outer dural covering of the brain. It is most commonly caused by a tear in the middle meningeal artery, in association with a skull fracture. The resultant bleeding leads to rapid compression of the brain stem, with consequences that are fatal unless the pressure is relieved and the bleeding is stopped. A **subdural hematoma** is an accumulation of blood in the subdural space. It is caused by a tear in the dural sinus veins. A **subarachnoid hemorrhage** is an intracranial hemorrhage that is confined to the surface of the brain. It is caused by disruption of the small meningeal blood vessels on the surface of the brain. In an athlete, it is usually due to rupture of a congenital aneurysm.

Intracerebral hemorrhage is bleeding within the substance of the brain. It is an injury that occurs secondary to tearing of small blood vessels within the brain tissues. **Cerebral edema** is an increase in pressure inside the skull, probably due to an increase in the amount of cerebrospinal fluid and, possibly, the occurrence of a self-limited intracranial bleeding.

Traumatic brain injury is permanent damage caused by concussion, contusion or hemorrhage sustained in vehicular accidents, assaults, falls and other kinds of traumas. Most of these are closed-head injuries. Traumatic brain injury is the leading cause of death and disability for persons under age 35 years. Over half of children who sustain traumatic brain injury have some degree of permanent spasticity and/or ataxia. Visual perception may be affected. Persons with traumatic brain injury typically have difficulty performing movements sequentially. As with autism, in the USA, traumatic brain injury was added as a separate category of disability in 1990 under P.L. 101-476, and is defined as an acquired injury to the brain caused by an external physical force, resulting in total or partial functional disability or psychosocial impairment, or both, that adversely affects a child's educational performance. Persons with traumatic brain injury are included in the US Cerebral Palsy Association.

Head trauma in soccer can occur in several ways including: heading; a single hard blow from the ball; contact with another player; striking the ground;

collision with goalposts; and, possibly, repeated heading. A soccer ball striking the head has about five-times lower impact than a typical boxing punch. Boxers can tolerate severe direct blows to the head provided their neck muscles are strong and they can keep their head still. Similarly, a soccer player should brace his neck muscles when heading the ball in order to keep the head rigid at impact. In heading a ball from either a standing jump or running jump, it is vital that the power is derived from a back-to-front movement starting at the hips. There is concern about soccer players' reports of increased neurologic symptoms such as headaches, heading-related migraine, neck pain and dizziness. However, research using electroencephalography, computerized tomography (sectional radiography), neurologic examinations and neuropsychological testing has not clearly established that heading is hazardous. Rutherford et al. (2003) concluded that there is exploratory evidence of subclinical neuro-psychological impairment as a consequence of soccer-related concussions, but there is no reliable or definitive evidence that such impairment occurs as a result of general soccer play or normal heading of a soccer ball. Current research shows that selected soccer players have some degree of cognitive dysfunction, but a player's history of concussive episodes is a more likely explanation for cognitive deficits. It is unlikely that the subconcussive impact of purposeful heading is a factor in the noted deficits, but it is not known whether multiple subconcussive impacts might have some lingering effects. In addition, it is unknown whether the noted deficits have any effect on daily life. The American Academy of Pediatrics (2001) concluded that there seems to be insufficient published data to support a recommendation that young soccer players completely refrain from heading the ball, but did recommend that adult supervisors of youth soccer minimize the use of heading until the potential for permanent cognitive impairment is further delineated.

Dementia pugilistica ('**punch-drunk syndrome**') is a set of symptoms including slurred speech, lack of coordination in movement and impaired mental functioning. It occurs in 17 to 55% of professional boxers, but is less common in amateur boxers. There is evidence that a knockout causes permanent structural damage to the brain. There is also evidence, however, that the number of bouts rather than the number of knockouts is related more strongly to chronic brain damage.

The finding of **cavum septi pellucidi** in a boxer is a sign of the presence of encephalopathy. The **septum pellucidum** forms the medial wall of the lateral cerebral ventricles. The posterior margin is the fornix and the rostral; the superior limits are formed by the corpus callosum. The **septum** consists of two leaves of tissue with both gray and white matter components, connected via the median forebrain bundle to the hippocampus and via the fornix to the limbic system. The functional role of the septum pellucidum is not completely established, but it does seem to take part in limbic functions involving moderation of rage and arousal. Cavum septi pellucidi in dementia pugilistica is believed to derive from the repeated delivery of blows to the head resulting in recurrent brief increases in intraventricular pressure, tearing of the leaves of the septum and the collection of cerebrospinal fluid within the space thus created. The prevalence of cavum septi pellucidi in the general adult population is probably less than 1%, but there is an increased prevalence among professional boxers, particularly those with symptoms of dementia pugilistica. Dementia pugilistica has been positively correlated with the length of career (number of bouts) and participation as a sparring partner, and negatively correlated with the boxer's skill.

Because amateur fights last only three rounds, compared to as many as 15 rounds in professional boxing, it is reasonable to expect that amateur boxers receive fewer blows to the head and thus, suffer fewer brain injuries. However, there is evidence that amateur boxers are still at risk of acquiring cognitive abnormalities and/or focal neurologic deficits. Prophylactic measures with helmets, unlimited lengths of hand bandage, and heavier gloves have not decreased the frequency of matches that are stopped for neurologic reasons.

Bungee jumping involves a person free-falling from a height of about 60 to 120 m, and being jerked to safety at the last moment by elastic recoil of an attached cord. Injury risk factors include natural forces, impact, technician error, equipment failure and repetitive strain. The person experiences a sudden deceleration, when acceleration of the body downwards is overcome by the cord at the end of the descent. This produces a rise in intrathoracic pressure and the negative acceleration causes a fluid shift towards the head. This may increase venous pressure of the eye, resulting in rupture of the small capillaries and subhyaloid hemorrhage, leading to detachment of the inner limiting membrane. Danger of irreversible damage from ocular hemorrhage seems unlikely, however. Hanging occurs when a person becomes entangled in the cord with the body suspended by the neck and ligature constriction imposed by the weight of the body. Increased elasticity of the cord, or shortening of the cord, minimizes the risk of hanging, because of a slower stop with a drop of distance and less recoil.

See also HELMET.

Chronology

•1719 • James Figg opened a boxing school in London and began to teach his style of bare-knuckle fighting. Figg's rules were brutal; boxers were required to fight without rest periods until one man could not continue.

•1722 • Elizabeth Wilkinson of Clerkenwell challenged Hannah Hyfield of Newgate Market to meet her on stage and box for a prize of three guineas. The women had to strike each other in the face while holding a half-crown coin in each fist and the first to drop the coin would be the loser.

•1743 • Jack Broughton, a British boxer, introduced the London Prize Ring Rules, which lasted until the 1860s. A fight would end when one man was knocked down and could not get up within 30 seconds. Bouts were still continuous.

•1811 • Tom Cribb of England beat Tom Molineaux, an African American, in what was actually a rematch after a disputed Cribb victory a year previous. Before the fight, Molineaux consumed a chicken, a large apple pie and seven pints of porter. He lost the fight in the 11th round when his jaw was broken. Molineaux was a slave, who gained his freedom by fighting on the Southern Plantation Circuit. He was trained by another freed slave, Bill Richmond, who had been beaten by Cribb in the 76th round of a fight in 1805.

•1865 • A new boxing code of 12 rules was formulated and required the use of gloves, rounds lasting three minutes, ten-second knockout counts, and prohibited wrestling holds. The rules were written by John G. Chambers, a member of the Amateur Athletic Club (AAC) of Great Britain, but they weren't published until 1867, with the patronage of John S. Douglas, the 8th Marquis of Queensberry. Chambers intended the rules for amateur boxing matches, such as those run by the AAC, but they weren't actually used for a truly amateur tournament (i.e. no prizes, no betting) until 1872. Prize fighting was allowed under these rules in place of the old London Prize Ring. In boxing, the Queensberry rules have survived with only slight changes to the present day.

•1894 • Louisiana banned boxing after the death of a New Orleans fighter.

•1896 • New York became the only state with legalized boxing when a bill, the Horton Act, passed the legislature and was approved, making 'sparring' matches of up to 10 rounds legal at licensed athletic clubs. The Horton Act was repealed in 1900, because of the sport's brutality, gambling and the influence of Tammany politicians. In 1912, the Democrats passed the Frawley Act, but it was repealed in 1917 by the Republicans.

•1904 • Women's boxing was a demonstration sport at the Olympic Games.

•1918 • Records were started on deaths in boxing. By 1998, 450 had died.

•1920 • New York passed the Walker Law, which permitted public prizefighting.

•1969 • In Britain, the Royal College of Physicians of London published their report on the medical aspects of boxing. The records of 250 ex-professional boxers (a random sample) were studied. From a final selection of 224 boxers, it was found that 37 showed some evidence of brain damage. In 13 cases this damage was disabling.

•1983 • An advisory panel of the American Medical Association concluded that banning boxing was impractical and unwarranted.

•1996 • In contrast to the stance taken by the British Medical Association, the Royal College of Nursing (RCN) voted overwhelmingly (75%) against a ban on boxing. Boxers who receive successive blows to the head may suffer irreversible brain damage. The RCN conceded that there were serious health risks, but decided that prohibition would infringe individual rights and make the sport more dangerous by driving it underground. In 1995, the Government had argued that boxing was an established, highly regulated sport that was part of Britain's sporting heritage.

•2002 • In the UK, an inquest into the death of former soccer player, Jeff Astle, who played for West Bromwich Albion, ruled that he died, aged 59 years, from a degenerative brain disease appeared to have been caused (or at least worsened) by heading heavy, leather soccer balls. Astle was regarded as one of the best exponents of the long-range header. The consultant neurological pathologist indicated that there was evidence of brain injury consistent with "repeated minor trauma" and that it was "quite probable that it was heading a heavy football that caused it." The coroner recorded a verdict of "death by industrial disease."

Bibliography

American Academy of Pediatrics (1997). Participation in boxing by children, adolescents, and young adults. *Pediatrics* 99(1), 134-135.

American Academy of Pediatrics (2001). Injuries in youth soccer. A subject review. *Pediatrics* 105(3), 659-661.

Asken, M.J. and Schwartz, R.C. (1998). Heading the ball in soccer: What's the risk of brain injury? *The Physician and Sportsmedicine*, 26(11) 37-44.

Bodensteiner, J.B. and Schaefer, G.B. (1997). Dementia pugilistica and cavum septi pellucidi: Born to box? *Sports Medicine* 24(6), 361-365.

Cantu, R.C. (1995, ed). *Boxing and medicine*. Champaign, IL: Human Kinetics.

Chalmers, D.J. (1998). Mouthguards. Protection for the mouth in rugby union. *Sports Medicine* 25(5), 339-349.

Guterman, A. and Smith, R.W. (1987). Neurological sequelae of boxing. *Sports Medicine* 4, 194-210.

Kirkendall, D.T., Jordan, S.E. and Garrett, W.E. (2001). Heading and head injuries in soccer. *Sports Medicine* 31(5), 369-386.

McCrory, P.R. and Berkovic, S.F. (1998). Concussive convulsions. Incidence in sport and treatment recommendations. *Sports Medicine* 25(2), 131-136.

Rutherford, A., Stephens, R. and Potter, D. (2003). The neuropsychology of heading and head trauma in association football (soccer): A review. *Neuropsychology Review* 13(3), 153-179.

Sturmi, J.E. Smith, C. and Lombardo, J.A. (1998). Mild brain trauma in sports. Diagnosis and treatment guidelines. *Sports Medicine* 25(6), 351-358.

Tysvaer, A.T. (1992). Head and neck injuries in soccer. Impact of minor trauma. *Sports Medicine* 14(3), 200-213.

Vanderford, L. and Myers, M (1995). Injuries and bungee jumping. *Sports Medicine* 20(6), 369-374.

Vines, G. (1986). Boxing takes a battering. *New Scientist*, 19 June.

HEAD-IN-SPACE RIGHTING REFLEX   *See* LABYRINTHINE RIGHTING REFLEX.

HEAD-RIGHTING REFLEX   A postural reflex that is normal from the first month of infancy through the 6th month, it is elicited by turning the baby's body in either direction when the infant is supine. This causes the head to turn to a front-facing position relative to the shoulder. Along with the body-righting reflex, the head-righting reflex is believed to play a role in the attainment of voluntary rolling movements. In forward or backward rolls, flexion of the head reinforces flexion of the trunk, arms and legs. In order to facilitate a one-armed pull, the head should be turned away in addition to being flexed. Conversely, to facilitate a one-armed push, the head should be turned toward the pushing arm as well as being extended. During a handstand, extension of the head reinforces extension in the arms. In archery, head rotation facilitates bow arm pushing on the chin side and bowstring arm pulling by the opposite side.

HEALING   A tissue effect resulting from repair. Healing is associated with minimal scarring, regeneration, freedom from pain, full range of movement, hypertrophy, normal movement patterns and no psychological after-effects.

HEALTH   It is the state of complete physical, mental and social well being, rather than simply freedom from disease and infirmity (World Health Organization, 1976). **Wellness** is defined as a state of optimal health that includes physical, emotional, intellectual, spiritual and social health. **Hygiene** was a term originally concerned with preserving one's health. Following World War I the term 'hygiene' became virtually obsolete and was replaced by terms such as health education.

Health behavior is the combination of knowledge, attitudes, and practices that contribute to motivate the actions people take regarding health and wellness. **Health promotion** is the science and art of helping people change their lifestyle and move toward a state of optimal health.

See also KINESIOLOGY; PHYSICAL EDUCATION; PHYSICAL FITNESS.

Chronology

•435 BC • Herodicus (Herodikus) of Selymbria originated the Valetudinarian school of 'medical gymnastics' and was the teacher of Hippocrates. Herodicus suffered from ill health and discovered from personal experience about treating disease by diet and exercise. Plato ridiculed Herodicus for corrupting the arts of gymnastics and medicine.

•420 BC • Hippocrates made many references to the value of exercise. He devoted considerable attention to diet and attempted to make scientific inquiry into the proper place, time, dosage and type of activity in which one should indulge.

•1569 • Hieronymus Mercurialis published his *De Arte Gymnastica*. In one section of the text, devoted to the therapeutic value of exercise, he established the following principles: (i) each exercise should preserve the existing healthy state; (ii) exercise should not disturb the harmony among the principal humors (body fluids); (iii) exercise should be suited to each part of the body; (iv) all healthy people should take exercise regularly; (v) sick people should not be given exercises that might exacerbate existing conditions; (vi) special individualized exercises should be prescribed for convalescing patients; and (vii) persons who lead sedentary lives urgently need exercise. With the exception of (ii), all of Mercurialis' principles are still widely accepted. During the Middle Ages, it was believed that health and temperament were regulated by four main body fluids (humors): blood; phlegm (a thick mucus from the respiratory passages), yellow bile and black bile.

•1745 • Benjamin Franklin reprinted John Armstrong's *Art of Preserving Health*, first published in London in 1644. Franklin was probably the first American to propose that physical training be part of the educational curriculum. In his pamphlet, *Proposals Relating to the Education of Youth in Pennsylvania* (1749), Franklin recommended regular physical activity, including running, swimming and basic forms of resistance training for health purposes.

•1854 • William A. Stearns, of Amherst College, announced the establishment of a department of hygiene and physical education, and the future appointment of a director trained in both medicine and gymnastics. This gave hygiene and physical education an academic status in the hierarchy of university disciplines and set a precedent for other higher education institutions.

•1866 • California became the first state in the USA to pass a law requiring a program of physical exercise in public elementary and secondary schools. Section 55 of the Revised School Law, written by John Swett, stated, "Instruction shall be given in all grades of schools, and in all classes, during the entire school course, in manners and morals, and the laws of health; and due attention shall be given to such physical exercises for the pupils as may be conducive to health and vigor of body, as well as mind; and to the ventilation and temperature of school rooms."

•1876 • At the convention of the German Gymnastic Teachers Association at Brunswick, August Hermann said that German people, like the English, must make gymnastics and participation in games a national habit if they were to combat the deteriorating effects of modern life.

•1878 • Dudley A. Sargent opened his Hygienic Institute and School of Physical Culture in New York City with the help of William Blaikie.

•1904 • G. Stanley Hall published his book on health and education of the adolescent that was reprinted five years later in a condensed form entitled *Youth, Its Education, Regime and Hygiene*. Hall felt that games and sports filled the health needs of too few youths and argued that gymnastics were still necessary.

•1909 • Thomas Storey claimed that the objectives of school hygiene and physical education are identical. In the following year, the theme of the American Physical Education Association Convention was "School Hygiene and Physical Education."

•1909 • The first bacterial studies of swimming pools in the USA led to the foundation of the American Association of Hygiene and Baths (1912).

•1910 • Thomas Wood, head of the department of physical education at Teacher's College, Columbia University, published *Health and Education* (Part I of the 9th *Yearbook of the National Society for the Study of Education*). Wood indicted the traditional physical education program that was based on the German and Swedish systems, believing in 'education through the physical' and that health should be a by-product of activity rather than the main aim.

•1911 • A. Mallwitz established a section on "Hygiene of Physical Exercise" at the World Hygiene Exposition in Dresden.

•1914 • In *Hygiene of the School Child*, Lewis M. Terman claimed that "…modern education has been influenced in its attitude toward the body by medieval rather than Greek and Roman ideals. Physical Education has played an insignificant part in modern educational theory and still less in educational practice."

•1918 • In the USA, the National Educational Association proclaimed its Seven Cardinal Principles of Education: health and safety; mastery of tools, techniques and spirit of learning; worthy home membership; vocational and economic effectiveness; citizenship; worthy use of leisure; and ethical character.

•1920 • The University of Oregon created the School of Health and Physical Education, the first such school in an American university.

•1922 • In the UK, a report was drawn up by a committee formed in the previous year at the instance of the College of Preceptors to consider the effect of physical education on girls. Representatives were appointed by the Royal College of Physicians, the Royal College of Surgeons, the British Medical Association, the Medical Women's Federation, the British Association for Physical Training, the National Union of Women's Teachers, the Association of Assistant Mistresses in Secondary Schools and the Private Schools Association. *The Times* of August 9 stated, "In this report, swimming, lawn tennis and cycling (in moderation) were seen as suitable for girls but football was another matter and hockey was seen by some as reasonable for only 'the older and stronger girls.' "

•1930 • Mary Stack founded the Women's League of Health and Beauty to promote her exercise program. The exercises were demonstrated by her daughter, Prunella, who came to be known as the 'Perfect Girl.' By 1939, the League, which gave demonstrations at the Royal Albert Hall in London, had 166,000 members. It was later renamed Health and Beauty Exercise.

•1937 • Prunella Stack was invited by the British Prime Minister to serve on the newly formed National Fitness Council.

•1937 • The American Physical Education Association (APEA) merged with the Department of School Health and Physical Education to form the American Association for Health and Physical Education (AAHPE). This reflects the integration of physical education with the total school curriculum. A year later its name was changed to the American Association for Health, Physical Education and Recreation (AAHPER).

•1939 • The Legislative Council of the American Association for Health, Physical Education and Recreation (AAHPER) passed a resolution for the establishment of a national committee to urge President Roosevelt and Congress to allocate federal funds in the pending National Health Bill to promote health, physical education and recreation programs in the nation's schools.

•1958 • The International Council for Health, Physical Education and Recreation (ICHPER) was founded.

•1966 • Jesse Owens, who won 4 gold medals in the 1936 Olympic Games, died at the age of 66. He was heavy smoker and died of lung cancer. As a child, Owens suffered chronic bronchial congestion and several bouts of pneumonia. Inadequate housing, food and clothing did not help his health.

•1979 • The "Healthy People" project was originated following a report by the US Surgeon General on Health Promotion and Disease Prevention that established five life-stage targets to be achieved over a ten-year period.

•1983 • The National Commission on Excellence in Education released a report, "A Nation at Risk: The Imperative for Education Reform." It warned that declining educational achievement, unhealthy lifestyles, drugs, alcohol abuse, teenage pregnancy and school failure undermined the ability of American people to achieve their full potential.

•1985 • The National Wellness Association was founded as a membership division of the National Wellness Institute in order to meet the growing needs of wellness and health promotion professionals for national leadership.

•1990 • In the USA, the Department of Health and Human Services released the report *Healthy People 2000*, which outlined three broad goals for public health: 1) to increase the span of healthy life; 2) to decrease disparities in health status among different populations; and 3) to provide access to preventive health-care services for all persons.

•1992 • The Outcomes Committee of the National Association for Sport and Physical Education (NASPE) developed and published a benchmark report, *Outcomes of Quality Physical Education,* providing a national framework for curriculum development. A Standards and Assessment Task Force was appointed to develop content standards and assessment material based on the outcomes document. The "Outcomes Project" culminated in the development of a definition of the physically educated person. This definition included five major focus areas, specifying that a physically educated person: i) has learned skills necessary to perform a variety of physical activities; ii) is physically fit; iii) does participate regularly in physical activity; iv) knows the implications and the benefits from involvement in physical activities; and v) values physical activity and its contribution to a healthful lifestyle.

•1994 • The Association for Research, Administration, Professional Councils and Societies (ARAPCS) of the American Alliance for Health, Physical Education, Recreation and Dance (AAHPERD) changed its name to the American Association for Active Lifestyles and Fitness (AAALF). The goal of AAALF is to promote active lifestyles and fitness for all populations through support of research, development of leaders, and dissemination of current information.

•1996 • *Physical Activity and Health: A Report of the Surgeon General* was the US Government's first comprehensive review of the health effects of exercise. The report concluded that regular physical activity has the following effects: i) greatly decreases the risk of dying of coronary artery disease; ii) decreases the risk of developing type II diabetes, hypertension and colon cancer; iii) enhances mental health; iv) fosters healthy muscles, bones and joints, and appears to decrease symptoms of osteoarthritis; v) helps older adults to maintain functional ability and preserve their independence; and iv) is an effective adjunct to dietary measures for avoiding weight gain or for losing weight. It was also concluded that people can gain these health benefits by doing some moderate activity (such as 30 minutes of brisk walking or 15 minutes of running) all or most days, and that longer or more vigorous bouts of activity yield greater benefits. It was found that 60% of Americans do not regularly exercise regularly, and of that group, 25% don't exercise at all.

•2000 • In the USA, *Healthy People 2010* was launched with its two primary goals being: i) increasing the quality and years of healthy life; and ii) the elimination of racial and ethnic disparities in health status. Also unveiled were the first-ever leading health indicators, comprising 10 areas of health status, based upon *Healthy People 2010* objectives: physical activity; overweight and obesity; tobacco use; substance abuse; mental health, injury and violence; environmental quality; immunization; responsible sexual behavior; and access to health care.

•2002 • In the USA, the Department of Health and Human Services' Office on Women's Health launched a new website (www.4girls.gov) to encourage adolescent girls to choose healthy behaviors.

•2002 • As an outgrowth of the "Healthy Schools Summit" held in Washington, DC, Action for Healthy Kids (AFHK) was developed as a nationwide initiative dedicated to improving the health and educational performance of children through better nutrition and physical activity in schools.

Bibliography

Anspaugh, D.J., Hamrick, M.H. and Rosato, F.D. (1997). *Wellness: Concepts and applications*. St Louis, MI: Mosby.

Cottrell, R.R., Girvan, J.T. and McKenzie, J.F. (2002). *Principles and foundations of health promotion and education*. 2nd ed. San Francisco, CA: Benjamin Cummings.

Cox, C.C. (2003, ed). *ACSM's worksite health promotion manual*. Champaign, IL: Human Kinetics.

Donatelle, R.J. and Davis, L.G. (2002). *Access to health*. 7th ed. San Francisco, CA: Benjamin Cummings.

Gerber, E.W. (1971). *Innovators and institutions in physical education*. Philadelphia: Lea & Febiger.

Hackensmith, C.W. (1966). *History of Physical Education*. New York: Harper and Row.

Mechikoff, R.A. and Estes, S.G. (2002). *A history and philosophy of sport and physical education. From ancient civilization to the modern world*. 3rd ed Boston, MA: McGraw-Hill.

Reagan, P.A. and Brookins-Fisher, J. (2002). *Community health in the 21st century*. 2nd ed. San Francisco, CA: Benjamin Cummings.

Rice, E.A., Hutchinson, J.L. and Lee, M. (1958). *A brief history of physical education*. 4th ed. New York: The Ronald Press Company.

HEALTH-RELATED FITNESS *See under* PHYSICAL FITNESS.

HEARING *See under* EAR.

HEART ATTACK *See* MYOCARDIAL INFARCTION.

HEART BLOCK A disease in the electrical system of the heart. A heart block can be a blockage at any level of the electrical conduction system of the heart. Blocks that occur within the atrioventricular node (AV node) are described as **AV nodal blocks**. Blocks that occur within the sinoatrial node (SA node) are described as **SA nodal blocks**. Blocks that occur below the AV node are known as **infra-Hisian blocks**.

HEART BURN *See under* ESOPHAGUS.

HEART DEFECTS The heart problems of children are mostly congenital. The incidence is 6 to 10 per 1,000 live births. Grouped according to impairment, the most common congenital heart defects are: ventricular septal defect, atrial septal defect and patent ductus arteriosus (left-to-right shunts, holes that raise blood pressure); pulmonic stenosis (valvular), aortic stenosis (valvular) and coarctation of the aorta obstructive lesions (impaired blood flow); and tetralogy of Fallot, transposition of the great vessels and tricuspid valve atresia (right to left shunts, cyanotic lesions). **Atresia** refers to congenital absence or poor development of a heart valve.

HEART FAILURE A condition that occurs when the heart becomes unable to maintain an adequate cardiac output. Heart failure usually develops slowly, often over years, as the heart gradually loses its pumping ability and works less efficiently. The loss of pumping action is usually a symptom of an underlying heart problem, such as coronary artery disease. Severe heart failure can interfere with daily life and prove fatal. There is evidence that ACE inhibitors may slow or even prevent the loss of pumping activity. **Congestion** (build up of fluid), leading to increased venous volume and pressure, is one characteristic of heart failure, but it does not occur in all patients.

Heart failure may be categorized as diastolic or systolic. **Systolic heart failure** occurs when the heart's ability to contract decreases. Blood flowing into the heart from the lungs may flow backwards, causing fluid to leak into the lungs (**pulmonary congestion**). **Diastolic heart failure** occurs when the heart has difficulty in relaxing and filling with blood. Fluid may accumulate, especially in the legs, ankles and feet.

Between 2 to 3 million Americans have heart failure, and 400,000 new cases are diagnosed each year. It is twice as common among African Americans as Caucasians. Risk factors include hypertension and diabetes. Symptoms of heart failure include dysnea - at rest or during exercise. Exercise is beneficial for most heart failure patients.

HEART HYPERTROPHY   *See* CARDIAC HYPERTROPHY.

HEART INJURY   **Cardiac contusions** result from a direct blow to the anterior chest wall in the heart region. A blunt blow to the anterior chest wall may cause **pericardial tamponade,** a life-threatening condition in which bleeding accumulates inside the pericardial sac that surrounds the heart. The bleeding gradually increases, causing external pressure on the heart, thereby producing a progressive decrease in ventricular diastolic filling leading to a decrease of stroke volume and cardiac output. Pericardial tamponade is the leading cause of death in youth baseball. It also occurs in softball, ice hockey and lacrosse. *See also* CATASTROPHIC INJURIES.

HEART MURMUR   *See under* MURMUR.

HEART RATE   The number of ventricular beats per minute. Heart rate is mainly controlled by a balance of the effects of the parasympathetic and sympathetic nervous systems, acting through the vagus and accelerator nerves, respectively. Sympathetic and parasympathetic effects on heart function are mediated by beta-adrenoceptors and muscarinic receptors, respectively.

Factors affecting resting heart rate include age, gender, size, posture, ingestion of food, emotion, body temperature, and drugs such as nicotine.

Before exercise, there is an anticipatory rise in heart rate. There is a further rise in heart rate due to inhibition of vagal activity, followed by another rise that is thought to be due to a combination of accelerator activity and increased activity of the adrenal glands.

In fitness training, heart rate is usually used to determine the intensity of exercise, because direct measurement of oxygen uptake is impractical without sophisticated equipment. The relationship between percentage of maximal oxygen uptake and percentage of maximal heart rate, regardless of age or sex, is such that one can be predicted from the other with an error of about 10%. 55% of maximal oxygen uptake corresponds to about 70% of maximal heart rate. In general, maximal heart rate can be estimated, regardless of age or sex, as 220 minus the individual's age. Children, endurance-trained athletes, and active older adults are among these who frequently evidence variations from predicted maximum heart rate response. Maximal heart rate is generally about 13 beats per minute lower in upper-body exercise (such as swimming) than in leg exercise (such as cycling) except among persons with severe arteriosclerosis of the lower extremities. The lower maximal heart rate for upper-body exercise is probably due mainly to the relatively smaller amount of muscle mass involved in upper-body exercise.

There is evidence that maximum heart rate is decreased following regular aerobic exercise by sedentary adults and endurance athletes, and can increase upon cessation of aerobic exercise. The decreased resting heart rate appears to be mainly the result of increased vagal parasympathetic activity and decreased cardiac sympathetic activity. There is also evidence suggesting that tapering/detraining can increase maximum heart rate.

Athletes often use the pulse in order to estimate their heart rate. The **pulse** is a wave of increased pressure that is propagated from the heart down all the arteries each time the ventricle pumps its blood into the aorta. The increased pressure causes a dilation of the arteries that can be felt on palpation of the artery at certain body sites, such as the radial artery at the wrist on the thumb side. Although the carotid pulse is often favored because it is easy to find during exercise, it may not be the best measure. The right and left common carotid arteries are located on the anterior portion of the neck in the groove formed by the larynx (Adam's apple) and the sternocleidomastoid muscles. Baroreceptors in the carotid sinus may be sensitive to pressure and result in a decrease in heart rate in some persons. When the artery is stretched from increased pressure, as when fingers are placed over the left carotid artery near the angle of the jaw, baroreceptors signal the brain to slow heart rate. In extreme cases, blood flow may be occluded to the point that light-headedness or fainting occurs. This is probably a concern when taking the pulse immediately after exercise, but is less of a concern at rest or during exercise.

The radial artery courses deep on the lateral (thumb) side of the forearm and becomes superficial near the distal head of the radius. Gently pressing the index and long fingers over this distal region palpates the radial pulse. Other arterial palpation sites include temporal (temple region of skull), popliteal (behind the knee), femoral (inguinal fold of the groin) and dorsal pedis (top of the foot).

For the highest precision in counting pulsations, if timing is initiated simultaneously with a pulsation, this first pulsation is counted as zero. If a second person is keeping time or if there is a lag between the initiation of timing and the first pulsation that is felt, the first pulse is counted as one. The pulse rate is determined by multiplying the number of pulsations by the number of counting intervals in one minute. Longer pulse counts afford greater accuracy and provide more time for detection of some dysrhythmias, but the heart rate of fit persons can decrease quite rapidly following exercise, possibly making long counts less accurate than short ones.

Many athletes use a heart rate monitor rather than their pulse to estimate their heart rate during training. This may involve telemetry. A radiotelemeter consists of a radio transmitter connected to the subject by electrodes and a radio receiver of the signals, which may be connected to an electrocardiograph. The telemeter is most useful for monitoring a single performance where rapid changes in heart rates are clearly observed. Many athletes now record their heart rate in the memory of a microcomputer, which can be carried on a wristwatch. In Polar® Heart Rate Monitors, the transmitter belt around the chest detects the electrocardiogram and sends an electromagnetic signal to a wrist receiver, where the heart rate can be read digitally. Recording the heart rate during a training session allows calculation of target heart rate. Three ways to calculate target heart rate are: i) the percentage difference between resting and maximum heart rate added to the resting heart rate; ii) percentage of the maximum heart rate calculated from zero to peak heart rate; and iii) the heart rate at a specified percentage of maximum oxygen uptake. Heart rate monitors are most useful under the following circumstances: i) as a check; ii) when an athlete's performance is expected to change; or iii) when a coach wants to control the effect of training in normal circumstances. *See* BRADYCARDIA.

Bibliography

Aubert, A., Seps, B. and Beckers, F. (2003). Heart rate variability in athletes. *Sports Medicine* 33(12), 889-919.

Karvonen, J. and Vuorimaa, T. (1988). Heart rate and exercise intensity during sports activities. *Sports Medicine* 5, 303-312.

Stamford, B. (1993). Tracking your heart rate for fitness. *The Physician and Sportsmedicine* 21(3), 227-228.

Zavorsky, G.S. (2000). Evidence and possible mechanisms of altered maximum heart rate with endurance training and tapering. *Sports Medicine* 29(1), 13-26.

HEART RATE DEFLECTION POINT It is a downward or upward change from the linear relationship between heart rate and work found during progressive incremental exercise testing.

Conconi et al. (1982) suggested that this phenomenon could be used as a non-invasive method to assess the anaerobic threshold. The degree of heart rate deflection point depends on the type of protocol used. The validity of heart rate deflection point to assess anaerobic threshold is uncertain, although a positive relationship exists between heart rate deflection point and the second lactate turnpoint. The mechanisms underlying the heart rate deflection point are not clearly understood, but there is a relationship between the degree and direction of heart rate deflection point and left ventricular function.

Bibliography

Bodner, M.E. and Rhodes, E.C. (2000). A review of the concept of the heart rate deflection point. *Sports Medicine* 30(1), 31-46.

Conconi, R. et al. (1982). Determination of the anaerobic threshold by a non-invasive field test in runners. *Journal of Applied Physiology* 52, 869-873.

HEART RATE RESERVE The difference between the predicted maximum heart rate attainable during maximal exercise and the actual maximum heart rate during maximal exercise. Heart rate reserve takes into account both maximum heart rate and resting heart rate, and is therefore more accurate than simply using heart rate training zone.

HEAT A form of energy associated with the motion of individual atoms or molecules of a body. **Sensible heat** is the heat gained or lost by a body resulting in a change in temperature. The amount of sensible heat gained or lost by a body is given by the product of its heat capacity (mass x specific heat capacity) and the temperature change. **Specific heat capacity** of a substance is defined as the amount of heat required to raise the temperature of a unit mass of it by 1 degree Celsius. Water has a specific heat capacity of 4.184 J/(g degrees Celsius). **Latent (hidden) heat** is the heat gained or lost by a body during a change of state when it does not result in any change in temperature. *See under* THERMODYNAMICS.

HEAT OF COMBUSTION *See under* ENERGY YIELD OF NUTRIENTS.

HEAT STRESS During heat stress, warm blood is redirected from the core to the periphery and heat is lost by radiation, convection, conduction and evaporation. As ambient temperature rises, the effectiveness of heat loss by radiation, convection and conduction diminishes. When ambient temperature exceeds body temperature, heat is gained by these mechanisms. The primary mechanism for maintaining normal body temperature during physical exercise in the heat is the evaporation of sweat. The rate of sweating increases as the ambient temperature increases. The most important factor determining the effectiveness of heat loss through sweating is relative humidity. In arid (dry) climates, sweat evaporates so rapidly from the skin that even the loss of large amounts of sweat may go unnoticed. With profuse sweating, water loss far exceeds electrolyte loss and dehydration may occur. Dehydration decreases the body's ability to produce sweat and causes a potentially lethal increase in core temperature. When relative humidity is high, the air is saturated with water vapor and the evaporation of sweat is slowed. It stops completely when the humidity reaches 100%. When exercise is prolonged and hydration is inadequate, venous return and central blood volume may be decreased, because of the greater proportion of blood volume being distributed to skin blood vessels as the core temperature rises. Lack of evaporation can cause core temperature to increase enough to cause heat illness.

If fainting occurs after exercise, when environmental conditions are mild, heat syncope per se is not involved. **Heat exhaustion** is a form of heat illness characterized by a weak and rapid pulse, low blood pressure while standing upright, headache, dizziness, fatigue and low sweat rate. Heavy sweating usually persists throughout the course of the illness. Core temperature remains below 40 degrees Celsius (104 degrees Fahrenheit) and there is no tissue injury. Heat exhaustion may progress to heat stroke. In non-athletic populations, the main cause of heat exhaustion is depletion of circulating fluid (e.g. plasma) that leads to inadequate cardiovascular compensation. Two types of heat exhaustion are commonly seen among athletes and soldiers: water depletion and salt depletion. **Water depletion heat exhaustion** occurs rapidly, usually within one day. It involves prominent thirst, because blood is concentrated due to excessive water loss in sweat. Dilute fluids or pure water are effective in bringing back the body's extracellular fluid to its normal homeostasis. **Salt depletion heat exhaustion** takes 3 to 5 days to develop, because salt losses in sweat and urine eventually exceed the dietary salt content. Thirst is seldom observed in salt depletion heat exhaustion, because body fluids are dilute and blood sodium levels are low. Muscle cramps, vomiting and progressive weaknesses are common.

Heat exhaustion can be distinguished from **exertional heatstroke**, a medical emergency and the most severe form of hyperthermia and heat illness. Core temperature rises above 41 degrees Celsius (105.9 degrees Fahrenheit), resulting in significant tissue injury. The skin may feel cool and the athlete often shivers. Unlike heat exhaustion, sweating may cease. There may be mental status changes and even convulsions and coma. Rhabdomyolysis, acute renal failure, hemolysis, myocardial infarction, hyperkalemia, and hepatic necrosis can also develop, and, if untreated, death often follows. The prognosis of heat stroke patients is directly related to the degree of hyperthermia and its duration. Heatstroke requires immediate treatment to decrease body temperature. Cooling should be initiated immediately at the time of collapse and should be based on feasible field measures including ice or tepid water (1 to 16 degrees Celsius), which are readily available. In the emergency department, management should be matched to the patient's age and medical background and include immersion in ice water (1 to 5 degrees Celsius) or evaporative cooling.

Individuals who are untrained are more susceptible to heat illness than are trained athletes. Obese individuals are at increased risk for heat illness, because the fat layer decreases heat loss. There are a number of medical conditions that increase the risk of heat illness, such as cystic fibrosis, sickle cell trait, malignant hyperthermia and neuroleptic malignant syndrome. **Malignant**

hyperthermia is inherited as an autosomal dominant trait. It causes muscle rigidity, resulting in elevation of body temperature due to the accelerated metabolism in skeletal muscle. **Neuroleptic malignant syndrome** is associated with the use of neuroleptic agents and anti-psychotic drugs and an unexpected idiopathic increase in core temperature during exercise.

Significant risk factors for heat illness include: dehydration; hot and humid climate; obesity; low physical fitness; lack of acclimatization; previous history of heat stroke; sleep deprivation; medication (especially diuretics or antidepressants); sweat gland dysfunction; and upper respiratory or gastro-intestinal illness. Dehydration, with fluid loss occasionally as high as 6 to 10% of bodyweight, appears to be one of the most common risk factors for heat illness in persons exercising in the heat. Core body temperature has been shown to rise an additional 0.15 to 0.2 degrees Celsius for every 1% of bodyweight lost to dehydration during exercise.

Prevention of heat illness is based on decreasing known risk factors. Exercise should be modified in the face of high ambient temperature and humidity. The athlete should begin exercise well hydrated and consume cold water frequently during exercise. After exercise, the athlete should continue drinking to replace fluid losses. If sweat loss exceeds six pounds, water containing one teaspoon of salt per gallon should be drunk. Salt tablets are not recommended, because they dissolve very slowly and may pass completely through the gastrointestinal system with little effect. Consumption of large amounts of salt can irritate the intestinal tract, which in turn can cause vomiting and/or diarrhea.

In warm weather, clothing should be loose enough to allow free circulation of air between the skin and the environment. This facilitates evaporation of sweat. Clothing should be lightweight. The more skin that is exposed, the greater is the available evaporative surface. A full football uniform prevents sweat evaporation from more than 60% of the body, thus is a risk factor for heat illness. Electromagnetic heat waves are absorbed by dark colors and reflected by light colors, thus light-colored clothing is preferable in a hot environment. Clothing can serve a protective function by decreasing radiant heat gain and thermal stress. Neither the inclusion of modest amounts of clothing, nor the clothing fabric alters thermoregulation or thermal comfort during exercise in warm conditions.

A pre-season conditioning program, when combined with a two-week period of acclimatization, further decreases the risk of heat injury. In extreme conditions, however, neither acclimatization nor fluid replacement will allow hard exercise to be performed without some risk of heat illness.

The American College of Sports Medicine (ACSM) advises that no long distance race should be run when the wet bulb globe thermometer (WBGT) is higher than 28 degrees Celsius, and that races should be staged early in the morning or late in the evening in areas where the daylight dry bulb temperature exceeds 27 degrees Celsius.

Heat acclimatization requires 10 to 14 days and involves physiological changes that improve heat tolerance, including decreased heart rate, decreased body temperature, improved blood flow to the skin (to transfer heat from the core to the periphery), improved distribution of cardiac output (so that blood pressure is more stable during exercise), a lowered threshold for the start of sweating (allowing heat loss from evaporation to start sooner), wider dispersion of sweat over the skin surface (giving a greater area for evaporation to occur), increased output of sweat, a lowered concentration of electrolytes in the sweat (thus decreasing the loss from extracellular fluid) and increased blood plasma volume. Adaptive responses to hormones such as aldosterone and vasopressin during heat acclimatization encourage the retention of fluids and electrolytes, in addition to promoting cardiovascular stability. Few differences exist in the ability of men and women to acclimatize to heat. Athletes with a high maximal oxygen uptake acclimatize to heat faster (and lose adaptations slower when they are inactive in a cool environment) than athletes with low maximal oxygen uptake.

Heat production relative to body mass at rest and during exercise is inversely related to age during childhood. In a thermoneutral environment,

children are characterized by a similar core temperature, but higher skin temperature than adults. The latter may reflect the higher reliance on dry heat loss compared with evaporative cooling in children. The main physical difference between children and adults affecting thermoregulation is the much higher surface-area-to-mass ratio of children. In extreme heat, the greater surface-area-to-mass ratio results in a higher rate of heat absorption, hence a greater risk of heat stress. The smaller blood volume in children compared with adults, even relative to body size, may limit the potential for heat transfer during heat exposure and may compromise exercise performance in the heat. The main physiological difference between children and adults is in the sweating mechanism affecting their thermoregulation in the heat (but not in the cold). The lower sweating rate characteristic of children is due to a lower sweating rate per gland, but not to a lower number of sweat glands (children actually have a higher density of heat-activated sweat glands). The lower sweating per gland may be explained by the smaller sweat gland size, a lower sensitivity of the sweating mechanism to thermal stimuli and, possibly, a lower sweat gland metabolic capacity. The higher metabolic cost of locomotion in children provides an added strain on the thermoregulatory system during exercise in the heat. The American Academy of Pediatrics (2001) provided the following advice regarding children and exercise in heat stress: "Before prolonged physical activity, the child should be well hydrated. During the activity, periodic drinking should be enforced (e.g. each 20 minutes 150 ml of cold tap water or flavored salted beverage for a child weighing 40 kg (88 lb) and 250 ml for an adolescent weighting 60 kg (132 lb), even if the child does not feel thirsty. Weighing before and after a training session can verify hydration status if the child is wearing little or no clothing." *See also under* CRAMP; FLUID REPLACEMENT.

Chronology

• 1954 • At the Empire Games marathon in Vancouver (Canada), in debilitating heat, Jim Peters attempted for 11 minutes to cover the last 385 meters of a race that he was leading by more than three miles. Dehydrated, he fell down about six times and began crawling along the track. He did not make it to the finishing line, nor did nine others from the field of sixteen runners. Only when it was clear that Peters was not going to cross the line, did his team mates (including Roger Bannister and Chris Brasher) go to his aid. Cinema newsreel shots of Peters showed his agony to the British public.

•1955 • Leading British runner Gordon Pirie's custom of not consuming fluids on the day of a race proved a disaster during the Amateur Athletics Association (AAA) 6-mile run. On the last lap, he accelerated into the lead, but crashed into the outside rail and collapsed. The temperature was 26 degrees Celsius.

•1960 • In the three months before the Olympic Games in Rome, British walker Don Thompson used his bathroom for training sessions. A kettle boiling on a stove was used to produce heat and humidity. With the room sealed, he would train in temperatures of c. 42 degrees Celsius; about 10 degrees higher than the day of the 50 km race in which he won a gold medal.

•1960 • In the Olympic Games, British runner Gordon Pirie finished 10th in the 10,000 meters. He argued that this resulted from the British Olympic Committee forbidding British athletes to travel early to Rome to acclimatize to the heat in Rome.

•2001 • Korey Stringer of the Minnesota Vikings collapsed during a training camp and died from heat stroke. Between 1995 and 2001, 21 athletes have died as a result of football-related heat stress. Of these, 16 athletes were at the high school level, 3 at collegiate level, and 2 were professionals.

•2003 • New rules from the National Collegiate Athletic Association (NCAA) empowered sports medicine staff at colleges and universities to cancel voluntary summer workouts if they are concerned about the heat. Teams were required to follow a new NCAA mandate to allow players to gradually acclimatize over the course of the first five days of workout for the season, with no team being permitted to hold two-a-day practices on successive days.

Bibliography

American Academy of Pediatrics (2000). Climatic heat stress and the exercising child and adolescent. *Pediatrics* 106, 158-159.

American College of Sports Medicine (1985). The prevention of thermal injuries during distance running. In: *American College of Sports Medicine. Position stands and opinion statements* (1975-1985). Indianapolis: American College of Sports Medicine.

Armstrong, L.E. (2000). *Performing in extreme environments*. Champaign, IL: Human Kinetics.

Armstrong, L.E. (2003, ed). *Exertional heat illnesses*. Champaign, IL: Human Kinetics.

Armstrong, L.E. and Maresh, C.M. (1991). The induction and decay of heat acclimatisation in trained athletes. *Sports Medicine* 12(5), 302-312.

Binkley, H.M. et al. (2002). National Athletic Trainers' Association Position Statement: Exertional Heat Illnesses. *Journal of Athletic Training* 37(3), 329-343.

Coris, E.E., Ramirez, A.M. and Van Durme, D.J. (2004). Heat illness in athletes: The dangerous combination of heat, humidity and exercise. *Sports Medicine* 34(1), 9-16.

DeBenedette, V. (1991). Sweat: Up close and personal. *The Physician and Sportsmedicine* 19(4), 103-107.

Falk, B. (1998). Effects of thermal stress during rest and exercise in the paediatric population. *Sports Medicine* 25(4), 221-240.

Fortney, S.M. and Vroman, N.B. (l985). Exercise, performance and temperature control: Temperature regulation during exercise and implications for sports performance and training. *Sports Medicine* 2, 8-20.

Gavin, T.P. (2003). Clothing and thermoregulation during exercise. *Sports Medicine* 33(13), 941-947.

Hadad, E. et al. (2004). Heat stroke: A review of cooling methods. *Sports Medicine* 34(8), 501-511.

Pascoe, D.D., Shanley, L.A. and Smith, E.W. (1994). Clothing and exercise. I: Biophysics of heat transfer between the individual, clothing and environment. *Sports Medicine* 18(1), 39-52.

Rowland, T.W. (1996). *Developmental exercise physiology*. Champaign, IL: Human Kinetics.

Sport Research Review. May/June 1989. High performance sports apparel. Nike, Inc. *The Physician and Sportsmedicine* 17(5), 141-144.

Stamford, B. (1986). Why do we sweat? *The Physician and Sportsmedicine* 16(7), 144.

Taylor, N.A.S. (1986). Eccrine sweat glands. Adaptations to physical training and heat acclimation. *Sports Medicine* 3, 387-397.

HEEL FAT PAD The heel fat pad is specialized adipose tissue (fat) that is anchored to the calcaneus and plantar fascia via a network of fibrous septae. It imparts shock-absorption properties and helps the heel to resist shear forces, but it starts to deteriorate by the age of 40 years. Overuse of the heel pad, such as from repeated jumping, can cause a rupture in the connective tissue bands. The fat compartments are pressed outwards from the area of the heel that makes contact with the running surface, and this causes the protective effect of the heel pad to be decreased. **Heel compression syndrome** involves atrophy of the fat pad.

HEEL SPUR   A bony growth on the calcaneus that causes inflammation of the accompanying soft tissue. It is aggravated by exercise.

HEIGHT   *See* STATURE.

HEIGHT-WEIGHT RATIO   *See* PONDERAL INDEX.

HELMET   Head-gear that is designed to decelerate a blow to the head at the point of impact, to absorb the forces, to distribute the focal impact over a large area, to withstand surface abrasion and to protect the bone and soft tissue of the head from injury.

Motor-sport helmets consist of a hard outer shell (usually made of fiberglass or polypropylene) with a large amount of internal padding that is designed to ensure a snug fit of the helmet and to prevent twisting of the helmet over the head.

Cycling helmets may be either 'hard shell' (with/without vents), 'racing shell' or 'soft shell' (with/without vents). Helmet use decreases the risk of head injury by 85%, brain injury by 88% and severe brain injury by at least 75%. Helmets are also protective against injuries to the upper- and mid-facial regions, decreasing injuries by two thirds. Both motor-sport helmets and cycling helmets are designed as 'single-impact use,' i.e. they should be discarded and replaced after an accident. An estimated 44.3 million persons younger than the age of 21 years ride bicycles in the USA. In 1998, an estimated 23,000 persons under the age of 21 years sustained head injuries (excluding the face) while bicycling in the USA. There were approximately 275 deaths and an estimated 430,000 visits to emergency departments. Reasons usually given for not using a helmet are discomfort (especially heat), perceived lack of importance for casual riding (in contrast to sport or race bicycling), lack of style and peer pressure. Two factors that are strongly associated with bicycle helmet use by young children are helmet use by an accompanying parent and a state mandatory use law or local ordinance. In Oregon,

enactment of a helmet law was associated with a doubling of observed helmet use to 49% among children and youth. In the USA, a bicycle helmet or multi-sport helmet intended for bicycle use manufactured after March 1999 must have certification that it met the Consumer Product Safety Commission (CPSC) standard, regardless of whether it met the standards of any other organization.

In snowmobiling, helmet designs need to be improved to minimize visor fogging and improve hearing protection. Between January 1992 and December 1997, the Death Certificate Data Files of the CPSC recorded 51 deaths in children younger than 16 years that were directly attributable to snowmobiles. According to the American Academy of Pediatrics (2000), this number is almost certainly an undercount because the CPSC does not routinely require certificates involving collisions with licensed motor vehicles.

Skateboard-related injuries account for an estimated 50,000 emergency department visits and 1,500 hospitalizations among children and adolescents in the USA each year. Nonpowered scooter-related injuries accounted for an estimated 9,400 emergency department visits between January and August 2000, and 90% of these patients were children younger than 15 years. Many of these injuries can be avoided if children and youths do not ride in traffic and if proper protective gear is worn. Children younger than 5 years should not use skateboards. According to the CPSC, approximately 90% of all children and adolescents treated for skateboard-related injuries in 1999 were males. The helmet should be a bicycle helmet that complies with the CPSC standard or a multi-sport helmet that complies with the N-94 standard established by the Snell Memorial Foundation. The N-94 standard requires that helmets pass multiple impact tests to the back during laboratory testing.

In rugby, headgear acts to protect the wearer from contact injuries such as laceration or skull fracture, and focal (point of impact) and/or diffuse (distance from the point of impact) injuries to the neural tissues that may result in concussion.

Chronology

•1986 • The US Cycling Federation made helmets compulsory for all its sanctioned races. As a result, race-related head injuries have declined. The Union Cycliste Internationale (UCI), however, did not require helmets for races in Europe. Most riders in the Tour de France do not wear helmets and one rider died of a head injury in the 1995 race.

•2003 • UCI ruled that helmets were compulsory following the death of Kazakh rider Andrei Kivilev, who died of head injuries sustained in a crash during the Paris-Nice race.

Bibliography

American Academy of Pediatrics (2000). Snowmobiling hazards. *Pediatrics* 106(5), 1142-1144.

American Academy of Pediatrics (2001). Bicycle helmets. *Pediatrics* 108(4), 1030-1032.

American Academy of Pediatrics (2002). Skateboard and scooter injuries. *Pediatrics* 109(3), 542-543.

Street, S.A. and Runkle, D. (2000). *Athletic protective equipment: Care, selection and fitting.* Boston, MA: McGraw-Hill.

Thompson, D.C. and Patterson, M.Q. (1998). Cycle helmets and the prevention of injuries. Recommendations for competitive sport. *Sports Medicine* 25(4), 213-219.

Thompson, R.S., Rivara, F.P. and Thompson, D.C. (1989). A case control study of the effectiveness of bicycle safety helmets. *New England Journal of Medicine* 320, 1361-1367.

Wilson, B.D. (1998). Protective headgear in rugby union. *Sports Medicine* 25(5), 333-337.

HEMANGIOMA   A vascular tumor or malformation that enlarges by rapid cellular proliferation and invariably regresses.

HEMATOCRIT   The percentage of blood volume that is comprised of red blood cells. The reference values are 41 to 55% for men; and 36 to 48% for women.

HEMATOMA   A localized mass of blood in tissue. It usually clots and becomes encapsulated by connective tissue. *See also* BLACK EYE; CAULIFLOWER EAR; HIP POINTER; HUMERUS; MUSCLE CONTUSION; TOE NAILS.

HEMATURIA   *See under* GENITO-URINARY INJURIES.

HEME   The part of hemoglobin, myoglobin and cytochromes that is responsible for their ability to transport and release oxygen and electrons. Heme is made from glycine and succinyl CoA.

HEME PROTEIN   A protein containing a special type of prosthetic group.

HEMIMELIA   Gross hypoplasia or aplasia of one or more of the long bones of one or more limbs.

HEMIPARESIS   Weakness affecting one side of the body.

HEMISPHERICITY   *See under* COGNITIVE STYLE.

HEMOCHROMATOSIS   An iron overload or storage disease. The extra iron builds up in organs and damages them. Without treatment, hemochromatosis can cause these organs to fail. Genetic or hereditary hemochromatosis is mainly associated with a defect in the HFE gene, which helps regulate the amount of iron absorbed from food. Two known mutations in HFE are C282Y and H63D. When C282Y is inherited from both parents, iron is overabsorbed from the diet and hemochromatosis can result. H63D usually causes little increase in iron absorption, but a person with H63D from one parent and C282Y from the other may rarely develop hemochromatosis. About 5 in 1,000 people of the US Caucasian population carry two copies of the hemochromatosis gene and are susceptible to developing the disease. One person in 8 to 12 is a carrier of the abnormal gene. It most often affects Caucasians of North European descent. The genetic defect of hemochromatosis is present at birth, but symptoms rarely appear before adulthood. Joint pain is the most common symptom of hemochromatosis. Other symptoms include fatigue, lack of energy, abdominal pain, loss of sex drive and heart problems. It is treated by phlebotomy ('blood letting').

 Juvenile hemochromatosis and **neonatal hemochromatosis** are two forms of the disease that are not caused by an HFE defect. Their cause is unknown. The juvenile form leads to severe iron overload, and liver and heart disease, in youths between the ages of 15 and 30 years. **Neonatal hemochromatosis** causes the same problems in infants.

Bibliography

Hemochromatosis Society. Http://www.americanhs.org

HEMOCONCENTRATION   An increase in the proportion of red blood cells in the blood. It is usually due to a decrease in plasma volume. It leads to an increase in the viscosity ('stickiness') of blood.

HEMODILUTION   A decrease in the proportion of red blood cells in the blood due to an increase in plasma volume. Moderate-to-intense exercise results in a decrease in blood and plasma volume, as water moves from the plasma compartment into both the interstitial and intracellular fluid compartments of contracting muscle. One of the effects of aerobic training is that it increases plasma volume acutely and perhaps chronically.

HEMODYNAMIC   Pertaining to the movements involved in the circulation of the blood.

HEMOGLOBIN   An iron-containing protein responsible for nearly all the oxygen transport in blood. Hemoglobin molecules are tetrameric (having four parts) and contain iron within a porphyrin heme structure. The oxygen-carrying capacity of blood is determined mainly by: hemoglobin concentration; the number of circulating erythrocytes; and the efficiency of the erythrocytes. When oxygenated, hemoglobin is referred to as **oxyhemoglobin**. The concentration of oxygen in the physically dissolved state in the blood plasma (partial pressure of oxygen) determines the extent to which hemoglobin is saturated with oxygen. This relationship is described by the **oxyhemoglobin dissociation curve**. The greater the absorption of oxygen by the blood plasma from the alveoli, the greater is the oxygen uptake by hemoglobin. Oxygenation of hemoglobin decreases its binding ability for carbon dioxide. This facilitates the removal of carbon dioxide in the lungs.

During exercise, when body temperature rises and pH falls, the affinity of hemoglobin for oxygen is decreased. The **Bohr effect** describes the decreased effectiveness of hemoglobin to hold oxygen under conditions of increased acidity, temperature or partial pressure of carbon dioxide. This causes the oxyhemoglobin dissociation curve to shift significantly downward and to the right.

Hemoglobin can act as a buffer, because it can bind or release hydrogen ions. Suboptimal hemoglobin levels (in terms of performance) are frequently observed in endurance athletes, even though only a small percentage have overt anemia. **Haptoglobin** is a serum protein that binds to hemoglobin. Its major role appears to be the conservation of body iron by binding hemoglobin and preventing its loss from the body. Free hemoglobin is rapidly bound by haptoglobin and metabolized in the liver. When plasma hemoglobin concentrations exceed 200 mg/dL, hemoglobin is directly excreted through the kidney.

There is at least one company that has hemoglobin-based products approved for both veterinary and human use. Hemopure™ is a product, commercially released for human use, which uses polymerized bovine hemoglobin. There are two separate views on the mechanism through which **hemoglobin-based oxygen carriers** influence vasoconstriction: nitric oxide scavenging and autoregulation. Ordinarily, cell-bound hemoglobin is unable to access the interstitial space. However, tetrameric hemoglobin, unfettered by the red cell membrane, can leave the vessels and bind nitric oxide. The affinity of hemoglobin for nitric oxide is 3,000 times higher than for oxygen. With nitric oxide widely present in vessel walls throughout the body, free hemoglobin results in a marked vasoconstrictor effects ('nitric oxide scavenging'). The nitric oxide scavenging function of free hemoglobin decreases the nitric-oxide mediated vasodilation in arterioles and capillaries. Nitric oxide scavenging is neither necessary nor sufficient, however, to cause an increase in mean arterial blood pressure.

Perfluorocarbons are chemically synthesized compounds that are able to dissolve large quantities of gases. Unlike hemoglobin, perfluorocarbons do not bind oxygen. It has been postulated that perfluorocarbons are able to improve oxygen delivery to small capillaries that are not usually penetrated by red blood cells. Perfluorocarbons may 'bridge' oxygen transport from red blood cells to the tissue by decreasing the diffusion distance between the cell and vessel endothelium. These effects might improve endurance performance through increased oxygenation.

Schumacher and Ashenden (2004) concluded that there is virtually no scientific evidence that artificial oxygen carriers truly improve exercise capacity in athletes. The potential adverse effects are severe and a serious risk to health. *See also* CARBAMINO EFFECT; GROWTH.

Bibliography
Schumacher, Y.O. and Ashenden, M. (2004). Doping with artificial oxygen carriers. *Sports Medicine* 34(3), 141-150.

HEMOGLOBINURIA The presence of hemoglobin in the urine, caused by the destruction of blood corpuscles in the blood vessels or urinary passages. It may be associated with prolonged walking or running and may be due to breakdown of muscle myoglobin in the legs or mechanical trauma on the soles of feet, damaging red blood cells that release their hemoglobin into the blood stream.

HEMOLYSIS Rupture of red blood cells. *See under* ANEMIA.

HEMOPHILIA It is a hereditary bleeding disorder. There are two types of hemophilia, A and B. People with hemophilia A lack the blood clotting protein, factor VIII, and those with hemophilia B lack factor IX. Of the 20,000 hemophilia patients in the USA, about 85% have hemophilia A and the remainder has hemophilia B. Hemophilia is caused by defects in the genes for factor VIII and factor IX. The severity of hemophilia is related to the amount of the clotting factor in the blood. About 70% of hemophilia patients have less than 1% of the normal amount and have severe hemophilia. A small increase in the blood level of the clotting factor, up to five percent of normal, results in mild hemophilia with

rare bleeding except after injuries or surgery. Internal bleeding, rather than external bleeding is the major problem in hemophilia. Common muscles for bleeding include those of the upper arm, forearm, upper leg and calf; common joints include ankle, knee, hip, shoulder and elbow. Bruising and swollen joints can cause significant limitation of movement.

Recent advances in screening of blood donors, laboratory testing of donated blood and techniques to inactivate viruses in blood and blood products have greatly increased the safety of blood products used to treat hemophilia. To ensure absolute safety from transfusion-transmitted viruses such as hepatitis A, hemophiliacs may now be treated with recombinant factor VIII, which is manufactured through biotechnology and is entirely free of blood products.

Some people with hemophilia do not exercise, because they think it may cause bleeds, but exercise actually helps prevent bleeds. Sports like swimming, badminton, cycling and walking are safe sports for most people with hemophilia.

Bibliography
World Federation of Hemophilia. Http://www.wfh.org

HEMOPROTEIN A conjugated protein that contains a heme as a prosthetic group. A **protoheme** is an iron-porphyrin complex that has a protoporphyrin nucleus, specifically one containing **protoporphyrin IX**, which is the oxygen-binding portion of the hemoglobin molecule.

HEMOPTYSIS Coughing up blood as a result of pulmonary or bronchial hemorrhage.

HEMORRHAGE *See under* HEAD INJURIES.

HEMOSTAT An instrument that is used for staunching (by compression) a bleeding vessel.

HEMOTHORAX Loss of blood, rather than air, into the pleural cavity. It may be caused by fractured ribs.

HENRY'S LAW *See under* GAS.

HEPARIN A mucopolysaccharide that is produced by the mast cells of connective tissue. It is secreted into the intercellular substance where it functions to prevent the formation of fibrin clots from the fibrinogen that escapes from capillaries. It also functions in the formation or activation of lipoprotein lipase.

HEPATIC Pertaining to the liver. A **hepatocyte** is a liver cell.

HEPATITIS B A major cause of viral infections that results in swelling, soreness and loss of normal function in liver. It is stronger and more durable than HIV. It can be spread more easily via sharp objects, open wounds or body fluids when compared to HIV.

HEPATITIS C It is a liver disease caused by the hepatitis C virus. It occurs when blood or body fluids from an infected person enter the body of a person who is not infected. The risk of infection is high among injecting drug users who share needles, but low from having sex with a partner with the disease and there is no evidence that it has been spread by oral sex. An estimated 3.9 million (1.8%) of Americans have been infected with hepatitis C, of whom 2.7 million are chronically infected. Persons at risk of hepatitis C might also be at risk of hepatitis B or HIV. Signs and symptoms include jaundice, fatigue, dark urine, abdominal pain, loss of appetite and nausea.

Bibliography
National Center for Infectious Diseases. Http://www.cdc.gov/ncidod/diseases

HEPATOSPLENOMEGALY Enlargement of the liver and spleen.

HERB Any plant used as medicine, seasoning or flavoring. In the USA, herbs can be defined as drugs, food or dietary supplements. Examples of herbs used as ergogenic aids are ginseng, ephedra and yohimbe.

Bibliography
Bucci, L.R. (2000). Selected herbals and human exercise performance. *American Journal of Clinical Nutrition* 72(2S), S624-S636.

HEREDITARY MOTOR AND SENSORY NEUROPATHY HMSN. Peroneal muscular atrophy. Charcot-Marie-Tooth disease. A group of conditions that give rise to weakness and wasting of the muscles. It appears between the ages of 5 and 30 years. It begins as weakness in the peroneal muscles, and gradually spreads to the posterior leg and small muscles of the hand. Weakness and atrophy of the peroneal muscles causes foot drop, which characterizes the steppage gait. Persons with this syndrome may be active for years, limited only by impaired gait and hand weakness. HMSN usually manifests itself between the ages of 5 and 15 years. It is the most common inherited neurologic disorder, affecting 1 in 2,000 people worldwide. In the USA, it affects around 115,000 persons.

More than a dozen genes have been implicated in HMSN, each one linked to a specific type of the disease. HMSN is caused by demyelination of spinal nerves and motor neurons in the spinal cord, is progressive, but sometimes arrests itself. The two most common forms of HMSN are categorized as type I and type II. **Type I HMSN** is the demyelinating type, where myelin genes cause a breakdown of myelin. **Type II HMSN** involves defective axon genes that cause an impairment of axon function (axonopathy). HMSN is inherited as an autosomal dominant (HMSN1 and possibly HMSN2), recessive, or X-linked fashion (HMSN1). About 75% of patients with HMSN have type Ia in which an abnormal gene (peripheral protein 22), which is involved in myelin formation, is located on chromosome 17.

Bibliography
Muscular Dystrophy Association. Http://www.mdausa.org
Stadler, T.S. and Ross, D. (2002). Charcot-Marie-Tooth disease in a high school tennis player. *The Physician and Sportsmedicine* 30(10). Http://www.physsportsmed.com

HEREDITY The biological transmission of genetic characteristics from parents to offspring. **Genetics**

is the study of heredity and variation. Biologically inherited traits are partly influenced by the environment. Organisms change genetically through generations in the process of biological evolution.

A **chromosome** is a thread-shaped body found in every cell and consists mainly of DNA (deoxyribonucleic acid) and protein. Each DNA molecule is subdivided into genes, which when transcribed or translated, produce the proteins necessary for life. A **gene** is the hereditary unit containing genetic information transcribed into an RNA molecule that is processed and either functions directly or is translated into a polypeptide chain. A gene can mutate into various, alternative forms (**alleles**).

All the genetic information of every species is contained in the structure of its DNA. In the Human Genome Project, completed in 2000, it was found that the entire human genome contains nearly 3 billion units of DNA. **Genetic code** is the relationship between the genetic information stored in the DNA of the chromosomes and that manifested in protein structure. The genetic code is a 'blueprint' that ensures continuity of life from parent to offspring is encoded in DNA.

The **genotype** is the set of genes the person possesses. The **phenotype** is the sum of characteristics manifested by a person. It refers to the observable properties of a cell or an organism, which result from the interaction of the genotype with the environment. It is possible for two people to have the same genotype, but different phenotypes (due to environmental effects) or the same phenotype with different genotypes. '**Nature versus nurture**' is usually a false dichotomy, because most traits are influenced by both genetic and environmental factors. It is thought that the genotype may be responsible for as much as 75% of the observed variation in response to regular exercise. A **risk factor** is any genetic or environmental agent that increases the risk of a particular phenotype, usually a disease.

Heritability is a measure of the degree to which a phenotypic trait can be modified by selection. In evolution, **selection** refers to intrinsic differences in the ability of genotypes to survive and reproduce.

In plant and animal breeding, selection is the choosing of organisms with certain phenotypes to be parents of the next generation. **Natural selection** is the process of evolutionary adaptation in which the genotypes genetically best suited to survive and reproduce in a particular environment give rise to a disproportionate share of the offspring and so gradually increase the overall ability of the population to survive and reproduce in that environment. By **population**, is meant a group of organisms of the same species. A **species** is a group of actually or potentially inbreeding organisms that is reproductively isolated from other such groups.

A **polymorphic** gene is a gene for which there is more than one relatively common form of a gene, chromosome or genetically determined trait. Chromosomal substructures include the centromere (center) and telomeres (ends). The **centromere** divides the chromosome into two arms. The **telomere** contains a DNA sequence required for stability of the chromosome end, and is the region that participates in normal chromosome movement during mitosis and meiosis. A gene can mutate to various forms called alleles. An **allele** (**allelomorph**) is one of two or more different forms of the same gene. Only one allele is carried on a chromosome.

A **genetic marker** is any pair of alleles whose inheritance can be traced through mating or through a pedigree. It is a segment of DNA that varies among individuals, has a known location on a chromosome, and can function as a genetic landmark for a gene involved in a physical or mental condition. Linkage studies look for patterns of inheritance of genetic markers in large families in which a particular condition is common. It was used, for example, to locate the gene responsible for Huntington's disease. Human cells have 23 matched pairs for a total of 46 chromosomes. Within each cell division, these 23 pairs of chromosomes should be passed on, each carrying the full DNA and genes to control further development. Of the 23 pairs in each cell, 22 are **autosomes** (important for specific genetic markers), and one is the **sex chromosome** pair, designated as XX (female) or XY (male), which determines sex. An **X-chromosome** is a chromosome that plays a role in sex determination. It is present in two copies in the homogametic sex (the female in humans) and in one copy in the heterogametic sex (the male in humans). A **Y-chromosome** is the sex chromosome present only in the heterogametic sex.

Meiosis is the process of nuclear division leading to progeny (off-spring) containing half the genetic complement of the parent cell; one replication of the chromosomes is followed by two successive divisions of the nucleus to produce four haploid nuclei. **Haploid** refers to a cell or organism of a species containing the set of chromosomes normally found in gametes. **Meiotic non-disjunction** involves a lack of chromosome separation; one sperm or egg cell will contain two members of a particular numbered chromosome while the other member will contain more. **Mitosis** is the ordered process by which a cell nucleus and cytoplasm divide into two identical progeny; daughter nuclei have the same chromosome number and genetic composition as the parent nucleus.

Monozygotic (identical) twins develop from a single ovum (egg) fertilized by a single sperm. The ovum splits into two embryos at an early division. **Dizygote (fraternal) twins** develop from two ova released within a few days of each other, and each ovum is fertilized by separate sperm. Fraternal twins have different genotypes. Identical twins have the same genotype, thus any difference in a given trait is presumably due to environmental or training factors. Research in which only one identical twin undergoes training has shown that the active twin improves fitness while the sedentary twin does not. But when the levels of activity are similar the physiological characteristics are similar. There is evidence that identical twins are more likely than fraternal twins to choose the same sport. In team competition, identical twins are likely to choose symmetrical roles. For example, in soccer, one twin may play on the left wing and the other on the right wing.

Chromosomal abnormalities affect about 7 in every 1,000 births. Abnormalities can occur in either autosomes or sex chromosomes, and usually result from chance errors in cell division shortly after an egg and a sperm unite.

Dominance is a condition in which a heterozygote expresses a trait in the same manner as the homozygote for one of the alleles. The allele or the corresponding phenotypic trait expressed in the heterozygote is said to be dominant. **Dominant inheritance** occurs when a single defective gene is inherited from one parent. Individuals with **autosomal dominant** diseases have a 50% chance of passing the mutant allele and hence the disorder onto their children.

Recessive refers to an allele, or the corresponding phenotypic trait, expressed only in homozygotes. **Recessive inheritance** occurs when both copies of the gene (one from each parent) are defective. For **autosomal recessive** diseases, when both parents are carriers of an autosomal recessive trait, there is a 25% chance of a child inheriting abnormal genes from both parents, and therefore of developing the disease.

Any syndrome that has X or O in its name (e.g. fragile X syndrome) is a **sex chromosome disorder**. A common sex-linked chromosome disorder is Turner syndrome. Most sex chromosome disorders are primarily characterized by height abnormalities and underdeveloped or overdeveloped genitalia.

In general, genetic influences are stronger on the structural components of the body than on the functional components, which can be influenced more by training and environmental factors. Genes have a large effect on: height, length of arms, muscle size, muscle fiber composition, heart size, lung size and volume, resting heart rate, muscular strength, flexibility. Genes have a moderate-to-large effect on: aerobic endurance and muscular endurance. Genes have a moderate effect on blood pressure, airflow in the lungs, movement speed and anaerobic power. Genes have a small-to-moderate effect on: waist girth, activities of muscle enzymes used to produce energy, reaction time and accuracy of movements. Genes have a small effect on mitochondria per gram of muscle and balance.

Cardiovascular endurance is even more strongly affected by genes than maximal oxygen uptake, probably because many physiological and biochemical variables determine endurance performance and genes can affect each of them.

Only a small percentage of the population has genetic levels of the phenotypes needed for success in sport, not all of these will train, and only a small percentage of those who do train will be superior responders (Skinner, 2001). Superior responders to sports participation probably have early success and feedback from competition. The potential use of genetic engineering as an ergogenic aid in sport is likely to be limited, because many genes are involved, there are interactions among different genes, and there are interactions among genes and the environment.

See also GENDER VERIFICATION.

Bibliography

Hart, D.L. and Jones, E.W. (2001). *Genetics. Analysis of genes and genomes*. Sudbury, MA: Jones and Bartlett Publishers.

Perusse, L. et al. (2003). The human gene map for performance and health-related fitness phenotypes: The 2002 update. *Medicine and Science in Sports and Exercise* 35(2), 1248-1264.

Skinner, J.S. (2001). Do genes determine champions? *Gatorade Sports Science Exchange* 14(4).

Vander, A., Sherman, J. and Luciano, D. (2001). *Human physiology. The mechanisms of body function*. 8th edition. Boston, MA: McGraw-Hill.

HERING-BREUER REFLEX *See under* RESPIRATION.

HERNIA It is a protrusion of the abdominal viscera through a weakened portion of the abdominal wall. It may be congenital or acquired. About 80% of all hernias are inguinal; 10% are femoral.

An **inguinal hernia** is a protrusion of abdominal contents through the peritoneum, in the groin region, as a result of weakness in muscles and connective tissues of the abdominal wall. Swelling appears along the inner half of a line between the pubic tubercle and the anterior superior iliac crest. An **indirect inguinal hernia** occurs when the small intestine extends into the scrotum and is the most common type of hernia in young athletes. A **direct inguinal hernia** occurs when the small intestine extends through a weakening in the inguinal ring, as a result of a weakness in an area of fascia

bounded by the *rectus abdominis* muscle, the inguinal ligament and the epigastric vessels. It is common in men over 40 years.

A **femoral hernia** involves a protrusion on the front of the upper thigh below the groin fold. Abdominal viscera protrude through the femoral ring into the femoral canal, compressing the lymph vessels, connective tissue, and the femoral artery and vein. Femoral hernias are more commonly seen in women.

Sports hernia (athletic pubalgia) is a syndrome of a weakness of the posterior inguinal wall without a readily palpable hernia causing chronic groin pain. Athletes who participate in sports that require repetitive twisting and turning at speed, such as soccer, may be at risk of developing a 'sports hernia.'

Most hernias are surgically repaired. Continued trauma and even increased intra-abdominal pressure can cause a hernia to twist on itself and produce a **strangulated hernia**, which can become gangrenous.

Bibliography

Kemp, S. and Batt, M.E. (1998). The 'sports hernia:' A common cause of groin pain. *The Physician and Sportsmedicine* 26(1), 36-44.

HETEROCYCLIC Of, or pertaining to, an organic compound that has a ring structure which consists of carbon atoms and one or more non-carbon atoms.

HETEROTOPIC OSSIFICATION The formation of lamellar bone, which may mature with time, where bone does not usually form in soft tissue. **Myositis ossificans** ('**Charley horse'**) is a condition in which heterotopic ossification occurs in muscles such as the *quadriceps femoris* in the area of a deep contusion. *See under* HUMERUS.

HETEROZYGOUS Carrying dissimilar alleles of one or more genes.

HICCUPS Sudden inspirations resulting from spasms of the diaphragm. Sound occurs when inspired air hits the vocal folds of a closed glottis.

Hiccups are a form of myoclonus.

One theory as to how hiccups are triggered is via the action of the diaphragm or phrenic nerves. Holding one's breath may be a remedy for hiccups, because it increases the carbon dioxide levels in the blood, decreasing the sensitivity of the vagus nerve that includes a branch to the diaphragm. When carbon dioxide accumulates in the blood, hiccups generally stop. Stimulating the vagus nerve by drinking water quickly or gently rubbing the eyeballs gently may also act as a remedy.

Persistent hiccups require more intensive treatment and various drugs may be prescribed (e.g. scopolamine). There are some serious diseases associated with hiccups, including pneumonia and heart attack.

HIGH DENSITY LIPOPROTEIN   *See under* CHOLESTEROL.

HIGH ENERGY COMPOUND A substance, the hydrolysis of which results in the release of a large amount of free energy. A high-energy compound has a negative free energy change of more than − 5 kcal/mol under standard conditions. The best-known high-energy compound is adenosine triphosphate (ATP).

HILTON'S LAW   Any nerve serving a muscle producing movement at a joint also innervates the joint itself and the skin over the joint.

HIP HEIGHT UNEVENNESS   *See under* LEG LENGTH.

HIP JOINT A ball and socket joint where the head of the femur fits into a cup (the **acetabulum**) on the lateral part of the pelvic girdle. The fibrocartilaginous **acetabular labrum** deepens the socket and further improves joint stability by joint cohesion. The joint capsule is reinforced by the iliofemoral, ischiofemoral and pubofemoral ligaments. The **transverse acetabular ligament** bridges the acetabular notch beneath which the ligamentum teres emerges on its way to the fovea of the femoral head. The movements of flexion,

extension, abduction, adduction, medial rotation and lateral rotation are permitted.

Flexion involves decreasing the angle between the femur and the pelvis. Muscles that produce **flexion** are: *Iliopsoas, rectus femoris, tensor fascia latae, sartorius, adductor longus, adductor brevis* and *pectineus*. Extension involves increasing the angle between the femur and the pelvis. Muscles that produce **extension** are: *Gluteus maximus, semimembranosus, semitendinosus, biceps femoris* (long head) and *adductor magnus*. Abduction involves sideways movement of the femur away from the midline of the body. Muscles that produce **abduction** are: *Gluteus medius, gluteus minimus, tensor fascia latae, piriformis, gluteus maximus* (upper part) and *sartorius*. Adduction is sideways movement of the femur towards the midline of the body. Muscles that produce **adduction** are: *Adductor magnus, adductor longus, adductor brevis, pectineus* (when hip is flexed), *gracilis and gluteus maximus* (lower part). Lateral rotation is rotation of the femur outward. Muscles that produce **lateral rotation** are: *Gluteus maximus, obturator internus, obturator externus, gemellus inferior, gemellus superior, quadratus femoris, piriformis* and *sartorius*. Medial rotation is rotation of the femur inward. Muscles that produce **medial rotation** are: *Adductor magnus* (lower part), *adductor longus, adductor brevis, tensor fascia latae, gluteus minimus, gluteus medius* and *gracilis* (when the hip is flexed).

HIP JOINT, BURSITIS   The most commonly affected bursae around the hip are the trochanteric, ischial and iliopectineal (or iliopsoas) bursae.

Trochanteric bursitis is an inflammation of the bursa over the greater trochanter region as a result of increased shear stress caused by the iliotibial band over the trochanter. It may result from direct trauma, overuse, or anatomical factors such as shortened hip abductors or external rotators.

Ischial apophysitis ('weaver's bottom,' **ischial bursitis**) and avulsion may be a result of excessive running, especially in adolescents. Repetitive strain is put upon the apophysis, compounded by tight hamstrings.

Iliopsoas bursitis is inflammation of the bursa located between the capsule of the hip joint and the *iliopsoas* muscle anteriorly. The three main causes of iliopsoas bursitis are rheumatoid arthritis, acute trauma and overuse injury. *See also* SNAPPING-HIP SYNDROME.

Bibliography
Johnston, C.A.M. et al. (1998). Iliopsoas bursitis and tendinitis. A review. *Sports Medicine* 25(4), 271-283.

HIP JOINT, DEFORMITIES *See* COXA VALGA; COXA VARA; HIP DISLOCATIONS; HIP HEIGHT UNEVENNESS.

HIP JOINT, DISLOCATION The head of the femur is separated from the hip socket. In most cases, the head of the femur becomes displaced upward and anteriorly. Hip dislocations may be either congenital or acquired.

Congenital hip dislocations result from deficits in prenatal development and abnormal birth conditions and encompass various degrees of dysplasia of the acetabulum and/or head of the femur. There may be decreased range of adduction of the hip on the affected side and asymmetrical fat folds on the upper legs. It has an incidence of about 1 to 3 per 1,000 births, is more common among girls than boys, and usually occurs in one hip rather than both. Non-surgical treatment involves repositioning, traction and casting. In the majority of cases in which the child is over 3 years, surgical reduction (repositioning) is used. After the age of 6 years, more complicated operative procedures such as osteotomy and arthroplasty are applied.

Hip dislocation conditions can be treated prior to the actual dislocation by surgery that cuts the muscles, tendon and/or nerves of the muscles exerting the inappropriate force on the joint. This usually involves the adductor muscles (and tendons) and the obturator nerve. After the hip has actually been dislocated, more extensive surgery is required involving restructuring of the hip joint. Dislocation of the hip is a problem commonly associated with persons unable to stand because of severe paralytic or neurological conditions such as polio or cerebral palsy. The incidence of dislocation in severely disabled non-ambulatory persons is 25%. Coxa valga is present in most normal infants before weight bearing begins; a gradual change in neck-shaft femoral angle accompanies normal motor development. Childhood coxa valga and associated hip dislocation thus sometimes characterize delayed or abnormal motor development.

Acquired hip dislocations can be either gradual or acute. Gradual dislocations are caused by a progressive deformation of the hip joint and are common in many children with neuromuscular conditions, such as cerebral palsy and spina bifida, who spend a majority of their time in wheelchairs. Acute dislocations are caused by trauma or injury to the hip. Because of the hip joint's strong support from muscles and ligaments, dislocations of the hip rarely occur and are caused by major trauma from external forces. In 90% of cases, hip dislocation is in a posteriosuperior direction as defined by the direction of the femoral head. Motor vehicle accidents ('**dashboard dislocation**'), falls from heights and skiing accidents are among the most common causes of hip dislocation. The most important ligament at the hip joint is the **iliofemoral ligament**, which is usually torn in hip dislocation, because it is intimately blended with the hip capsule. *See also* FEMUR; OSTEITIS PUBIS; PELVIS; SLIPPED CAPITAL FEMORAL EPIPHYSIS; SKIER'S HIP; STRESS FRACTURES;

HIP JOINT, NERVES Nerve entrapment at the hip usually involves the ilioinguinal nerve, obturator nerve, genitofemoral nerve or lateral cutaneous nerve of the thigh. Common causes of nerve entrapment are scarring and muscle hypertrophy (e.g. ilioinguinal nerve entrapped by the abdominal muscles).

HIP POINTER A contusion injury that results from a direct blow to the iliac crest, anterior superior iliac spine or both. A subperiosteal hematoma is consequently formed. It is common in collision and contact sports, such as American football.

HIRSUTISM Excessive hair growth in an androgen-dependent pattern. It is seen in females with hair growth in the beard area, around the nipples and in a male pattern on the abdomen. Androgens induce the transformation of fine vellus hair into coarse terminal hair. Hirsutism should not be confused with **hypertrichosis**, which is the growth of hair on any part of the body in excess of the amount usually present in persons of the same age, race and sex.

See also HYPERANDROGENISM.

HISTAMINE A substance derived from the amino acid histidine. As a dilator of arterioles and capillaries, it is responsible for the outbreak of urticaria. It is a powerful stimulant of gastric juice and also a constrictor of smooth muscle (including that of the bronchi). Histamine causes itchy, runny noses and watery eyes in hay fever sufferers. It dilates the walls of blood vessels, allowing fluids to leak into the surrounding tissues. Swelling and itching occur as a consequence.

See also ALLERGY; ANTIHISTAMINES.

HISTIDINE A glycogenic (glucogenic), six-carbon amino acid. It forms part of the active center of many enzymes, is an important component of hemoglobin and is also used as a buffer.

HISTIOCYTE *See under* LEUKOCYTE.

HISTOCOMPATIBILITY Acceptance by a recipient of transplanted tissue from a donor.

HISTOCOMPATIBILITY PROTEINS A special class of protein in body cells, different in each individual except for identical twins, which is recognized by the immune system as 'safe.' **Major histocompatibility complex** is the group of closely linked genes coding for antigens that play a major role in tissue incompatibility and that function in regulation and other aspects of the immune response.

HISTONE Any of the small basic proteins bound to DNA in chromatin.

HISTORY *See* SPORTS HISTORY.

HITTING THE WALL *See under* GLUCOSE.

HIV *See under* AIDS.

HOFFA'S DISEASE Infrapatellar fat pad syndrome. Synovial lipomastosis. It involves hypertrophy and inflammation of the infrapatellar fat pad. It is typically caused by direct trauma (a blow to the anterior knee) or repeated microtrauma to the infrapatellar fat pad during exercise that involves maximal, repetitive extension/hyperextension of the knee. The fat pad becomes trapped and compressed between the femoral condyles and the tibial plateau upon extension of the knee. It occurs most commonly from jumping and kicking.

HOFFMAN REFLEX H-reflex. A monosynaptic reflex elicited by electrical stimulation of afferent 1a axons of a nerve, especially the tibial nerve. The H-reflex is used in experimental research, such as investigations of spinal cord circuitry. The H-reflex is different from a tendon tap response in two ways. First, the stimulus is an electrical shock to sensory fibers coming from muscle spindles rather than a mechanical stretching of those receptors. Second, the response is electromyographic activity recorded from the muscle, rather than the mechanical contraction that follows the electrical activity. Otherwise the anatomy and physiology are the same. The H-reflex enables better control of the stimulus and more precise measurement of the response.

HOLLOW FOOT *See* PES CAVUS.

HOME ADVANTAGE Home-field advantage. It is an audience-related phenomenon in sport. From archival data from 20 seasons (1974-1993) of professional ice hockey, Bray (1999) found that a home-game winning average of 52% was present in the league. Individual teams were found to have won 17.3% more games at home than away. The magnitude of home/away winning percentage differential was consistent across teams regardless of team quality. A small percentage of teams were also found to have a home disadvantage in their regular season play.

Crowd factors, and especially the ability of the crowd to influence the officials to subconsciously favor the home team, appear to provide the most dominant causes of home advantage. Professional baseball teams playing in domed stadiums have an advantage over team using open-air fields because noise levels are higher in domes. The home advantage in Major League baseball has been found to increase as crowd density increases, even when team quality is accounted for (Schwartz and Barsky, 1977). Contrarily, Baumeister and Steinhilber (1984) hypothesized that supportive audiences interfere with the execution of skillful responses during important performances, because the players become more self-conscious. Furthermore, it is hypothesized that home teams tend to lose decisive championship games in professional sport. Results from National Basketball Association (1967-1982) and World Series baseball matches (1924-1982) show that home teams tend to win early games, but lose final ones. The scores of contending home players in a golf tournament were found to deteriorate more than those of contending foreign players from the first to the last round (Wright et al, 1991). According to Benjafield et al (1989), the general home-field disadvantage appears only in series involving teams that have developed a reputation for being winners. Because the home audiences of recurrent champions expect their teams to win, there is increased pressure that is not only communicated to the members of the team, but is also the source of their performance decrements in home championship losses.

From a study of 19 baseball teams on the east and west coasts of the USA, it has been found that West coast teams do significantly worse in away games that involve a long flight. The severity of jet lag and the time needed to recover depend on the number of time zones crossed and the direction of travel. Traveling from west to east is worse, requiring longer recovery time. For the three seasons between 1991 and 1993, home teams won 56% and 62% of their total games, and games against teams that had just traveled westward and eastward, respectively. Furthermore, it was found that the home team could, on average, expect to score 1.24 more runs than usual when their opponent had just completed eastward travel.

Basketball consistently shows an advantage for the home team. Varca (1980) proposed that functional aggressive play results in more blocked shots, rebounds and steals by the home team. Visiting teams committed more dysfunctional aggression as represented by the number of fouls.

In general, home advantage is greater in college athletics than in professional sports. Recent changes in professional sports suggest that home support may not be as strong as once expected as structural conditions producing the home advantage have shifted. Distancing of players from fans via free agency and rapid salary escalation, coupled with marketing designed to create national publics, can produce declines in the home advantage.

In the North Atlantic Conference (1988-1989), a measles epidemic resulted in a quarantine that prevented having spectators at 11 high-school basketball games between Siena and Hartford. It was found that performance was improved under the no spectator condition. The authors concluded that it was difficult to explain the findings in terms of present theories.

See also TEAM PERFORMANCE.

Bibliography

Baumeister, R.F. and Steinhilber, A. (1984). Paradoxical effects of supportive audiences on performance under pressure: The home field disadvantage in sports championships. *Journal of Personality and Social Psychology* 47, 85-93.

Benjafield, J., Liddell, W.W. and Benjafield, I. (1989). Is there a home field disadvantage in professional sports championships? *Social Behavior and Personality* 17(1), 45-50.

Bray, S.R. (1999). The home advantage from an individual team perspective. *Journal of Applied Sport Psychology* 11, 116-125.

Courneya, K.S. and Carron, A.V. (1992). The home advantage in sport competition: A literature review. *Journal of Sport and Exercise Psychology* 14(1), 13-27.

Moore, J.C. and Brylinsky, J.A. (1993). Spectator effects on team performance in college basketball. *Journal of Sport Behavior* 16, 77-83.

Nevill, A.M. and Holder, R.L. (1999). Home advantage in sport. An overview of studies on the advantage of playing at home. *Sports Medicine* 28(4), 221-236.

Pollard, R. (1986). Home advantage in soccer: A retrospective analysis. *Journal of Sports Sciences* 4, 237-248.

Schwartz, B. and Barsky, S.R. (1977). The home advantage. *Social Forces* 55, 641-661.

Smith, D.R. (2003). The home advantage revisited. Winning and crowd support in an era of national publics. *Journal of Sport & Social Issues* 27(4), 346-371.

Varca, P. (1980). An analysis of home and away game performances of male college basketball teams. *Journal of Sport Psychology* 2, 245-257.

Wright, E.F. et al (1991). The home-course disadvantage in golf championships: Further evidence for the undermining effect of supportive audiences on performance under pressure. *Journal of Sport Behavior* 14(1), 51-60.

HOMEOSTASIS   The condition in which the body's internal environment remains relatively constant, within physiological limits. Most physiological systems are under **negative feedback control** - the response of the system (e.g. fall in temperature) is opposite in direction to the change that set it in motion (a rise in temperature). With **positive feedback control**, the response of the system goes in the same direction as the change in motion. The luteinizing hormone surge in females, that triggers ovulation, is an example of positive feedback control. The pituitary gland secretes luteinizing hormone that stimulates the ovaries to secrete estrogens. Under certain conditions, a rise in plasma estrogen can trigger an increase in secretion of luteinizing hormone that stimulates estrogen secretion, which enhances luteinizing hormone secretion even more. Negative feedback minimizes changes in physiological variables; positive feedback allows a variable to change rapidly in response to a stimulus. But there is always some factor to terminate the positive feedback loop: during an luteinizing hormone surge, for example, the concentration of luteinizing hormone increases rapidly to a peak, and then begins to fall as the surge triggers ovulation, which temporarily inhibits the ability of the ovaries to secrete estrogen. The resulting decrease in plasma estrogen removes the stimulus that caused luteinizing hormone secretion to increase in the first place, thereby allowing luteinizing hormone levels to

return to normal.

See also STEADY STATE.

HOMOCYSTEINE   A sulfur-containing intermediary in the metabolism of the essential amino acid methionine. Normally, excess methionine converts to homocysteine that, in turn, converts to cysteine and eventually degrades and is voided in the urine. Homocysteine can also recycle back to methionine. Folic acid, vitamin B_6 and vitamin B_{12} facilitate enzymes that affect these inter-conversions.

 If the conversion slows because of a genetic defect or vitamin insufficiency, homocysteine levels increase and promote cholesterol's damaging effects on the arterial lumen. Excessive homocysteine in the blood (**hyperhomocysteinemia**) is a metabolic abnormality present in nearly 30% of patients with cardiovascular disease and 40% of patients with cerebrovascular disease. There is debate as to whether an elevated homocysteine level is a risk factor for, or a cause of, cardiovascular disease. One theory is that excess homocysteine causes blood platelets to clump, fostering blood clots and deterioration of smooth muscle cells that line the arterial walls. Chronic homocysteine exposure eventually scars and thickens arteries, and provides a fertile medium for circulating LDL cholesterol to initiate cell damage.

 Other diseases and disorders that have been linked to elevated plasma homocysteine levels are: stroke, dementia from Alzheimer's disease, venous thrombosis, osteoporosis, recurrent early miscarriage, birth defects, premature delivery and abnormally low birth weights.

 Homocystinuria is a rare genetic error of metabolism that causes homocysteine levels to increase to hundreds of micromoles and produce premature hardening of the arteries and early death from heart attack or stroke. It is inherited as an autosomal recessive trait. There is no specific cure for homocystinuria, but about 50% of patients respond to high doses of vitamin B_6. Little is known about the effects of regular exercise on homocysteine regulation.

HOMOPHOBIA   *See under* GENDER.

HOMOZYGOUS Having the same allele of a gene in homologous chromosomes. **Homologous chromosomes** (**homologs**) are chromosomes that pair in meiosis and have the same genetic loci and structure. *See also* HETEROZYGOUS.

HOOKE'S LAW *See under* STIFFNESS.

HOPPING A form of locomotion that involves a one-foot takeoff with a landing on the same foot. Motor milestones are as follows: hopping up to three times on the preferred foot (3 years), hopping from four to six times on the same foot (4 years), hopping from eight to ten times on the same foot (5 years), hopping a distance of 50 feet in about 11 seconds (5 years) and hopping skillfully with rhythmical alteration (6 years).

Bibliography

Gallahue, D.L. (1976). *Motor development experiences for young children*. New York: John Wiley & Sons.

HORMONE REPLACEMENT THERAPY *See under* ESTROGENS.

HORMONES Substances released into the blood stream by endocrine glands. An **endocrine system** consists of a host organ (endocrine gland), chemical messengers (hormones) and a target (receptor) organ. There are 6 recognized endocrine glands: the thyroid, parathyroid, adrenals, pituitary, testes or ovaries, and pancreas. Endocrine glands have no secretory ducts and secrete hormones directly into the extracellular spaces around the gland. The hormone then diffuses into the blood for transport throughout the body.

Examples of hormones produced by minor endocrine organs are: prostaglandins, gastrin, enterogastrin, secretin, cholecystokinin, erythropoietin, active vitamin D_3 and atrial natriuretic peptide. Gastrin, enterogastrin, secretin, cholecystokinin and active vitamin D_3 are involved in the gastro-intestinal system.

Hormones have a regulatory effect on such processes as the activity of specific enzyme systems in cells of specific organs (target organs) or in cells widely distributed throughout the body. The effect a hormone exerts on a tissue is directly related to the concentration of the hormone and the number of receptor sites on the tissue. Hormone concentration is determined by the rate of secretion of the hormone from the endocrine gland, the rate of inactivation or excretion of the hormone, the quantity of transport protein in the plasma (for some hormones) and the changes in plasma volume.

There are two types of hormones. First, there are hormones that are proteins, peptides or derivatives of amino acids. In this case, the hormone binds to a receptor site on the surface of the cell membrane and activates an enzyme in the cytoplasm to convert ATP to cyclic AMP that, in turn, induces a change in some cellular process. The binding hormone can be thought of as a 'first messenger,' and cyclic AMP can be thought of as a 'second messenger.' Second, there are steroid hormones (gonad and adrenal cortical hormones), where the hormone binds with a cytoplasmic receptor protein, which migrates into the nucleus of the cell and induces gene transcription (copying). This leads to the synthesis of proteins, most of which function as enzymes.

A **hormonal axis** involves a sequence of hormone actions. The **sympathetic-adrenal-medullary axis** and **hypothalamic-pituitary-adrenocortical axis** both involve the adrenal glands. These hormonal axes are involved in the stress response.

Exercise training has the potential to alter the secretion of hormones by changing the stimuli that release hormones, the ability of cells to respond to hormones, or the maximal capacity of endocrine tissues to release hormones.

Factors which modify hormonal response to exercise include the following: the intensity of exercise, circadian rhythms, the menstrual cycle, body temperature, obesity, hypoxia, diet, and psychological factors such as competition.

The response of the following hormones is increased during exercise: catecholamines, growth hormone, corticotropin, thyrotropin, thyroxine, luteinizing hormone, testosterone, estradiol, progesterone, glucagon, renin, angiotensin, aldosterone, vasopressin and cortisol. The response of insulin is decreased.

Trained individuals generally show elevated hormone response during exercise for corticotropin and cortisol; and lowered values for growth hormone, prolactin, gonadotropic hormones, testosterone, vasopressin, thyroxine, catecholamines and insulin. There does not appear to be a training response for aldosterone, renin and angiotensin. *See also under* EICOSANOIDS.

Bibliography

Borer, K.T. (2003). *Exercise endocrinology*. Champaign, IL: Human Kinetics.

Bunt, J.C. (1986). Hormonal alterations due to exercise. *Sports Medicine* 3, 331-345.

Deschenes, M.R., Kraemer, W.J., Maresh, C.M. and Crivello, J.F. (1991). Exercise-induced hormonal changes and their effects upon skeletal muscle tissue. *Sports Medicine* 12(2), 80-93.

HOUSEMAID'S KNEE   *See under* KNEE, BURSAE.

H-REFLEX   *See* HOFFMAN REFLEX.

HUMAN CHORIONIC GONADOTROPIN

Human chorionic gonadotrophin. It is a glycoprotein hormone that is produced in large amounts by the placenta during pregnancy and also by certain types of tumor. The biological action of human chorionic gonadotropin is identical to that of luteinizing hormone. Some male athletes use pharmaceutical preparations of human chorionic gonadotropin to stimulate testosterone production before competition and/or to prevent testicular shutdown and atrophy during and after prolonged courses of androgen administration. The injection or ingestion of human chorionic gonadotropin is regarded as doping by the World Anti-Doping Agency (WADA). In contrast to testosterone, administration of human chorionic gonadotropin stimulates the endogenous production of both testosterone and epitestosterone without increasing the urinary testosterone/epitestosterone (T/E) ratio above normal values.

Bibliography

Kicman, A.T., Brooks, R.V. and Cowan, D.A. (1991). Human chorionic gonadotrophin and sport. *British Journal of Sports Medicine* 25(2), 73-80.

World Anti-Doping Agency. Http://www.wada-ama.org

HUMAN MOVEMENT   A philosophy that emphasizes the ability to move as a means for expressing, exploring, developing and interpreting one's own self and one's relationship to the world. Following the seminal work of Rudolf Laban, it gained a following between 1955 and 1975. The human movement philosophy includes '**movement education**,' which aims to teach the student to: move effectively and efficiently; become aware of the meaning, significance, feeling and joy of movement; and acquire and apply principles of human movement (Logsdon et al, 1977, cited in Siedentop, 2004). *See also* KINESIOLOGY; PHYSICAL EDUCATION.

Chronology

•1946 • Ruth Morison, a tutor at I.M. Marsh College of Physical Education in Liverpool, had abandoned the Swedish system of gymnastics and tried to apply Laban's principles of movement to gymnastics. Morison later produced a small booklet, *Educational Gymnastics*, showing how Laban's basic concepts of space, time, weight and flow could be applied to gymnastics with and without apparatus. In order to develop his concept of 'human movement,' Rudolf Laban was forced to leave Nazi Germany for England. His revolutionary ideas were described in his classic *Die Welt des Tanzers* (The World of Dancers) published in 1922. His daughter later stated that her father "not only valued dance for contributing both to artistic growth and to the search for individual worth, for its scientific benefits and educational implications, but also to effect the discovery of self – a synthesis of existence achieved through movement" (DeLaban, 1964, quoted by Estes & Meichikoff, 1999). Laban's human movement theory appealed to a small group of British physical educators. The women's colleges often saw new ideas and approaches as an opportunity to assert the independence of women. Laban's emphasis on the development of the 'self' was an attractive argument for women who were working to promote the status of women (Estes & Meichikoff, 1999, p195).

•1958 • Physical education faculty at UCLA began to define and develop an undergraduate curriculum in human movement.

•1963 • In *Theory in Physical Education: A Guide to Program Change*, Camille Brown and Rosalind Cassidy laid the theoretical basis for a curriculum in human movement.

Bibliography

DeLaban, J. (1964). Modus operandi. *Quest 2*, 15-18.

Estes, S.G. and Mechikoff, R.A. (1999). *Knowing human movement*. Boston, MA: Allyn & Bacon.

Logsdon, B. et al. (1977). *Physical education for children: A focus on the teaching process*. Philadelphia, PA: Lea & Febiger.

Siedentop, D. (2004). *Introduction to physical education, fitness and sport*. 5th ed. Boston, MA: McGraw-Hill.

HUMANISTIC PSYCHOLOGY   A school of thought in psychology which views human beings as free willed, creative, capable of self change and striving to express their full potential. It de-emphasizes theistic or environmental control.

Positive psychology focuses on the qualities that enable people to be happy, optimistic and resilient in times of stress. Health and wellness appear to depend on having some optimistic 'positive illusions' about oneself and one's circumstances. Optimistic people maintain a positive outlook while recognizing life's realities and limitations. Optimism is related to having an internal locus of control. Gould (2002) argues that, "[positive psychology] is what we have been doing in sport psychology for the last 25 years."

The **humanistic approach to coaching** is a person-centered philosophy that emphasizes the empowerment of the individual towards achieving personal goals within a facilitative interpersonal relationship. *See* ATTRIBUTION THEORY; PEAK EXPERIENCE.

Chronology

•1933 • In the aftermath of the Great Depression in the USA, Bernarr Macfadden captured the Zeitgeist by subtitling *Physical Culture*, "The Personal Problem Magazine," and presenting American middle class readers with optimistic self-help articles.

•1973 • In *Humanistic Physical Education*, Donald Hellison advocated an approach to physical education in schools that emphasized personal development, self-expression and interpersonal relationships.

Bibliography

Fredrickson, B.L. (2001). The role of positive emotions in positive psychology: The broaden-and-build theory of positive emotions. *American Psychologist* 56(3), 218-226.

Gould, D. (2002). Sport psychology in the new millennium: The psychology of athletic excellence and beyond. *Journal of Applied Sport Psychology* 14, 137-139.

Green, J. (1986). *Fit for America. Health, fitness, sport and American society*. New York: Pantheon Books.

Lyle, J. (2002). *Sports coaching concepts. A framework for coaches' behavior*. London: Routledge.

Seligman, M.E.P. and Czikszentmihalyi, M. (2000). Positive psychology: An introduction. *American Psychologist* 55, 5-14.

HUMERO-RADIAL JOINT   *See under* ELBOW JOINT COMPLEX.

HUMERO-ULNAR JOINT   *See under* ELBOW JOINT COMPLEX.

HUMERUS   The long bone of the upper arm. The lateral aspect of the humerus is very vulnerable to direct blows, because the bone is close to the surface and there is little protection from muscle. **'Linebacker's spur'** results from repeated contusions to the outer aspect of the mid-humerus, with the development of a hematoma and subsequent calcification. Wearing a pad or protector over the vulnerable area when playing a sport such as American football can help prevent the hematoma. It is not a true myositis because the ectopic formation is not infiltrated into the muscle, but rather is an irritative exostosis arising from the bone. In the throwing athlete, the humerus of the throwing arm undergoes hypertrophy. The main muscles of the throwing arm that undergo hypertrophy are *pectoralis major* and *latissimus dorsi*. With hypertrophy, there is a relative decrease in the size of the olecranon and, in a baseball pitcher, inability to extend the dominant arm because the olecranon jams into the olecranon fossa.

HUMIDITY   The measure of water vapor present in the air. **Absolute humidity** is the weight of water contained in a unit volume of air and is usually expressed as percentage of vapor by weight. The water vapor is saturated when the concentration of the vapor, or the absolute humidity, is such that the partial pressure is equal to the vapor pressure. The ratio of the partial pressure to the vapor pressure at the same temperature is called the **relative**

humidity and is usually expressed as a percentage. The temperature at which the water vapor in a given sample of air becomes saturated is called the **dew point**. Measurement of the dew point is the most accurate way of determining relative humidity. A less accurate, but easy way of determining relative humidity is using a **wet and dry bulb thermometer**. This consists of two thermometers. The bulb of one thermometer is kept wet and thus cooled by evaporation. The difference in temperature between the two thermometers is used as a measure of relative humidity.

High humidity stimulates the growth of bacteria, dust mites, molds and other fungi, which may cause allergy and bad smells. Low humidity causes dryness and facilitates irritation of skin and mucous membranes in some individuals.

HUMPHREY'S LIGAMENTS *See under* KNEE LIGAMENTS.

HUNGER The physiological need to eat. *See also* ANOREXIA; APPETITE; SATIETY.

HUNTER'S SYNDROME MPS II. It is the only mucopolysaccharidosis that is inherited as an X-linked recessive trait. Mild and severe forms of the disorder result from mutations of the IDS gene that regulates the production of the iduronate sulfatase enzyme (IDS). The IDS gene is located on the long arm (q) of chromosome X (Xq28). Initial symptoms and findings associated with Hunter syndrome usually become apparent between the age of 2 and 4 years. Abnormalities may include progressive growth delays, resulting in short stature; joint stiffness, with associated restriction of movements; and coarsening of facial features, including thickening of the lips, tongue and nostrils. Affected children may also have an abnormally large head (macrocephaly), a short neck and broad chest, delayed tooth eruption, progressive hearing loss, and enlargement of the liver and spleen (hepatosplenomegaly).

Two relatively distinct clinical forms of Hunter syndrome have been recognized. In the mild form of the disease (MPS IIB), intelligence may be normal or only slightly impaired. In the more severe form of

the disease, profound mental retardation may be apparent by late childhood.

Bibliography
National Organization for Rare Disorders. Http://www.rarediseases.org

HUNTING REACTION *See under* CYRO-THERAPY.

HUNTINGTON'S CHOREA Huntington's disease. A progressive disease that typically begins between the ages of 30 and 45 years, though onset may occur as early as the age of 2 years. Due to loss of the inhibitory output of the basal ganglia to the thalamus, it is characterized by hypotonia and involuntary hyperkinesia. There are jerky movements of the limbs (rapid, irregular flow and flicking motions), which can look purposeful. Voluntary movements are slowed. During the early stages of Huntington's disease, people can blend the spontaneous abnormal movements into the intentional ones so that they're barely noticeable. With time, the abnormal movements become more obvious. There is a rapid deterioration in cognitive functioning and dementia caused by cortical degeneration.

It is inherited as an autosomal dominant trait. Genetically, Huntingdon's disease is a trinucleotide repeat-expansion on chromosome 4. There is mutation in a protein called huntingtin that accumulates and causes defective GABAergic and cholinergic transmission in the interneurons of the striatum, globus pallidus and cerebral cortex. In the USA, the prevalence is approximately 5 cases per 100,000 persons.

Bibliography
The Huntington's Disease Society of America. Http://www.hdsa.org

HURLER'S SYNDROME Alpha-L-iduronate deficiency. Gargoylism. A rare hereditary and congenital metabolic disease that belongs to a group of diseases called mucopolysaccharidoses. It is associated with an inability to synthesize an enzyme called lyosomal alpha-L-iduronate. It is inherited as an autosomal recessive trait. Characteristics of Hurler's syndrome include dwarfism, hunchback, thick and coarse facial features (gargoylism) with low nasal bridge, severe mental retardation and cardiac abnormalities. About 1 in 150,000 infants are affected by Hurler's syndrome. Newborn infants appear normal, but by the end of the first years, signs and symptoms begin to develop.

Bibliography

National Mucopolysaccharide Syndrome Society, Inc. Http://www.mpssociety.org

HYALURONIC ACID   A highly soluble polysaccharide formed by repeating disaccharide units. It is a natural component of connective tissues and acts as a lubricant and shock absorber.

HYDRATION STATUS   *See under* DEHYDRATION.

HYDRIDE ION   A hydrogen atom with an additional electron so it has a negative charge.

HYDROCEPHALUS   *See under* BRAIN; SPINA BIFIDA.

HYDROGEN   It is an element that has one proton and one electron. It is the lightest element and it is inflammable and explosive when mixed with air. It is found in water and in almost all organic compounds. Its ion is the active constituent of all acids in the water system. It has an atomic number of 1, an atom weight of 1.00797 and a specific gravity of 0.069.

Hydrogen exists in three isotopes: ordinary (light) hydrogen is the mass 1 isotope (**protium**), heavy hydrogen is the mass 2 isotope (**deuterium**) and the mass 3 istotope is **tritium**.

HYDROGENATION   *See under* FATTY ACIDS.

HYDROGEN ION   Proton. It is a positively charged atom of hydrogen. Hydrogen ions do not exist on their own in body fluids, but are combined with water to form **hydronium (hydroxonium)**

ions. The quantity of hydrogen ions in the dilute solutions present in the human body can usually be considered as equal to the concentration of hydrogen ions. The **pH** of a solution is defined as the negative logarithm to the base 10 of the hydrogen ion concentration. The concentration of free hydrogen ions, i.e. the concentration of hydrogen ions, $[H^+]$, increases 10-fold for each unit increase of pH. A pH of 7 is neutral, acids have a pH of less than 7 and bases have a pH of greater than 7. The pH of water is 7, but blood is about 7.3.

See ACID-BASE BALANCE.

HYDROLASES   *See under* ENZYME.

HYDROLYSIS   The process by which a molecule is broken apart with the addition of water. Hydrolysis occurs under the action of enzymes known as hydrolases. During hydrolysis, the hydroxyl ion of an ionized water molecule is added to the 'residue' on one side of a bond while a hydrogen ion is added to the 'residue' on the other side. It is the reverse of condensation.

HYDRONIUM ION   *See under* HYDROGEN ION.

HYDROSTATIC PRESSURE   *See under* PRESSURE.

HYDROSTATIC WEIGHING   It is the 'gold standard' of indirect measurement of body density. *See under* BODY COMPOSITION.

HYDROXONIUM ION   *See under* HYDROGEN ION.

HYOID BONE   A small bone that lies just inferior to the mandible in the anterior neck. It is the only bone in the body that does not articulate directly with any other bone. It serves as an attachment point for neck muscles that raise and lower the larynx during swallowing and speech.

HYPERANDROGENISM   Excess male hormones in females. Symptoms and signs include hirsutism, deepening of the voice, acne vulgaris, clitoromegaly (enlargement of the clitoris), menstrual irregularity, infertility and increased libido (sexual desire). Differential diagnoses of hyperandrogenism include: non-tumor related endogenous androgen overproduction that may be adrenal (e.g. congenital adrenal hyperplasia, Cushing's syndrome) or ovarian causes (e.g. polycystic ovary disease); and tumor-related endogenous androgen overproduction that may be adrenal, ovarian, or pituitary.

Female athletes who engage in sports that emphasize strength may be characterized by a distinct hormonal profile characterized by hyperandrogenism.

Bibliography

Warren, M.P. and Perlroth, N. (2001). Hormones and sport: The effects of intense exercise on the female reproductive system. *Journal of Endocrinology* 170(1), 3-11.

HYPERBARIA   Increased barometric pressure.

HYPERBARIC PHYSIOLOGY   The branch of physiology concerned with high-pressure environments. When the body is submerged in seawater, the pressure increases one atmosphere (760 mm Hg) every 10 m. In fresh water, the increase in pressure is not as great because of the lower water density; it approximates 1 atmosphere every 10.4 m of depth.

In skin diving, the ideal snorkel is about 38 cm in length with an inside diameter of about 1.6 cm. Increasing the length of a snorkel does not enable one to swim deeper in the water and still breathe ambient air through the top of the snorkel. Using a snorkel, in effect, increases the volume of anatomic dead space. In addition to the increased water pressure on the chest cavity as one submerges, there is an increased pulmonary dead space brought about by enlarging the snorkel. At a depth of about 1 meter, the compressive force of water against the chest cavity becomes so large that the inspiratory muscles are usually unable to overcome the external pressure in order to increase the thoracic volume. Consequently, inspiration is impossible unless air is supplied at a pressure sufficient to counter the compressive force of water at the particular depth.

When the body is submerged in water to the level of the neck, acute cardiovascular adaptations occur in response to the increased compressive forces exerted on the skin, resulting in decreased cutaneous blood flow, increased central blood volume, increased venous return and a lowered heart rate. During immersion of the face in water an additional neurologic reflex (the **mammalian diving reflex**) is excited that also lowers heart rate.

Diving mammals have a number of special adaptations that allow them to stay submerged, including greater volume of blood and proportion of red blood cells. Heart rate is decreased and blood supply to tissues that are tolerant of oxygen deprivation (such as skeletal muscle) is decreased to less than 10% of normal. Most of the blood is directed to the heart and brain, whose cells would die after four minutes without oxygen. Humans display weak diving responses, but do not exhibit the oxygen conservation function of marine mammals. It is greater in children than adults.

Prolonged water immersion may decrease plasma volume, because of an increased urine volume and this may be detrimental to exercise performance when returning to dry land.

When exercise in water is compared with exercise on land, the increased resistance provided by the water causes a higher oxygen uptake for a given amount of physical power output. For a given oxygen uptake, however, heart rate is lower when underwater. During breath holding when diving to increased depths, the increasing water pressure actually increases alveolar partial pressure of oxygen despite continued metabolic activity of the body. However, on return to the surface, the decreasing pressure can rapidly decrease alveolar partial pressure of oxygen to dangerous levels, increasing the risk for syncope.

During diving to increased pressures, decreases in lung volumes can be tolerated to the point at which lung volume equals residual volume. Thereafter, continued increases in pressure are exerted on what is now a closed-lung volume, which in turn risks the eventual rupturing of the alveoli. Thus the depth limit for breath-hold diving depends on the residual volume relative to total lung capacity. Generally, individuals have a lung capacity to residual volume of 4:1 to 5:1, which can be calculated from the known increase in pressure at increased depths and Boyle's law, to limit the depth of breath-hold dives to between 30 to 40 m.

In a closed-circuit **scuba** (self-contained underwater breathing apparatus) system, a diver breathes either pure oxygen (which limits depth because of potential oxygen poisoning) or a gas mixture containing oxygen and an inert gas (e.g. helium); the expired gas is re-circulated rather than released to the surrounding water. A chemical filter removes carbon dioxide, while oxygen is added slowly from the tank. When a person breathes self-contained air through a regulator that equilibrates air pressure to that of the environment, the increasing depth increases the pressure of the air inhaled. This phenomenon increases the density of the gas, which in turn increases the work of breathing. This change causes divers to hypoventilate, which can cause altered acid-base balance, headache and impaired cognitive function. At depths causing pressures to exceed 6 atmospheres, air mixtures should be altered by adding helium and lowering the nitrogen content, which decreases the density of the gas. The nitrogen content of scuba-compressed gas should be decreased also in order to lower the risks associated with nitrogen retention by the body. Such risks include neurologic impairment (i.e. 'raptures of the deep') and decompression sickness. **Barotrauma** is tissue injury caused by changing pressure.

Decompression sickness (the **'bends'**) is an illness that afflicts divers and can be fatal. It is caused by nitrogen bubble formation in the tissues and venous blood as a result of rapid ascent. During ascent to the surface from deep water, nitrogen leaves body tissues in proportion to the decrease in barometric pressure. If a diver ascends at a slow rate, the risk of getting bubbles in the circulation is lower, because most of the body's excess nitrogen will diffuse from the tissues into the blood and be exhaled through the lungs. It takes a longer time for nitrogen to leave certain tissue (e.g. fat) than others (e.g. blood). **Arterial gas embolism** results from the introduction of bubbles directly into the arterial circulation. Decompression tables provide rates of ascent, depths and the duration of rest periods. Decompression treatment involves a compression chamber in which the patient is compressed to a simulated depth of 18 m and breathes 100% oxygen. To decrease the risk of oxygen toxicity, the decompression period is interspersed with short intervals of breathing air.

The volume of gases decreases or increases as a diver descends or ascends, respectively (Boyle's Law). On descent, the volume decreases in enclosed spaces such as the sinuses, lungs, middle ear, teeth and facemask. This creates a negative pressure. Unless this pressure is allowed to equalize with air from outside the space, barotrauma can occur. Preventive measures include a slow descent rate. Scuba diving with a gas supply that is insufficient relative to the rate of descent, or breath-hold diving at extreme depth, can cause **pulmonary descent barotrauma (pulmonary squeeze)**. Lung volume is decreased to the point where negative intrathoracic pressure is created, and pulmonary hemorrhage is increased. **Pulmonary ascent barotrauma** occurs when divers hold their breath during the ascent from depths even as low as four feet. There is overdistention and rupture of the lungs as the gas volume expands. When a diver descends to a depth at which total lung volume becomes less than normal residual volume, insufficient air volume exists in the lung to balance the pressure across the lung tissue. Thus, the internal pressure (from blood to alveoli) exceeds the pressure within the alveoli. This results in a movement of fluid into the lung, and greatly decreases oxygen diffusion across the pleural membrane from the lung to the blood.

Middle ear squeeze affects more than 40% of all breath-hold and scuba divers. It occurs because the eustachian tube is closed due to a mucus plug or inflammation. Consequently, the pressure in the middle ear cannot equilibrate with air in the lungs via the trachea and the external water pressure exceeds the pressure in the middle ear. In order to prevent middle ear squeeze, the middle ear should be inflated immediately on submerging using the **Frenzel maneuver**, either with the mouth open or with a mouthpiece and demand regulator in place.

The diver increases pressure within the pharynx by occluding the nose, closing the glottis and contracting the pharynx muscle. Air is thus forced through the eustachian tubes without altering thoracic pressure and venous return to the heart is not inhibited.

Earplugs should never be worn during diving, because hydrostatic pressure pushes the earplug deep into the external ear canal. This makes it impossible for water to enter the external ear canal in order to equalize pressure on both sides of the tymphanic membrane.

Critical hypoxia is often reached on ascent from a dive, near the surface, hence the term 'shallow-water blackout.' It can occur at any depth, but being in deep water is somewhat protective because the pressure of oxygen in the lungs and blood is higher than it would be at the surface with the same breath-holding time. As the breath-hold diver ascends, the pressure of oxygen in the lungs falls because his body continues to utilize oxygen and the pressure from the water falls too.

Bibliography

Armstrong, L.E. (2000). *Performing in extreme environments.* Champaign, IL: Human Kinetics.

Ferretti, G. (2001). Extreme human breath-hold diving. *European Journal of Applied Physiology* 84(4), 254-271.

Gorman, D.F. (1989). Decompression sickness and arterial gas embolism in sports scuba divers. *Sports Medicine* 8(1), 32-42.

Lin, Y.C. (1988). Applied physiology of diving. *Sports Medicine* 5, 41-56.

Manley, L. (1990). Apneic heart rate response in humans: A review. *Sports Medicine* 9 (5), 286-310.

Strauss, M.B. and Aksenov, I.V. (2004). Diving science. *Essential physiology and medicine for divers.* Champaign, IL: Human Kinetics.

HYPERCAPNIA   Excessive carbon dioxide in body fluids.

HYPERCHOLESTEROLEMIA   *See under* HYPERLIPIDEMIA.

HYPEREMIA   Engorgement. Increased blood supply to an organ. It may be active or passive.

Active hyperemia is increased blood in a part due to local or general relaxation of the arterioles. **Passive hyperemia** is increased blood in a part resulting from obstruction to its outflow from the area.

HYPERESTROGENISM   An excess of estrogen in the body. Hyperestrogenism is a risk factor for male breast cancer. *See* GYNECOMASTIA.

HYPERFLEXIBILITY   Excessive flexibility. This may be due to the connective tissues failing to limit movement about a joint. This particularly refers to joint laxity or lax ligaments, which can be a cause of genu varus and genu valgus. Both the latter can predispose an individual to knee injuries. Extreme hyperflexibility may be due to osteogenesis imperfecta. It may also be caused by intense training before calcification of the epiphyseal growth plates. In a particular individual, hyperflexibility may be specific to one joint or a characteristic of a number of joints.

HYPERGLYCEMIA   Abnormally high concentration of glucose in the blood (greater than 5 mmol/L). *See* HYPOGLYCEMIA.

HYPERINSULINEMIA   *See under* INSULIN RESISTANCE.

HYPERKALEMIA   Excessive potassium in the blood.

HYPERKINESIA   Hyperactivity. Abnormally increased motor function or activity.

HYPEROPIA   'Far-sightedness.' The focusing point is behind the retina resulting in straining to focus correctly, particularly at close distances. Hyperopia can result from shortness of the eyeball, a lens that is weak, or a cornea that is relatively flat.

HYPERPLASIA   An increase in the number of cells.

HYPERLIPIDEMIA   Elevation of lipids in the

blood, which are transported as part of lipoproteins. These lipids include cholesterol, cholesterol esters, phospholipids and triglycerides. There are five major classes of blood (plasma) lipoproteins: chylomicrons, very low-density lipoproteins (VLDL), intermediate-density lipoproteins (IDL), low-density lipoproteins (LDL), and high-density lipoproteins (HDL). When hyperlipidemia is defined in terms of a class or classes of elevated lipoproteins in the blood, the term **hyperlipoproteinemia** is used.

There are various types of hyperlipidemia, which are differentiated by the type(s) of lipids that are elevated in the blood. Some types may be caused by a primary disorder, such as familial hyperlipidemia, and others are due to secondary causes. Secondary causes of hyperlipidemia are related to disease risk factors, dietary risk factors, and drugs associated with hyperlipidemia. Disease risk factors include: type-1 diabetes mellitus; type-2 diabetes mellitus; hypothyroidism; Cushing's syndrome; and certain types of renal failure. Dietary risk factors include: dietary fat intake of greater than 40% of total calories; saturated fat intake of greater than 10% of total calories; cholesterol intake of greater than 300 milligrams per day; habitual excessive alcohol use; and obesity. Drugs include: birth control pills; hormones, such as estrogen and corticosteroids; certain diuretics; and beta-blockers. Cigarette smoking with hyperlipidemia increases the risk of heart disease.

Type 1 hyperlipidemia is a relatively rare inherited deficiency of either lipoprotein lipase activity or the lipase-activating protein apolipoprotein C-II, causing an inability to effectively remove chylomicrons and very low-density lipoprotein (VLDL) triglycerides from the blood. It is characterized by: eruptive xanthomas, especially over pressure points and extensor surfaces; lipemia retinalis; and hepatosplenomegaly. Increased dietary fat accumulates in the circulation as chylomicrons. There is no evidence that type 1 hyperlipidemia predisposes to atherosclerosis.

Type II hyperlipidemia involves an elevation of low-density lipoprotein (LDL), which may be primary or secondary. Primary type II

hyperlipidemia includes several genetic conditions that lead to elevation of LDL, including familial hypercholesterolemia, familial combined hyperlipidemia, familial defective apolipoprotein B, and polygenic hypercholesterolemia.

Hypercholesterolemia refers to excess cholesterol in the blood. The guidelines of the American Heart Association (AHA) and the National Cholesterol Education Program (NCEP) Adult Treatment Panel III define hypercholesterolemia as a blood cholesterol concentration greater than or equal to 240 mg of cholesterol per decilitre of blood (mg/dL). The normal or desirable cholesterol level is defined as less than 200 mg/dL. The National Health and Nutrition Examination Survey III, carried out from 1988-1991, found that 26% of American adults had high blood cholesterol concentrations and 49% had desirable values. Total cholesterol can be measured at any time of day; fasting is not required. For LDL cholesterol, a desirable level is less than 130 mg/dL, or less than 100 mg/dL in patients who have had coronary heart disease in the past; 130 to 159 mg/dL is intermediate risk; and 160 mg/dL or above is high risk of coronary heart disease. The LDL cholesterol can only be determined accurately on a blood test after fasting for 12 to 14 hours. **Hypertriglyceridemia** refers to high triglyceride levels in the blood. Levels for triglycerides are: less than 150 mg/dL (desirable); less than 200 mg/dL (normal); 200 to 400 mg/dL (borderline high); 400 to 1000 mg/dL (high); and greater than 1000 mg/dL (very high). Triglycerides can only be determined accurately on a blood test after fasting for 12 to 14 hours. A very high level of HDL cholesterol (at least 60 mg/dL) is a considered a 'negative' risk factor for coronary heart disease, i.e. this level of HDL cholesterol removes one risk factor for coronary heart disease from the overall cardiac risk profile. Less than 40 mg/dL is considered a low level of HDL cholesterol.

Familial hypercholesterolemia is a disorder characterized by consistently high levels of LDL cholesterol and total cholesterol. It is a disorder of absent or grossly malfunctioning LDL receptors. The LDL receptor is the primary determinant of hepatic LDL uptake, which normally processes approximately 70% of circulating LDL. This defect in the LDL receptors is caused by a mutation in the gene coding for the ligand of the LDL receptor, apolipoprotein B-100. It is inherited as an autosomal dominant trait. The LDL receptor also binds another ligand, apolipoprotein E, which is found on most lipoproteins other than LDL. The LDL receptor binds apolipoprotein E with higher affinity than apolipoprotein B-100, and some mutations in the LDL receptor may spare binding to apolipoprotein E. Both forms of familial hypercholesterolemia, heterozygous and homozygous, are caused by a mutation in either the LDL receptor or the apolipoprotein B protein. There is one known apolipoprotein B defect (R3500Q) and a multitude of LDL receptor defects. The LDL-receptor gene is located on the short arm of chromosome 19. In the **heterozygous form**, only one of the two alleles is damaged and there will be at least 50% of the normal LDL receptor activity. The heterozygous form occurs in 1 in 500 or 1 in 1,000 persons, depending on the population. Total cholesterol is approximately 350 to 500 mg/dL and coronary artery disease usually becomes clinically apparent during the fourth or fifth decade of life. In the **homozygous form**, however, both alleles are damaged to some degree, which can lead to extremely high levels of LDL. LDL-receptor gene defects can be identified with genetic testing. Total cholesterol concentrations can exceed 600 mg/dL, resulting in very early development of atherosclerosis and coronary artery disease. The prevalence of homozygous familial hypercholesterolemia is 1 case per 1 million persons. The incidence of the homozygous form is 1 in 1 million. LDL normally circulates in the body for 2.5 days, after which it is cleared for the liver. In familial hypercholesterolemia, the half-life of an LDL particle is 4.5 days. The excess LDL is taken up from the circulation by cells all over the body. The degree of atherosclerosis depends on the amount of LDL receptors still produced in the liver and the functionality of these receptors.

Familial combined hyperlipidemia is a genetic disorder of lipid metabolism, characterized by elevated serum total cholesterol and a variety of lipoprotein patterns (excess LDL, VLDL or both). It is inherited as an autosomal dominant trait. The disorder appears to be due to excessive hepatic production of apolipoprotein B. Xanthomas are rare in familial combined hyperlipidemia, but there is a marked predisposition for premature coronary artery disease. Familial combined hyperlipidemia responds well to weight reduction and restriction of saturated fat and cholesterol, followed when necessary by drug therapy.

Familial ligand defective apolipoprotein B-100 (familial defective apolipoprotein B-100) is responsible for a syndrome almost indistinguishable from heterozygous familial hypercholesterolemia. This defect is caused by a mutation in the gene coding for the ligand for the LDL receptor, apolipoprotein B-100. Although the receptors are normal in both number and function, LDL cholesterol is taken up inefficiently, leading to elevated LDL cholesterol. The levels of LDL cholesterol are lower than in familial hypercholesterolemia. Xanthomas are uncommon, but patients are at increased risk of coronary artery disease.

Polygenic hypercholesterolemia (non-familial hypercholesterolemia) is the most common form of elevated serum cholesterol concentrations. It results from a relative deficiency of functioning LDL receptors, which leads to elevated LDL cholesterol in the setting of a high fat, high cholesterol diet. It is a moderate hypercholesterolemia (240 to 350 mg/dL) with serum triglyceride concentrations within the reference range. Unlike familial hypercholesterolemia, tendon xanthomas are not present in patients with nonfamilial hypercholesterolemia. It is associated with increased risk of coronary heart disease. Some patients with polygenic hypercholesterolemia are sensitive to dietary restriction of saturated fat and cholesterol. When this fails, therapy with a statin, cholestyramine or niacin (see below) will usually lower the elevated LDL to normal levels.

Type III hyperlipidemia (dysbetalipo-proteinemia) is a rare familial disorder, characterized by the accumulation in plasma of a beta-migrating VLDL, which is rich in triglycerides and total cholesterol. It is nearly always associated with abnormalities of apolipoprotein E and defective conversion and removal of VLDL from the plasma. The disorder usually appears in early adulthood in men, and 10 to 15 years later in women. Peripheral vascular disease manifested by claudication or xanthomas on the elbows and knees may be the first sign. There is a marked predisposition to severe, premature atherosclerosis. It responds to drug therapy (e.g. statins).

Type IV hyperlipidemia is a common disorder, often with a familial distribution, characterized by variable elevations of plasma triglyceride contained predominantly in VLDL. It is frequently associated with mild insulin resistance and obesity. It may be associated with premature coronary artery disease. Weight reduction and limitation of alcohol consumption, when applicable, are the most effective treatments.

Type V hyperlipidemia (**mixed hyper-triglyceridemia**; **mixed hyperlipidemia**) is a rare disorder, sometimes familial, associated with defective clearance of exogenous and endogenous triglycerides. It usually first appears in early adulthood with xanthomas over the extensor surfaces of the extremities, lipemia retinalis, hepatosplenomegaly, and abdominal pain. Weight reduction is effective and should be followed with a maintenance diet restricting all fats to less than 50 g per day and stopping all alcohol.

Familial lecithin cholesterol acyl-transferase deficiency is a rare disorder, inherited as a recessive trait, characterized by lack of the enzyme that normally esterifies cholesterol in the plasma, and manifested by marked hypercholesterolemia and hyperphospholipidemia, together with hypertriglyceridemia. Renal and hepatic failure, anemia, and lens opacities are common.

Statins are a class of drugs that have been found to lower cholesterol more than other types of drugs. Examples are lovastatin (Mevacor) and simvastatin (Zocor). Statins inhibit the enzyme, **hydroxymethylglutaryl CoA reductase** (**HMG-CoA reductase**), which controls the rate of cholesterol production in the body. Studies using statins have reported 20 to 60% lower LDL-cholesterol levels in patients on these drugs, and also produce a modest increase in high-density lipoprotein (HDL) and a decrease in elevated triglyceride levels. Statins have not been shown to provide an overall health benefit in primary prevention trials, however. With homozygous familial hypercholesterolemia, LDL levels are much higher and most effective statins require at least one copy of the functional LDL receptor gene. Therefore, high amounts of bile acid sequestrants are often given. Occasionally, high-dosed statins can help express a dysfunctional (but working) LDL receptor. In the last resort, liver cells can be supplied with working LDL receptors. Heterozygous familial hypercholesterolemia can be treated effectively with statins. Statins typically have fewer side effects than other cholesterol-lowering medications. On rare occasions, however, they have been associated with muscle or liver injury. Certain statins cannot be used in people with kidney disease.

Bile acid sequestrants, such as cholestyramine and colestipol, combine with bile acids in the intestine, interfering with dietary cholesterol absorption. Bile acid sequestrants are prescribed for the treatment of mild to moderate elevations of LDL cholesterol. Bile acid sequestrants can interact with the actions of some medications, such as digoxin and warfarin (coumadin), which are used to treat heart disease, and also interact with the absorption of fat-soluble vitamins. Timing when these medications are taken can solve these problems in some cases.

Nicotinic acid lowers levels of both VLDL and LDL cholesterol and raises HDL cholesterol levels. Nicotinic acid is prescribed for the treatment of high cholesterol levels and some types of familial hyperlipidemia. It has several possible side effects, including flushing, itching, nausea, and numbness and tingling. This medication can also injure the liver and its use therefore requires regular monitoring of liver function.

Fibrates, such as gemfibrozil and fenofibrate, increase acyl-coenzyme A synthase and fatty acid transporter protein; this facilitates intracellular transport, acylation and beta-oxidation of fatty acids, with the net effect of decreasing the availability of fatty acids for triglyceride synthesis and hepatic apolipoprotein-B secretion. Fibrates are prescribed for treatment of elevated triglyceride levels and combined hyperlipidemia. The dose of fibrates needs to be adjusted in people with kidney disease and in those taking warfarin or cyclosporine.

Neomycin is an antibiotic that has a beneficial effect on blood lipids, but is rarely used. It lowers LDL cholesterol by binding bile acids and by altering the liver's role in lipid processing. Neomycin is associated with a risk of kidney and ear damage at high doses.

Bibliography

American Heart Association. Http://www.americanheart.org

Citkowitz, E. (2004). Hypercholesterolemia, familial. Http://www.emedicine.com

Citkowitz, E. (2004). Hypertriglyceridemia. Http://www.emedicine.com

Isley, W.L. (2003). Hypercholesterolemia, Polygenic. Http://www.emedicine.com

The Merck Manual. Http://www.merck.com

The National Institutes of Health. Http://www.nlm.nih.gov

HYPERPNEA *See under* BREATHING.

HYPERTENSION A disorder characterized by high arterial blood pressure. Various criteria for its threshold have been suggested, ranging from 140 mmHg (systolic) and 90 mmHg (diastolic) to as high as 200 mmHg (systolic) and 110 mmHg (diastolic). It is a risk factor of atherosclerosis, heart failure and kidney disease. In the USA, hypertension is the most common cardiovascular disease, with about more than 50% of people greater than 65 being afflicted. The majority of hypertensive persons in the general population suffer mild hypertension (diastolic blood pressure between 90 and 104 mm Hg and/or systolic blood pressure between 140 and 159 mm Hg). Approximately 50 million adults in the USA have systolic blood pressure of at least 140 mmHg and/or diastolic blood pressure of at least 90 mmHg. African Americans have more severe high blood pressure than Caucasians and a higher risk of heart disease.

A distinction can be made between **primary hypertension** (**essential hypertension**, **idiopathic hypertension**) that has no identifiable cause, and **secondary hypertension** when the cause is known. About 95% of hypertensive individuals have primary hypertension. These people seem to develop pathologic elevations in blood pressure, because of an increase in total peripheral resistance that is probably mediated by plasma epinephrine and norepinephrine in conjunction with effects from the kidneys and the renin-angiotensin system. There are many causes of secondary hypertension, including adrenal gland tumors, alcohol, arteriosclerosis, Cushing's syndrome, diabetes mellitus, glomerulonephritis, oral contraceptives and stress. There is some evidence that accumulation of intra-abdominal visceral fat and hyperinsulinemia play a role in the pathogenesis of hypertension.

Hypertension accelerates atherosclerosis by scarring, narrowing and decreasing elasticity of the arteries and arterioles. This may limit the heart's ability to supply nutrients to oxygen, and limit the functional capacity of the organs and tissues. A narrowed and less elastic artery is also at risk for blockage by a blood clot, which could result in a heart attack or stroke.

Dynamic and static exercise produce similar hemodynamic responses in hypertensive persons and these responses differ in some respects from those of normotensive individuals. The most important difference is that hypertensive patients generally demonstrate exercise-induced increases in total peripheral resistance. Myocardial oxygen consumption increases, and impaired vasodilation with exercise may result in exaggerated blood pressure elevations.

Cardiovascular exercise training is the most effective mode of exercise in the prevention and treatment of hypertension (20 to 60 minutes of exercise at 40 to 70% of maximal oxygen uptake, 3 to 5 days per week). High-intensity exercise (greater than 75% of maximal oxygen uptake) may not be as effective as low-intensity exercise (less than 70% of maximal oxygen uptake) in decreasing elevated blood pressures. Exercise can be effective without a change in bodyweight or body fat. Not all hypertensive patients respond to exercise treatment.

The specific mechanisms for this benefit are not understood, but it is probably not caused by a single mechanism. Furthermore, different mechanisms are possible for different types of hypertension or in different hypertensive populations. It is possible that the decrease in blood pressure is related to an effect similar to that of beta-blockade on the sympathetic nervous system. It is a different effect, however, from the beta-blockade achieved with an anti-hypertensive drug (beta blocker). Both exercise and medication result in a decrease of resting heart rate and left ventricular output at a given amount of work. Unlike beta-blocker drugs, however, exercise does not place an upper limit on heart rate.

Endurance training will elicit a 10 mmHg average decrease in both systolic and diastolic blood pressures in individuals with mild essential hypertension. Individuals with hypertension of greater than 180 mmHg (systolic) and 105 mmHg (diastolic) should include endurance exercise training in their treatment regimen only after initiating drug therapy. The goals of drug therapy are to decrease elevated resting blood pressure, to lower increases in systolic and diastolic blood pressure during exercise, and to preserve central hemodynamics and exercise work capacity. Anti-hypertensive drugs include beta-blockers, angiotensin-converting enzyme (ACE) inhibitors, diuretics, calcium-channel blockers and nitrates. In general, drugs that decrease total peripheral resistance affect exercise performance the least. All commonly used anti-hypertensives, except for non-selective beta-blockers and diuretics, allow for essentially normal exercise capacity.

Many experts believe that a major cause of hypertension in many cases is a high-sodium diet combined with a genetic predisposition to hypertension. There is no evidence that moderate sodium presents any hazards. There is also evidence that low intake of potassium, calcium, and possibly magnesium may also contribute to the development of hypertension. The Dietary Approaches to Stop Hypertension (DASH) diet is high in low-fat dairy products and fiber, including fruits and vegetables.

Bibliography

American College of Sports Medicine (1993). Position stand: Physical activity, physical fitness and hypertension. *Medicine and Science in Sports and Exercise* 25(10), i-x.

American College of Sports Medicine (2000). *ACSM's guidelines for exercise testing and prescription*. 6th ed. Philadelphia, PA: Lippincott Williams and Wilkins.

Bacon, S.L. et al. (2004). Effects of exercise, diet and weight loss on high blood pressure. *Sports Medicine* 34(5), 307-316.

MacKnight, J.M. (1999). Hypertension in athletes and active patients. *The Physician and Sportsmedicine* 27(4), 35-44.

Massie, B.M. (1992). To combat hypertension, increase activity. *The Physician and Sportsmedicine* 20(5), 89-111.

Tanji, J.L. (1990). Hypertension. Part 1: How exercise helps. *The Physician and Sportsmedicine* 18(7), 77-82.

Tanji, J.L. (1990). Hypertension. Part 2: The role of medication. *The Physician and Sportsmedicine* 18(8), 87-91.

Wallace, J.P. (2003). Exercise in hypertension. A clinical review. *Sports Medicine* 33(8), 585-598.

HYPERTENSIVE   Characterized by increased tension or pressure.

HYPERTHERMIA   *See under* HEAT STRESS.

HYPERTHYROID MYOPATHY   An endocrine myopathy that is caused by the thyroid gland producing too much thyroxine. Symptoms include weakening and atrophy of muscles, especially in the shoulders and hips.

HYPERTELORISM   Excessive width between two bodily parts of organs (eyes; ocular hypertelorism).

HYPERTONIA   Excess tension in skeletal muscles, a stiff appearance and decreased range of movement. It is most commonly associated with spastic cerebral palsy, but it is also associated with spinal cord paralysis, traumatic brain injury and many *les autres* conditions such as multiple sclerosis. **Fluctuating tonus** is involuntary shifting between hypertonia and hypotonia; it is usually associated with athetoid cerebral palsy.

HYPERTRIGLYCERIDEMIA   *See under* HYPER-LIPIDEMIA.

HYPERTROPHIC CARDIOMYOPATHY   *See under* SUDDEN DEATH.

HYPERTROPHY   An increase in size of an organ or tissue as a result of an increase in the size of its cells.

HYPERVENTILATION   A higher rate of ventilation than is necessary to meet the demands of the body. This leads to a decrease in alveolar and arterial partial pressure of carbon dioxide and an increased pH in the blood and cerebrospinal fluid (respiratory alkalosis). Episodes are generally self-limiting, but if they last long enough symptoms such as dizziness and trembling can occur. Previously considered to be an underlying cause of panic attack, hyperventilation does actually occur in a substantial number of panic attacks. The panic attack may be a cause or result of anxiety, but sometimes there is no obvious trigger. Drug options for the treatment of hyperventilation and panic include selective serotonin reuptake inhibitors, benzodiazepines, tricyclic antidepressants and monoamine oxidase inhibitors.

Hyperventilation before swimming allows a greater distance to be covered before breathing becomes necessary. Such use of hyperventilation is dangerous, because rapid use of the limited supply of oxygen during swimming (and increased tolerance to carbon dioxide) can result in unconsciousness and drowning.

See also ALTITUDE; ASTHMA; HYPERBARIC PHYSIOLOGY.

Bibliography

Rubin, A. and Chassay, C.M. (1996). When anxiety attacks: Treating hyperventilation and panic. *The Physician and Sportsmedicine* 24(12), 55-65.

Stamford, B. (1986). A talk about breathing. *The Physician and sportsmedicine* 14(5), 252.

HYPNOSIS   A state of mind that is more receptive than usual to suggestions. It is often described as an altered state of consciousness. The term hypnosis was first used in the nineteenth century with regard to a trance-like state observed in patients before entering a surgical operation after they had been subjected to certain procedures aimed at inducing such a state in them. Hypnosis is still used in medicine and dentistry to overcome patients' fear of injections. It has been applied to sport for use with imagery and mental practice in addition to dealing with stress, phobias and other psychological problems.

A hypnotic state can be induced by staring at an object, attending to a monotonous or repetitive noise, and through the use of relaxation, verbal and imagery techniques. **Heterohypnosis** involves a hypnotist who hypnotizes the subject. **Self-hypnosis** involves the subject inducing hypnosis without directly using a hypnotist. A **post-hypnotic suggestion** is a suggestion received by a person under hypnosis that he or she will attempt to carry out in the future (either immediately after coming out of the hypnotic trance or sometime later).

Three theories that have been proposed to explain hypnosis are Neodissociation, Hemispheric and Cognitive-Behavioral theories. The **Neodissociation theory** is based on the premise that, during hypnosis, normally linked cognitive subsystems such as perception and memory become dissociated from central control. Through this dissociation, hypnotized individuals are enabled access to processes that are normally outside conscious awareness. The **Hemispheric theory** is based on the premise that the process of hypnosis inhibits the functions of the left hemisphere and facilitates the functions of the right hemisphere. The **Cognitive-Behavioral theory** emphasizes the personality of the subject and is based on the premise that subjects carry out hypnotic behaviors because they have positive attitudes, motivations and expectations that lead to a willingness to think and imagine with the themes suggested by the hypnotist or by themselves. This viewpoint seems plausible in light of the fact that only about 10% of subjects who go through the process of hypnotic induction can reach a deep trance.

A research review by Johnson (1961) concluded that the deeper the hypnotic trance, the more likely it is that suggestions will work. It was also found that arousal-altering techniques, such as 'psyching up,' are more useful in enhancing muscular strength and endurance than hypnotic suggestions. Morgan (1972) concluded that positive suggestions were effective in facilitating performance regardless of whether or not the athlete was hypnotized and that negative suggestions almost always caused a decrement in performance.

In athletes, hypnosis may substantially enhance imagery intensity and effectiveness.

Chronology

•1973 • Before a heavyweight boxing match against Muhammad Ali, Ken Norton hired a professional hypnotist to help overcome flaws in his fighting. Norton won the fight.

Bibliography

Johnson, W.R. (1961). Hypnosis and muscular performance. *Journal of Sports Medicine and Physical Fitness* 1, 71-79.

Liggett, D.R. (2000). *Sport hypnosis*. Champaign, IL: Human Kinetics.

Liggett, D.R. (2000). Enhancing imagery through hypnosis: *A performance aid for athletes. American Journal of Clinical Hypnosis* 43(2), 149-157.

Morgan, W.P. (1972). Hypnosis and muscular performance. In: Morgan, W.P. (ed). *Ergogenic aids and muscular performance.* pp193-233. New York: Academic Press.

Nash, M.R. (2002). Hypnosis, the brain and sports: Salient findings. *International Journal of Clinical and Experimental Hypnosis* 50(3), 282-285.

Taylor, J., Horevitz, R., Balague, G. (1993). The use of hypnosis in applied sport psychology. *Sport Psychologist* 7, 58-78.

HYPOCHONDROPLASIA
A common disorder of cartilage development, transmitted as an autosomal dominant trait. Clinical features resemble those of achondroplasia but are milder, such as short stature, with long trunk and short limbs, broad and short fingers; the face is normal in appearance.

HYPOESTROGENISM
A condition of subnormal estrogen production with resultant atrophy or failure of development of estrogen-dependent tissues. In sports emphasizing leanness, nutritional restriction and negative energy balance may be an important causal factor in hypoestrogenism. In premenopausal women, the most severe menstrual dysfunction is amenorrhea, which is associated with chronic hypoestrogenism. In postmenopausal women, hypoestrogenism is associated with a number of clinical sequelae related to cardiovascular health.

Bibliography

O'Donnell, E. and De Souza, M.J. (2004). The cardiovascular effects of chronic hypoestrogenism in amenorrhoeic athletes: A critical review. *Sports Medicine* 34(9), 601-627.

HYPOFLEXIBILITY
Lack of flexibility. This may be caused by restrictions to movement imposed by bone or cartilage, or the joint capsule and ligaments not being able to lengthen sufficiently to allow a normal range of movement about the joint. Hypoflexibility increases the risk of injuries such as strains and sprains.

HYPOGLYCEMIA
Abnormally low concentration of glucose in the blood (less than 3.5 mmol/L). In nondiabetic people, two types of hypoglycemia occur: reactive hypoglycemia and fasting hypoglycemia. **Reactive hypoglycemia** occurs about one hour after eating food that is rich in carbohydrate; the body overreacts and produces too much insulin. Individuals can prevent reactive hypoglycemia by eating frequent, smaller meals to smooth out blood glucose responses to food. **Fasting hypoglycemia** occurs when the body produces too much insulin, even when no food is eaten. It may be caused by pancreatic tumors.

Exercise hypoglycemia is a cause of fatigue or exercise cessation, and also impairs thermoregulatory adaptation. In persons with acute and chronic increases in glucose effectiveness and insulin sensitivity, hypoglycemia during exercise is a common event due to an imbalance between training volume, nutrition and external influences such as temperature. Adequate training induces resistance to hypoglycemia via a shift in the balance of oxidized substrates and marked hormonal adaptations. Overtraining, however, partially reverses the resistance to hypoglycemia.

See also BLOOD GLUCOSE; DIABETES MELLITUS; DIET; HYPERGLYCEMIA.

Bibliography

Brun, J.F., Dumortier, M., Fedou, C. and Mercier, J. (2001). Exercise hypoglycemia in nondiabetic subjects. *Diabetes Metabolism* 27(2), 92-106.

HYPOGONADISM   Decreased or absent secretion of hormones from the sex glands (gonads). In **primary hypogonadism**, the ovaries or testes themselves do not function properly. Some causes include: surgery; radiation; genetic and developmental disorders; liver and kidney disease; infection; and certain autoimmune disorders. The most common genetic disorders are Turner syndrome (in women) and Klinefelter syndrome (in men). In **central hypogonadism**, the centers in the brain the control the gonads (hypothalamus and pituitary) do not function properly. Some causes of central hypogonadism include tumors (growths); surgery and radiation; infections; trauma; bleeding; genetic problems; nutritional deficiencies; and hemochromatosis.

HYPOHYDRATION   *See* DEHYDRATION.

HYPONATREMIA   An illness in which there is a low concentration of sodium in the blood plasma. It exists when serum sodium concentration falls below 136 mmol/l. A sustained decrease in plasma sodium concentration disrupts the osmotic balance across the blood-brain barrier, resulting in a rapid influx of water into the brain. This causes brain swelling and a cascade of increasingly severe neurological responses (confusion, seizure and coma) that can culminate in death from rupture of the brainstem. The faster and lower the blood sodium falls, the greater the risk of life-threatening consequences. A decrease in plasma sodium concentration to 125 to 135 mmol/l usually results in either no noticeable symptoms or in relatively modest gastrointestinal disturbances such as bloating or mild nausea. Below 125 mmol/l, the symptoms become more severe and include throbbing headache, vomiting, wheezy breathing, swollen hands and feet, restlessness, unusual fatigue, confusion and disorientation. When plasma sodium concentration drops below 120 mmol/l, seizure, respiratory arrest, coma, permanent brain damage

and death become more likely. Some athletes have survived hyponatremia of less than 115 mmmol/l, whereas others have died at 120 mmol/l.

There are many causes of hyponatremia other than exercise including: sodium depletion from an inadequate diet; inappropriate secretion of vasopressin; and the effects of certain drugs, such as alcohol. In athletes, however, the hyponatremia that occurs most often is characterized by hypo-osmolality (hypotonicity) of plasma. This condition is known as **hypotonic (dilutional) hypo-natremia**, i.e. more water than normal for the amount of substances dissolved in the plasma. **Hypertonic hyponatremia** (less water than normal for the amount of substances dissolved in plasma) can occur with severe hyperglycemia or with glycerol loading when water retained in the vascular space is sufficient to temporarily decrease blood sodium concentration.

Athletes who start already hyponatremic from excessive drinking in the days or hours before the race are at particular risk of more severe hyponatremia during the race, because less fluid is required to drop plasma sodium to dangerous levels.

29% of athletes in the 1984 Ironman triathlon were found to be hyponatremic upon completion of the race. As the number of endurance and ultra-endurance athletic events grew during the 1980s, so did periodic reports of hyponatremic athletes developing seizures, slipping into comas and dying. Davis et al. (2001) described 26 cases of symptomatic hyponatremia from the 1998 and 1999 San Diego Marathons. The average finish time for the 26 runners was 5 hours, 38 minutes (range 4:00 to 6:34), and many runners admitted drinking as much fluid as possible during and after the event. Plasma sodium values ranged from 117 to 134 mmol/l. A post-race blood study done on 481 participants who ran the 2002 Boston Marathon found that 13% experienced hyponatremia. Risk factors included female gender, slower finishing times and excess fluid consumption.

The clinical outcome for females is worse than for males. This may be because estrogen inhibits the enzyme responsible for moving potassium out of brain cells. The response to the swelling caused by hyponatremia is to transport potassium out of the cell, thereby decreasing intracellular osmolality and offsetting the influx of more water into the cell. Accordingly, if the sodium-potassium ATPase enzyme is inhibited by estrogen, the clinical outcome of hyponatremia may be more serious. Young women, who have relatively high levels of estrogen, are 25 times more likely to die or have permanent brain damage as a result of postoperative hyponatremic brain swelling than men or postmenopausal women, who have relatively low levels of estrogen.

Since its first description in 1985, two opposing theories have been proposed to explain the etiology of symptomatic hyponatremia of exercise. One theory is that the condition occurs only in athletes who lose both water and sodium during exercise, and fail to fully replace their sodium losses. The other theory holds that the symptomatic form of hyponatremia occurs in athletes who generate a whole body fluid overload as a result of an excessive fluid intake during prolonged exercise. There is no evidence that, in the absence of fluid overload, the usual sodium deficits generated during exercise can cause this condition. Noakes (2000) argues that hyponatremic runners are overhydrated rather than dehydrated (hence the term 'water intoxication' to describe exercise-induced hyponatremia), although hyponatremia can occur with relatively modest fluid intakes, and that loss of sodium is not an etiological factor.

Armstrong (2003) suggests that four factors may account for the increased incidence of exertional hyponatremia. Due to increased emphasis on fluid replacement during exercise, some competitors may attempt to 'drink as much as possible,' thereby increasing their risk of exertional hyponatremia. Directors of ultraendurance events may have become more aware of the need for aid stations, making water more readily available during races than it was previously. A slower running pace is acknowledged as an important predisposing factor for exertional hyponatremia, because triathletes and runners are on the course for many hours. Non-steroidal anti-inflammatory drugs are known to potentiate the effect of vasopressin on the kidney (i.e. the collecting ducts) and reportedly have been associated with hyponatremia because they impair water diuresis. Davis et al. (2001) reported that three hyponatremic runners used non-steroidal anti-inflammatory during a 42 km race.

In a study carried out in the Nevada desert during World War II, groups of army conscripts exercised for as long as they could, usually up to 8 hours, without any fluid ingestion whatsoever. During this time they would cover up to 34 km. The conscripts were able to recover from 'dehydration exhaustion' within minutes of drinking fluid orally. Up to 1969, endurance athletes were encouraged not to drink during exercise. Wyndham (1977) mentions only one case of heatstroke in a competitive marathon runner, i.e. Jim Peters in the 1954 Empire Games Marathon in Vancouver. Noakes (1991) describes reasons other than dehydration to explain Peters' collapse. Noakes (2000) argues that dehydration is not a diagnosis of a specific medical condition, as is commonly believed, and that there is no proven relationship between dehydration and any condition associated with collapse in distance runners.

Exercise-associated collapse is the sudden onset of postural hypotension. This typically occurs after an athlete completes an endurance event. Formerly this condition was called heat exhaustion (see under HEAT STRESS). Exercise-associated collapse is the most common reason that athletes are treated in the medical tent following an endurance event. It is postural hypotension that results when the loss of muscle pumping action caused by the cessation of exercise is combined with cutaneous vasodilation. The inactivation of the calf muscle pump immediately after the cessation of endurance exercise results in blood pooling in the compliant veins of the lower limbs, causing a decreased atrial filling pressure and subsequent syncope. This circulatory decompensation is often exacerbated by heat-induced increases in muscle and cutaneous venous capacitance. Another factor may be a right atrial reflex that causes a paradoxical skeletal muscle vasodilation when the right atrial pressure falls dramatically (the Barcroft-Edholm reflex). Training-induced adaptations to the autonomic nervous system have been postulated as contributing to the postural hypotension of exercise-associated collapse.

If an athlete collapses before finishing a race in heat, the diagnosis of exercise-associated collapse is excluded. Noakes has found that athletes who are fully conscious and whose rectal temperatures are below 40 degrees Celsius do not require active cooling, because their body temperatures will normalize without intervention. Nor are their symptoms of collapse caused by their (normally) elevated body temperatures. Rather, they are likely to be suffering from postural hypotension and will recover rapidly when treated in the head-down position. Mental changes in an exerciser whose rectal temperature is less than 40 degrees Celsius should only be ascribed to a heat injury if hyponatremia and hypoglycemia have been excluded by appropriate blood testing. According to Hsieh (2004), most athletes suffering from exercise-associated collapse can be treated simply by continued ambulation after finishing or elevation of legs while in a supine position for those who cannot walk. Care providers should consider the use of intravenous hydration with normal saline carefully since it is not needed by most collapsed athletes and may worsen the conditions of patients with unsuspected hyponatremia.

Noakes (2000) discusses a case of acute exertional hyponatremia (originally reported by Flinn and Sherer, 2000) of a military recruit who suffered a generalized tonic-clonic seizure following 9 hours of moderate military exercises in a hot, humid environment. He had been actively encouraged to drink water, presumably in copious amounts, to prevent exertional heat injury. Heat stroke was excluded by expeditious measurement of rectal temperature, and the correct diagnosis – exertional hyponatremia – was immediately established by the equally rapid measurement of the serum sodium concentration. He had drunk at least 6 L of plain water before the seizure and his serum sodium concentration was 113 mmol/L. Although the symptoms of acute exertional hyponatremia overlap those of heat injury, hyponatremia is distinguishable by the serum sodium level. The rapid intake of large quantities of fluids appears to be the major cause of acute exertional hyponatremia and results in a lowering of plasma sodium concentrations to

dangerous levels. It appears that the kidneys preferentially try to maintain the intravascular volume and retain free water despite decreasing plasma sodium levels, but the mechanism for this phenomenon is unclear.

Noakes (2002) recommends that athletes restrict fluid intake to no more than 400 to 800 ml per hour during exercise to decrease the risk of hyponatremia. Murray and Stofan (2003) argue that this is sound advice for those athletes who sweat at low rates, but faulty advice for those who sweat substantially more. Those athletes can benefit from rate of fluid intake that more closely match their sweat losses, without increasing their risk of hyponatremia, provided that sodium is also ingested during exercise.

The recommendation by Noakes (2002) was made in response to position statements such as: "It is recommended that individuals drink about 500 ml of fluid about 2 hours before exercise to promote adequate hydration and allow time for the excretion of excess ingested water. During exercise, athletes should start drinking early and at regular intervals in an attempt to consume fluids at a rate sufficient to replace all the water lost through sweating (i.e. body weight loss), or to consume the maximal amount that can be tolerated." (American College of Sports Medicine, 1996) and "Athletes should drink enough fluid to balance their fluid losses. Two hours before exercise, 400 to 600 ml (14 to 22 oz) of fluid should be consumed, and during exercise, 150 to 350 ml (6 to 12 oz) of fluid should be consumed every 15 to 20 minutes depending on tolerance." (American Dietetics Association, Dieticians of Canada, and American College of Sports Medicine, 2000). According to Murray and Stofan (2003), these guidelines recognize that drinking adequately during exercise improves performance and decreases the risk of heat-related illness, but none suggests that athletes 'drink as much fluid as possible during exercise.'

Bibliography

Almond, C.S. et al. (2003). Risk factors for hyponatremia among runners in the Boston Marathon. *Academic Emergency Medicine* 10(5), 534-535.

American College of Sports Medicine (1996). Position stand on exercise and fluid replacement. *Medicine and Science in Sports* and Exercise 28, i-vii.

American Dietetic Association, Dietitians of Canada, and American College of Sports Medicine (2000). Nutrition and athletic performance. *Journal of the American Dietetic Association* 100, 1542-1556.

Armstrong, L.E. (2000). *Performing in extreme environments.* Champaign, IL: Human Kinetics.

Armstrong, L.E. (2004). Exertional hyponatremia. *Journal of Sports Sciences* 22, 144-145.

Davis, D.P. et al. (2001). Exercise associated hyponatremia in marathon runners: A two-year experience. *Journal of Emergency Medicine* 21, 47-57.

Eichner, E.R., Laird, R., Hiller, D., Nadel, E. and Noakes, T. (1993). Hyponatremia in sport: Symptoms and prevention. Roundtable. *Gatorade Sports Science Exchange* 4(2).

Flinn, S.D. and Sherer, R.J. (2000). Seizure after exercise in the heat: Recognizing life-threatening hyponatremia. *The Physician and Sportsmedicine* 28(9), 61-67.

Hsieh, M. (2004). Recommendations for treatment of hyponatremia at endurance events. *Sports Medicine* 34(4), 231-238.

Montain, S.J., Sawka, M.N. and Wenger, C.B. (2001). Hyponatremia associated with exercise: Risk factors and pathogenesis. *Exercise and Sport Sciences Reviews* 29(3), 113-117.

Murray, R. and Stofan, J. (2003). Hyponatremia in athletes. *Gatorade Sports Science Exchange* 16(1).

New, T.D. et al. (2003). The incidence, risk factors and clinical manifestations of hyponatremia in marathon runners. *Clinical Journal of Sports Medicine* 13(1), 41-47.

Noakes, T.D. (2000). Hyponatremia in distance athletes. Pulling the IV on the 'dehydration myth.' *The Physician and Sportsmedicine* 28(9), 71-76.

Noakes, T. (2002). IMMDA-AIMS advisory statement on guidelines for fluid replacement during marathon running. *New Studies in Athletics: IAAF Technical Quarterly* 17(1), 7-11.

Noakes, T. (2002). Hyponatremia in distance runners: Fluid and sodium balance during exercise. *Current Sports Medicine Reports* 1(4), 197-207.

Noakes, T.D. (2003). *The lore of running.* 4th ed. Champaign, IL: Human Kinetics.

Noakes, T.D. et al. (1985). Water intoxication: A possible complication during endurance exercise. *Medicine and Science in Sports and Exercise* 17, 370-375.

Noakes, T.D. et al. (1991). Collapsed runners: Blood biochemical changes after iv fluid therapy. *The Physician and Sportsmedicine* 19(7), 70-80.

Speedy, D.B., Noakes, T.D. and Schneider, C. (2001). Exercise-associated hyponatremia: A review. *Emergency Medicine* 13(1), 17-27.

Speedy, D.B., Noakes, T.D. and Holzhausen, L-M. (2003). Exercise-associated collapse. Postural hypotension, or something deadlier? *The Physician and Sportsmedicine* 31(3), 23-29.

Wyndham, C.H. (1977). Heat stroke and hyperthermia in marathon runners. *Annals of the New York Academy of Science* 301, 128-138.

HYPOPLASTIC   Underdeveloped.

HYPOPLASTIC LEFT HEART SYNDROME   A rare type of congenital heart disease in which there is inadequate growth of the left ventricle and associated structures such as the aortic and mitral valves. The left side of the heart is completely unable to support the circulation required by the body's organs, but the right side of the heart is typically normally developed. Blood returning from the lungs to the left atrium must pass through an atrial septal defect to the right side of the heart. The right ventricle must then pump blood both to the lungs and out to the body via a patent ductus arteriosus, which is often the only pathway through which blood can reach the body from the heart. When the ductus arteriosus begins to close, as it typically does in the first days of life, the blood flow to the body will severely diminish. This results in dangerously poor perfusion of vital organs and shock.

Bibliography

American Heart Association. Http://www.americanheart.org

HYPOTENSION   Arterial systolic blood pressure that is below normal. After a period of sustained submaximal exercise, systolic blood pressure is temporarily decreased below pre-exercise levels for both normotensive and hypertensive individuals. This hypotensive response to previous exercise can last for up to 12 hours into recovery and occurs in response to aerobic exercise of low/moderate intensity. When aerobic exercise ceases, there is a prolonged period during which a significant quantity of blood remains in the visceral organs and/or lower limbs. This decreases the central blood volume, which causes a lowering of systemic arterial blood pressure. *See also* HYPONATREMIA; ORTHOSTATIC TOLERANCE.

HYPOTHALAMIC-PITUITARY-ADRENOCORTICAL AXIS *See under* HORMONES.

HYPOTHALAMUS *See under* BRAIN.

HYPOTHENAR EMINENCE *See under* HAND MUSCLES.

HYPOTHENAR HAMMER SYNDROME Traumatic thrombosis of the distal ulnar artery. It may be caused by repetitive blunt trauma or single severe trauma to the hypothenar region. It is a condition of the hand in which the blood flow to the fingers is decreased, with symptoms that include pain, paresthesia and loss of sensation in the affected hand. The fingers become sensitive to the cold and they change color. Occupationally, it typically afflicts persons who use vibrating hands tools or who hammer objects with the hypothenar aspect. However, it may occur in sports, such as baseball (catching baseballs), softball (sliding on the heel of the hand) and karate (direct punches).

HYPOTHERMIA Body core temperature below 36 degrees Celsius (96 degrees Fahrenheit) occurs when heat loss is greater than metabolic heat production. Early signs and symptoms of hypothermia include shivering, euphoria, confusion, and behavior similar to intoxication. Lethargy, muscle weakness, disorientation, hallucinations, depression, or combative behavior may occur as core temperature continues to fall. *See* COLD STRESS.

HYPOTHYROID MYOPATHY An endocrine myopathy that is caused by the thyroid gland producing insufficient thyroxine. Symptoms include weakening of muscles in the legs and arms.

HYPOTONIA Flaccidity. Low muscle tone. It is associated with damage of nuclei deep in the cerebellum that, in turn, affect functioning of the motor cortex and brain stem. It is a manifestation of muscle weakness that is present in many infants, toddlers and young children with disabilities. It is particularly associated with Down syndrome and may be the major reason that these children are delayed in acquiring locomotor skills. Problems in persons with hypotonia include: poor head and trunk control; absence of postural and protective reactions; shallow breathing; and hypermobility. In time, the motor cortex may compensate by increasing facilitatory impulses. An extreme state of hypotonia is a **vegetative state** (when persons cannot sit or move unaided). *See also* HYPERTONIA.

HYPOVENTILATION This occurs when the metabolic requirements of the body cells exceed ventilation, carbon dioxide accumulates and hypercapnia occurs. It is caused by abnormal conditions such as airway obstruction. The most common form of central hypoventilation, Pickwickian syndrome, occurs in association with morbid obesity.

HYPOVOLEMIA Low blood volume. *See under* DEHYDRATION.

HYPOXEMIA A lack of oxygen in the blood. **Exercise-induced arterial hypoxemia** is a condition found especially in endurance athletes in which the amount of oxygen carried in the blood is severely decreased. It may result from a fall in arterial partial pressure of oxygen (and thus also arterial oxygen saturation), from a rightward shift of the oxygen dissociation curve without a fall in arterial partial pressure of oxygen or from a combination of these processes. Habitually active subjects are the only healthy subjects who have demonstrated exercise-induced arterial hypoxemia in appreciable numbers. The prevalence of exercise-induced arterial hypoxemia near sea level has been estimated at 50% of young, adult, highly fit male athletes. In highly-trained endurance athletes, pulmonary capillary blood volume reaches its maximum at relatively low workloads. Instead of a subsequent expansion of pulmonary capillary blood volume, it seems that there may be an increase in blood flow velocity and a decrease in red blood cell transit time such that there is incomplete diffusion and equilibrium of gases. Arterial desaturation becomes more apparent as the duration of exercise increases. In humans, exercise-induced arterial hypoxemia severity correlates most consistently and inversely with alveolar-to-arterial oxygen difference.

Bibliography

Dempsey, J.A. and Wagner, P.D. (1999). Exercise-induced arterial hypoxemia. *Journal of Applied Physiology* 87(6), 1997-2006.

Prefaut, C. et al. (2000). Exercise-induced arterial hypoxaemia in athletes: A review. *Sports Medicine* 30(1), 47-61.

HYPOXIA   A lack of oxygen. It is sometimes used interchangeably with anoxia, although the latter indicates an absence rather than a deficiency of oxygen. In swimming, **hypoxic training** involves decreasing the number of breaths that are taken. Hypoxic training is based on the premise that it increases the ability of muscles to work without oxygen. It is also believed that decreasing the number of breaths per lap will increase the swimmer's speed, because changing the body position to take a breath tends to increase drag. There is evidence that it can improve swimming mechanics, and thus swimming speed, but there is no evidence that swimming without oxygen necessarily trains the anaerobic system.

HYSTERESIS   *See under* RESILIENCE.